Osteoporosis: A Growing Concern

Osteoporosis: A Growing Concern

Editor: Reed Spears

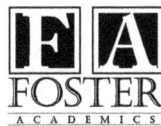

FA
FOSTER
ACADEMICS

www.fosteracademics.com

www.fosteracademics.com

FA
FOSTER
A C A D E M I C S

Cataloging-in-Publication Data

Osteoporosis : a growing concern / edited by Reed Spears.
    p. cm.
Includes bibliographical references and index.
ISBN 978-1-63242-859-2
1. Osteoporosis. 2. Osteoporosis--Prevention. 3. Bones--Diseases. 4. Vitamin D deficiency. I. Spears, Reed.
RC931.O73 O88 2019
616.716--dc23

Foster Academics,
118-35 Queens Blvd., Suite 400,
Forest Hills, NY 11375, USA

ISBN 978-1-63242-859-2 (Hardback)

Contents

Preface

The world is advancing at a fast pace like never before. Therefore, the need is to keep up with the latest developments. This book was an idea that came to fruition when the specialists in the area realized the need to coordinate together and document essential themes in the subject. That's when I was requested to be the editor. Editing this book has been an honour as it brings together diverse authors researching on different streams of the field. The book collates essential materials contributed by veterans in the area which can be utilized by students and researchers alike.

The disease in which increased bone weakness aggravates the risk of a broken bone is known as osteoporosis. If the bone breaks, it leads to chronic pain and difficulties in carrying out normal activities. Osteoporosis is commonly associated with the bones of the forearm, the vertebrae in the spine and the hip. It may occur due to either lower or greater than normal bone mass. It may also occur due to alcoholism, surgical removal of ovaries, anorexia, kidney disease, chemotherapy, etc. Dual-ray X-ray absorptiometry is the most common method to measure it. The imbalance between bone resorption and bone formation is the underlying mechanism in most cases. This book aims to shed light on some of the unexplored aspects of osteoporosis and the recent researches related to it. Different approaches, evaluation and advanced studies on the disease have been included herein. The extensive content of this book provides the readers with a thorough understanding of osteoporosis.

Each chapter is a sole-standing publication that reflects each author's interpretation. Thus, the book displays a multi-facetted picture of our current understanding of application, resources and aspects of the field. I would like to thank the contributors of this book and my family for their endless support.

Editor

Association between Secreted Phosphoprotein-1 (*SPP1*) Polymorphisms and Low Bone Mineral Density in Women

Jen-Hau Chen[1,2,3], Yen-Ching Chen[3], Chien-Lin Mao[3], Jeng-Min Chiou[4], Chwen Keng Tsao[5], Keh-Sung Tsai[1,2,6]*

1 Department of Geriatrics and Gerontology, National Taiwan University Hospital, No. 1, Taipei, Taiwan, 2 Department of Internal Medicine, National Taiwan University Hospital, No. 7, Taipei, Taiwan, 3 Institute of Epidemiology and Preventive Medicine, College of Public Health, National Taiwan University, Taipei, Taiwan, 4 Institute of Statistical Science, Academia Sinica, Nankang, Taipei, Taiwan, 5 MJ Health Management Institution, 12F., No. 413, Section 4, Taipei, Taiwan, 6 Department of Laboratory Medicine, National Taiwan University Hospital, No. 7, Taipei, Taiwan,

Abstract

Background: A recent meta-analysis found that secreted phosphoprotein-1 (SPP1) can predict the risk of both osteoporosis and fracture. No study has explored the association of *SPP1* haplotype-tagging single nucleotide polymorphisms (htSNPs) and haplotypes with bone mineral density (BMD).

Methods: This is a cross-sectional study. A total of 1,313 healthy Taiwanese women aged 40 to 55 years were recruited from MJ Health Management Institute from 2009 to 2010. BMD was dichotomized into high and low BMD groups. Three common (allele frequency ≥5%) htSNPs were selected to examine the association between sequence variants of *SPP1* and BMD.

Results: Homozygosity for the T allele of rs4754 were protective from low BMD [TT vs. CC: adjusted OR (AOR) = 0.58, 95% confidence interval (CI) = 0.83–0.89]. A protective effect was also found for women carrying 2 copies of Hap3 TCT (AOR = 0.57, 95% CI = 0.34–0.95). Menopausal status marginally interacted with *SPP1* rs6839524 on BMD ($p = 0.049$). Postmenopausal women carrying variant rs6839524 (GG+GC vs. CC: AOR = 2.35, 95% CI = 1.06–5.20) or Hap1 TGC (AOR = 2.36, 95% CI = 1.06–5.24) were associated with 2.4-fold risk of low BMD. For women with low BMI (<18.5 kg/m^2), variant rs6839524 (AOR = 7.64) and Hap1 (AOR = 6.42) were associated with increased risk of low BMD. These findings did not reach statistical significance after correction for multiple tests.

Conclusions: SPP1 htSNP protected against low BMD in middle-aged women. *SPP1* genetic markers may be important for the prediction of osteoporosis at an early age.

Editor: Maria Eugenia Saez, CAEBi, Spain

Funding: Funding for the study was provided by National Science Council grants 98-2314-B-002-081, 99-2314-B-002-128, and 101-2118-M-001-011-MY3. The funders had no role in study design, data collection and analysis, decision to publish, or preparation of the manuscript.

Competing Interests: The authors have declared that no competing interests exist.

* E-mail: kstsaimd1128@ntuh.gov.tw

Introduction

Osteoporosis, characterized by low bone mass and propensity to fracture, has become a global health issue as the rapid growth of aging population [1,2]. About 21% of women aged 50 to 84 years has osteoporosis, which is three times higher than that in men [3]. In the US (1988–1994), the prevalence of osteoporosis was highest among white (19%), followed by Mexican American (16%) and black (7%) [4], which in part correspondence to the levels of bone mineral density (BMD) ranged from lowest in Asian, followed by native Americans, Hispanic, and then African American [5]. This may be explained by different lifestyle in the East and West. Compared with other Asian countries, Japanese and Korean, but not Taiwanese, women showed clear age-dependent loss of BMD [6]. Osteoporosis is a "silent disease" until a sudden strain, twist, fall, or fracture, which is associated with increased mortality in later life [1]. Therefore, it is important to identify osteoporosis risk at an early age to prevent fall and fracture risk in late life.

Secreted phosphoprotein-1 (SPP1) is known as osteopontin. It is a glycoprotein related to bone formation and anchoring of osteoclasts to the bone remodeling matrix via binding with vitronectin receptor [7,8]. SPP1 exists in osteoblasts and mineralized bone matrix and intramembranous ossification [7], which enhances osteoblastic differentiation and proliferation [9,10]. SPP1 modulates both bone formation and resorption [11]. As compared to wildtype mice, *SPP1* gene knockout mice are resistant to bone resorption [12]. A Chinese study found that the heritability of BMD was quite high (0.6 to 0.9, vary by body site and sex) [13], therefore, genetic difference may pay a role on BMD level. Because SPP1 is involved in osteogenesis and bone remodeling, *SPP1* polymorphisms may play an important role in the pathogenesis of osteoporosis. Variation on functional single nucleotide polymorphisms (SNPs) may affect the production of *SPP1* protein and then bone formation; intronic SNPs may affect BMD via regulating the alternative splicing and the subsequent protein production [14,15].

Few epidemiologic studies have explored the association between *SPP1* polymorphisms and osteoporosis or BMD. One study found that increased plasma SPP1 level was associated with low BMD [16]. The other candidate-gene study including white and African Americans reported no difference between average hip or spine BMD level by genotypes of *SPP1* rs11730582 or rs4754 [17]. However, the selection of these two SNPs only captured limited genetic information in *SPP1* gene ($r^2 = 0.62$). In addition, these studies did not assess the association between *SPP1* genetic polymorphisms and low BMD or osteoporosis. A meta-analysis study, included 5 genome-wide association studies [GWASs, using data mining approach to explore a massive number of SNPs for specific outcome(s)] on BMD and fracture, found that polymorphisms of 9 genes (*ESR1*, *LRP4*, *ITGA1*, *LRP5*, *SOST*, *SPP1*, *TNFRSF11A*, *TNFRSF11B*, and *TNFSF11*) were significantly associated with BMD level; and *SPP1*, *SOST*, *LRP5*, and *TNFRSF11A* were also related to elevated risk of fracture [18]. Another recent meta-analysis, included 17 GWASs on BMD, found that polymorphisms of *FAM210A*, *SLC25A13*, *LRP5*, *MEPE/SPP1*, *SPTBN1*, and *DKK1* were significantly associated with both BMD and fracture risk [19]. Among the genes that can predict both BMD and fracture risk, *SPP1* is the only one that modulates both osteoblast and bone resorption [8], and associated with the risk of both vertebral and non-vertebral fracture [18]. In addition, no studies have explored how *SPP1* genetic polymorphisms affect the risk of low BMD by using representative haplotype-tagging single nucleotide polymorphisms (htSNPs) and haplotypes. Data in Asian is also lacking.

Because of the above research gap, this study was aimed to explore the association between *SPP1* polymorphisms and the risk of low BMD in middle-aged women. A systematic approach was used to select representative htSNPs in *SPP1* to capture sufficient genetic information and to identify SNPs representative for Asian population. We also evaluated the interactions between *SPP1* polymorphisms and menopausal status or body mass index (BMI) on BMD, which has not been explored previously.

Materials and Methods

Study population

This is a cross-sectional study. A total of 1,567 healthy Taiwanese (Chinese ethnicity) women, aged 40 to 55 years, were recruited from MJ Health Management Institution from October 2009 to August 2010. The outcome of this study is spinal BMD (g/cm^2). Spinal BMD is the major site measured at the MJ Health Management Institute. Participants with the following conditions or diseases were excluded (n = 254): (1) diseases known to affect BMD levels (e.g., hyperparathyroidism, hyperthyroidism, type 1 diabetes, inflammatory bowel disease, chronic active hepatitis, liver cirrhosis, chronic cholestatic diseases, and multiple myeloma), (2) took medications for osteoporosis (e.g., raloxifene), (3) received hormone replacement therapy or other medications (e.g., steroid, oral contraceptive agents) that may affect BMD, (4) lack of BMD at lumbar spine, (5) lack of blood samples or genotyping data. A total of 1,313 women were included for data analyses.

A questionnaire was administered to collect information on demography, lifestyle (e.g., smoking status, alcohol consumption, and exercise), and disease history, etc. A blood sample was collected in an 8 ml EDTA tube from each participant. Genomic DNA was extracted by using QuickGene-Mini80 kit (Fujifilm, Tokyo, Japan). Participants with the following conditions were excluded: BMD was measured at sites other than spine (n = 85), lack of blood sample (n = 113), or genotyping data (n = 2), and had

steroid or hormone therapy (n = 70). Some participants may lack of two or more information above.

Ethics Statement

The study protocol has been approved by the Institutional Review Boards of National Taiwan University and MJ Health Management Institution. Written informed consent was obtained from each study participant. The consent from the legal guardian/next of kin was obtained when patients had serious cognitive impairment. This research carried out with human subjects complies with the World Medical Association Declaration of Helsinki - Ethical Principles for Medical Research Involving Human Subjects.

Measurement of bone mineral density

The BMD (g/cm^2) of the lumbar spine (L1-L4) was measured by a dual-energy X-ray absorptiometry densitometer (DXA, General Electric Lunar Health Care, DPX-L, USA). Calibration of BMD measurement was performed daily. The long-term coefficient of variation in BMD was around 1%. This healthy population included few participants with osteoporosis (<1%). Instead of using osteoporosis as the outcome variable, BMD was tertiled (i.e. T1, T2, and T3) on the basis of the data of the whole population in order to identify the subgroup with an elevated risk of low BMD. Previous studies [20,21] and our recent study [22] have used similar approaches that involve BMD tertiles. The high BMD group comprised participants in T2 plus T3 (i.e., the reference group) and the low BMD group comprised participants in T1 (i.e., the comparison group) with a BMD cut-off point of 1.27 g/cm^2.

SNP selection and genotyping assays

Common (frequency ≥ 0.05) SNPs in *SPP1* were identified from genotyping data of Han Chinese in Beijing, China (CHB) of the International HapMap Project (http://hapmap.ncbi.nlm.nih.gov). Haplotype block was defined by Haploview program (http://www.broadinstitute.org/haploview/haploview) using modified Gabriel algorithm [23,24]. Three representative htSNPs [rs11730582 in 5'untranslated region (UTR), rs6839524 in intron, and rs4754 in exon] were selected from 12 common SNPs using tagSNP program [25] based on the common disease/common variant hypothesis [26]. TaqMan Assay was used to determine genotypes using HT7900 (Applied Biosystems Inc., CA, USA). Genotyping success rate was greater than 95% for each SNP. Quality control samples were replicates of 5% study participants and the concordance rate was 100%.

Statistical analyses

Hardy-Weinberg equilibrium (HWE) test was performed for each SNP to check genotyping error. The expectation-maximization algorithm was used to estimate haplotype frequencies in the haplotype block using tagSNP program [25]. High and low BMD was defined as above. Power analysis was performed by using QUANTO program (http://hydra.usc.edu/GxE/).

Logistic regression model was used to estimate the adjusted odds ratio (AOR) and 95% confidence interval (CI) for the risk of low BMD in participants carrying either 1 or 2 versus 0 copies of minor allele of each SNP and each multilocus haplotype. Haplotype trend regression [27] was used to test the global association between *SPP1* haplotypes and low BMD. Given a significant global test, haplotype-specific tests can provide some guidance as to which variant(s) contributes to the significant global test. The association between *SPP1* genetic polymorphisms and continuous BMD were also assessed by using general linear model (GLM). After stepwise model selection and the inclusion of variables with biological importance, age, menopausal status (yes/no), BMI (kg/m^2), alkaline phosphatase (ALP, IU/L), uric acid (UA, mg/dL), low-density lipoprotein (LDL, mg/dL), and exercise (frequency × duration × intensity) were adjusted in the models. All participants had normal creatinine level (<1.3 mg/dL) and thus this variable was not explored in this study.

A likelihood ratio test was used to evaluate how menopausal status (pre- and post-menopause) and BMI groups (<18.5, 18.5 to <24, ≥24 kg/m^2) modified the association between *SPP1* polymorphisms and risk of low BMD. Stratified analyses were performed by menopausal status and BMI groups. Correction for multiple tests was performed by false discovery rate (FDR) using method of Benjamini and Hochberg (1995) [28]. Statistical analyses were performed by using SAS 9.2 (SAS Institute, Cary, NC) and all statistical tests were two-sided.

Results

Characteristics of the study population

This study included 1,313 participants. The differences between participants with low and high BMD are summarized in Table 1

SPP1 polymorphisms and BMD

Three *SPP1* htSNPs [rs11730582 (5′ UTR), rs6829524 (intron), and rs4754 (exon)] were genotyped. The minor allele frequencies (MAFs) of these SNPs ranged from 31% to 42%, which were similar to the MAFs of CHB data from International HapMap Project (29 to 38%). All *SPP1* SNPs were in HWE among participants with low BMD, high BMD, or the whole population. Power analysis showed that given 881 and 432 participants with low and high BMD, respectively, rs4754 (MAF = 0.31) has over 0.99 of power to detect an OR at 0.58. Because of the modest effect and high MAF, the power is low (<0.7) for rs11730582 (MAF = 0.33) and rs6829524 (MAF = 0.42) to detect an OR at 1.14 and 0.91, respectively.

Homozygosity for the T allele of rs4754 were protective from low BMD (TT vs. CC: AOR = 0.58, 95% CI = 0.83–0.89, $p = 0.005$, Table 2). This association did not reach statistical significance after correction for multiple tests. The other two htSNPs did not show significant relationship with the outcome.

Three common htSNPs (rs11730582, rs6839524, and rs4754) spanning *SPP1* gene formed one block using the modified Gabriel algorithm [23,24]. Four common (frequency ≥0.05) haplotypes were identified (cumulative frequency, 97.9%); the global test for the association between *SPP1* haplotypes and low BMD was significant ($p<0.0001$, Table 2). Two copies of Hap3 TCT were protective from low BMD (AOR = 0.57, 95% CI = 0.34–0.95, $p = 0.03$, Table 2). Other haplotypes were not associated with the outcome. The conditional haplotype analysis was performed conditioning on other haplotypes and the results did not reach statistical significance (Hap1: ref; Hap2: AOR = 1.14, 95% CI = 0.90–1.44; Hap3: AOR = 0.93, 95% CI = 0.74–1.17; Hap4: AOR = 0.85, 95% CI = 0.59–1.24). These findings did not remain significant after correction for multiple tests.

We also kept only participants with the lowest and the highest BMD tertile and compared them for the same analyses above. Because of removing one-third of the study population (the 2nd tertile), the statistical power decreased and the protective effect for rs4754 and Hap3 no longer reached statistical significance.

Interactions between menopausal status and SPP1 polymorphisms

Menopausal status has known as an important modifier for BMD. Interaction between menopausal status and *SPP1* htSNPs or haplotypes for low BMD did not reach statistical significance. After stratification by menopausal status, postmenopausal women carrying variant rs6839524 were associated with low BMD (GG+GC vs. CC: AOR = 2.35, 95% CI = 1.06–5.20, $p = 0.03$). Postmenopausal women carrying Hap1 TGC was associated with low BMD (AOR = 2.36, 95% CI = 1.06–5.24, $p = 0.03$). These findings did not reach statistical significance after correction for multiple tests. No significant association was found in other subgroups or for other *SPP1* htSNPs/haplotypes after stratification by menopausal status.

Interaction between BMI and SPP1 polymorphisms

No significant interaction was observed between *SPP1* SNPs or haplotypes and low BMD. After stratification by BMI groups (< 18.5, 18.5 to <24, ≥24 kg/m^2), women with low BMI (<18.5 kg/m^2) carrying rs6839524 variant were associated with low BMD (GG+GC vs. CC: AOR = 7.64, 95% CI = 1.42–40.97, $p = 0.02$). Women with low BMI (<18.5 kg/m^2) carrying Hap1 TGC were associated with low BMD (AOR = 6.42, 95% CI = 1.23–33.60, $p = 0.03$). These findings did not reach statistical significance after correction for multiple tests.

The power for assessing interaction between *SPP1* SNPs and menopausal status or BMI is low because of the smaller sample size in subgroup analysis and the results should be interpreted with caution.

Discussion

To the best of our knowledge, this is the first study exploring the association between *SPP1* polymorphisms and low BMD using htSNPs in Asian population. We found that homozygosity for the T allele of *SPP1* rs4754 (TT) and Hap3 TCT were associated with low BMD; the former result remained significant after correction for multiple tests for SNP analysis but lost significance after correction for multiple tests for SNP and haplotype analysis. The only candidate-gene study [17], which included white and black populations, only compared mean BMD by *SPP1* genotypes of 2 SNPs (i.e., no estimation of multivariable OR and 95% CI) and no significant difference was observed. Previous GWASs and meta-analysis [18,19,29–33] for BMD or fracture risk mainly focused on white population. In addition, haplotype analysis, which offers more information than single-locus SNPs, has not been performed previously. Therefore, our results provide important information because of the estimation of outcome risk by using multivariable OR, large sample size (n>1,300), selection of representative htSNP, and performing haplotype analysis.

Among 3 htSNPs genotyped in this study, rs4754 is a synonymous SNP. That is, rs4754 does not lead to the change of amino acid but may affect BMD level via its influence on translational efficiency. Interestingly, C allele is the major allele of rs4754 in Chinese (MAF: C = 0.66, T = 0.34) but the minor allele in white (MAF: C = 0.23, T = 0.77, http://hapmap.ncbi.nlm.nih.gov). Therefore, the inconsistent findings were observed between this Asian study and previous studies focused on whites [18,19,29–33]. Hap3 TCT also showed significant association with high BMD, which may be attributable to the only SNP rs4754 with the minor allele in Hap3. Three htSNPs were in one haplotype block and strong linkage disequilibrium (LD) were observed between rs11730582 and rs6839524 (|D′| = 0.98) as well as between rs6839524 and rs4754 (|D′| = 0.96). However, the pairwise r^2 for

Table 1. Characteristics of the study population.

Variables	Low BMD (<1.27 g/cm²)	High BMD (≥1.27 g/cm²)	p
	n = 881	n = 432	
	Mean ± SE		
Age	46.8±0.2	45.6±0.2	**<0.001**
Alkaline phosphatase (IU/L)	61.5±0.6	55.5±0.7	**<0.001**
	n (%)		
Menopause			**<0.001**
Yes	227 (26)	45 (11)	
No	647 (74)	381 (89)	
Cigarette smoking			0.45
Yes	63 (8)	39 (9)	
No	777 (92)	378 (91)	
Alcohol consumption			0.84
Yes	50 (6)	27 (7)	
No	775 (94)	379 (93)	
Body mass index (kg/m²)			**<0.0001**
<18.5	56 (6)	15 (3)	
≥18.5 to <24	652 (74)	279 (65)	
≥24	172 (20)	137 (32)	
High-density lipoprotein (mg/dL)			0.71
≥50	808 (92)	396 (92)	
<50	73 (8)	33 (8)	
Low-density lipoprotein (mg/dL)			**0.0001**
<130	670 (76)	366 (85)	
≥130	211 (24)	63 (15)	
Triglyceride (mg/dL)			0.28
<150	794 (90)	381 (88)	
≥150	87 (10)	51 (12)	
Uric acid (mg/dL)			**0.006**
<6	806 (91)	374 (87)	
≥6	75 (9)	58 (13)	
Hypertension			0.48
Yes	88 (10)	49 (11)	
No	793 (90)	382 (89)	
Diabetes			0.05
Yes	262 (30)	151 (35)	
No	619 (70)	281 (65)	
Regular exercise			0.39
Yes	368 (47)	194 (50)	
No	412 (53)	195 (50)	

Abbreviations: BMD, bone mineral density; BMI, body mass index; hypertension, systolic blood pressure >140 mmHg or diastolic blood pressure >90 mmHg or had medication for controlling blood pressure; diabetes, fasting glucose ≥126 mg/dl or using medication for diabetes; regular exercise: walking or hiking ≥30 mins/2 to 3 days.
Numbers in bold indicate significant findings (p<0.05).

any two SNPs were low (0.02 to 0.34). Especially, both D' (0.30) and r² (0.02) were low between rs11730582 and rs4754, this may explain the non-significant association between SPP1 rs11730582 and BMD.

SPP1 plays a role in a wide spectrum of physiologic and pathologic processes [34–37]. First, it mediates the attachment of

osteoclasts to bone matrix and then regulates bone resorption and normal bone development [37]. The polymorphisms of SPP1 gene may regulate SPP1 structure, decrease serum SPP1 level, change or reduce SPP1 protein, which may affect bone formation, resorption and the osteoclastic process. The downgrading of osteoclastic process may slow BMD decline and thus prevent

Table 2. Association of *SPP1* common htSNPs and haplotypes with low BMD.

| | Freq. | Codominant Model | | | | | | | | |
| | | 0 copies | | 1 copy | | | 2 copies | | |
SNP	(%)	BMD (L/H)	AOR	BMD (L/H)	AOR (95% CI)	p	BMD (L/H)	AOR (95% CI)	p
rs11730582		394/206	1.00	385/177	1.17 (0.89–1.53)	0.54	102/49	1.13 (0.73–1.74)	0.83
rs6839524		295/157	1.00	429/197	1.25 (0.94–1.67)	0.05	158/78	0.91 (0.63–1.32)	0.22
rs4754		439/195	1.00	368/179	1.07 (0.81–1.41)	0.02	74/57	**0.58 (0.83–0.89)**	**0.005**
Haplotype (Global test *P*<0.0001)									
Hap1 TGC	41.2	299/162	1.00	431/193	1.30 (0.97–1.73)	0.08	151/77	0.90 (0.62–1.31)	0.58
Hap2 CCC	26.3	466/248	1.00	351/160	1.18 (0.90–1.55)	0.24	64/24	1.45 (0.83–2.53)	0.20
Hap3 TCT	23.9	522/243	1.00	317/153	1.08 (0.82–1.43)	0.60	42/36	**0.57 (0.34–0.95)**	**0.03**
Hap4 CCT	6.5	782/371	1.00	92/59	0.73 (0.49–1.09)	0.13	7/2	1.81 (0.35–9.34)	0.48
Total	97.9								

Abbreviations: SNP, single nucleotide polymorphism; Freq., haplotype frequency; BMD, bone mineral density; AOR, adjusted odds ratio; CI, confidence interval; L, low BMD; H, high BMD.
All models were adjusted for age, menopausal status, BMI (kg/m²), serum ALP (IU/L), UA (mg/dL), LDL (mg/dL), and exercise (frequency × duration × intensity).
The SNPs with underscore indicate variant allele.
Numbers in bold indicated significant findings (*p*<0.05).

osteoporosis. Second, SPP1 plays an important role in regulating immune response [38]. Therefore, polymorphisms of *SPP1* may block or reduce the inflammation responses and thus showed increased BMD. In addition, *SPP1* polymorphisms may also interact with two important modifiers, menopausal status or BMI, on BMD as detailed below.

It has been known that sex hormone plays an important role in maintaining bone strength [39]. For most of women, BMD decreases rapidly during the first few years after menopause [40] as a result of excessive osteoclastic activities via unopposed osteoclastic activation after rapid declination of estrogen. Because SPP1 modulates osteoclast and thus sequence variants of *SPP1* may affect bone resorption. This may explain our finding that postmenopausal women carrying 1 or 2 copies of variant rs6839524 were associated with low BMD (AOR = 2.35), which did not reach statistical significance after correction of multiple tests. An association was also observed for Hap1, which rs6839524 is the only SNP with minor allele. It is possible that variant rs6839524 affects bone formation and this effect becomes more evident after menopause. In addition, rs6839524 is an intronic SNP and its variation may affect the alternative splicing, e.g., altering mRNA folding or the stability of mRNA structure, and then the subsequent protein production [14,15]. All these may explain the associations, which did not reach statistical significance after correction of multiple tests, between rs6839524 or Hap1 and low BMD in postmenopausal women.

BMI has been related to BMD previously. Low BMI has been associated with increased risk of osteoporosis and fracture [41] and the association varied by ethnic groups, e.g., positive association between one unit increase of BMI and BMD in white women but negative association was observed in African American women [42]. Because of different diet and lifestyle, body shape can be quite different between people in Western and Eastern countries. However, relevant data and research in Asian population are sparse. Our research, for the first time, explored that among women with low BMI (<18.5 kg/m^2), variant carriers of rs6839524 (AOR = 7.64) or Hap1 TGC (AOR = 6.42) were associated with low BMD, which did not reach statistical significance after correction for multiple tests. The application of these polymorphisms will help us to identify women with low BMD.

This study has several strengths. First, the selections of a set of representative htSNPs for Asian captured the majority of genetic

information of *SPP1* ($r^2 = 0.82$, estimated by tagSNP program) as compared with that ($r^2 = 0.65$) of the only candidate-gene study [17]. Second, haplotypes capture unknown variants via LD between these SNPs and thus provide more information than single SNP. In addition, unlike most previous studies, this study included premenopausal women (n~1000) that allowed us to assess how menopausal status interacted with *SPP1* polymorphisms on BMD and, importantly, to predict outcome risk at an early age.

This study had some limitations. First, this is a cross-sectional study, which causal inference is usually not available. Functional analysis will be needed to unravel the underlying mechanism between *SPP1* polymorphisms and BMD. In addition, the original questionnaire did not collect fracture information. Because this population is healthy, fracture frequency is low. We also assessed the association between *SPP1* genetic polymorphisms and continuous BMD by using GLM and no significant findings were observed. Because the aim of this study is to identify a high-risk population of low BMD, no further analyses were performed by using continuous BMD as outcome.

SPP1 plays a role in bone formation and resorption. This study has some first findings. Homozygosity for the T allele of rs4754 and Hap3 TCT in *SPP1* were significantly associated with low BMD in this Asian population. rs6839524 and haplotypes in *SPP1* have not been explored before. Variant carriers of rs6839524 and Hap 1 TGC were associated with low BMD in menopausal women or women with low BMI. These findings did not reach statistical significance after correction for multiple tests. Because of the complex role of *SPP1* in bone physiology, functional and larger studies are warranted to confirm our findings.

Acknowledgments

The authors gratefully acknowledge Dr. Wen-Chung Lee for epidemiological consultation.

Author Contributions

Conceived and designed the experiments: KST YCC JHC. Performed the experiments: CLM. Analyzed the data: CLM JMC YCC JHC. Contributed reagents/materials/analysis tools: JHC YCC KST. Wrote the paper: CLM JHC JMC YCC CKT KST. Approval of the final version of the manuscript: CLM JHC JMC YCC CKT KST.

References

1. Sànchez-Riera L, Wilson N, Kamalaraj N, Nolla JM, Kok C, et al. (2010) Osteoporosis and fragility fractures. Best Pract Res Clin Rheumatol 24: 793–810.

2. Vestergaard P, Rejnmark L, Mosekilde L (2007) Increased mortality in patients with a hip fracture-effect of pre-morbid conditions and post-fracture complications. Osteoporos Int 18: 1583–1593.

3. Kanis JA, Johnell O, Oden A, Jonsson B, De Laet C, et al. (2000) Risk of hip fracture according to the World Health Organization criteria for osteopenia and osteoporosis. Bone 27: 585–590.

4. Dawson-Hughes B, Looker AC, Tosteson ANA, Johansson H, Kanis JA, et al. (2011) The potential impact of the National Osteoporosis Foundation guidance on treatment eligibility in the USA: an update in NHANES 2005–2008. Osteoporos Int.

5. Barrett-Connor E, Siris ES, Wehren LE, Miller PD, Abbott TA, et al. (2005) Osteoporosis and fracture risk in women of different ethnic groups. J Bone Miner Res 20: 185–194.

6. Sugimoto T, Tsutsumi M, Fujii Y, Kawakatsu M, Negishi H, et al. (1992) Comparison of bone mineral content among Japanese, Koreans, and Taiwanese assessed by dual-photon absorptiometry. Journal of Bone and Mineral Research 7: 153–159.

7. Denhardt D, Noda M (1998) Osteopontin expression and function: Role in bone remodeling. J Cell Biochem: 92–102.

8. Choi ST, Kim JH, Kang E-J, Lee S-W, Park M-C, et al. (2008) Osteopontin might be involved in bone remodelling rather than in inflammation in ankylosing spondylitis. Rheumatology (Oxford) 47: 1775–1779.

9. Moore M, Gotoh Y, Rafidi K (1991) Characterization of a cDNA for chicken osteopontin: expression during bone development, osteoblast differentiation, and tissue distribution. Biochemistry.

10. Zohar R, Cheifetz S, McCulloch C (1998) Analysis of intracellular osteopontin as a marker of osteoblastic cell differentiation and mesenchymal cell migration. European Journal of Oral Sciences 106: 401–407.

11. Standal T, Borset M, Sundan A (2004) Role of osteopontin in adhesion, migration, cell survival and bone remodeling. Exp Oncol 26: 179–184.

12. Rittling SR, Matsumoto HN, Mckee MD, Nanci A, An X-R, et al. (1998) Mice Lacking Osteopontin Show Normal Development and Bone Structure but Display Altered Osteoclast Formation In Vitro. J Bone Miner Res 13: 1101–1111.

13. Feng Y, Hsu Y, Terwedow H, Chen C, Xu X, et al. (2005) Familial aggregation of bone mineral density and bone mineral content in a Chinese population. Osteoporos Int 16: 1917–1923.

14. Moyer RA, Wang D, Papp AC, Smith RM, Duque L, et al. (2011) Intronic polymorphisms affecting alternative splicing of human dopamine D2 receptor are associated with cocaine abuse. Neuropsychopharmacology 36: 753–762.

15. Kawase T, Akatsuka Y, Torikai H, Morishima S, Oka A, et al. (2007) Alternative splicing due to an intronic SNP in HMSD generates a novel minor histocompatibility antigen. Blood 110: 1055–1063.

16. Chang IC, Chiang TI, Yeh KT, Lee H, Cheng YW (2010) Increased serum osteopontin is a risk factor for osteoporosis in menopausal women. Osteoporos Int 21: 1401–1409.

17. Taylor BC, Schreiner PJ, Doherty TM, Fornage M, Carr JJ, et al. (2005) Matrix Gla protein and osteopontin genetic associations with coronary artery calcification and bone density: the CARDIA study. Hum Genet 116: 525–528.

18. Richards JB, Kavvoura FK, Rivadeneira F, Styrkarsdottir U, Estrada K, et al. (2009) Collaborative meta-analysis: associations of 150 candidate genes with osteoporosis and osteoporotic fracture. Ann Intern Med 151: 528–537.

19. Estrada K, Styrkarsdottir U, Evangelou E, Hsu YH, Duncan EL, et al. (2012) Genome-wide meta-analysis identifies 56 bone mineral density loci and reveals 14 loci associated with risk of fracture. Nat Genet 44: 491–501.

20. Bidoli E, Schinella D, Franceschi S (1998) Physical activity and bone mineral density in Italian middle-aged women. Eur J Epidemiol 14: 153–157.

21. Nock NL, Patrick-Melin A, Cook M, Thompson C, Kirwan JP, et al. (2011) Higher bone mineral density is associated with a decreased risk of colorectal adenomas. Int J Cancer 129: 956–964.

22. You YS, Lin CY, Liang HJ, Lee S, Tsai KS, et al (2013(Epub ahead of Print)) Association between Metabolome and Low Bone Mineral Density in Taiwanese Women Determined by 1H NMR Spectroscopy. Journal of Bone and Mineral Research.

23. Chen YC, Giovannucci E, Lazarus R, Kraft P, Ketkar S, et al. (2005) Sequence variants of Toll-like receptor 4 and susceptibility to prostate cancer. Cancer Res 65: 11771–11778.

24. Gabriel SB, Schaffner SF, Nguyen H, Moore JM, Roy J, et al. (2002) The structure of haplotype blocks in the human genome. Science 296: 2225–2229.

25. Stram DO, Leigh Pearce C, Bretsky P, Freedman M, Hirschhorn JN, et al. (2003) Modeling and E-M Estimation of Haplotype-Specific Relative Risks from Genotype Data for a Case-Control Study of Unrelated Individuals. Hum Hered 55: 179–190.

26. (2001) Challenges for the 21st century. Nat Genet 29: 353–354.

27. Zaykin DV, Westfall PH, Young SS, Karnoub MA, Wagner MJ, et al. (2002) Testing association of statistically inferred haplotypes with discrete and continuous traits in samples of unrelated individuals. Hum Hered 53: 79–91.

28. Benjamini Y, Hochberg Y (1995) Controlling the false discovery rate: a practical and powerful approach to multiple testing. J R Statist Soc B 57: 289–300.

29. Hofman A, Breteler MMB, van Duijn CM, Krestin GP, Pols HA, et al. (2007) The Rotterdam Study: objectives and design update. Eur J Epidemiol 22: 819–829.

30. Sayed-Tabatabaei FA, van Rijn MJE, Schut AFC, Aulchenko YS, Croes EA, et al. (2005) Heritability of the function and structure of the arterial wall: findings of the Erasmus Rucphen Family (ERF) study. Stroke 36: 2351–2356.

31. Richards JB, Rivadeneira F, Inouye M, Pastinen TM, Soranzo N, et al. (2008) Bone mineral density, osteoporosis, and osteoporotic fractures: a genome-wide association study. Lancet 371: 1505–1512.

32. Styrkarsdottir U, Halldorsson BV, Gretarsdottir S, Gudbjartsson DF, Walters GB, et al. (2009) New sequence variants associated with bone mineral density. Nat Genet 41: 15–17.

33. Kiel DP, Demissie S, Dupuis J, Lunetta KL, Murabito JM, et al. (2007) Genome-wide association with bone mass and geometry in the Framingham Heart Study. BMC Med Genet 8 Suppl 1: S14.

34. Gravallese EM (2003) Osteopontin: a bridge between bone and the immune system. Journal of Clinical Investigation 112: 147–149.

35. Reinholt FP, Hultenby K, Oldberg A, Heinegard D (1990) Osteopontin—a possible anchor of osteoclasts to bone. Proceedings of the National Academy of Sciences of the United States of America 87: 4473–4475.

36. Denhardt D (1993) Osteopontin: a protein with diverse functions. The FASEB journal.

37. O'Regan AW, Chupp GL, Lowry JA, Goetschkes M, Mulligan N, et al. (1999) Osteopontin is associated with T cells in sarcoid granulomas and has T cell adhesive and cytokine-like properties in vitro. Journal of Immunology 162: 1024–1031.

38. Denhardt DT, Noda M, O'Regan AW, Pavlin D, Berman JS (2001) Osteopontin as a means to cope with environmental insults: regulation of inflammation, tissue remodeling, and cell survival. Journal of Clinical Investigation 107: 1055–1061.

39. Satoh Y, Soeda Y, Dokou S (1995) Analysis of Relationships Between Sex-Hormone Dynamics and Bone Metabolism and Changes in Bone Mass in Surgically Induced Menopause. Calcif Tissue Int 57: 258–266.

40. Saarelainen J, Kiviniemi V, Kröger H, Tuppurainen M, Niskanen L, et al. (2011) Body mass index and bone loss among postmenopausal women: the 10-year follow-up of the OSTPRE cohort. J Bone Miner Metab.

41. Morin S, Tsang JF, Leslie WD (2009) Weight and body mass index predict bone mineral density and fractures in women aged 40 to 59 years. Osteoporosis International 20: 363–370.

42. Castro JP, Joseph LA, Shin JJ, Arora SK, Nicasio J, et al. (2005) Differential effect of obesity on bone mineral density in White, Hispanic and African American women: a cross sectional study. Nutr Metab (Lond) 2: 9.

2

Do Premenopausal Women with Major Depression Have Low Bone Mineral Density? A 36-Month Prospective Study

Giovanni Cizza[1]*, Sima Mistry[2], Vi T. Nguyen[1], Farideh Eskandari[1], Pedro Martinez[3], Sara Torvik[1], James C. Reynolds[4], Philip W. Gold[3], Ninet Sinai[4], Gyorgy Csako[4], for the POWER Study Group

1 Section on Neuroendocrinology of Obesity, National Institutes of Diabetes and Digestive Kidney Diseases (NIDDK), National Institutes of Health, Bethesda, Maryland, United States of America, 2 Tulane University Internal Medicine-Pediatrics Residency Program, Tulane University School of Medicine, New Orleans, Louisiana, United States of America, 3 Behavioral Endocrinology Branch, National Institute of Mental Health, National Institutes of Health, Bethesda, Maryland, United States of America, 4 Clinical Center, National Institutes of Health, Bethesda, Maryland, United States of America

Abstract

Background: An inverse relationship between major depressive disorder (MDD) and bone mineral density (BMD) has been suggested, but prospective evaluation in premenopausal women is lacking.

Methods: Participants of this prospective study were 21 to 45 year-old premenopausal women with MDD (n = 92) and healthy controls (n = 44). We measured BMD at the anteroposterior lumbar spine, femoral neck, total hip, mid-distal radius, trochanter, and Ward's triangle, as well as serum intact parathyroid hormone (iPTH), ionized calcium, plasma adrenocorticotropic hormone (ACTH), serum cortisol, and 24-hour urinary-free cortisol levels at 0, 6, 12, 24, and 36 months. 25-hydroxyvitamin D was measured at baseline.

Results: At baseline, BMD tended to be lower in women with MDD compared to controls and BMD remained stable over time in both groups. At baseline, 6, 12, and 24 months intact PTH levels were significantly higher in women with MDD *vs.* controls. At baseline, ionized calcium and 25-hydroxyvitamin D levels were significantly lower in women with MDD compared to controls. At baseline and 12 months, bone-specific alkaline phosphatase, a marker of bone formation, was significantly higher in women with MDD *vs.* controls. Plasma ACTH was also higher in women with MDD at baseline and 6 months. Serum osteocalcin, urinary N-telopeptide, serum cortisol, and urinary free cortisol levels were not different between the two groups throughout the study.

Conclusion: Women with MDD tended to have lower BMD than controls over time. Larger and longer studies are necessary to extend these observations with the possibility of prophylactic therapy for osteoporosis.

Trial Registration: ClinicalTrials.gov NCT 00006180

Editor: Massimo Federici, University of Tor Vergata, Italy

Funding: This study was fully supported by the National Institutes of Health (NIH), Intramural Research Program: National Institute of Mental Health (NIMH), National Institute of Diabetes and Digestive and Kidney Diseases (NIDDK). Alendronate and Placebo were generously provided by Merck Research Laboratories, Rahway, NJ. The funders had no role in study design, data collection and analysis, decision to publish, or preparation of the manuscript.

Competing Interests: Alendronate and Placebo were generously provided by Merck Research Laboratories, Rahway, NJ. The informatics support for this study was provided by Mr. Frank Pierce from ®Esprit Health. Giovanni Cizza was a former Merck Employee and currently owns Merck stock options. This does not alter the authors' adherence to all the PLoS ONE policies on sharing data and materials.

* E-mail: cizzag@intra.niddk.nih.gov

Introduction

Major Depressive Disorder (MDD) is a common condition affecting 98.7 million people globally [1] and nearly 35 million adults in the United States [2]. This chronic condition, characterized by depressed mood and/or anhedonia that interfere with activities of daily living, is a major cause of disability worldwide. By the year 2020, MDD will become second only to ischemic heart disease in the amount of disability experienced by sufferers of all ages according to the World Health Organization Global Burden of Disease Survey. The economic impact of depression is estimated in the tens of billions of dollars: depression cost employers over $40 billion dollars annually in lost productive work time [3]. MDD, once considered a disease only of the psyche, is now known to be associated with a number of medical conditions including cardiovascular disease [4–8], immune alterations [9–12], insulin resistance [13–16], diabetes mellitus [17–20], and obesity [21–24]. We and others have shown that depression is also associated with osteoporosis [25–42], yet depression is rarely listed as a risk factor for osteoporosis.

Unlike most physical illnesses observed in conjunction with MDD, osteoporosis is primarily asymptomatic and often remains undiagnosed until patients sustain pathologic fractures later in their lives. Due to the insidious presentation of osteoporosis, any concomitant mood change is unlikely to be reactive in nature. Although a few cross-sectional and cohort studies examining the relationship between depression and low bone mineral density (BMD) have been reported in pre- and post-menopausal women, there has been no prospective evaluation in premenopausal women [30]. Therefore, to investigate over time the association between BMD and depression in this population, we conducted a three-year prospective study by monitoring BMD over time in premenopausal women with MDD and healthy controls.

Materials and Methods

Participants

Participants of the *P*remenopausal, *O*steoporosis, *W*omen, Alendronat*e*, Dep*r*ession (POWER) study were 21- to 45-year-old premenopausal women with current or recent MDD (n = 92) and healthy control women (n = 44). Recruitment took place from July 1, 2001, to February 28, 2003, in the Washington, DC, metropolitan area by newspaper and radio. Internet and flyer advertisement [27]. Women with MDD were enrolled if they met the Diagnostic and Statistical Manual of Mental Disorders, 4th. Edition (*DSM*-IV) criteria for MDD and experienced a depressive episode in the preceding three years; a limit chosen to minimize recall bias associated with more remote depressive episodes.

Exclusion criteria for women with MDD included eating disorders, bipolar disorders, schizophrenia, schizoaffective disorder, and suicidal risk. Patients with anxiety disorders or a history of drug or alcohol dependence in remission for at least five years were eligible. Subjects were allowed to continue their antidepressant treatments under the care of their physician. Hyperthyroidism, vitamin D deficiency and other conditions and treatments that affect bone turnover were additional exclusion criteria. Exclusion criteria for controls were a T-score equal to or lower than −1.5 at the anterior-posterior (AP) lumbar spine, femoral neck or total hip and a history of any DSM-IV diagnosis apart from prior alcohol abuse. Pregnancy and menopause were additional exclusion criteria [27].

The health status of each subject was evaluated by medical history and physical examination. Screening electrocardiogram, serum pregnancy test, complete metabolic panel, complete blood count, 25-hydroxyvitamin D, intact parathyroid hormone (iPTH), thyrotropin, and free thyroxine and urine toxicology screen were obtained. Figure 1 describes the number of individuals screened and the reasons for exclusion. Of note, none of the control subject screened had a T-score equal to or lower than −1.5 at the anterior-posterior (AP) lumbar spine, femoral neck or total hip. The National Institute of Mental Health's Institutional Review Board and the Scientific Review Board approved the original 12 month study and its subsequent extension to 36 month. In addition, all subjects provided written informed consent. The trial was registered in ClinicalTrials.gov, NCT 00006180.

Study design

The POWER Study was designed as a 12-month investigation consisting of: 1) a longitudinal follow-up comparison of BMD in women with MDD and controls (Natural History Arm) and; 2) a randomized, double-blind, placebo-controlled, 12- month trial of alendronate in women with MDD with moderate osteopenia (Clinical Trial Arm). Further details on study design have been previously reported [27]. In the Clinical Trial Arm women with MDD, who at baseline had a T-score equal to or lower than −1.5 at the anterior-posterior (AP) lumbar spine, femoral neck or total

hip (n = 14), were randomized to 70 mg of alendronate (n = 7) or matching placebo tablets (n = 7) orally once a week (Merck & Co., Inc., Rahway, NJ). In addition, both groups in the Clinical Trial Arm received 500 mg daily of elemental calcium and 400 IU of vitamin D.

We subsequently extended the study to a total of 36 months (Figure 1). At the end of the 12-month main study, subjects from the Natural History Arm and those subjects in the Clinical Trial Arm that were randomized to placebo were offered continued participation in an additional 24-month study extension to assess bone mineral density and biochemical markers of bone turnover at yearly intervals ("Extended Natural History Arm").

Procedures

BMD, biochemical markers of bone turnover, and hormonal measurements. BMD was measured by dual-energy x-ray absorptiometry (DXA QDR 4500 machine; Hologic Inc., Bedford, MA) at the following sites: anteroposterior lumbar (L1–L4) spine, total hip, femoral neck, trochanter, Ward's triangle, and mid-distal radius. The coefficient of variation was <0.4% at each site. DXAs were analyzed by the study radiologist, J.R., blinded to group allocation. Two markers of bone formation, serum bone-specific alkaline phosphatase and 8:00 AM osteocalcin, and a marker of bone resorption, urinary N-telopeptide, were assessed. 8:00 AM plasma adrenocorticotropic hormone (ACTH), 8:00 AM serum cortisol, 24-hour urinary-free cortisol, serum iPTH, plasma 25-hydroxyvitamin D and ionized serum calcium were also obtained. These measurements were obtained at 0, 6, 12, 24 and 36 month. 25-Hydroxyvitamin D plasma levels were only measured at baseline.

Psychiatric evaluation. We administered the structured clinical interview (SCID) for DSM-IV Axis I disorders and enrolled subjects if they met DSM-IV criteria for MDD and had an episode of major depression in the past three years (SCID). The Hamilton Depression Scale (HAM-D) and Hamilton Anxiety Scales (HAM-A) were used to determine the severity of depression and anxiety in study participants at baseline, 12, 24 and 36 months.

Life style risk factors for osteoporosis. Calcium from food and supplements, caffeine, and alcohol intake were assessed using a food frequency questionnaire. A nutritionist informed the subjects of their calcium intake and recommended to consume 1000 mg/day of calcium [27]. Cigarette smoking history and oral contraceptive use were also recorded. The Cooper test (12-minute walk/run test) was administered as an indirect index of physical fitness, and was measured in meters traversed within 12-minutes on a standardized treadmill [27].

Anthropometric measurements. As previously described, height was measured to the nearest 0.1 cm using a stadiometer and weight to the nearest 0.1 kg using a digital scale [27]. BMI was calculated as kg/m^2.

Statistical analyses

Data are reported as mean (SD) or by frequencies and percents, unless otherwise indicated. Differences between groups (MDD and control subjects, or between the clinical trial treatment arms) were tested by the *t*-test (or non-parametric parallel, as necessary) and Fisher exact test, as appropriate. Paired data between time intervals utilized the paired *t*-test (or non-parametric parallel, as necessary) for continuous variables or McNemar test for categorical ones. The relationship between depression and BMD was assessed by analysis of covariance, adjusting for BMI. In women with MDD, the association of BMD with clinical parameters of depression and anxiety was assessed by linear regression.

Main Study

Screened (*n* = 186)

Screened for MDD (*n* = 123) — Screened for Control (*n* = 63)

Not enrolled (*n* = 31)
No MDD Episode in 3 years: 10
Other psychiatric diagnosis: 7
Depressive Disorder NOS: 5
Incomplete screening: 5
Postmenopausal: 1
Vitamin D Deficiency: 1
Medication Use: 2

Not enrolled (*n* = 19)
History of MDD: 7
Other psychiatric dx: 4
Depressive Disorder NOS: 5
Vitamin D deficiency: 2
Hyperthyroidism: 1
Hyperparathyroidism: 1
Back Pain: 1
Medication use: 1
Withdrew consent: 1

Enrolled (*n* = 92) — Enrolled (*n* = 44)

Not completed (*n* = 14)
Withdrew: 7
Lost to follow-up: 6
Missed visit: 1

Natural History Arm (*n* = 74) — Randomized Control Trial (*n* = 18)

Not completed (*n* = 19)
Withdrew: 9
Lost to follow-up: 9
Missed visit: 1

Placebo (*n* = 9)

Not completed (*n* = 2)
Lost to follow-up: 1
Gastric stapling: 1

Alendronate (*n* = 9)

Not completed (*n* = 2)
Lost to follow-up: 1
Rash: 1

Completed 12-M (*n* = 55) | Placebo (*n* = 7) 12-M | Alendronate (*n* = 7) 12-M | Completed 12-M (*n* = 30)

2-yr Extension

Completed 24-M (*n* = 33) | Placebo (*n* = 3) 24-M | Completed 24-M (*n* = 23)

Completed 36-M (*n* = 20) | Placebo (*n* = 3) 36-M | Completed 36-M (*n* = 7)

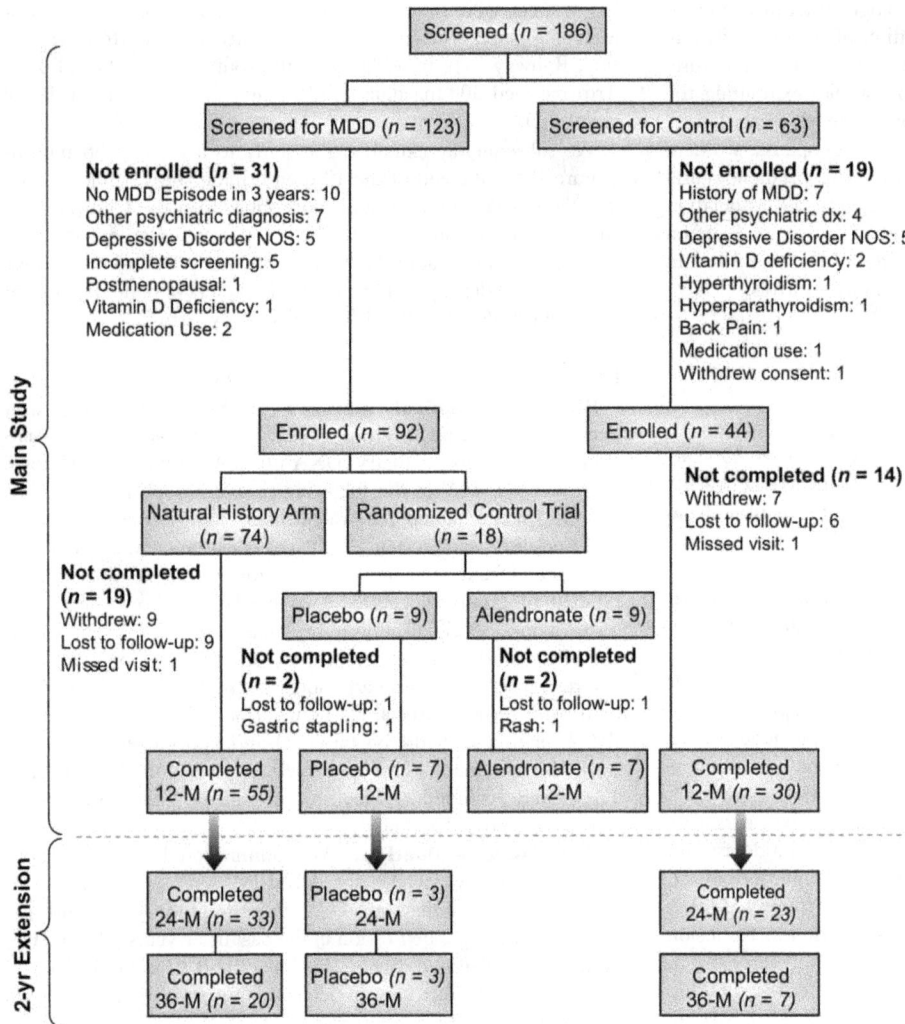

Figure 1. Study flow diagram. Note: The number of exclusions does not match the number of people as some participants were found to have more than one exclusionary criterion.

Repeated-measures analysis of variance (ANOVA) using mixed modeling was used to compare changes in BMD over time, and was adjusted for BMI. All analyses were done using SAS v9.2 (SAS Institute Inc, Cary, NC), and all tests were 2-sided with a significance level of 0.05.

Results

Clinical characteristics of study participants over time

Participant retention rate over the course of the main study was not significantly different between groups (women with MDD 78%; control women 68%; P = 0.211). The subjects who elected to enroll in the study extension did not differ in demographic characteristics from those who did not (data not shown). Of note, only 2 of the 18 women with depression participating in the Clinical Trial Arm were lost to follow-up.

Our sample was composed of mostly white, college-educated women (Table 1). Demographic characteristics were not different between women with MDD and controls at any of the study follow-up phases, but women with MDD tended to have a higher BMI and tended to be less often married than control women. Women with MDD reached menarche one year earlier than

controls but had a similar number of pregnancies and a similar current use of OCP than controls. Alcohol use was less common in women with MDD.

At baseline, only one-fifth of women with MDD (17/92) had current depression defined as a major episode within the last month. This sample of women with MDD however, had a considerable lifetime burden of depression, as indicated by cumulative history (68.6±77.9 months) and total number of depressive episodes (5.9±11.4). Age of onset was in the late teens (19±9 years old). Approximately half (52%) of the women had other *DSM-IV* axis I diagnoses, mostly anxiety disorders (not shown). Finally, 81 out of 92 women were taking antidepressants, 70% a selective serotonin reuptake inhibitor (SSRI), and 30% another antidepressant. Hamilton anxiety and depression scores were relatively low in women with depression consistent with their remission state, and remained stable over time (Figure 2).

BMD over time in the Extended Natural History Arm

At baseline, BMD was between 2% and 3% lower in women with MDD at the main skeletal sites, however, these differences did not reach statistical significance (Table 2). The prevalence of osteopenia appeared consistently greater in women with MDD

Table 1. Baseline demographic, lifestyle and clinical characteristics of study participants included at various study follow-up phases.*

Characteristics	BASELINE			12-MONTH STUDY			24- MONTH EXTENSION STUDY		
	MDD Women (n=92)	Control Women (n=44)	P	MDD Women (n=72)	Control Women (n=30)	P	MDD Women (n=36)	Control Women (n=23)	P
Age, y	36.0 (6.9)	35.3 (6.9)	0.50	36.0 (6.9)	36.0 (6.8)	0.91	38.2 (6.3)	36.6 (7.1)	0.41
BMI, kgm²	26.4 (6.2)	24.1 (3.7)	0.10	25.8 (5.6)	23.8 (3.4)	0.23	26.3 (5.1)	23.6 (2.9)	0.06
Race (White), %	87	86	1.00	88	90	1.00	94	96	1.00
Education, y	16.4 (2.1)	16.3 (2.1)	0.66	16.7 (2.0)	16.7 (2.1)	0.94	16.5 (1.8)	16.4 (1.9)	0.85
Married, %	36	48	0.26	35	53	0.12	39	61	0.12
Age Menarche, y	12.5 (1.6)	13.0 (1.6)	0.11	12.6 (1.5)	13.1 (1.6)	0.17	12.7 (1.3)	13.0 (1.3)	0.71
No. Pregnancies	1.2 (1.6)	1.2 (1.3)	0.59	1.0 (1.5)	1.3 (1.5)	0.32	1.3 (1.7)	1.4 (1.5)	0.81
Current OCP, %	32	34	0.85	32	30	1.00	19	22	1.00
Alcohol Use, %	70	98	<0.001	81	97	0.06	89	100	0.15
History of smoking, %	40	34	0.58	41	27	0.26	44	22	0.10
Calcium intake, mg/d‡	1396 (663)	1385 (734)	0.71	1356 (627)	1461 (810)	0.78	1392 (618)	1550 (856)	0.61
Caffeine intake, mg/d	215 (261)	217 (164)	0.43	193 (251)	219 (164)	0.27	208 (282)	202 (155)	0.53
Cooper test§, m/12 min	1316 (385)	1400 (254)	0.12	1328 (386)	1398 (273)	0.23	1236 (356)	1402 (247)	**0.03**

Abbreviations: BMI, body mass index (calculated as weight in kilograms divided by height in meters squared); MDD, major depressive disorder; OCP, oral contraceptive pill.

*All values expressed as mean (SD), unless otherwise specified.

‡Calcium intake calculated from dietary and supplement sources.

§Index of physical fitness, meters covered in 12-minut

A

B

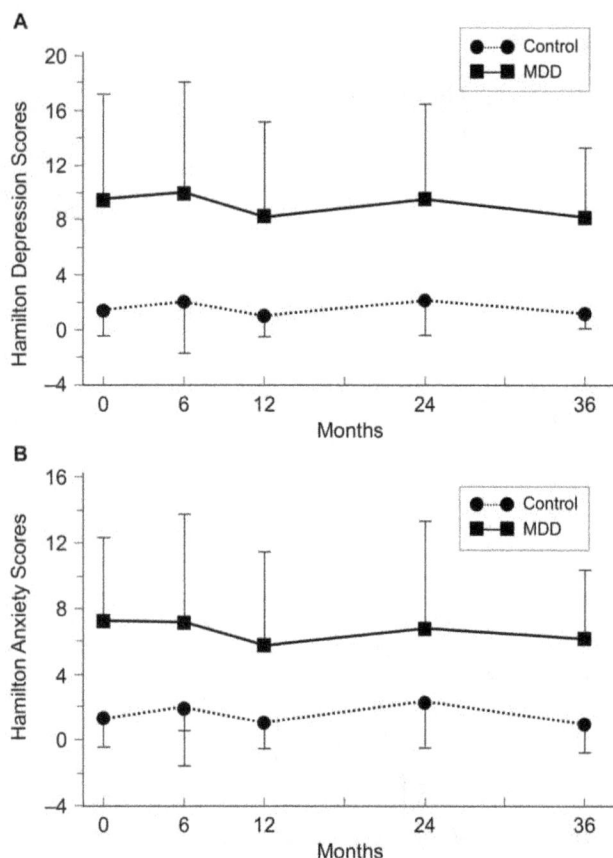

Figure 2. Hamilton depression (upper panel) and anxiety (lower panel) scores in women with MDD and control women over time. Both depression and anxiety scores were relatively low and remained stable over time in women with MDD. As expected, scores for depression and anxiety were much higher in women with MDD vs. control women.

compared to control women at the total hip and femoral neck. Over 36 months, there was no decline in BMD in either group.

Biochemical markers of bone turnover and hormones of hypothalamic-pituitary-adrenal (HPA) axis in the Extended Natural History Arm

Intact PTH levels were significantly higher in women with MDD vs. control women and generally remained higher up to 36 months (Table 3). Ionized calcium was lower in women with MDD at baseline and this difference was maintained across study duration. Vitamin D levels at baseline were significantly lower in women with MDD. Bone specific alkaline phosphatase, a marker of bone formation, was significantly higher in women with MDD at baseline and remained higher in this group across study duration, although only statistically significantly different at 12 months. Another marker of bone formation, serum osteocalcin, was not different between groups and neither was urinary N-telopeptide, a marker of bone resorption. The 8 am plasma ACTH was higher in women with MDD at baseline and 6 months only. The 8 am serum cortisol and urinary free cortisol levels were not different between groups at any time point.

Relationship between plasma cortisol and indices of clinical severity of depression and anxiety and BMD over time in the Extended Natural History Arm

There was no relationship between current depression, current treatment or current SSRI treatment vs. BMD and biochemical markers of bone turnover. Surprisingly, in women with MDD, both depression and anxiety scores were slightly positively related with BMD at the AP spine (BMD values after adjustment for BMI versus depression and anxiety scores, respectively: $r = 0.173$; $p = 0.005$; $r = 0.136$; $p = 0.029$) and trochanter (data not shown).

BMD over time in the Clinical Trial Arm

Fourteen out of 92 of women with MDD (20%) and none of the controls exhibited a T-score lower than -1.5 in at least one skeletal site. Thirteen of these women with MDD participated in the Clinical Trial Arm of the study (Figure 3). Patients in the placebo group compared to those randomized to alendronate had similar characteristics. Treatment with alendronate significantly increased BMD at the lumbar spine (0.8525 ± 0.0312 g/cm^2 vs. 0.8792 ± 0.0379 g/cm^2, P = 0.003; C.I., 0.01 to 0.04, baseline vs. 12-month) and tended to increase BMD at the femoral neck (0.7423 ± 0.0735 vs. 0.7588 ± 0.0709 g/cm^2, P = 0.06). No changes over time were observed in the placebo group. Alendronate treatment decreased osteocalcin concentration (4.2 ± 1.6 vs. 2.1 ± 1.1 ng/ml, P = 0.04; C.I., -4.0 to -0.2, baseline vs. 12-month), but did not significantly affect bone-specific alkaline phosphatase or urinary N-telopeptide. There were no changes in biochemical markers in the placebo group.

Discussion

Osteoporosis is a significant cause of morbidity and mortality in the US and costs approximately $17 billion dollars annually [43]. It results in over two million fractures annually in the US, 71% of which occur in women [43]. Therefore, investigation and identification of risk factors are of great importance. There have been several studies with conflicting findings regarding the possible influence of depression on BMD [25–42]; most of these studies were retrospective analyses conducted in post-menopausal women. In this study, we followed a group of premenopausal women with MDD and healthy controls prospectively and measured their BMD at regular intervals. Our finding that neither group exhibited a substantial change in BMD at any skeletal site over time may not be surprising since BMD has been reported to remain relatively stable in healthy premenopausal women [44–47]. The observation that women with MDD maintained their BMD throughout the study is reassuring as it implies that little, if any, bone loss was associated with MDD in this age range and time span. It should be however noted that these subjects were aware that they were participating in a clinical experiment, thus we cannot exclude a non specific "Hawthorne effect". In this particular case, regular encounters with the research team may have positively influenced their mood and induced improvements in life style conditions. Our observation allows for considering prophylactic treatment of these women to prevent osteoporosis after menopause, when their risk is magnified. Women reach peak bone mass by their third decade [48,49] and BMD remains relatively stable until menopause where women begin to lose up to 1–2% of the BMD annually [44–47].

Alterations in the HPA axis are significant findings in biological psychiatry [50]. Several studies have investigated the possible pathophysiology of osteoporosis in psychiatric patients and have hypothesized a link between depression and low BMD [28]. Elevated ACTH and cortisol levels, and enhanced cortisol

Table 2. BMD values adjusted by BMI in women with depression versus control women at each main skeletal site.[*]

Site	BASELINE Control	MDD	P	6-MONTH Control	MDD	P	12-MONTH Control	MDD	P	24-MONTH Control	MDD	P	36-MONTH Control	MDD	P
AP Spine															
Density, g/cm²	1.053 (0.016)	1.021 (0.011)	0.10	1.072 (0.015)	1.040 (0.011)	0.10	1.067 (0.017)	1.041 (0.012)	0.22	1.063 (0.022)	1.051 (0.018)	0.69	1.103 (0.042)	1.052 (0.023)	0.30
T-score	−0.014 (0.143)	−0.266 (0.098)	0.44	0.132 (0.137)	−0.090 (0.103)	0.20	0.148 (0.154)	−0.067 (0.107)	0.26	0.146 (0.194)	0.068 (0.153)	0.76	0.482 (0.369)	0.085 (0.199)	0.36
Percent Osteopenia, %	15.9	18.9	0.81	14.7	15.0	1.00	16.7	16.4	1.00	17.4	11.1	0.70	00	17.4	0.55
Total hip															
Density, g/cm²	0.986 (0.0163)	0.956 (0.011)	0.13	0.991 (0.019)	0.970 (0.014)	0.38	0.982 (0.020)	0.965 (0.014)	0.48	0.969 (0.020)	0.968 (0.016)	0.97	0.998 (0.037)	0.965 (0.020)	0.45
T-score	0.294 (0.130)	0.058 (0.089)	0.14	0.306 (0.146)	0.209 (0.109)	0.60	0.303 (0.158)	0.157 (0.110)	0.45	0.203 (0.166)	0.193 (0.130)	0.96	0.400 (0.312)	0.157 (0.168)	0.51
Percent Osteopenia, %	2.3	15.2	**0.04**	2.9	11.7	0.25	0	14.8	**0.03**	4.4	11.1	0.64	14.3	13.0	1.005
Femoral neck															
Density, g/cm²	0.878 (0.016)	0.843 (0.011)	0.13	0.878 (0.0178)	0.852 (0.013)	0.39	0.858 (0.019)	0.850 (0.013)	0.25	0.838 (0.021)	0.845 (0.017)	0.72	0.857 (0.041)	0.831 (0.022)	0.59
T score	0.179 (0.135)	−0.116 (0.093)	0.37	0.174 (0.154)	−0.025 (0.115)	0.37	0.046 (0.168)	−0.033 (0.117)	0.31	−0.113 (0.188)	−0.014 (0.925)	0.71	−0.003 (0.360)	−0.210 (0.193)	0.62
Percent Osteopenia, %	4.6	17.4	0.06	8.8	15.0	0.53	13.3	13.1	1.00	30.4	11.1	0.09	28.6	13.0	0.57
Radius															
Density, g/cm²	0.712 (0.008)	0.695 (0.005)	0.13	0.711 (0.008)	0.670 (0.006)	0.19	0.710 (0.009)	0.694 (0.006)	0.14	0.715 (0.011)	0.698 (0.008)	0.24	0.719 (0.020)	0.706 (0.011)	0.57
T score	0.344 (0.124)	−0.003 (0.085)	0.053	0.291 (0.134)	0.115 (0.100)	0.30	0.236 (0.143)	0.002 (0.098)	0.18	0.343 (0.175)	0.064 (0.137)	0.23	0.398 (0.329)	0.195 (0.177)	0.60
Percent Osteopenia, %	9.1	10.9	1.00	8.8	6.7	0.70	6.9	13.1	0.49	8.7	11.1	1.00	0	8.7	1.00

Table 3. Calcium metabolism, bone turnover markers, and hormonal measurements in women with depression compared to control women.*

Variable	BASELINE			6-MONTH			12-MONTH			24-MONTH			36-MONTHS		
	Control	MDD	P	Control	MDD	P	Control	MDD	P	Control	MDD	P	Control	MDD	P
iPTH, pg/mL	37.00 (16.67)	43.84 (18.91)	**0.04**	31.85 (11.72)	41.71 (18.40)	**<0.01**	24.45 (5.704)	38.80 (18.51)	**<0.001**	25.35 (9.369)	31.28 (12.56)	0.07	26.26 (6.509)	37.64 (13.74)	**0.04**
Ionized calcium, mmol/L	1.261 (0.04139)	1.242 (0.04755)	**0.03**	1.256 (0.03606)	1.242 (0.04800)	0.16	1.254 (0.03118)	1.262 (0.05033)	0.43	1.267 (0.02739)	1.265 (0.04738)	0.91	1.271 (0.03934)	1.272 (0.04695)	0.96
25-Hydroxy-vitamin D, ng/mL‡	34.20 (2.267)	27.57 (1.112)	**<0.01**	N/A	N/A	N/A	N/A	N/A	N/A	N/A	N/A	N/A	N/A	N/A	N/A
Bone-specific alkaline phosphatase, µg/L	8.567 (2.201)	9.710 (2.726)	**0.03**	8.852 (2.099)	9.901 (3.054)	0.08	9.231 (2.526)	10.63 (3.190)	**0.04**	9.640 (2.395)	10.72 (3.716)	0.24	8.314 (1.878)	10.70 (3.623)	0.10
8am Osteocalcin, ng/mL	4.383 (1.822)	4.665 (3.593)	0.66	4.377 (1.222)	3.924 (1.863)	0.22	4.597 (1.379)	4.447 (1.620)	0.66	4.280 (1.084)	4.250 (2.175)	0.95	3.357 (1.391)	5.297 (3.653)	0.18
Urinary N-telopeptide, nmol/mmol of creatinine	24.08 (10.34)	21.18 (7.849)	0.09	23.06 (8.534)	24.99 (13.27)	0.46	24.04 (12.13)	23.11 (8.866)	0.68	20.19 (8.118)	23.88 (10.51)	0.21	17.00 (6.261)	26.04 (13.15)	0.11
8am plasma ACTH pg/mL	23.54 (8.410)	33.91 (27.30)	**0.02**	20.57 (7.365)	27.01 (16.05)	**0.03**	19.72 (7.005)	23.55 (13.84)	0.16	13.46 (6.291)	19.38 (14.25)	0.10	14.27 (6.434)	17.45 (8.912)	0.38
8am serum cortisol, µg/dL	19.52 (8.498)	20.36 (6.400)	0.54	18.37 (7.869)	18.33 (7.549)	0.98	17.40 (9.328)	17.23 (7.163)	0.93	11.85 (6.729)	14.50 (8.453)	0.22	10.60 (2.871)	13.08 (7.360)	0.39
Urinary-free cortisol, µg/24 h	62.19 (22.58)	57.57 (26.91)	0.35	44.95 (21.96)	49.47 (23.89)	0.38	50.04 (22.71)	47.13 (22.72)	0.58	43.82 (19.91)	41.69 (18.15)	0.72	52.33 (11.02)	42.30 (18.17)	0.36

*All values expressed as mean (SD), unless otherwise specified.
‡25-Hydroxyvitamin D, ng/mL levels were only obtained at baseline.
Sample size indicated in Table 1.

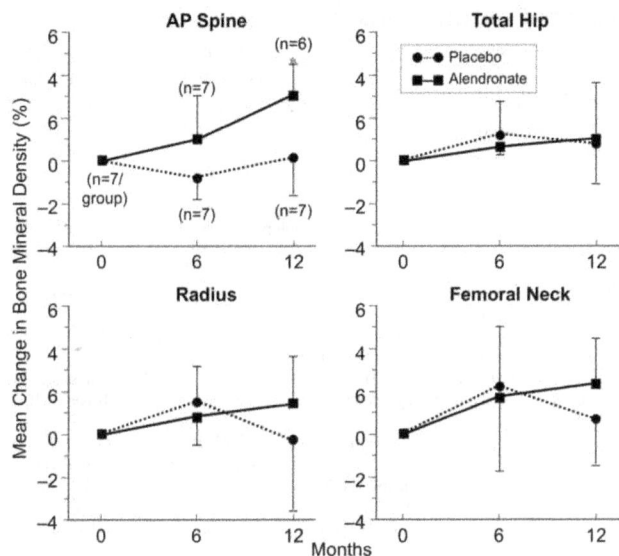

Figure 3. Bone mineral density measurements in women with MDD and moderate osteopenia or osteoporosis randomized to alendronate *vs.* placebo. Over 12 months, the Alendronate group showed a significant increase in BMD at the lumbar spine (P = 0.003), and there was a trend for increased BMD at the femoral neck (P = 0.06). No changes over time were observed in the Placebo group.

responsiveness have been demonstrated in depressed individuals [25,32,41,51–53]. Similar to the bone loss observed in Cushing syndrome as a result of hypercortisolemia, women with depression could thus have decreased BMD, albeit not as pronounced as in Cushing syndrome. We found that ACTH levels and bone-specific alkaline phosphatase levels tended to be elevated in women with depression compared to controls. Serum and urinary free cortisol, osteocalcin, and urinary N-telopeptide levels were not different between participants with depression and controls throughout the study.

In an ancillary investigation, we reported that women with depression had a greater prevalence of *Bcl1* polymorphism, which is associated with glucocorticoid hypersensitivity [54–56]. Therefore, women with MDD may also have a greater HPA activity at tissue level. The cortisol plasma levels were not elevated in our study of women with MDD, but hyperactivity of the HPA axis is not always accompanied by hypercortisolism [57]. Alterations in the HPA axis tend to occur during acute depressive states and normalize after treatment [51,53]. Given that the majority of the subjects with depression were being pharmacologically treated throughout the duration of the study as previously reported [27], increases in cortisol levels may not have occurred, as these patients were likely to be in clinical remission. As we have recently reported in greater detail in a related manuscript [58], approximately half of the sample was comprised of women with melancholic depression, and the remaining subjects suffered either from undifferentiated or atypical depression. Women with atypical features of depression had higher ACTH levels during the night and women with undifferentiated depression had a significantly higher prevalence of low BMD at the femoral neck than controls. Thus, the clinical subtype of depression may influence bone and endocrine features, among other parameters.

In the women with MDD and moderate osteopenia or osteoporosis, weekly alendronate was effective in increasing BMD. This is the first pharmacotherapeutic study of osteoporosis in younger women with MDD and one of the few controlled studies of alendronate treatment in premenopausal women [59–61]. Of note, in this arm the drop-out rate was only 10%, much smaller than in the overall cohort. In future research, it would be interesting to identify the predictors of drop-out rate in studies of women with depression. It is possible that the women participating in the randomized controlled arm of this trial may have been more motivated to remain in the study than the women with depression in the natural history arm and the normal controls, possibly because of the therapeutic advantages of the drug being received. As estrogens are not a treatment option in this population, our study supports the possible use of alendronate in this population. Recently the use of selective serotonin reuptake inhibitors has been linked to an increased risk of fractures and bone loss [62]. As reported [27], in our study the use of selective serotonin reuptake inhibitors was not associated with low BMD.

Vitamin D levels were lower in women with MDD than controls. Consistent with decreased vitamin D levels, women with MDD had significantly higher iPTH and ionized calcium levels, highly suggestive of secondary hyperparathyroidism. PTH levels remained elevated in women with MDD compared to controls. While elevated PTH levels have been demonstrated in depressed elderly women and young men [36,63,64], to the best of our knowledge, this is the first time elevated PTH plasma levels are observed in premenopausal women with MDD. Future studies should be conducted to evaluate the pathogenetic role of secondary hyperparathyroidism in subjects with depression.

Study limitations and merits

The small sample size, together with a drop-out rate of approximately 30% in the first year, may have reduced our ability to detect some associations. Vitamin D levels were only measured at baseline. Furthermore, since there is little bone loss in this age range [44–47], the duration of the study and the age of the participants may have limited our ability to identify a subtle decrease in BMD. Our results may have failed to detect significant changes in biochemical markers and hormones in patients who were in remission since abnormalities in many of these parameters might only be apparent during acute disease states [51,53]. Our sample was well characterized and homogeneous, and the length of follow-up was longer than most studies of this kind.

Conclusion

Premenopausal women with MDD had lower BMD than controls over a sustained period of time. Larger and longer studies are needed to confirm and extend these observations. The effects of antidepressants and other psychotropic medications on bone mass *per se* should be assessed. The reversibility of bone loss due to successful behavioral or pharmacologic interventions or to spontaneous resolution of depression should be considered. Lastly, studies examining the role of genetics leading to enhanced susceptibility to reductions in BMD need to be conducted.

Acknowledgments

Alendronate and Placebo were generously provided by Merck Research Laboratories, Rahway, NJ. The informatics support for this study was provided by Mr. Frank Pierce from ®Esprit Health. The following individuals were investigators of the POWER Protocol: (Premenopausal Osteoporosis Women Alendronate Depression): Giovanni Cizza (Principal Investigator), Ann Berger, Marc R. Blackman, Karim A. Calis, Gyorgy Csako, Bart Drinkard, Farideh Eskandari, Philip W. Gold, McDonald Horne, Christine Kotila, Pedro Martinez, Kate Musallam, Terry M. Phillips, James. C. Reynolds, Nancy G. Sebring, Esther Sternberg and Sara Torvik.

We wish to thank: all the subjects participating in this study and the NIMH nurses who supported these studies. The informatics support for this study was provided by Mr. Frank Pierce from ®Esprit Health.

Author Contributions

Conceived and designed the experiments: G. Cizza PWG G. Csako. Performed the experiments: G. Cizza FE PM ST JCR. Analyzed the data: G. Cizza SM VTN FE ST NS G. Csako. Wrote the paper: G. Cizza SM PM ST G. Csako.

References

1. World Health Organization (2008) The global burden of disease: 2004 update. Geneva: World Health Organization ISBN 92 4 156257 9
2. Kessler RC, Berglund P, Demler O, Jin R, Koretz D, et al. (2003) The epidemiology of major depressive disorder: results from the national comorbidity survey replication (NCS-R). JAMA 289:3095–3105.
3. Stewart WF, Ricci JA, Chee E, Hahn SR, Morganstein D (2003) Cost of lost productive work time among US workers with depression. JAMA 289:3135–3144.
4. Licinio J, Wong ML (1999) The role of inflammatory mediators in the biology of major depression: central nervous system cytokines modulate the biological substrate of depressive symptoms, regulate stress-responsive systems, and contribute to neurotoxicity and neuroprotection. Mol Psychiatry 4:317–327.
5. Barth J, Schumacher M, Herrmann-Lingen C (2004) Depression as a risk factor for mortality in patients with coronary heart disease: a meta-analysis. Psychosom Med 66:802–813.
6. Lett HS, Blumenthal JA, Babyak MA, Sherwood A, Strauman T, et al. (2004) Depression as a risk factor for coronary artery disease: evidence, mechanisms, and treatment. Psychosom Med 66:305–315.
7. Whang W, Kubzansky LD, Kawachi I, Rexrode KM, Kroenke CH, et al. (2009) Depression and risk of sudden cardiac death and coronary heart disease in women: results from the Nurses' Health Study. J Am Coll Cardiol 53:950–958.
8. Rubinow DR, Girdler S (2011) Hormones, heart disease, and health: individualized medicine versus throwing the baby out with the bathwater. Depress Anxiety 28:E1–E15.
9. Alesci S, Martinez PE, Kelkar S, Ilias I, Ronsaville DS, et al. (2005) Major depression is associated with significant diurnal elevations in plasma interleukin-6 levels, a shift of its circadian rhythm, and loss of physiological complexity in its secretion: clinical implications. J Clin Endocrinol Metab 90:2522–2530.
10. Anisman H, Merali Z, Hayley S (2008) Neurotransmitter, peptide and cytokine processes in relation to depressive disorder: comorbidity between depression and neurodegenerative disorders. Prog Neurobiol 85:1–74.
11. Dantzer R, O'Connor JC, Freund GG, Johnson RW, Kelley KW (2008) From inflammation to sickness and depression: when the immune system subjugates the brain. Nat Rev Neurosci 9:46–56.
12. Blume J, Douglas SD, Evans DL (2011) Immune suppression and immune activation in depression. Brain Behav Immun 25:221–229.
13. Brown ES, Varghese FP, McEwen BS (2004) Association of depression with medical illness: does cortisol play a role? Biol Psychiatry 55:1–9.
14. Timonen M, Laakso M, Jokelainen J, Rajala U, Meyer-Rochow VB, et al. (2005) Insulin resistance and depression: cross sectional study. BMJ 330:17–18.
15. Adriaanse MC, Dekker JM, Nijpels G, Heine RJ, Snoek FJ, et al. (2006) Associations between depressive symptoms and insulin resistance: the Hoorn Study. Diabetologia 49:2874–2877.
16. Skilton MR, Moulin P, Terra JL, Bonnet F (2007) Associations between anxiety, depression, and the metabolic syndrome. Biol Psychiatry 62:1251–1257.
17. Everson-Rose SA, Meyer PM, Powell LH, Pandey D, Torréns JI, et al. (2004) Depressive symptoms, insulin resistance, and risk of diabetes in women at midlife. Diabetes Care 27:2856–2862.
18. Mezuk B, Eaton WW, Albrecht S, Golden SH (2008) Depression and type 2 diabetes over the lifespan: a meta-analysis. Diabetes Care 31:2383–90.
19. Golden SH, Lazo M, Carnethon M, Bertoni AG, Schreiner PJ, et al. (2008) Examining a bidirectional association between depressive symptoms and diabetes. JAMA 299:2751–2759.
20. Pan A, Lucas M, Sun Q, van Dam RM, Franco OH, et al. (2010) Bidirectional association between depression and type 2 diabetes mellitus in women. Arch Intern Med 170:1884–1891
21. Onyike CI, Crum RM, Lee HB, Lyketsos CG, Eaton WW (2003) Is obesity associated with major depression? results from the Third National Health and Nutrition Examination Survey. Am J Epidemiol 158:1139–1147.
22. Blaine B (2008) Does depression cause obesity? A meta-analysis of longitudinal studies of depression and weight control. J Health Psychol 13:1190–1197.
23. Simon GE, Ludman EJ, Linde JA, Operskalski BH, Ichikawa L, et al. (2008) Association between obesity and depression in middle-aged women. Gen Hosp Psychiatry 30:32–39.
24. Allison DB, Newcomer JW, Dunn AL, Blumenthal JA, Fabricatore AN, et al. (2009) Obesity among those with mental disorders: a National Institute of Mental Health meeting report. Am J Prev Med 36:341–350.
25. Amsterdam J, Hooper M (1998) Bone density measurement in major depression. Prog Neuropsychopharmacol Biol Psychiatry 22:267–277.
26. Cizza G, Ravn P, Chrousos GP, Gold PW (2001) Depression: a major, unrecognized risk factor for osteoporosis? Trends Endocrinol Metab 12:198–203.
27. Eskandari F, Martinez PE, Torvik S, Phillips TM, Sternberg EM, et al. (2007) Low bone mass in premenopausal women with depression. Arch Intern Med 167:2329–2336.
28. Cizza G, Primma S, Csako G (2009) Depression as a risk factor for osteoporosis. Trends Endocrinol Metab 20:367–373.
29. Yirmiya R, Bab I (2009) Major depression is a risk factor for low bone mineral density: a meta-analysis. Biol Psychiatry 66:423–43.
30. Cizza G, Primma S, Coyle M, Gourgiotis L, Csako G (2010) Depression and osteoporosis: a research synthesis with meta-analysis. Horm Metab Re 42,467–482.
31. Williams IJ, Bjerkeset O, Langhammer A, Berk M, Pasco JA, et al. (2011) The association between depressive and anxiety symptoms and bone mineral density in the general population: the HUNT Study. J Affect Disord 131:164–171.
32. Mussolino ME, Jonas BS, Looker AC (2004) Depression and bone mineral density in young adults: results from NHANES III. Psychosom Med 66:533–537.
33. Mussolino ME (2005) Depression and hip fracture risk: the NHANES I epidemiologic follow-up study. Public Health Rep 120:71–75
34. Kahl KG, Greggersen W, Rudolf S, Stoeckelhuber BM, Bergmann-Koester CU, et al. (2006) Bone mineral density, bone turnover, and osteoprotegerin in depressed women with and without borderline personality disorder. Psychosom Med 68:669–674.
35. Petronijevic M, Petronijevic N, Ivkovic M, Stefanović D, Radonjić N, et al. (2008) Low bone mineral density and high bone metabolism turnover in premenopausal women with unipolar depression. Bone 42:582–590.
36. Michelson D, Stratakis C, Hill L, Reynolds J, Galliven E, et al. (1996) Bone mineral density in women with depression. N Engl J Med 335:1176–1181.
37. Ozsoy S, Esel E, Turan MT, Kula M, Demir H, et al. (2005) Is there any alteration in bone mineral density in patients with depression? Turk Psikiyatri Derg 16:77–82.
38. Reginster JY, Deroisy R, Paul I, Hansenne M, Ansseau M (1999) Depressive vulnerability is not an independent risk factor for osteoporosis in postmenopausal women. Maturitas 33:133–137.
39. Whooley MA, Cauley JA, Zmuda JM, Haney EM, Glynn NW (2004) Depressive symptoms and bone mineral density in older men. J Geriatr Psychiatry Neurol 17:88–92.
40. Yazici AE, Bagis S, Tot S, Sahin G, Yazici K, et al. (2005) Bone mineral density in premenopausal women with major depression. Joint Bone Spine 72:540–543.
41. Halbreich U, Rojansky N, Palter S, Hreshchyshyn M, Kreeger J, et al. (1995) Decreased bone mineral density in medicated psychiatric patients. Psychosom Med 57:485–491.
42. Michelson D, Stratakis C, Hill L, Reynolds J, Galliven E, et al. (1996) Bone mineral density in women with depression. N Engl J Med 16:1176–1181.
43. Burge R, Dawson-Hughes B, Solomon DH, Wong JB, King A, et al. (2007) Incidence and economic burden of osteoporosis-related fractures in the United States, 2005–2025. J Bone Miner Res 22:465–475.
44. Bouxsein ML, Myburgh KH, van der Meulen MC, Lindenberger E, Marcus R (1994) Age-related differences in cross-sectional geometry of the forearm bones in healthy women. Calcif Tissue Int 54:113–118.
45. Burger H, van Daele PLA, Algra D, van den Ouweland FA, Grobbee DE, et al. (1994) The association between age and bone mineral density in men and women aged 55 years and over: The Rotterdam Study. Bone Miner 25:1–13.
46. Ahlborg HG, Johnell O, Turner CH, Rannevik G, Karlsson MK (2003) Bone loss and bone size after menopause. N Engl J Med 349:327–334.
47. Emaus N, Berntsen GK, Joakimsen RM, Fønnebø V (2005) Longitudinal changes in forearm bone mineral density in women and men aged 25–44 years: the Tromsø study: a population-based study. Am J Epidemiol 162:633–643.
48. Matkovic V, Jelic T, Wardlaw GM, Ilich JZ, Goel PK, et al. (1994) Timing of peak bone mass in Caucasian females and its implication for the prevention of osteoporosis. J Clin Invest 93:799–808.
49. Heaney RP, Abrams S, Dawson-Hughes B, Looker A, Marcus R, et al. (2000) Peak bone mass. Osteoporos Int 11:985–1009.
50. Stetler C, Miller GE (2011) Depression and hypothalamic-pituitary-adrenal activation: a quantitative summary of four decades of research. Psychosom Med 73:114–126.
51. Aihara M, Ida I, Yuuki N, Oshima A, Kumano H, et al. (2007) HPA axis dysfunction in unmedicated major depressive disorder and its normalization by pharmacotherapy correlates with alteration of neural activity in prefrontal cortex and limbic/paralimbic regions. Neuroimaging 155:245–256.
52. Heuser I, Yassouridis A, Holsboer F (1994) The combined dexamethasone/CRH test: a refined laboratory test for psychiatric disorders. J Psychiatr Res 28:341–356.
53. Kunugi H, Ida I, Owashi T, Kimura M, Inoue Y, et al. (2006) Assessment of the dexamethasone/CRH test as a state-dependent marker for hypothalamic-

pituitaryadrenal (HPA) axis abnormalities in major depressive episode: a multicenter study. Neuropsychopharmacology 31:212–220.

54. Krishnamurthy P, Romagni P, Torvik S, Gold PW, Charney DS, et al. (2008) Glucocorticoid receptor gene polymorphisms in premenopausal women with depression. Horm Metab Res 40:194–198.

55. van Rossum EF, Koper JW, van den Beld AW, Uitterlinden AG, Arp P, et al. (2003) Identification of the BclI polymorphism in the glucocorticoid receptor gene: association with sensitivity to glucocorticoids in vivo and body mass index. Clin Endocrinol 59:585–592.

56. van Rossum EF, Binder EB, Majer M, Koper JW, Ising M, et al. (2006) Polymorphisms of the glucocorticoid receptor gene and major depression. Biol Psychiatry 59:681–688.

57. Nemeroff CB (1996) The corticotropin-releasing factor (CRF) hypothesis of depression: new findings and new directions. Mol Psychiatry 1:336–342.

58. Cizza G, Ronsaville DS, Kleitz H, Eskandari F, Mistry S, et al. (2012) Clinical subtypes of depression are associated with specific metabolic parameters and circadian endocrine profiles in women: the power study. PLoS One 7(1):e28912.

59. Adachi JD, Saag KG, Delmas PD, Liberman UA, Emkey RD, et al. (2001) Two-year effects of alendronate on bone mineral density and vertebral fracture in patients receiving glucocorticoids. Arthritis Rheum 4444:202–211.

60. Gourlay M, Brown SA (2004) Clinical considerations in premenopausal osteoporosis. Arch Intern Med 164:603–614.

61. Bhalla A (2010) Management of osteoporosis in a pre-menopausal woman. Best Pract Res Clin Rheumatol 24:313–332.

62. Wu Q, Bencaz AF, Hentz JG, Crowell MD (2012) Selective serotonin reuptake inhibitor treatment and risk of fractures: a meta-analysis of cohort and case-control studies. Osteoporos Int 23:365–375.

63. Hoogendijk WJG, Lips P, Dik MG, Deeg DJ, Beekman AT, et al. (2008) Depression is associated with decreased 25-hydroxyvitamin D and increased parathyroid hormone levels in older adults. Arch Gen Psychiatry 65:508–512.

64. Zhao G, Ford ES, Li C, Balluz LS (2010) No associations between serum concentrations of 25-hydroxyvitamin D and parathyroid hormone and depression among US adults. Br J Nutr 104:1696–1702.

3

The Risk of Stroke after Percutaneous Vertebroplasty for Osteoporosis

Ching-Lan Wu[1,9], Jau-Ching Wu[2,3,4,9], Wen-Cheng Huang[2,3], Hung-Ta H. Wu[1,3], Hong-Jen Chiou[1,3], Laura Liu[5,6], Yu-Chun Chen[7]*, Tzeng-Ji Chen[8], Henrich Cheng[2,3,4], Cheng-Yen Chang[1,3]

1 Department of Radiology, Taipei Veterans General Hospital, Taipei, Taiwan, 2 Department of Neurosurgery, Neurological Institute, Taipei Veterans General Hospital, Taipei, Taiwan, 3 School of Medicine, National Yang-Ming University, Taipei, Taiwan, 4 Institute of Pharmacology, National Yang-Ming University, Taipei, Taiwan, 5 Department of Ophthalmology, Chang Gung Memorial Hospital, Taoyuan, Taiwan, 6 College of Medicine, Chang Gung University, Taoyuan, Taiwan, 7 Department of Medical Research and Education, National Yang-Ming University Hospital, I-Lan, Taiwan, 8 Institute of Hospital and Health Care Administration, National Yang-Ming University School of Medicine, Taipei, Taiwan

Abstract

Purpose: To investigate the incidence and risk of stroke after percutaneous vertebroplasty in patients with osteoporosis.

Methods: A group of 334 patients with osteoporosis, and who underwent percutaneous vertebroplasty during the study period, was compared to 1,655 age-, sex- and propensity score-matched patients who did not undergo vertebroplasty. All demographic covariates and co-morbidities were deliberately matched between the two groups to avoid selection bias. Every subject was followed-up for up to five years for stroke. Adjustments using a Cox regression model and Kaplan-Meier analyses were conducted.

Results: A total of 1,989 osteoporotic patients were followed up for 3,760.13 person-years. Overall, the incidence rates of any stroke, hemorrhagic stroke and ischemic stroke were 22.6, 4.2 and 19.6 per 1,000 person-years, respectively. Patients who underwent vertebroplasty were not more likely to have any stroke (crude hazard ratio = 1.13, $p = 0.693$), hemorrhagic stroke (HR = 2.21, $p = 0.170$), or ischemic stroke (HR = 0.96, $p = 0.90$). After adjusting for demographics, co-morbidities and medications, the vertebroplasty group had no significant difference with the comparison group in terms of any, hemorrhagic and ischemic strokes (adjusted HR = 1.22, 3.17, and 0.96, $p = 0.518$, 0.055, and 0.91, respectively).

Conclusions: Osteoporotic patients who undergo percutaneous vertebroplasty are not at higher risk of any stroke in the next five years after the procedure.

Editor: Giuseppe Biondi-Zoccai, University of Modena and Reggio Emilia, Italy

Funding: The authors have no support or funding to report.

Competing Interests: The authors have declared that no competing interests exist.

* E-mail: yuchn.chen@googlemail.com

9 These authors contributed equally to this work.

Introduction

Stroke is a major cause of disability and death worldwide [1,2]. Osteoporosis, as a known consequence of stroke, causes increased risk of fractures due to loss of bone desnity and falls [3,4,5,6,7,8,9]. The inter-relationship of stroke, physical inactivity, osteoporosis and fracture is mutually implicative and constitutes a vicious cycle for the elderly. An intervention that ameliorates any of these four components may significantly promote health in this population. Vertebroplasty is now a common surgical procedure for osteoporotic vertebral fractures. Aside from being popular among spine care specialists, its effect of pain relief has been demonstrated by randomized control studies [10,11,12]. Pulmonary, venous and cerebrovascular embolism with or without symptoms has been reported as complications [13,14,15,16]. Moreover, the long-term effect of vertebroplasty regarding the incidence of stroke in osteoporotic patients remains elusive.

Although very rare, stroke can happen soon or long after percutaneous vertebroplasty in osteoporotic patients [13,17,18,19].

There is increased risk of stroke after hip fractures and osteoporotic vertebral fractures [20]. This study hypothesized that the risk of stroke in osteoporotic patients did not increase after percutaneous vertebroplasty. The study also aimed to investigate the incidence and risk ratios of stroke after percutaneous vertebroplasty, as well as the differences in specific types (i.e. hemorrhagic or ischemic) of strokes.

In order to investigate such infrequent events and their correlation with surgery, a large number of patients with an extremely high follow-up rate was required. Thus, the National Health Insurance Research Database (NHIRD) was used so that follow-up would not be affected by patients seeking medical services across institutions. In Taiwan, hindrance to medical care is extremely low; this therefore enhanced the completeness and accuracy of identifying strokes, especially for those that did not happen immediately post-operation. This cohort study was deliberately designed to investigate the correlation of percutaneous vertebroplasty and subsequent strokes by applying a prudently matched comparison group with very similar disease profiles.

Materials and Methods

Data source

The National Health Insurance Research Database (NHIRD) of Taiwan contains 26 million administered insurants, accumulated between January 1996 and December 2008. A unique feature of the database is its comprehensive coverage of 99% of the population [21], who has unrestricted access to any healthcare provider of the patient's choice [22]. NHIRD data are de-identified and encrypted before their release for medical research. Thus, this study was exempted from full review by the Institutional Review Board.

The National Health Research Institute (NHRI) recompiles the medical claims and makes the database publicly available for research purposes. To protect privacy, individual and hospital identifiers are unique to the research database and can not be used to trace back to each individual patient or healthcare provider. Moreover, regular cross-checks and validation of the medical charts and claims are performed by the Bureau of National Health Insurance (NHI) of Taiwan to ensure the accuracy of diagnosis coding of the NHIRD. Fraudulent coding, overcharging, or malpractice by physicians and institutions are subject to penalties or suspension. Therefore, the fidelity of coding in the database is reliable; this was confirmed by a validation study [23].

Study cohort

This cohort study used a representative cohort composed of one million of Taiwan's cumulative population during the period January 1, 2000 to December 31, 2008. The representative cohort was provided by the NHRI through a random selection for scientific purposes, with no significant differences in age, gender or healthcare costs between the representative group and all beneficiaries under the NHI program. Many studies using this representative cohort have been published [20,24,25,26]. Extraction of the vertebroplasty and comparison groups from the database is illustrated in Figure 1. All original claims data of the extracted subjects were analyzed.

Identification of the vertebroplasty and medical treatment groups

A total of 58,703 persons with the International Classification of Disease, 9th Version (ICD-9) diagnostic code for osteoporosis (733.0) were identified from the database. First-time hospitaliza-

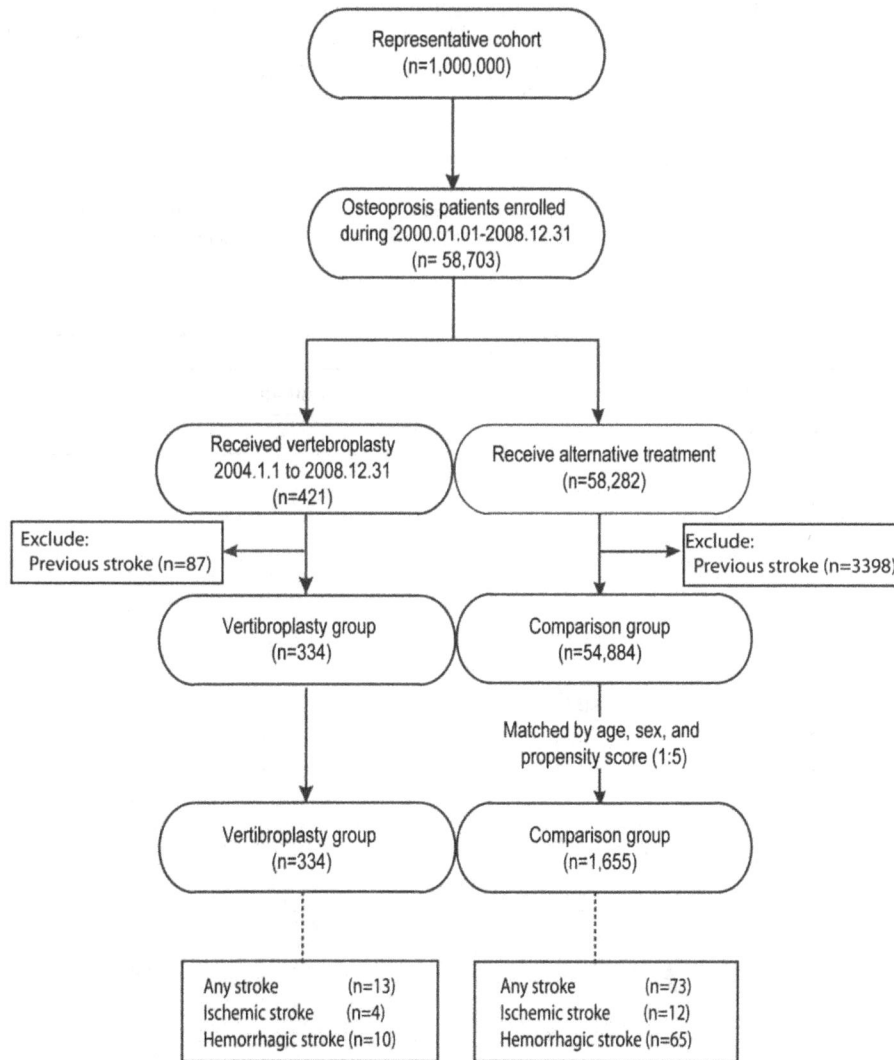

Figure 1. Flow of data processing. From an osteoporotic cohort of 58,703 patients in a nationwide representative cohort of one million people, 421 patients had percutaneous vertebroplasty (vertebroplasty group; n = 421), while age-, sex- and propensity score-matched patients comprised the comparison group (n = 1,655). The two groups were compared and followed-up for up to five years for subsequent stroke events.

tion with the ICD-9 procedure codes of percutaneous vertebro-plasty (81.65) and percutaneous vertebral augmentation (81.66) from January 1, 2004 to December 31, 2008 were identified and enrolled as the vertebroplasty group. The first day of follow-up (entry date) was defined as the date of vertebroplasty.

A carefully designed one-to-five comparison was conducted. The osteoporotic cohort also included all enrollees not exposed to vertebroplasty during the study period. For every subject in the vertebroplasty group, five subjects who received medical treatment (but not vertebroplasty) were randomly assigned as the comparison control group. This group had prudently matched characteristics, (i.e., propensity scores), as described below.

Propensity scores (i.e., the predicted probability that a person would receive vertebroplasty) were used to capture the comparison group in order to adjust for confounding factors associated with receiving vertebroplasty. The propensity scores were calculated by medical co-morbidities (i.e., history of hypertension, diabetes, dyslipidemia, chronic obstructive pulmonary disease, chronic renal failure, and Parkinson's disease), demographic characteristics (e.g., age, sex, insurance level, geographic location of residence, and urbanization level of residence), and other spinal diseases (e.g. spondylosis, spondylolithesis, spinal stenosis, intervertebral disc disorders, and inflammatory spondylopathies).

The first matched visit date of those in the comparison group was designated as their first day of follow-up (entry date). Every subject in the study cohort was tracked back from enrolment date to January 1, 2000 to ensure no previous vertebroplasty or stroke events. Each subject was followed-up for up to five years. The cohort study censored follow-up only on the following conditions: when the subjects expired, on the dates of outcome

incidence (i.e. stroke), or at the end of this cohort (December 31, 2008) (Fig. 1).

Ascertainment of covariates

There are known and unknown risk factors of stroke [27,28]. This study attempted to include influential covariates of stroke incidence for adjustment, including co-morbidities, exposure to medications, and baseline demographic characteristics. Co-morbidities included: hypertension (ICD-9 code, 401-5.x), diabetes mellitus (250.x), dyslipidemia (272.0-4), chronic obstructive pulmonary diseases (COPD) (490, 491.0-1, 491.20-2,491.8-9, 492.0, 492.8, 494, 494.0-1, and 496), chronic renal failure (585.x), Parkinson disease (332.0), atrial fibrillation (426-7.x), coronary heart disease (410-4.x), and valvular heart disease (394-7.x, 424.x). These were determined by the presence of either diagnostic codes of outpatient records or discharge codes of hospitalization records six months before the entry dates to the date of the outcome event or the end of follow-up. Adjustments for exposure to medications were defined as more than 90 days cumulative exposure to the medications of aspirin, lipid-lowering drugs, nitrates, anti-coagulants and non-steroid anti-inflammatory drugs (NSAIDs) between the entry dates and end of follow-up.

The demographic characteristics of each patient were adjusted by Charlson's co-morbidity index, age, sex and socio-economic status [29,30,31]. Socio-economic status was estimated by insurance level, and geographic location or residency, and urbanization level, used a similar method as previous NHIRD studies [22,32,33]. The income level of each subject was grouped into one of four categories according to the premium paid (NTD$ ≥40,000, 20,000–39,999, 1–19,999, and dependents). In the NHI

Table 1. Comparison for demographics and socio-economic status (n = 1989).

	Comparison group		Vertebroplasty group		
	n = 1655	(%)	n = 334	(%)	p value
Gender					0.975
Female	1292	(78.1)	261	(78.1)	
Male	363	(21.9)	73	(21.9)	
Age, Mean (SD)	75.1	(9.0)	75.0	(9.3)	0.859
Demographic characteristics					
Insurance levels (NTD$)					0.427
40,000-	20	(1.2)	2	(.6)	
20,000–39,999	625	(37.8)	139	(41.6)	
1–19,999	382	(23.1)	69	(20.7)	
Dependent	628	(37.9)	124	(37.1)	
Geographic locations					0.065
Northern area	712	(43.0)	165	(49.4)	
Central area	306	(18.5)	44	(13.2)	
Southern area	587	(35.5)	114	(34.1)	
Eastern area	50	(3.0)	11	(3.3)	
Urbanization levels					0.435
1 (most urbanization)	407	(24.6)	71	(21.3)	
2	409	(24.7)	75	(22.5)	
3	235	(14.2)	54	(16.2)	
4	294	(17.8)	68	(20.4)	
5 (least urbanization)	310	(18.7)	66	(19.8)	

of Taiwan, premiums are mostly determined by the insured wage and premium rate. Thus, the higher the premium, the implied higher income. Those without salaries, such as the unemployed, students, children or the elderly, are designated as dependents by the Bureau of NHI (BNHI), and the government or their foster families cover their insurance premiums.

The geographic locations of residency were grouped into four categories of northern, central, southern and eastern. More economic and political centers were located in the northern areas. The urbanization of the locations of NHI registration was also used as a proxy parameter for socio-economic status. According to previous reports using the NHIRD [34], urbanization levels are divided into 7 strata, in which level 1 is referred to as the "most urbanized" and level 7 as the "least urbanized". However, in our study, given that there were fewer numbers in levels 5, 6 and 7, these three were combined into a single group and thereafter referred to as level 5 [31].

Stroke incidences: hemorrhagic vs. ischemic

Any stroke event during the study period, determined by the date of hospitalization records with the discharge diagnostic code

Table 2. Comparison of co-morbidities (n = 1989).

	Comparison group		Vertebroplasty group		
	n = 1655	(%)	n = 334	(%)	p value
Comorbidities					
Hypertension					0.413
Yes	1157	(69.9)	241	(72.2)	
No	498	(30.1)	93	(27.8)	
Diabetes					0.609
Yes	679	(41.0)	132	(39.5)	
No	976	(59.0)	202	(60.5)	
Dyslipidemia					0.964
Yes	800	(48.3)	161	(48.2)	
No	855	(51.7)	173	(51.8)	
COPD					0.288
Yes	874	(52.8)	187	(56.0)	
No	781	(47.2)	147	(44.0)	
Chronic renal failure					0.659
Yes	141	(8.5)	26	(7.8)	
No	1514	(91.5)	308	(92.2)	
Parkinson's disease					0.163
Yes	62	(3.7)	18	(5.4)	
No	1593	(96.3)	316	(94.6)	
Charlson's comorbidity index, Mean (SD)	4.01	(2.7)	4.16	(2.8)	0.358
Spinal diseases					
Inflammatory spondylopathies					0.991
Yes	10	(.6)	2	(.6)	
No	1645	(99.4)	332	(99.4)	
Spondylosis					0.747
Yes	224	(13.5)	43	(12.9)	
No	1431	(86.5)	291	(87.1)	
Spondylolisthesis					0.194
Yes	182	(11.0)	45	(13.5)	
No	1473	(89.0)	289	(86.5)	
Spinal stenosis					0.009*
Yes	251	(15.2)	70	(21.0)	
No	1404	(84.8)	264	(79.0)	
Intervertebral disc disorders					0.462
Yes	199	(12.0)	45	(13.5)	
No	1456	(88.0)	289	(86.5)	
Propensity score, Mean (SD)	0.56	(0.2)	0.58	(0.2)	0.066

*p<0.05.

of stroke (ICD-9 code, 430–435) after the entry date, was identified. The first event of stroke was considered as the outcome in patients who had more than one stroke. To further analyze the characteristics of these strokes, all stroke events were further separated into hemorrhagic strokes, including sub-arachnoid hemorrhage (ICD- 9 code, 430) and intra-cerebral hemorrhage (ICD- 9 code, 431–432), and ischemic strokes (ICD- 9 code, 432–435).

Statistical analysis

All of the data were linked using the SQL server 2008 (Microsoft Corp.) and analyzed by SPSS software (SPSS, Inc., Chicago, IL). Chi-square and independent t-tests were used to compare differences between the vertebroplasty and comparison groups. The Kaplan-Meier method and log-rank test were used to estimate the incidence rates of strokes. The Cox proportional hazard model with propensity scores was used to compare the stroke incidence rates between the two groups after adjusting for covariates. A two-tailed level of 0.05 was considered statistically significant.

Results

A total of 1,989 patients with osteoporosis (i.e. 331 who received vertebroplasty and 1,655 who did not) were followed-up for 3,760.1 person-years. There were 74 ischemic and 16 hemorrhagic stroke events in 85 patients. The overall incidence rates of any, ischemic and hemorrhagic stroke were 22.6, 4.2 and 19.6 per 1,000 person-years, respectively.

Similar demographics and co-morbidities

The gender distribution (78.1% female), mean age (75 years), and other parameters of socio-economic status were all very similar between the vertebroplasty and comparison groups (Table 1).

The co-morbidities were similar between the two groups, including hypertension ($p = 0.413$), diabetes ($p = 0.609$), dyslipidemia ($p = 0.964$), chronic pulmonary obstructive disease ($p = 0.288$), chronic renal failure ($p = 0.659$), and Parkinson's disease ($p = 0.163$). There were no differences in the Charlson's co-morbidity index between the vertebroplasty and comparison groups (2.8 vs. 2.7, $p = 0.358$). Spinal diseases, including inflammatory spondylopathies, spondylosis, spondylolisthesis and intervertebral disc disorders, were also similar except for spinal stenosis, which was significantly more evident in the vertebroplasty group (21.0% vs. 15.2%, $p = 0.009$). There were no differences in the propensity scores between the vertebroplasty and comparison groups (0.56 vs. 0.58, $p = 0.066$) (Table 2).

Incidence of stroke

There were no significant differences in stroke incidence rates after vertebroplasty among osteoporosis patients. Among the 334 subjects in the vertebroplasty group, the incidence rates (95% confidence interval) were 25.9 (15.0–44.6), 7.7 (2.9–20.6) and 19.7 (10.6–36.7) per 1,000 person-years for any stroke, hemorrhagic and ischemic strokes, respectively. On the other hand, for the 1,655 subjects without vertebroplasty in the comparison group, the incidence rates were 22.1 (17.5–27.8), 3.6 (2.0–6.3) and 19.6 (15.4–25.1) per 1,000 person-years for any stroke, hemorrhagic and ischemic strokes, respectively. There were no statistical differences in stroke incidence rates for stroke sub-types between the two groups ($p = 0.585$, 0.211, and 0.956, respectively) (Fig. 2).

The accumulated incidence of each stroke sub-type showed no significant difference between the vertebroplasty and comparison groups (Fig. 3).

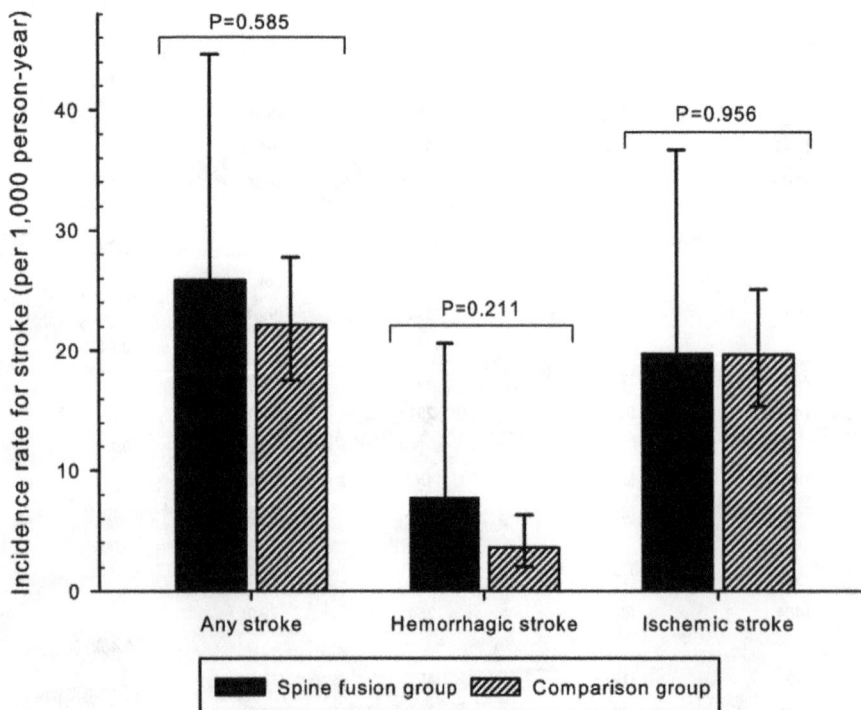

Figure 2. Comparison of stroke incidence rates. The vertebroplasty group had similar incidence rates of any, hemorrhagic and ischemic strokes to that of the comparison group.

A. Any stroke event

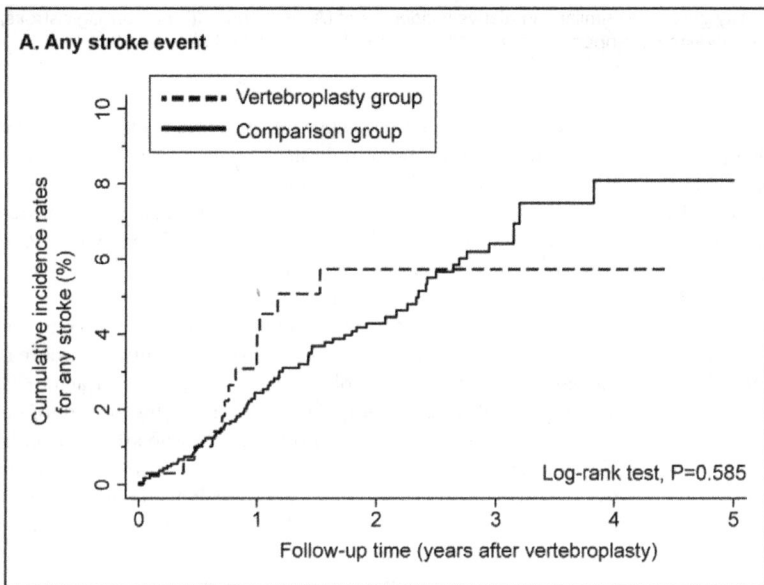

B. Hemorrhagic stroke event

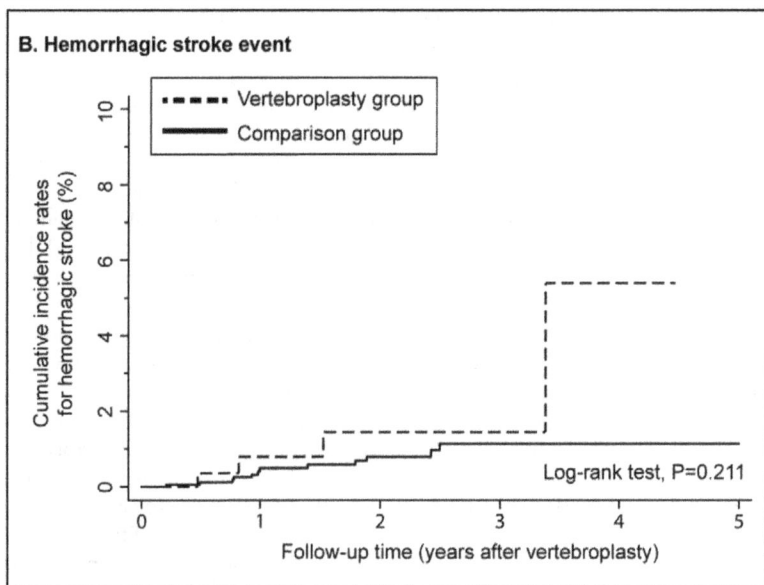

C. Ischemic stroke event

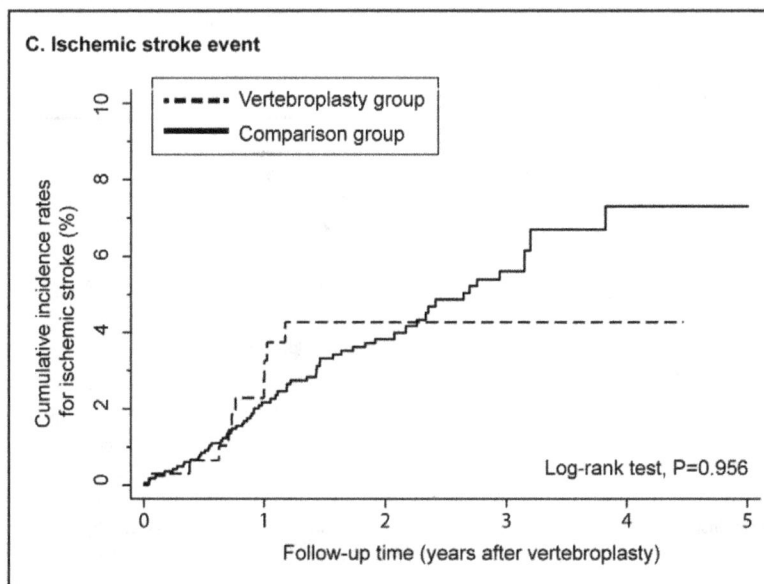

Figure 3. Cumulative incidence of stroke. The vertebroplasty group had similar cumulative incidences of (**A**) any stroke, (**B**) hemorrhagic stroke, and (**C**) ischemic stroke as the comparison group from the immediate post-operative period till the end of the five-year follow-up.

Hazard ratios of strokes.

Patients in the vertebroplasty group were insignificantly more or less likely to have stroke compared to the comparison group. The vertebroplasty group had crude hazard ratios (95% CI) of 1.13 (0.62–2.04), 2.21 (0.71–6.86), and 0.96 (0.49–1.91) for any stroke, hemorrhagic stroke and ischemic stroke ($p = 0.693$, 0.170, and 0.90, respectively) compared to the comparison group (Table 3). After adjustments for demographic characteristics, co-morbidities and medications, the adjusted hazard ratios of the vertebroplasty group were 1.22 (0.67–2.24), 3.17 (0.97–10.3), and 0.96 (0.49–1.91) for any stroke, hemorrhagic stroke and ischemic stroke ($p = 0.518$, 0.055, and 0.91, respectively). Thus, osteoporotic patients who received vertebroplasty did not have an increased risk of stroke in the five years post-operation.

Discussion

In the last decade, percutaneous vertebroplasty has been accepted as an option for spinal compression fractures for elderly patients with osteoporosis. Numerous reports have demonstrated its rapid pain relief [10,11,35]. However, in spite of the escalating number of vertebroplasty procedures performed worldwide, there is a lack of robust evidence about the long-term effects [10,11,12,36,37,38]. Stroke is rare after vertebroplasty but can cause severe neurologic consequences or death [17,18,19]. To date, the actual incidence and risk of stroke after percutaneous vertebroplasty remain elusive in the literature.

The current study used a comprehensive nationwide database, NHIRD, to investigate the risk and incidence of stroke in patients with osteoporosis, but who were treated differently. A total of 334 vertebroplasty patients and 1,655 medically treated patients were extracted from an osteoporotic cohort. In a follow-up of five years, the group of patients who had vertebroplasty was compared to the well-matched (i.e. age, sex and co-morbidities) group of patients not treated with vertebroplasty. There were no significant differences in the incidence and risk of stroke between the two groups. Thus, percutaneous vertebroplasty does not alter the chances of stroke in osteoporotic patients. This data also corroborates the safety of vertebroplasty and long-term medical outcome.

Several reports of prospective randomized control studies of vertebroplasty have been published recently [10,11,12]. Most clinicians agree that in selected patients with acute osteoporotic vertebral compression fractures and persistent pain, percutaneous vertebroplasty appears to be an effective and safe procedure. Pain relief is immediate and sustainable for at least a year, and is significantly greater than that achieved with conservative treatments [10]. However, the actual long-term outcome of vertebroplasty is uncertain. The most common concern of this procedure is the possible increased risk of vertebral compression fracture at adjacent spinal levels [39,40]. Other effects of this procedure on the medical condition of osteoporotic patients who are particularly old and at a high risk of cardiovascular and other systemic diseases, are not addressed in the literature. This report is the first investigation focused on the risk of subsequent stroke after percutaneous vertebroplasty.

The complication rate of vertebroplasty is low but very serious, and irreversible complications have been reported, including spinal cord injury, nerve root compression, venous and pulmonary embolism, and cardiovascular collapse [13,14,15,16,35,41,42,43]. The elderly, in whom most osteoporotic vertebral compression fractures occur, are particularly at higher risk of stroke. The database used in this study is uniquely appropriate to investigate the risks of stroke after vertebroplasty. Because the monopolistic government-operated health insurance system offers unlimited access to health care for the entire population of Taiwan and does not restrict health service providers, the universal coverage of health insurance yields an opportunity for an extremely high follow-up rate. This health insurance system even reimburses health care services provided by some overseas institutions. Theoretically, all subsequent stroke events were captured during the study period. Loss of follow up would only occur if the patient refused to seek medical attention at all upon having a stroke and still stayed in the system for a long time, which is very unlikely. Therefore, the incidence rates computed here are very accurate.

The strength of this report is its demonstration of the rarity and unlikelihood of stroke after vertebroplasty, even in patients with osteoporosis, who are older and potentially of a higher risk of stroke. The well-matched comparative group of patients amelio-

Table 3. Hazard ratios of subsequent strokes post-vertebroplasty (2004.1.1–2008.12.31, n = 1989).

Stroke during 5-year-follow-up	Comparison group	Vertebroplasty group	(95% CI)	p value
Any stroke				
Crude hazard ratio	1.00	1.13	(0.62–2.04)	0.693
Adjusted hazard ratio[a]	1.00	1.22	(0.67–2.24)	0.518
Hemorrhagic stroke				
Crude hazard ratio	1.00	2.21	(0.71–6.86)	0.170
Adjusted hazard ratio[a]	1.00	3.17	(0.97–10.3)	0.055
Ischemic stroke				
Crude hazard ratio	1.00	0.96	(0.49–1.91)	0.90
Adjusted hazard ratio[a]	1.00	0.96	(0.49–1.91)	0.91

[a]Adjustments were made for demographic characteristics (i.e., age, sex, insurance level, geographic location, and urbanization level), co-morbidities (e.g., hypertension, diabetes, valvular heart disease, arrhythmia, cardiovascular disease and Charlson's co-morbidity index), medications (e.g., aspirin, nitrates, lipid lowering drugs, anti-coagulants, and NSAIDs), and baseline propensity scores.

rates most of the confounders, rendering as valid this study that was specifically aimed at the correlation of vertebroplasty and stroke. The results indicating the safety of this procedure, although may be anticipated by most spine surgeons, is proven for the first time. One can infer that the increased risk of stroke brought on by osteoporotic spinal compression fracture is likely to be offset by this procedure. But this inference remains uncertain and its causes also need further investigation to corroborate.

Furthermore, after the strokes were divided into hemorrhagic stroke and ischemic stroke, there was still little difference between the patients who underwent vertebroplasty and others (Fig. 2). The Kaplan-Meier analysis and adjustment of all other confounding factors for stroke allowed for a valid estimation of the risks of any, hemorrhagic and ischemic strokes (Fig. 3). This information may be valuable in peri-operative management of vertebroplasty for elderly osteoporotic patients.

This study has several limitations. First, the detailed operative notes of vertebroplasty were not available for analysis. The levels of procedure, amount of cement injected, indications of surgery, and severity of pre-operative symptoms were not analyzed. Second, the comparison group was composed of osteoporotic patients with similar medical conditions but not treated by vertebroplasty; the percentage of acute vertebral compression fracture in the comparison group may not be as high as those treated by vertebroplasty. This issue could be a major difference

between the groups (e.g. less severe osteoporosis could imply less likelihood of stoke). A randomized study of patients with acute osteoporotic compression fracture may overcome this limitation. Third, stroke is relatively rare (22.6 per 1,000 person-years) in these osteoporotic patients. Although the extremely high follow-up rate substantially compensated for this, a larger scale study with longer follow-up could further corroborate it.

In conclusion, osteoporotic patients who undergo percutaneous vertebroplasty are not at higher risk of any stroke in the five years after the surgery.

Acknowledgments

This study was based partly on data from the NHRI database provided by the BNHI, Department of Health, and managed by NHRI in Taiwan. The interpretation and conclusions contained herein do not represent those of the BNHI, the Department of Health, or NHRI.

Author Contributions

Conceived and designed the experiments: J-CW C-LW LL Y-CC. Performed the experiments: J-CW C-LW LL Y-CC. Analyzed the data: J-CW C-LW LL Y-CC. Contributed reagents/materials/analysis tools: J-CW C-LW LL Y-CC W-CH. Wrote the paper: J-CW C-LW LL Y-CC W-CH. Database and administrative support: W-CH H-THW H-JC T-JC HC C-YC.

References

1. Feigin VL (2005) Stroke epidemiology in the developing world. Lancet 365: 2160–2161.
2. Bonita R (1992) Epidemiology of stroke. Lancet 339: 342–344.
3. Brown DL, Morgenstern LB, Majersik JJ, Kleerekoper M, Lisabeth LD (2008) Risk of fractures after stroke. Cerebrovasc Dis 25: 95–99.
4. Ramnemark A, Nyberg L, Borssen B, Olsson T, Gustafson Y (1998) Fractures after stroke. Osteoporos Int 8: 92–95.
5. Dennis MS, Lo KM, McDowall M, West T (2002) Fractures after stroke: frequency, types, and associations. Stroke 33: 728–734.
6. Poole KE, Reeve J, Warburton EA (2002) Falls, fractures, and osteoporosis after stroke: time to think about protection? Stroke 33: 1432–1436.
7. Kanis J, Oden A, Johnell O (2001) Acute and long-term increase in fracture risk after hospitalization for stroke. Stroke 32: 702–706.
8. Pang MY, Eng JJ, McKay HA, Dawson AS (2005) Reduced hip bone mineral density is related to physical fitness and leg lean mass in ambulatory individuals with chronic stroke. Osteoporos Int 16: 1769–1779.
9. del Puente A, Pappone N, Mandes MG, Mantova D, Scarpa R, et al. (1996) Determinants of bone mineral density in immobilization: a study on hemiplegic patients. Osteoporos Int 6: 50–54.
10. Klazen CA, Lohle PN, de Vries J, Jansen FH, Tielbeek AV, et al. (2010) Vertebroplasty versus conservative treatment in acute osteoporotic vertebral compression fractures (Vertos II): an open-label randomised trial. Lancet 376: 1085–1092.
11. Kallmes DF, Comstock BA, Heagerty PJ, Turner JA, Wilson DJ, et al. (2009) A randomized trial of vertebroplasty for osteoporotic spinal fractures. N Engl J Med 361: 569–579.
12. Buchbinder R, Osborne RH, Ebeling PR, Wark JD, Mitchell P, et al. (2009) A randomized trial of vertebroplasty for painful osteoporotic vertebral fractures. N Engl J Med 361: 557–568.
13. Lee MJ, Dumonski M, Cahill P, Stanley T, Park D, et al. (2009) Percutaneous treatment of vertebral compression fractures: a meta-analysis of complications. Spine 34: 1228–1232.
14. Luetmer MT, Bartholmai BJ, Rad AE, Kallmes DF (2011) Asymptomatic and unrecognized cement pulmonary embolism commonly occurs with vertebroplasty. AJNR American journal of neuroradiology 32: 654–657.
15. Rollinghoff M, Siewe J, Eysel P, Delank KS (2010) Pulmonary cement embolism after augmentation of pedicle screws with bone cement. Acta orthopaedica Belgica 76: 269–273.
16. Syed MI, Jan S, Patel NA, Shaikh A, Marsh RA, et al. (2006) Fatal fat embolism after vertebroplasty: identification of the high-risk patient. AJNR American journal of neuroradiology 27: 343–345.
17. Lim JB, Park JS, Kim E (2009) Nonaneurysmal subarachnoid hemorrhage : rare complication of vertebroplasty. Journal of Korean Neurosurgical Society 45: 386–389.
18. Marden FA, Putman CM (2008) Cement-embolic stroke associated with vertebroplasty. AJNR American journal of neuroradiology 29: 1986–1988.
19. Amar AP, Larsen DW, Esnaashari N, Albuquerque FC, Lavine SD, et al. (2001) Percutaneous transpedicular polymethylmethacrylate vertebroplasty for the treatment of spinal compression fractures. Neurosurgery 49: 1105–1114. discussion 1114-1105.
20. Kang JH, Chung SD, Xirasagar S, Jaw FS, Lin HC (2011) Increased risk of stroke in the year after a hip fracture: a population-based follow-up study. Stroke 42: 336–341.
21. Wen CP, Tsai SP, Chung WS (2008) A 10-year experience with universal health insurance in Taiwan: measuring changes in health and health disparity. Ann Intern Med 148: 258–267.
22. Wu JC, Liu L, Chen YC, Huang WC, Chen TJ, et al. (2011) Ossification of the posterior longitudinal ligament in the cervical spine: an 11-year comprehensive national epidemiology study. Neurosurgical focus 30: E5.
23. Cheng CL, Kao YH, Lin SJ, Lee CH, Lai ML (2010) Validation of the national health insurance research database with ischemic stroke cases in Taiwan. Pharmacoepidemiol Drug Saf.
24. Yang YW, Chen YH, Xirasagar S, Lin HC (2011) Increased risk of stroke in patients with bullous pemphigoid: a population-based follow-up study. Stroke 42: 319–323.
25. Ho JD, Hu CC, Lin HC (2009) Open-angle glaucoma and the risk of stroke development: a 5-year population-based follow-up study. Stroke 40: 2685–2690.
26. Lin HC, Chien CW, Ho JD (2010) Herpes zoster ophthalmicus and the risk of stroke: a population-based follow-up study. Neurology 74: 792–797.
27. Goldstein LB, Adams R, Alberts MJ, Appel LJ, Brass LM, et al. (2006) Primary prevention of ischemic stroke: a guideline from the American Heart Association/American Stroke Association Stroke Council. Stroke 37: 1583–1633.
28. Goldstein LB, Bushnell CD, Adams RJ, Appel LJ, Braun LT, et al. (2011) Guidelines for the primary prevention of stroke: a guideline for healthcare professionals from the American Heart Association/American Stroke Association. Stroke 42: 517–584.
29. Elixhauser A, Steiner C, Harris DR, Coffey RM (1998) Comorbidity measures for use with administrative data. Medical care 36: 8–27.
30. Halfon P, Eggli Y, van Melle G, Chevalier J, Wasserfallen JB, et al. (2002) Measuring potentially avoidable hospital readmissions. Journal of clinical epidemiology 55: 573–587.
31. Wu JC, Chen YC, Liu L, Chen TJ, Huang WC, et al. (2011) Effects of Age, Gender, and Socio-economic Status on the Incidence of Spinal Cord Injury: An Assessment Using the Eleven-Year Comprehensive Nationwide Database of Taiwan. Journal of neurotrauma.
32. Sheu JJ, Chiou HY, Kang JH, Chen YH, Lin HC (2010) Tuberculosis and the risk of ischemic stroke: a 3-year follow-up study. Stroke 41: 244–249.
33. Ho JD, Liou SW, Lin HC (2009) Retinal vein occlusion and the risk of stroke development: a five-year follow-up study. American journal of ophthalmology 147: 283–290 e282.
34. Lin HC, Chao PZ, Lee HC (2008) Sudden sensorineural hearing loss increases the risk of stroke: a 5-year follow-up study. Stroke 39: 2744–2748.
35. Burton AW, Rhines LD, Mendel E (2005) Vertebroplasty and kyphoplasty: a comprehensive review. Neurosurgical focus 18: e1.
36. Do HM, Kim BS, Marcellus ML, Curtis L, Marks MP (2005) Prospective analysis of clinical outcomes after percutaneous vertebroplasty for painful

osteoporotic vertebral body fractures. AJNR American journal of neuroradiology 26: 1623–1628.

37. Watts NB, Harris ST, Genant HK (2001) Treatment of painful osteoporotic vertebral fractures with percutaneous vertebroplasty or kyphoplasty. Osteoporos Int 12: 429–437.

38. Buchbinder R, Kallmes DF (2010) Vertebroplasty: when randomized placebo-controlled trial results clash with common belief. The spine journal 10: 241–243.

39. Cortet B, Cotten A, Boutry N, Flipo RM, Duquesnoy B, et al. (1999) Percutaneous vertebroplasty in the treatment of osteoporotic vertebral compression fractures: an open prospective study. The Journal of rheumatology 26: 2222–2228.

40. Lin EP, Ekholm S, Hiwatashi A, Westesson PL (2004) Vertebroplasty: cement leakage into the disc increases the risk of new fracture of adjacent vertebral body. AJNR American journal of neuroradiology 25: 175–180.

41. Teng MM, Cheng H, Ho DM, Chang CY (2006) Intraspinal leakage of bone cement after vertebroplasty: a report of 3 cases. AJNR American journal of neuroradiology 27: 224–229.

42. Kim YJ, Lee JW, Park KW, Yeom JS, Jeong HS, et al. (2009) Pulmonary cement embolism after percutaneous vertebroplasty in osteoporotic vertebral compression fractures: incidence, characteristics, and risk factors. Radiology 251: 250–259.

43. Baumann A, Tauss J, Baumann G, Tomka M, Hessinger M, et al. (2006) Cement embolization into the vena cava and pulmonal arteries after vertebroplasty: interdisciplinary management. Eur J Vasc Endovasc Surg 31: 558–561.

Cortical Thickness Mapping to Identify Focal Osteoporosis in Patients with Hip Fracture

Kenneth E. S. Poole[1]*, Graham M. Treece[2], Paul M. Mayhew[1], Jan Vaculík[3], Pavel Dungl[3], Martin Horák[4], Jan J. Štěpán[5], Andrew H. Gee[2]

1 Department of Medicine, University of Cambridge, Cambridge, Cambridgeshire, United Kingdom, 2 Department of Engineering, University of Cambridge, Cambridge, Cambridgeshire, United Kingdom, 3 Department of Orthopaedics, Faculty of Medicine, Charles University Prague and Bulovka Hospital, Prague, Czech Republic, 4 Department of Radiology, Homolka Hospital, Prague, Czech Republic, 5 Department of Rheumatology, Faculty of Medicine 1, Charles University Prague and Institute of Rheumatology, Prague, Czech Republic

Abstract

Background: Individuals with osteoporosis are predisposed to hip fracture during trips, stumbles or falls, but half of all hip fractures occur in those without generalised osteoporosis. By analysing ordinary clinical CT scans using a novel cortical thickness mapping technique, we discovered patches of markedly thinner bone at fracture-prone regions in the femurs of women with acute hip fracture compared with controls.

Methods: We analysed CT scans from 75 female volunteers with acute fracture and 75 age- and sex-matched controls. We classified the fracture location as femoral neck or trochanteric before creating bone thickness maps of the outer 'cortical' shell of the intact contra-lateral hip. After registration of each bone to an average femur shape and statistical parametric mapping, we were able to visualise and quantify statistically significant foci of thinner cortical bone associated with each fracture type, assuming good symmetry of bone structure between the intact and fractured hip. The technique allowed us to pinpoint systematic differences and display the results on a 3D average femur shape model.

Findings: The cortex was generally thinner in femoral neck fracture cases than controls. More striking were several discrete patches of statistically significant thinner bone of up to 30%, which coincided with common sites of fracture initiation (femoral neck or trochanteric).

Interpretation: Femoral neck fracture patients had a thumbnail-sized patch of focal osteoporosis at the upper head-neck junction. This region coincided with a weak part of the femur, prone to both spontaneous 'tensile' fractures of the femoral neck, and as a site of crack initiation when falling sideways. Current hip fracture prevention strategies are based on case finding: they involve clinical risk factor estimation to determine the need for single-plane bone density measurement within a standard region of interest (ROI) of the femoral neck. The precise sites of focal osteoporosis that we have identified are overlooked by current 2D bone densitometry methods.

Editor: Xing-Ming Shi, Georgia Health Sciences University, United States of America

Funding: This analysis was funded by Arthritis Research UK via a Clinician Scientist Fellowship award to KESP. Cambridge National Institute for Health Research Biomedical Research Centre funded PMM. The Evelyn Trust funded GMT. The funders had no role in study design, data collection and analysis, decision to publish, or preparation of the manuscript.

Competing Interests: GMT and KESP are co-inventors on a related GB patent application A method of determining the cortical thickness of a patients bone (GB0917524.1 Accurate cortical thickness measurement from clinical CT data, A method of determining the cortical thickness of a patients bone. International (PCT) Patent Application No PCT/GB2010/051671, CU ref: TRE-2326-09-01, International search ref: PC925159WO. Title: Image data processing systems, Inventors: G.M. Treece & K.E.S Poole). The other authors have declared that no competing interests exist. This does not alter the authors' adherence to all the PLoS ONE policies on sharing data and materials.

* E-mail: kp254@nhs.net

Introduction

The annual incidence of hip fractures is projected to rise fourfold to 6.3 million worldwide by 2050, because of the exponentially increasing risk of fracture as people live longer. Studying femoral neck and trochanteric fractures is therefore a health priority [1]. In older people, the proximal femur breaks when the loads placed on it overcome its strength, with common loading scenarios being sideways falls, stumbles or sudden unusual movements [2]. However, a spontaneous or 'impact-free' mechanism accounts for up to 6% of hip fractures (fig. 1) [3,4]. We know that women with osteoporosis (who have generally thinner and more porous bones) are more likely to suffer hip fracture, but most people who will sustain hip fracture do not have generalised osteoporosis [5]. We also know that the outer 'cortical' bone of the femur where fractures initiate [6] thins rapidly with age [7,8], is a key determinant of bone strength and fracture risk [9–13] and responds well to certain osteoporosis drugs [14,15]. Here we ask; Is there a pattern of femoral bone thinning common to hip fracture patients and, if so, is it generalised or focal? Could focal osteoporosis of the femur be a cause of hip fracture in the elderly? The answer to these questions might illuminate why hip fractures tend to initiate in particular zones (fig. 1).

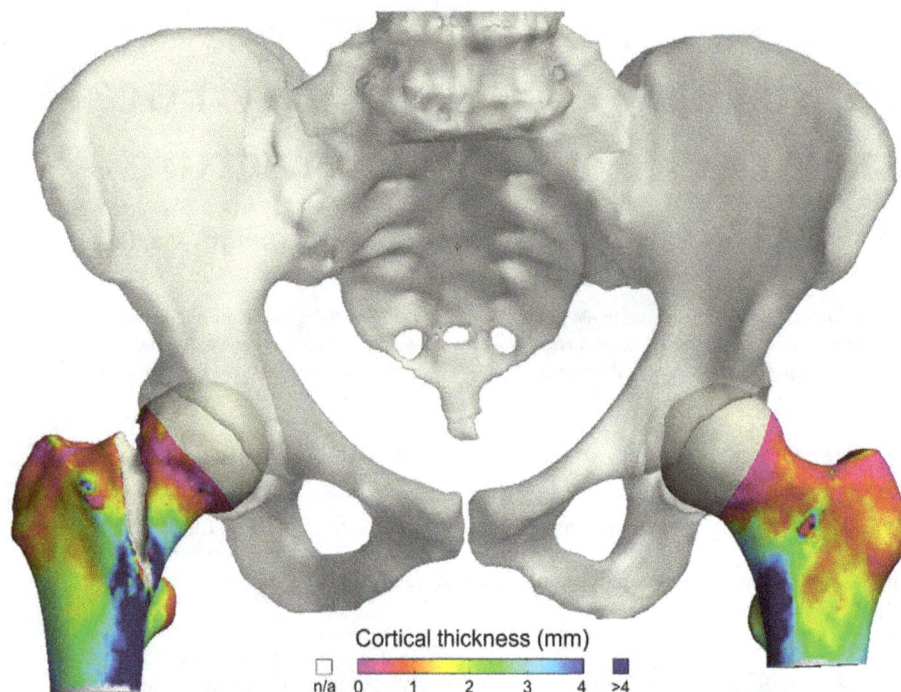

Figure 1. Cortical Thickness Colour Mapping using ordinary clinical CT data. Femora and pelvis from an 84-year-old osteoporotic female who sustained a fracture without falling. She felt her right hip break as she placed her right foot on a low step. Femoral neck BMD was 0.46 g/cm2, T score −3.3. From the Arthritis Research UK FEMCO study (07/H0305/61).

A new CT image processing technique [16] allows us to display cortical thickness as a colour map over the bone surface, with several thousand independent measurements across each proximal femur and sufficient sensitivity to detect even small differences (~30 microns) when expressed systematically by a suitably sized cohort. We use it here to pinpoint differences in bone thickness between women with and without hip fracture. We examined the contra-lateral side as a surrogate for the broken hip in these female fracture patients, having previously identified symmetry in femoral neck cortical thickness [8].

Methods

From 2006 to 2009, women admitted to Bulovka University Hospital, Prague with an acute hip fracture were consented to the pragmatic 'Surgical treatment of the hip joint in trauma' study (PI Professor P Dungl), part of which involved a clinical CT scan of both hips before surgical fixation [17]. Participants were positioned on the Siemens two-compartment Osteo phantom and a single CT scan (either Siemens Sensation 40 or 16 detector, B10/20 kernel, ≤1 mm reconstructed slice thickness) was performed including both hips from above the acetabulum to just below the lesser trochanter. Women were aged over 50, were awaiting surgical repair of a cervical or trochanteric fracture and had sustained a low energy injury. Women were excluded if they had metalwork in either hip, high trauma injury, metastatic cancer, unilateral bone disease, subtrochanteric fracture or terminal illness. Using the same criteria, a convenience control sample of older women without fracture was recruited by invitation at rheumatology clinics and two residential care centres in the same districts of Prague. From 204 invitations, 108 fracture-free women responded of whom 81 were eligible for CT scanning at Homolka hospital, Prague (Siemens Sensation 16 detector B20 kernel, ≤1mm reconstructed slice thickness). At the image quality

control step, 6 scans were excluded (due to insufficient scan length or undisclosed metalwork) leaving 75 female controls. One age-matched case was selected for each of the 75 eligible control participants, from the total sample of 242 women with hip fracture. Where precise birth year age matching was not possible, the next nearest matching case was selected up to a maximum 5-year age difference. The final sample taken forward for cortical thickness mapping comprised 150 femurs from 75 women in each group (mean ages of femoral neck fracture cases 78.1+/−7.1 years, trochanteric fracture cases 75.2+/−7.9, controls 76.6+/−7.3 years). There were 36 femoral neck fractures and 39 trochanteric fractures.

The analysis method is illustrated in figure 2. Anonymised axial dicom images were received in Cambridge via the secure DICOM internet connection ePACS (ICZ, Brno, Czech Rep.) where they were reconstructed to classify fracture side and site according to AO criteria. Standard clinical hip bone density (2D areal DXA-equivalent) was measured in the 'total hip' region of interest (ROI) of each femur using QCTpro software (v4.2.3 Mindways, Austin, Texas, USA). The unfractured contralateral hip (or matching side in controls) was segmented semi-automatically in Stradwin v4.2 software (Treece, Gee, Cambridge) before mapping cortical thickness at approximately 6000 surface points per femur. Cortical thickness was estimated from the CT data using the method described by Treece et al. [16]. By making reasonable assumptions about both the anatomy and the imaging blur, thickness can be measured to super-resolution accuracy across the entire proximal femur, apart from at the femoral head where the proximity of the acetabulum is problematic. The methodology has been validated against thickness measurements obtained from high resolution micro-CT scans of cadaveric femurs [16]. Analysis of the 150 thickness maps followed established practice within the neuroim-aging community, who have pioneered techniques for statistical inference from dense, spatially correlated data. To account for variations in inter-subject morphology, each map was spatially realigned with a canonical femur surface using a B-spline free-form deformation calculated by the iterative closest point registration algorithm [18]. The spatially normalized maps were then smoothed with a 10 mm full-width-half-maximum filter. We investigated differences in cortical thickness between i) femoral neck fractures (n36) and all controls or ii) trochanteric fractures (n39) and all controls. Formal inference was accomplished by statistical parametric mapping (SPM) [19], as implemented in the SurfStat package [20]. Model effects were group (case*control), age, height and weight. Missing height and weight values (2 fracture cases) were replaced with group mean values. T-statistics were calculated to test the significance of the group term. Random field theory then furnished p-values, corrected for multiple comparisons to control the overall image-wise chance of false positives. Figure 3 shows corrected p maps based on the magnitude of peaks (sensitive to focal effects) and on the extent of connected clusters exceeding an uncorrected p-value threshold of 0.001 (sensitive to distributed effects). All participants with fracture gave written informed consent. Control participants gave verbal consent which was documented in the medical notes as agreed with the Ethics Committee. Ethics committees approved the study in the Czech Republic (Ethical Committee of the Institute of Rheumatology and Ethical Committee of Bulovka Hospital, ref IRB0002384101) and in the UK (Cambridgeshire 4, ref 07/H0305/61).

Results

Percentage differences in cortical thickness between each hip fracture group and the control group were displayed on an average right femur surface map using a colour scale. Views from several anatomical planes were chosen to illustrate the differences (femoral neck fractures vs. controls; fig. 3 *left upper panel* and trochanteric fractures vs controls; fig. 3 *right upper panel*). Similar maps were created to visualise the statistical significance of differences (fig 3. *lower panels*). Several distinct patches of up to 30% thinner cortical bone were identified in fracture cases which coincided with typical sites of hip fracture. No regions of statistically significant thicker bone were seen in fracture cases. WHO-defined osteoporosis (a total hip DXA-equivalent bone mineral density T score <-2.5) was present in less than half of hip fracture patients (31/75, 41.3%) and 9/75 (12%) controls. The age, height and weight adjusted values for the clusters of thinner bone associated with each fracture type are shown in table 1. The mean, unadjusted value of whole proximal femur cortical thickness among femoral neck fracture

patients was 1.20 mm±0.17 mm, compared with a value of 1.25 mm±0.20 mm among trochanteric fracture patients and 1.30 mm±0.21 mm among controls (ANOVA p = 0.0388). Whole femur cortical thickness was statistically significantly lower in femoral neck fracture compared with control (Dunnett's values* were 0.012 for neck fracture, p = 0.024, and −0.04 for trochanteric fracture, p = 0.34; *[absolute difference in sample means] - [least significant difference]). The age and weight terms were significant within the 150 femurs (age range 55–98 and weight range 40–89 kg). Significant thinning of approximately 0.02 mm per year from age 55–98 was apparent in the infero-medial region. Significant thickening of approximately 0.02 mm per kilogram was evident in a similar infero-medial region.

Discussion

We used cortical thickness mapping to explore differences between women with and without recent hip fracture and identified generalised thinning of the femoral cortex in fracture patients. We also discovered focal differences manifest as several well-defined patches of markedly thinner femoral cortex in hip fracture patients compared to controls. Since osteoporosis is defined as microarchitectural deterioration of bone tissue, we consider that these areas of focally thinner bone are best described as patches of focal osteoporosis (fig. 4, right panel). The patches were evident at common sites involved in fracture, the most severe being a thumbnail-sized patch of up to 30% thinner bone at the head-neck junction in patients with femoral neck fracture (figs. 3, 4 and 5). Focal osteoporosis at the head-neck junction may play an important role in fractures associated with falls, and might even be involved in 'spontaneous' hip fracture on rare occasions. While the locations of the patches of focal osteoporosis appear to be critical in determining fracture type, we cannot judge whether they are involved in causing hip fracture, which requires prospective research. However it is noteworthy that among all the bone structural parameters measured in the largest prospective study of hip CT in older men and women conducted to date, cortical thickness estimates from a supero-anterior part of the femoral neck were the best predictor of subsequent hip fracture [9].

We assume that a fall onto or near the hip was the principal fracture mechanism in these women, but we did not routinely collect information on how these women fell, a priority for future work. The largest patch of thinner femoral cortex that we identified (fig 3c) appears to correspond to a key site of fracture initiation in a simulation of femoral neck fracture during a sideways fall to the ground [21]. Although the women we studied with trochanteric fracture also had patches of thinner bone in

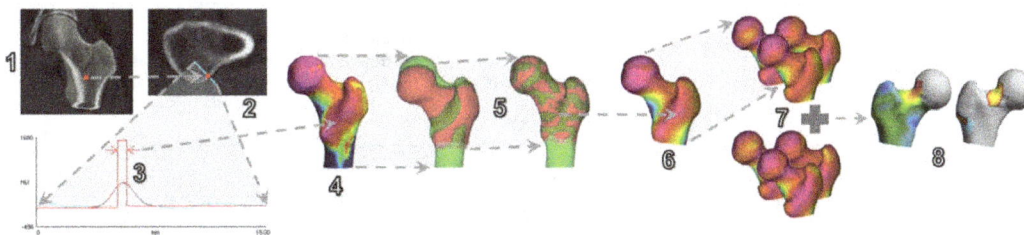

Figure 2. Cortical thickness analysis. 1. Measurements are performed at every vertex in an approximate segmentation of the hip. 2. At each vertex, the CT data is sampled on a line passing through the cortex. 3. A model-based fit is used to estimate the cortical thickness, allowing for image blur. 4. The thickness is mapped back to the surface (here blue is thick, pink is thin). 5. An average femur (red) is deformed to match the current femur (green). 6. Thickness estimates are then transferred to the average femoral surface and smoothed. 7. This process is repeated for all subjects, producing subject-specific thickness estimates all mapped to the same, average surface. 8. The data is analysed using statistical parametric mapping, to obtain mean thickness differences between groups and also the significance of these differences.

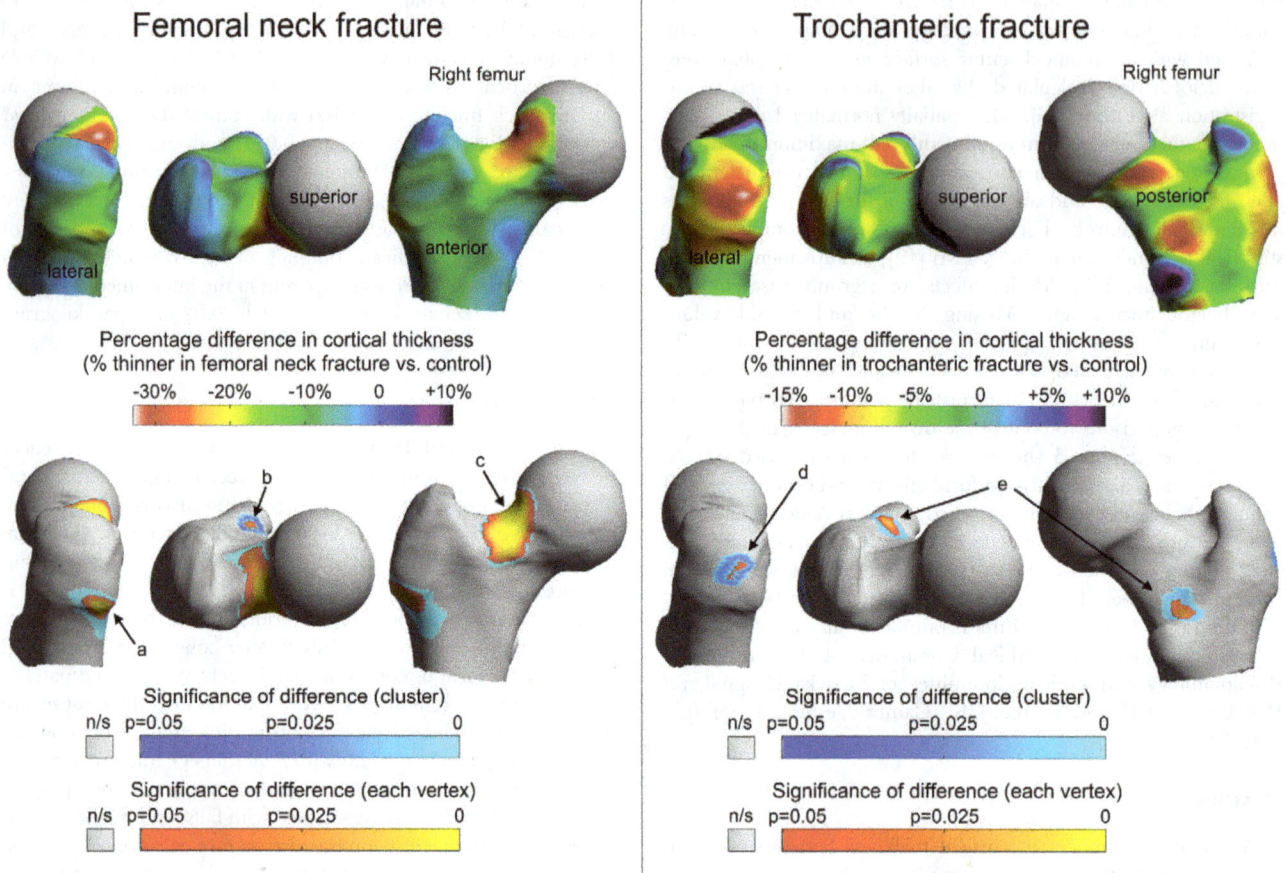

Figure 3. Results for femoral neck fracture (left) and trochanteric fracture (right). Upper colour maps show the average percentage difference in cortical thickness for each fracture type versus control (displayed on an average right femur model). The lower colour maps are the significance of the differences adjusted for age, height and weight, either point by point (vertex) or as a whole patch (blue clusters). Note that all the blue clusters extend uninterrupted beneath their respective orange/yellow vertices. Table 1 gives adjusted thickness values and significance of the clusters a–e.

fracture-relevant zones (fig. 3d and 3e), it is not clear whether they correspond to trochanteric fracture initiation sites in the relevant simulations [21]. Nevertheless, it is interesting to note that the focally thin bone in the lateral facet of the greater trochanter (fig. 3d) in the trochanteric fracture patients coincided with one of

the insertion sites of gluteus medius, which receives considerable force during locomotion.

While most hip fractures in the elderly are a result of injurious falls, spontaneous fractures of the femoral neck prior to falls have been implicated in up to 6% of cases, translating to more than

Table 1. Details of thinner patches of femoral cortex in hip fracture.

Hip fracture type	Location of 'cluster' Patch where bone cortex was thinner in hip fracture cases	Mean adjusted cortical thickness in cluster (Cases)		Mean adjusted cortical thickness in cluster (Cluster)		p value for difference
		Millimetres	±SD	Millimetres	±SD	
Femoral neck fractures						
Patch a (fig.3a)	Greater trochanter	1.14	0.15	1.34	0.26	0.00407
Patch b (fig.3b)	Lesser trochanter	0.85	0.16	0.98	0.19	0.0319
Patch c (fig.3c)	Head-neck junction	0.62	0.10	0.77	0.14	0.00000350
Trochanteric fractures						
Patch d (fig.3d)	Greater trochanter	1.05	0.25	1.21	0.27	0.0237
Patch e (fig.3e)	Lesser trochanter	0.78	0.15	0.88	0.17	0.0108

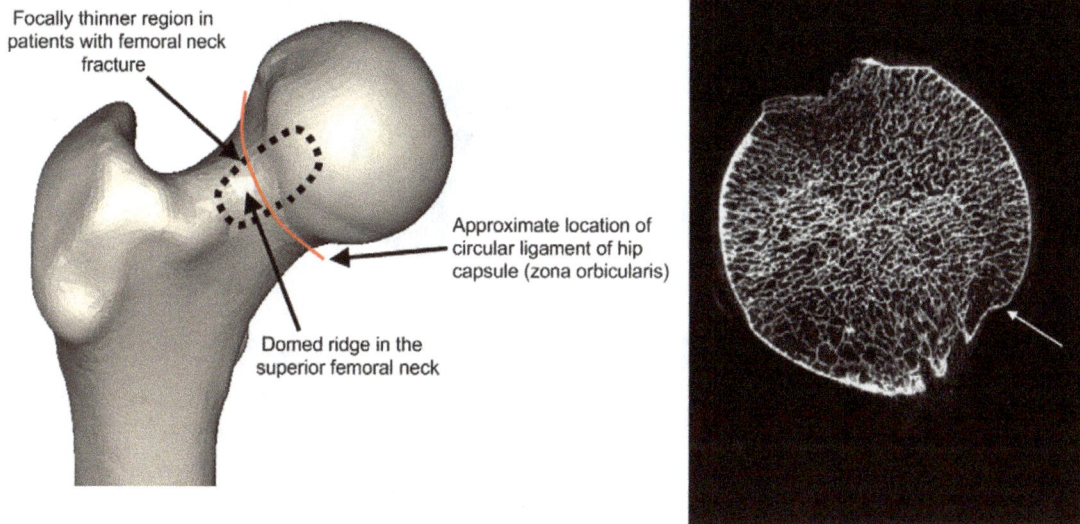

Figure 4. Anatomical context of focal thinning in women with femoral neck fracture. The left pane is a right proximal femur model seen from the front. The thin patch of cortex (fig 3c) in femoral neck fracture patients occurs on the domed ridge called the femoral neck eminence [25]. The right pane is a high resolution CT image through the femoral head of a 90 year old female (aBMD total hip T-score −1.9) which suggests that the patch is osteoporotic with microarchitectural thinning (white arrow). Femur courtesy of the Melbourne Femur Collection, Chairman Professor John Clement (Melbourne Dental School).

4000 hip fractures annually in the UK [22]. Previously, several research groups have reproduced these impact-free hip fractures in cadaveric femurs by simulating either the effects of increasing loads in stance or sudden large hip flexor muscle contractions. In Cristofolini's specimens, increasing the load by simulating one-legged stance (as in fig. 5b), led to crack initiation at the junction between the femoral head and neck, with the subsequent catastrophic failure of the femur closely resembling that observed in our patient with impact-free fracture (fig. 1) [3]. Likewise simulating sudden psoas muscle contraction (as happens when a person attempts to stabilise their trunk on a fixed leg during a slip or stumble) led to subcapital fracture in a similar location [23]. The conserved patch of focal osteoporosis we identified among our femoral neck fracture patients (fig. 3c) appears to correspond with the sites of high tensile stress induced in those simulations. In the light of our findings we wonder what effect osteoporosis medicines might have on the thin patches of bone and in particular if strengthening the thin areas could prevent stumbling-induced or spontaneous hip fractures. Analysis of large clinical trials with serial CT is needed to address this question.

We are currently unable to answer a key question generated by these results; namely how did the focal patches of thin cortex arise? Several intriguing ideas come from histological and macroscopic studies of the head-neck junction in patients with fracture and from cadavers. Freeman et al. discovered that in fracture specimens, the underlying bone from the head-neck junction frequently contains microcallus, considered to be evidence of tensile fatigue damage [24]. Modelling the behaviour of the head-neck junction during habitual locomotion and falls is therefore a priority for biomechanics research. Although there were marked age and weight effects within the women we studied, the decreasing cortical thickness associated with age and increasing thickness associated with weight affected the inferior femur; i.e. on the opposite side of the femoral neck to the patch of focally thin bone. Thus we assume that neither younger nor heavier women were necessarily protected from having a thin cortex at the head-

neck junction. The patch of focal osteoporosis in femoral neck fracture patients corresponds macroscopically with the junction between femoral head cartilage and bone, and tracks along the domed ridge running along the top of the femoral neck (called the femoral neck eminentia, or eminence [25], fig. 4). Since the thin cortical bone is so well circumscribed at this site, we concur with Panzer et al. in describing the differences as 'focal osteoporosis', but acknowledge that higher resolution and histological studies would be useful to further characterise the cortical and sub-cortical bone [26]. The circular fibres of the hip capsule (the zona orbicularis) also encircle the femoral neck at the focally thin patch. Pitt and others described a mechanical, abrasive action of the overlying hip capsule, ligaments and psoas muscle at this patch that commonly results in a 'reaction area' with occasional underlying radiolucency. This lucency can be appreciated on plain x-rays and is known to radiologists as 'Pitt's Pit' [27]. Studies of the underlying histology of this zone in femoral neck fracture cases are clearly warranted [28,29], and Pitt suggested that the zone could be involved in hip fracture pathogenesis.

This work has several weaknesses, namely pragmatic case selection, the use of a convenience sample of controls and reliance on the intact hip as a surrogate for the fractured hip. The results need replication in a better-characterised population sample, with particular attention to recalled injury mechanism. Statistical Parametric Mapping does not indicate causality; for instance it is possible (but unlikely) that controls could have substantial thickening of bone at various sites through unknown mechanisms. Finally, although studying the cortex is important in determining bone strength, alternative methods such as finite element (FE) models use whole bone biomechanics, and can therefore be informative in determining how and why individuals fracture their hips (as reviewed recently by Cristofolini et al [30]). In this regard, it is interesting to note that our cortical thickness maps have the potential to be converted into inner and outer surfaces for optimal delineation of cortical and trabecular compartments, which may

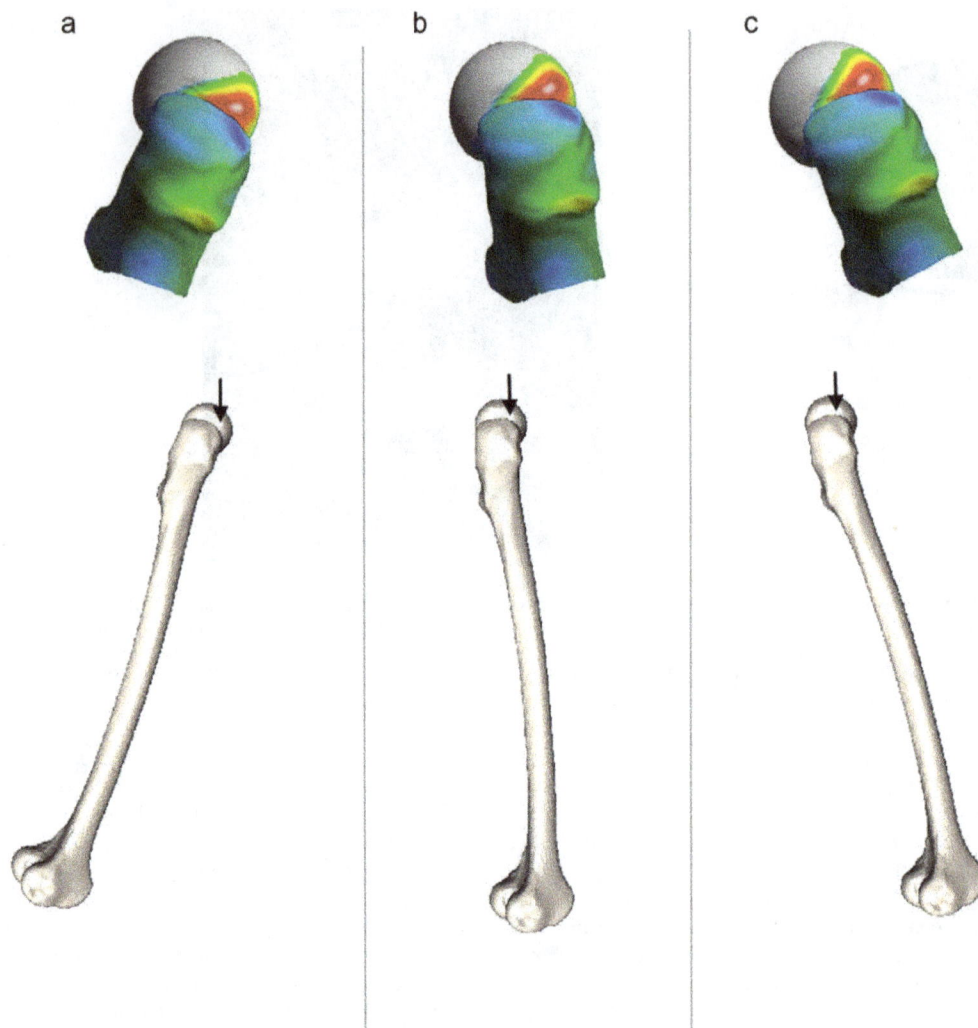

Figure 5. Approximate orientation of the focally thin (red) zone during the different phases of gait. Right femur (a) toe-off, (b) single leg stance and (c) heel strike. A slightly modified stance position (b) conferred the greatest risk of spontaneous femoral neck fracture in the laboratory simulations of Cristofolini et al [3]. The focally thin patch we identified coincides with a region of high tensile stress during simulations of spontaneous fracture.

help to improve the FE methods that currently assume a constant cortical thickness throughout the bone.

In related work, Li et al applied SPM to 3D density maps of femurs and discovered focal regions where clustered voxels of bone density differed significantly between hip fracture cases and controls [31]. In their analysis, several fracture-relevant density ROI's showed promise in defining a hip fracture phenotype. The fact that Li's head-neck junction femoral ROI based on volumetric density appears to coincide with the focally thinner femoral cortex we find at the head-neck junction suggests that having poor quality bone here is particularly concerning for future fracture risk. Previous prospective studies indicated that combining measures (e.g one measure of density, one of cortical thickness and one of bone shape) resulted in the optimum prediction of incident hip fracture [11,32]. However, large prospective studies are necessary to determine what thresholds of cortical thickness or density in these newly discovered zones are predictive of hip fracture and might be a trigger for intervention in an individual. Our work is useful in defining ROI's for cortical bone analysis that can then be taken forward for testing in prospective studies. Current hip

fracture prevention strategies are based on case finding: they involve clinical risk factor estimation to determine the need for single plane bone density measurement within a standard femoral neck ROI. The precise sites of focal osteoporosis that we have now identified are overlooked by current 2D bone densitometry methods.

Acknowledgments

We thank Dr Jonathan Reeve, Department of Medicine, University of Cambridge, UK for his help with the Prague-Cambridge collaboration and for guidance on the selection of appropriate control participants.

Author Contributions

Conceived and designed the experiments: KESP PMM JS MH JV PD GMT AHG. Performed the experiments: KESP PMM GMT AHG. Analyzed the data: KESP AHG GMT. Contributed reagents/materials/analysis tools: JS MH JV PD PMM. Wrote the paper: KESP GMT AHG PMM JS MH JV PD. Designed the study to recruit patients with hip fracture in Prague: JV PD. Methods section critical review: JV PD.

References

1. Pulkkinen P, Gluer CC, Jamsa T (2011) Investigation of differences between hip fracture types: a worthy strategy for improved risk assessment and fracture prevention. Bone 49: 600–604.
2. Sievanen H, Kannus P, Jarvinen TL (2007) Bone quality: an empty term. PLoS Med 4: e27.
3. Cristofolini L, Juszczyk M, Martelli S, Taddei F, Viceconti M (2007) In vitro replication of spontaneous fractures of the proximal human femur. J Biomech 40: 2837–2845.
4. Yli-Kyyny T, Tamminen I, Syri J, Venesmaa P, Kröger H (2011) Bilateral hip pain. The Lancet 377: 2248.
5. Wainwright SA, Marshall LM, Ensrud KE, Cauley JA, Black DM, et al. (2005) Hip fracture in women without osteoporosis. J Clin Endocrinol Metab 90: 2787–2793.
6. de Bakker PM, Manske SL, Ebacher V, Oxland TR, Cripton PA, et al. (2009) During sideways falls proximal femur fractures initiate in the superolateral cortex: evidence from high-speed video of simulated fractures. J Biomech 42: 1917–1925.
7. Feik SA, Thomas CD, Clement JG (1997) Age-related changes in cortical porosity of the midshaft of the human femur. J Anat 191 (Pt 3): 407–416.
8. Poole KE, Mayhew PM, Rose CM, Brown JK, Bearcroft PJ, et al. (2010) Changing structure of the femoral neck across the adult female lifespan. J Bone Miner Res 25: 482–491.
9. Johannesdottir F, Poole KE, Reeve J, Siggeirsdottir K, Aspelund T, et al. (2011) Distribution of cortical bone in the femoral neck and hip fracture: a prospective case-control analysis of 143 incident hip fractures; the AGES-REYKJAVIK Study. Bone 48: 1268–1276.
10. Mayhew PM, Thomas CD, Clement JG, Loveridge N, Beck TJ, et al. (2005) Relation between age, femoral neck cortical stability, and hip fracture risk. Lancet 366: 129–135.
11. Gluer CC, Cummings SR, Pressman A, Li J, Gluer K, et al. (1994) Prediction of hip fractures from pelvic radiographs: the study of osteoporotic fractures. The Study of Osteoporotic Fractures Research Group. J Bone Miner Res 9: 671–677.
12. Hansen S, Jensen JE, Ahrberg F, Hauge EM, Brixen K (2011) The combination of structural parameters and areal bone mineral density improves relation to proximal femur strength: an in vitro study with high-resolution peripheral quantitative computed tomography. Calcif Tissue Int 89: 335–346.
13. Holzer G, von Skrbensky G, Holzer LA, Pichl W (2009) Hip fractures and the contribution of cortical versus trabecular bone to femoral neck strength. J Bone Miner Res 24: 468–474.
14. Borggrefe J, Graeff C, Nickelsen TN, Marin F, Gluer CC (2009) Quantitative Computed Tomography Assessment of the Effects of 24 months of Teriparatide Treatment on 3-D Femoral Neck Bone Distribution, Geometry and Bone Strength: Results from the EUROFORS Study. J Bone Miner Res 25: 472–481.
15. Poole KE, Treece GM, Ridgway GR, Mayhew PM, Borggrefe J, et al. (2011) Targeted regeneration of bone in the osteoporotic human femur. PLoS One 6: e16190.
16. Treece GM, Gee AH, Mayhew PM, Poole KE (2010) High resolution cortical bone thickness measurement from clinical CT data. Med Image Anal 14: 276–290.
17. Vaculík J, Malkus T, Majerníček M, Podškubka A, Dungl P (2007) Incidence of proximal femoral fractures. Ortopedie 1: 62–68.
18. Rueckert D, Frangi AF, Schnabel JA (2003) Automatic construction of 3-D statistical deformation models of the brain using nonrigid registration. IEEE Trans Med Imaging 22: 1014–1025.
19. Friston KJ, Holmes AP, Worsley KJ, Poline J-P, Frith CD, et al. (1994) Statistical parametric maps in functional imaging: A general linear approach. Human Brain Mapping 2: 189–210.
20. Worsley K, Taylor J, Carbonell F, Chung M, Duerden E, et al. (2009) SurfStat: A Matlab toolbox for the statistical analysis of univariate and multivariate surface and volumetric data using linear mixed effects models and random field theory. NeuroImage Organization for Human Brain Mapping 2009 Annual Meeting 47: S102.
21. Bessho M, Ohnishi I, Matsumoto T, Ohashi S, Matsuyama J, et al. (2009) Prediction of proximal femur strength using a CT-based nonlinear finite element method: differences in predicted fracture load and site with changing load and boundary conditions. Bone 45: 226–231.
22. Parker MJ, Twemlow TR (1997) Spontaneous hip fractures, 44/872 in a prospective study. Acta Orthop Scand 68: 325–326.
23. Yang KH, Shen KL, Demetropoulos CK, King AI, Kolodziej P, et al. (1996) The relationship between loading conditions and fracture patterns of the proximal femur. Journal of Biomechanical Engineering-Transactions of the Asme 118: 575–578.
24. Freeman MA, Todd RC, Pirie CJ (1974) The role of fatigue in the pathogenesis of senile femoral neck fractures. J Bone Joint Surg Br 56-B: 698–702.
25. Odgers PNB (1931) Two details about the neck of the femur: (1) The eminentia. (2) The empreinte. Journal of Anatomy 65: 352–U321.
26. Panzer S, Esch U, Abdulazim AN, Augat P (2010) Herniation pits and cystic-appearing lesions at the anterior femoral neck: an anatomical study by MSCT and microCT. Skeletal Radiol 39: 645–654.
27. Pitt M, Graham A, Shipman J, Birkby W (1982) Herniation pit of the femoral neck American Journal of Roentgenology 138 1115–1121.
28. Zebaze RM, Ghasem-Zadeh A, Bohte A, Iuliano-Burns S, Mirams M, et al. (2010) Intracortical remodelling and porosity in the distal radius and post-mortem femurs of women: a cross-sectional study. Lancet 375: 1729–1736.
29. Bell KL, Loveridge N, Power J, Garrahan N, Meggitt BF, et al. (1999) Regional differences in cortical porosity in the fractured femoral neck. Bone 24: 57–64.
30. Cristofolini L, Schileo E, Juszczyk M, Taddei F, Martelli S, et al. (2010) Mechanical testing of bones: the positive synergy of finite-element models and in vitro experiments. Philos Transact A Math Phys Eng Sci 368: 2725–2763.
31. Li W, Kornak J, Harris T, Keyak J, Li C, et al. (2009) Identify fracture-critical regions inside the proximal femur using statistical parametric mapping. Bone 44: 596–602.
32. Kaptoge S, Beck TJ, Reeve J, Stone KL, Hillier TA, et al. (2008) Prediction of incident hip fracture risk by femur geometry variables measured by hip structural analysis in the study of osteoporotic fractures. J Bone Miner Res 23: 1892–1904.

5

Human Umbilical Cord Blood-Derived CD34⁺ Cells Reverse Osteoporosis in NOD/SCID Mice by Altering Osteoblastic and Osteoclastic Activities

Reeva Aggarwal[1], Jingwei Lu[1], Suman Kanji[1], Matthew Joseph[1], Manjusri Das[1], Garrett J. Noble[2], Brooke K. McMichael[3], Sudha Agarwal[4], Richard T. Hart[2], Zongyang Sun[4], Beth S. Lee[3], Thomas J. Rosol[5], Rebecca Jackson[6], Hai-Quan Mao[7], Vincent J. Pompili[1], Hiranmoy Das[1]*

1 Cardiovascular Stem Cell Research Laboratory, Davis Heart and Lung Research Institute, The Ohio State University Medical Center, Columbus, Ohio, United States of America, 2 Department of Biomedical Engineering, College of Engineering, The Ohio State University, Columbus, Ohio, United States of America, 3 Department of Physiology and Cell Biology, College of Medicine, The Ohio State University, Columbus, Ohio, United States of America, 4 Division of Oral Biology, Department of Orthopedics, College of Dentistry, The Ohio State University, Columbus, Ohio, United States of America, 5 Department of Veterinary Clinical Sciences, College of Veterinary Medicine, The Ohio State University, Columbus, Ohio, United States of America, 6 Division of Endocrinology, Diabetes and Metabolism, College of Medicine, The Ohio State University, Columbus, Ohio, United States of America, 7 Department of Materials Science and Engineering, John's Hopkins University, Baltimore, Maryland, United States of America

Abstract

Background: Osteoporosis is a bone disorder associated with loss of bone mineral density and micro architecture. A balance of osteoblasts and osteoclasts activities maintains bone homeostasis. Increased bone loss due to increased osteoclast and decreased osteoblast activities is considered as an underlying cause of osteoporosis.

Methods and Findings: The cures for osteoporosis are limited, consequently the potential of CD34+ cell therapies is currently being considered. We developed a nanofiber-based expansion technology to obtain adequate numbers of CD34⁺ cells isolated from human umbilical cord blood, for therapeutic applications. Herein, we show that CD34⁺ cells could be differentiated into osteoblastic lineage, *in vitro*. Systemically delivered CD34⁺ cells home to the bone marrow and significantly improve bone deposition, bone mineral density and bone micro-architecture in osteoporotic mice. The elevated levels of osteocalcin, IL-10, GM-CSF, and decreased levels of MCP-1 in serum parallel the improvements in bone micro-architecture. Furthermore, CD34⁺ cells improved osteoblast activity and concurrently impaired osteoclast differentiation, maturation and functionality.

Conclusions: These findings demonstrate a novel approach utilizing nanofiber-expanded CD34⁺ cells as a therapeutic application for the treatment of osteoporosis.

Editor: Zoran Ivanovic, French Blood Institute, France

Funding: This work was supported by National Institutes of Health grants, K01 AR054114 (NIAMS), SBIR R44 HL092706-01 (NHLBI), R21 CA143787 (NCI) and The Ohio State University start-up fund. The funders had no role in study design, data collection and analysis, decision to publish or preparation of the manuscript.

Competing Interests: The authors have read the journal's policy and have the following conflicts: Dr. Pompili has equity interests with Arteriocyte Inc., Cleveland. Hiranmoy Das is a PLoS ONE Editorial Board member. This does not alter the authors' adherence to all the PLoS ONE policies on sharing data and materials. No other conflicts to declare.

* E-mail: hiranmoy.das@osumc.edu

Introduction

Osteoporosis is a systemic bone disorder, affecting more than 200 million people worldwide [1]. Bone is a dynamic organ that undergoes constant remodeling via cycles of bone formation and resorption, by osteoblasts and osteoclasts [2]. Imbalance of osteoclastic and/or osteoblastic activities generally results in low bone mineral density (BMD), loss of bone mass and mechanical strength, leading to increased risk of fractures, typical of osteoporosis [3]. Impaired osteoblastic differentiation of bone marrow progenitor cells may also play a significant role in developing osteoporosis. Age, endocrine malfunction or deficiency, nutrition, or lack of physical activity, all can imbalance the osteoblasts and osteoclasts activities, affecting both trabecular and cortical bone at molecular, cellular and structural levels [4,5]. It has been shown that reduction in trabecular bone in osteoporosis is associated with increased adiposity in bone marrow, which could be due to transcriptional switch in favor of adipogenesis instead of osteoblastogenesis of bone marrow precursor cells [6,7].

The mesenchymal progenitor cells in the bone marrow give rise to osteoblasts under the influence of multiple osteogenic signals specific for their proliferation and differentiation [8]. Osteoblastic differentiation is initiated by binding of bone morphogenetic proteins (BMPs) to their receptors that activate transcription factors, Runx2 and Osterix, and subsequent expression of downstream osteoblast specific genes such as alkaline phosphatase, collagen type 1, osteonectin, osteocalcin and bone sialoprotein

[9,10,11]. BMPs upregulate osteoblastic genes *via* activation of Smad1/5/8 signaling molecules and regulate mineralization of osteoblastic cells via Wnt in an autocrine signaling loop [12]. Runx2 is a potent inhibitor of adipogenesis, and is required for the differentiation of adipocytes to osteogenic lineage [13]. Additionally, balance of osteoprotegrin (OPG): receptor activator of nuclear factor kappa-B ligand (RANKL) ratio, osteocalcin and cytokines such as interleukin (IL)-1 IL-4, IL-6, monocyte chemotactic protein (MCP)-1 and granulocyte macrophage colony stimulating factor (GM-CSF) have been shown to regulate the activities of osteoblastic and osteoclastic cells [14,15].

Although, associated with side effects, anti-resorptive and anabolic therapies are currently available for osteoporosis [3,16]. Furthermore, these therapies have temporary effects, and the decrease in fracture incidences in long-term is debatable [17,18]. Recently, much effort has been expended to understand the therapeutic effectiveness of CD34+ cells in various degenerative diseases. However, the major hurdles are the unavailability of sufficient number of biologically functional CD34+ cells and maintaining their regenerative potential for therapeutic applications.

We previously reported that human $CD133^+/CD34^+$ cells could be expanded *in vitro* up to 250-fold in a serum-free medium on aminated poly-ether sulfone (PES) nanofiber coated plates within 10 days, while preserving stem cell phenotype and biological functionality [19]. These cells are considered biologically superior as they exhibit better engraftment capabilities, express homing markers (CXCR4 and LFA-1) towards bone marrow and maintain their multipotency. This allows them to differentiate into multiple lineages such as endothelial, and hematopoietic lineages. Here we show that nanofiber-expanded $CD34^+$ cells could be differentiated towards osteoblastic lineage, *in vitro*. Furthermore, $CD34^+$ cell transplantation into an osteoporotic NOD/SCID murine model augments bone formation rate, bone mineral density and improves bone micro-architecture. These improvements correlate with the elevated serum levels of osteocalcin, interleukin (IL)-10 and granulocyte-macrophage colony stimulating factor (GM-CSF), and decreased level of monocyte chemotactic protein-1 (MCP-1). $CD34^+$ cell transplantation not only improved osteoblast functionality but also concurrently impaired differentiation and maturation of osteoclasts, thereby reducing osteoclast activity in osteoporotic mice. The findings demonstrate a novel potential of nanofiber-expanded $CD34^+$ cells in reverting osteoporosis.

Results

Differentiation of nanofiber-expanded $CD34^+$ cells towards osteoblastic lineage

Our previous studies showed that nanofiber expanded human umbilical cord blood (hUCB) $CD34^+$ cells retain multipotency as evident by their ability to differentiate into endothelial or smooth muscle cells [19,20]. Here we sought, whether these cells could also be differentiated towards osteoblastic lineage *in vitro*. To test that, $CD133^+$ cells were isolated from hUCB and expanded on nanofiber coated plates in serum-free expansion medium with supplements for 10 days, *in vitro* [19]. The cell phenotype was confirmed by the expression of CD34, CD45, CXCR4, LFA-1, MHC-I & II, CD14, CD11a and absence of CD69, CD117, CD105 using flowcytometric analyses (data not shown). CD34+ cells were then induced to osteoblastic differentiation in the presence of ascorbic acid and b-glycerophosphate, *in vitro*. Remarkable cellular changes in shape and size were observed within 7 days and mineralized nodules were apparent at 21 days in more than 95% of the cells (Figure 1A, upper right panel). The

mineral deposition by induced $CD34^+$ cells was confirmed by the presence of calcium in Alizarin red stained cells. $CD34^+$ cells cultured in tissue culture media (TCM) lacking ascorbic acid and b-glycerophosphate, also showed few randomly scattered cells with faint intracellular alizarin red staining (Figure 1A, lower left panel). However, the intensity of stain was markedly higher in cells induced to differentiate into osteoblastic lineages (Figure 1A, lower right panel).

Molecular evidences for osteoblastic differentiation of $CD34^+$ cells

To further investigate the differentiation of $CD34^+$ cells into osteoblastic lineage, the expression of osteoblast specific genes and proteins were analyzed. Semi quantitative RT-PCR analysis revealed that differentiated nanofiber-expanded cells upregulated expression of transcription factor Runx2, and bone associated proteins such as alkaline phosphatase, osteocalcin, osteonectin and collagen type 1A1 at various time points during the course of differentiation (Figure 1B). The expression of osteocalcin in freshly isolated $CD133^+$ cells was consistent with earlier reports [21]. Fold increase for the gene expressions at mRNA level compared to undifferentiated control was analyzed, as follows: Runx2; Day 7, 0.84 ± 0.14; Day 21, 1.18 ± 0.1; Alk Phos; Day 7, 0.9 ± 0.05; Day 21, 1.7 ± 0.13; Osteocalcin; Day 7, 1.02 ± 0.05; Day 21, 1.56 ± 0.1; Osteonectin; Day 7, 1.16 ± 0.04; Day 21, 1.51 ± 0.48; Collagen 1A1; Day 7, 0.61 ± 0.13; Day 21, 1.79 ± 0.27. Additionally, immunocytochemical analysis revealed that $CD34^+$ cells stained positive with Smad1/5/8 and osteocalcin upto 21 days of differentiation (Figure 1C). Western blots showed an increase in protein levels of BMP2, BMP4, dishevelled protein (DVL) 2, DVL3 and Smad1/5/8 in differentiated cells at all time points during the course of differentiation. GAPDH was used as loading control and MC3T3 cells differentiated into osteoblasts were used as a positive control (Figure 1D). Fold increase of the protein level compared to undifferentiated control was analyzed, as follows BMP2; Day 7, 0.78 ± 0.24; Day 21, 1.2 ± 0.01; BMP4; Day 7, 0.45 ± 0.2; Day 21, 1.7 ± 0.61; Smad 1/5/8; Day 7, 1.46 ± 0.04; Day 21, 1.01 ± 0.12; DVL2; Day 7, 0.72 ± 0.09; Day 21, 1.1 ± 0.12; DVL3; Day 7, 1.24 ± 0.04; Day 21, 1.0 ± 0.12. Collectively, these data confirm osteoblastic differentiation of nanofiber expanded hUCB $CD34^+$ cells.

Nanofiber-expanded $CD34^+$ cells induce bone formation in a murine model of osteoporosis

We further investigated the therapeutic potential of nanofiber-expanded human $CD34^+$ in a mouse model of dexamethasone-induced osteoporosis in immunocompromised NOD/SCID mice. Mice (n = 6/group) injected with dexamethasone for 21 consecutive days, followed by withdrawal for 5 days with tapering dose, and subsequently were either not treated and sacrificed (Op), treated with $CD34^+$ cells via intra-cardio-ventricular injection (Op+ Cells; 0.5×10^6/mouse), or treated with DMEM alone (Op+Med). Mice in all groups did not exhibit weight loss or gain during the course of experimentation. Hematoxylin and eosin (H & E) staining of longitudinal sections of femurs showed a decrease in the number of trabecular bone spicules in Op and Op+Med mice, as compared to untreated controls. However, after 28 days of $CD34^+$ cell transplantation, an increase in the numbers of trabecular bone spicules was observed (Figure 2B, arrows). The number of adipocytes was significantly increased in Op and Op+Med mice, as compared to untreated control (Figure 2B, arrowheads). Further, the number of adipocytes was evaluated in each group and a marked reduction in adipocytes was observed in

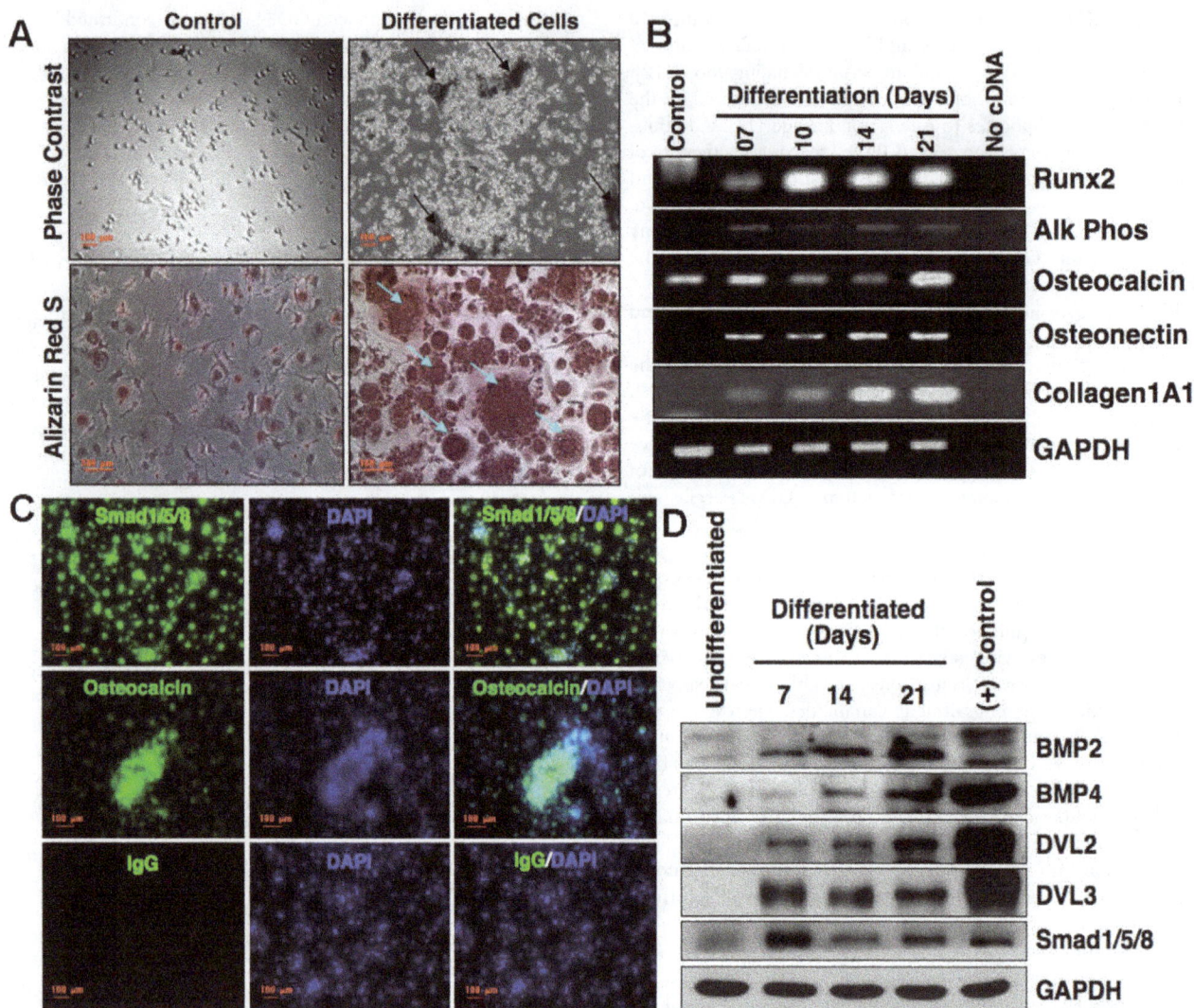

Figure 1. Osteoblastic differentiation of nanofiber-expanded CD34+ cells. (A). Morphology of the cells was visualized under phase contrast microscope at day 1 (control, upper panel) after seeding of nanofiber-expanded CD34+ cells (10 days expansion of CD133+/CD34+ cells on nanofiber) and at day 14 after differentiation of cells with osteoblast specific stimulants (b-glycerophosphate and ascorbic acid) in DMEM complete medium cultured on a 24-well tissue culture plate. Arrowheads indicate the clusters that formed after differentiation. Alizarin Red S staining (lower panel) was performed to the cells cultured for 21 days either with osteoblast specific differentiation medium (differentiated cells) or DMEM complete medium only (control). Red stains in the control image indicate the intracellular calcium in random differentiated cells and arrowheads indicate higher level of mineral depositions in differentiated cells. The experiment was repeated at least three times and representative images are shown. **(B).** RNA was isolated from differentiated cells during the course of osteoblastic differentiation at various time points as stated, and one microgram of RNA was used to make cDNA. One micro liter of cDNA was used to perform semi-quantitative RT-PCR analysis for Runx2, alkaline (Alk) phosphate, osteocalcin, osteonectin, collagen Type 1A1 and GAPDH as a loading control. Nanofiber expanded cells (10 days) were used as a control. **(C).** Detection of osteoblast specific proteins in differentiated cells. Immunocytochemical staining was performed with the 21 days-differentiated cells using either Sma and Mad related proteins (Smad 1/5/8) or osteocalcin specific antibodies, and IgG isotype as control. Green fluorescence indicates positive staining and blue fluorescence indicate DAPI (nuclear) staining. **(D).** Protein levels were evaluated for various signaling molecules of BMP, Wnt and Smad pathways during the course of osteoblastic differentiation of nanofiber-expanded CD34+ cells. Undifferentiated nanofiber-expanded cells and differentiated MC3T3 cell line were used as controls. Representative of three sets of experiments is shown here.

Op+Cells mice, as compared to Op mice. The number of adipocytes/high power field (HPF) was: control, 9.5±2.7; Op, 34.25±7.5; Op+Media, 29.75±3.9; Op+Cells, 13.75±1.7 (Figure 2C, lower panel).

CD34+ cells home to the bone marrow

The chemokine receptor, CXCR4 binds to SDF-1, a chemotactic ligand expressed by bone marrow cells. Additionally, the presence of lymphocyte adhesion molecules (LFA-1) is required for

the bone marrow homing of CD34+ cells. Since, we observed that both CXCR4 and LFA1 are highly expressed on CD34+ cells after 10 day of expansion on nanofibers, we next sought to examine the homing of these cells in the osteoporotic mice. Although delivered systemically, via intra-cardio-ventricular injection, CD34+ cells home to bone marrow (Figure 2D) as well as other organs such as lung, liver and spleen (data not shown). In the bone marrow, CD34+ were detected near the endosteal sites and around the bone marrow sinusoids, as well as at the surface of trabecular bone

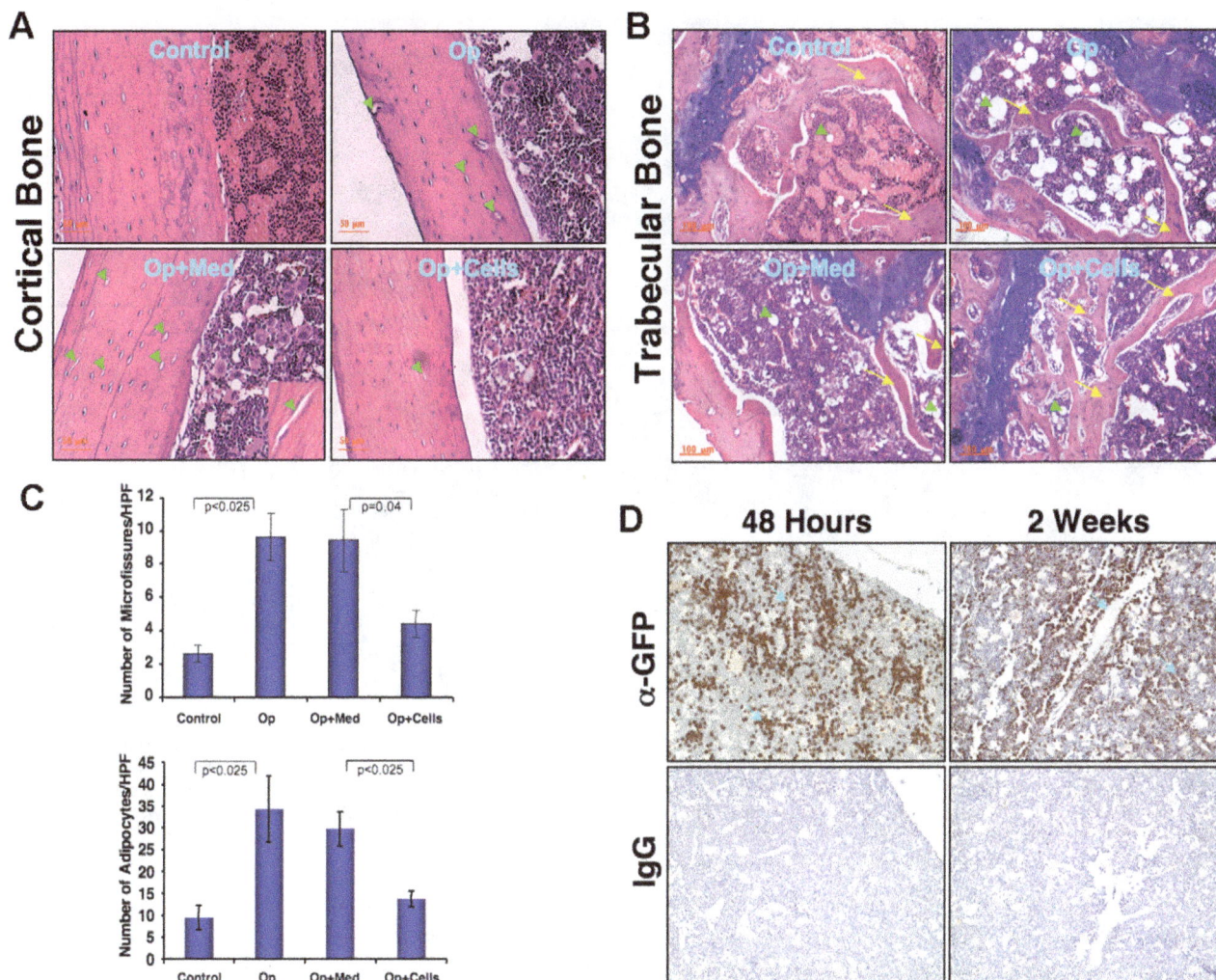

Figure 2. Effect of CD34$^+$ cells on bone histomorphology in femurs of osteoporotic NOD/SCID mice. Osteoporosis (Op) was developed by injection of dexamethasone (for 21 days and 5 days for withdrawal) or saline as a control (Control) in seven month-old female NOD/SCID mice. Nanofiber-expanded CD34$^+$ cells (half a million per mouse) were injected to the osteoporotic mice (Op+Cells) and serum-free medium was used as a media control (Op+Med). Femurs were harvested after 28 days of CD34+ cell injection, fixed, embed and H & E staining was performed. (**A**). An increased number of cortical bone micro fissures (arrowheads) were found in Op mice compared to control and numbers were reduced in Op+Cells animals. (**B**). A decreased number of trabecular bone spicules (arrows) and increased numbers of adipocytes (arrowheads) were found in Op mice compare to control under the growth plate region. In Op+Cells animals increased number of trabecular bone spicules and a decreased number of adipocyes were observed (n = 6/each group). (**C**). Evaluated numbers of microfissures and adipocytes per high-power field (HPF) in femur bone sections were shown in a graphical form (n = 6, four HPF/section). (**D**). Detection of systemically delivered GFP+ nanofiber-expanded human CD34$^+$ cell in the bone marrow after 48 h and two weeks. Arrows indicate trabecular bone and sinusoids within the bone marrow.

spicules after 48 hours (Figure 2D, upper left panel), as well as after 2 weeks (Figure 2D, upper right panel).

Mineral apposition rate in response to CD34$^+$ cell transplantation

To determine the effect of CD34$^+$ cell transplantation on the mineral apposition rate (MAR), calcium binding fluorescent dye calcein (green) was injected at 17 days post CD34+ cell or medium injection. Subsequently, on day 24, fluorescent dye alizarin (red), and femurs were harvested on day 28. The inter-label distance between the two dyes was narrower at cortical and trabecular regions of the Op+Med mice compared to the Op+Cells mice indicating limited bone deposition in Op+Med mice. The values for mineral apposition rate were assessed in plastic embedded femur bone sections of Op+Med and Op+ Cells on the endosteal surface of metaphysial region of the femur, distal to the growth

plate (Cortical MAR, μm/day; Op+Med, 0.47±0.04; Op+Cells, 3.07±0.29). Similarly, significant increase in trabecular MAR was observed in Op+Cells compared to Op+Med at the growth plate region (Trabecular MAR, μmm/day; Op+Med, 0.49±0.05; Op+Cells, 1.35±0.09) (Figure 3).

Ultra structural analysis of bones after CD34$^+$ cell transplantation

To evaluate the extent of trabecular and cortical bone repair/regeneration and to image the differences in bone quality at the ultrastructural level, femurs from Op, Op+Med, Op+Cells were examined by micro computed tomography (MicroCT) (Figure 4A–1B, left panels). Quantitative analyses showed an increase in trabecular number in Op+Cells as compared to Op+Med mice (trabecular number, 1/mm; control, 0.46±0.1; Op, 0.11±0.1; Op+Med, 0.23±0.1; Op+Cells, 0.64±0.1) (Figure 4A, upper right

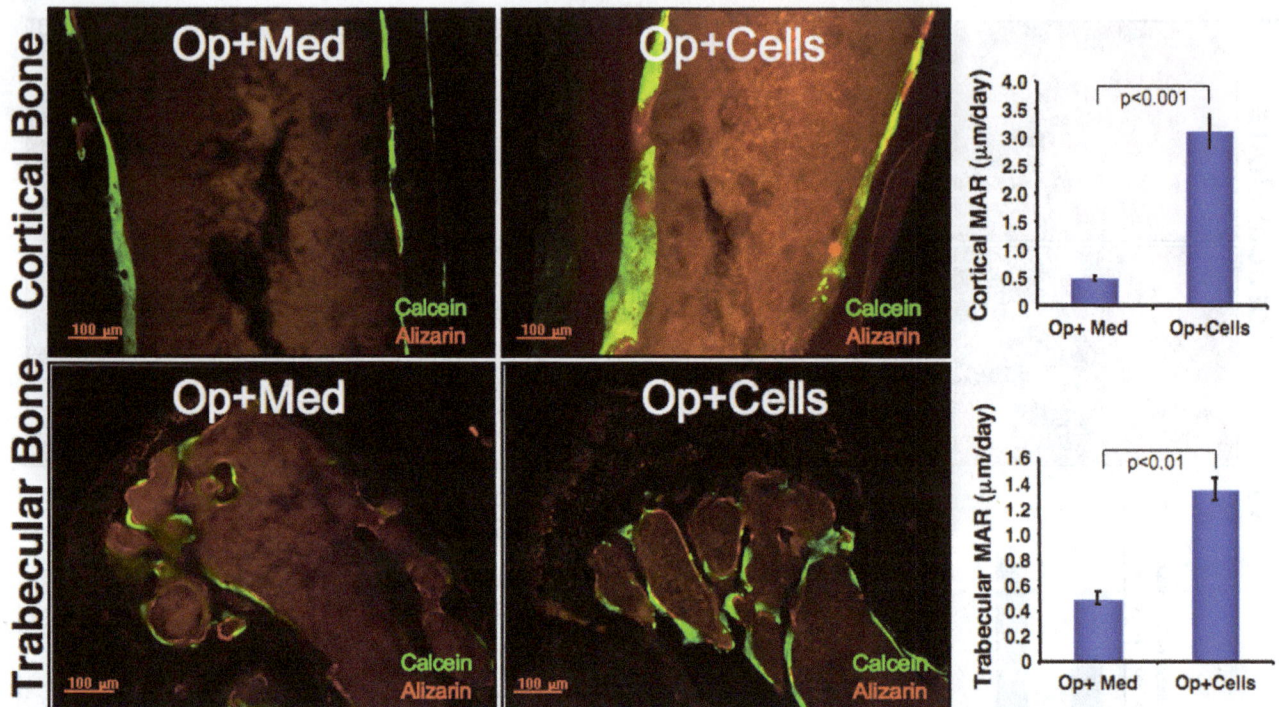

Figure 3. Detection of *in vivo* bone regeneration. *In vivo* immunolabeling with calcein (green) and alizarin (red) was performed in osteoporotic mice that received CD34+ cell (Op+Cells) or medium (Op+Media) as a control 10 and 3 days respectively before sacrifice of the mice. Femurs were harvested, formalin fixed and then embedded in methylmethacrylate resin. Thirty μm thick sections were mounted on the slides and observed under a fluorescence microscope. Increased mineral apposition rate (MAR) was observed in the endosteal sites of the cortical bone as well as trabeculae, distal from the growth plate, as detected by green fluorescence in mice that received CD34+ cells compared to control (n = 3/group). The values of MAR (μm/day) for the cortical and trabecular bone are shown graphically.

panel). Similar trend was observed for trabecular thickness (mm): control, 0.63 ± 0.06; Op, 0.45 ± 0.02; Op+Med, 0.46 ± 0.09; Op+Cells, 0.59 ± 0.04. A significant increase in trabecular bone volume/ total volume was observed in Op+Cells mice, as compared to Op+Med mice, i.e., trabecular bone volume/total volume in control, 4.67 ± 1.5; Op, 0.55 ± 0.4; Op+Med, 1.59 ± 1.1; Op+Cells, 10.22 ± 3.8 (Figure 4A, lower right, panel). Similarly, similar pattern was observed for bone mineral density (BMD) of the trabeculae. BMD was significantly increased in Op+Cells mice compared to Op +Med (BMD, g/cm^3; control, 0.223 ± 0.02; Op, 0.121 ± 0.02; Op+Med, 0.129 ± 0.02; Op+Cells, 0.21 ± 0.01). The reductions in BMD in Op mice indicated that dexamethasone treatments effectively decreased mineral density, and BMD was increased after CD34+ cell transplantation indicated reversal of the osteoporotic phenotype. Similarly, significant decrease in the degree of anisotropy (DA) was observed in the Op+Cells mice compared to Op+ Med mice (DA; control, 2.2 ± 0.29; Op, 3 ± 0.28; Op+Med, 2.6 ± 0.23; Op+Cells, 1.75 ± 0.1). Our data correlates with the previously reported results where higher degree of anisotropy was observed in osteoporotic bone compared to their healthy controls [22,23]. Similarly, structure model index (SMI) of the trabeculae bone was reported to be an important predictor of changes in micro-architecture of trabeculae in osteoporotic conditions. SMI indicates three-dimensional shape of the trabecular bone. Value of SMI for ideal plate is 0 and for ideal rod is 3 [24]. Transition from plate to rod shape has been reported in osteoporotic and aged bones when compared to the healthy controls [25]. Similarly, our data showed a transition from more rod like structures in Op, Op+Med mice and more plate like in

Op+Cells mice (SMI; control, 0.2 ± 0.22; Op, 1.0 ± 0.017; Op+Med, 1.13 ± 0.25; Op+Cells, 0.27 ± 0.08).

Metaphysial bones were also analyzed for cortical porosity, ratio of total bone volume to tissue volume and bone mineral density (BMD). MicroCT analysis of cortical bones revealed significant decrease in BMD in Op+Cells mice as compared to Op+Med mice, (BMD, g/cm^3; control, 0.28 ± 0.02; Op, 0.2 ± 0.01; Op+Med, 0.19 ± 0.02; Op+Cells, 0.33 ± 0.01). Similar results were obtained for ratio of cortical bone volume/tissue volumes (control, 79.64 ± 2.13; Op, 66.4 ± 0.86; Op+Med, 67 ± 1.34; Op+Cells, 77.9 ± 4), suggesting a marked increase in cortical bone volume/ tissue volume in Op+Cells mice as compared to Op+Med mice. Furthermore, results for cortical bone revealed a non-significant decrease in porosity of cortical bones in Op+Cells mice as compared to Op+Med mice, (cortical bone porosity (%); control, 17.17 ± 1.3; Op, 35.52 ± 0.5; Op+Med, 29.35 ± 4.9; Op+Cells, 25.03 ± 1.77) (Figure 4B, upper right panel).

CD34+ cell transplantation elevated serum levels of osteocalcin

As osteocalcin is the characteristic marker of osteoblast function, the levels of osteocalcin in the serum were evaluated to investigate *in vivo* effects of CD34+ cell therapy on osteoporotic mice. As shown in Figure 5, after osteoporosis, the serum levels of osteocalcin decreased as compared to untreated control mice. However, after CD34+cell transplantation, the levels of serum osteocalcin (ng/ml) were elevated, as follows: control, 30.5 ± 1.1; Op, 24.2 ± 0.04; Op+Med, $27.5 \pm$ and Op+Cells, 30.72 ± 1.7. This increase in the levels of serum osteocalcin indicates potential

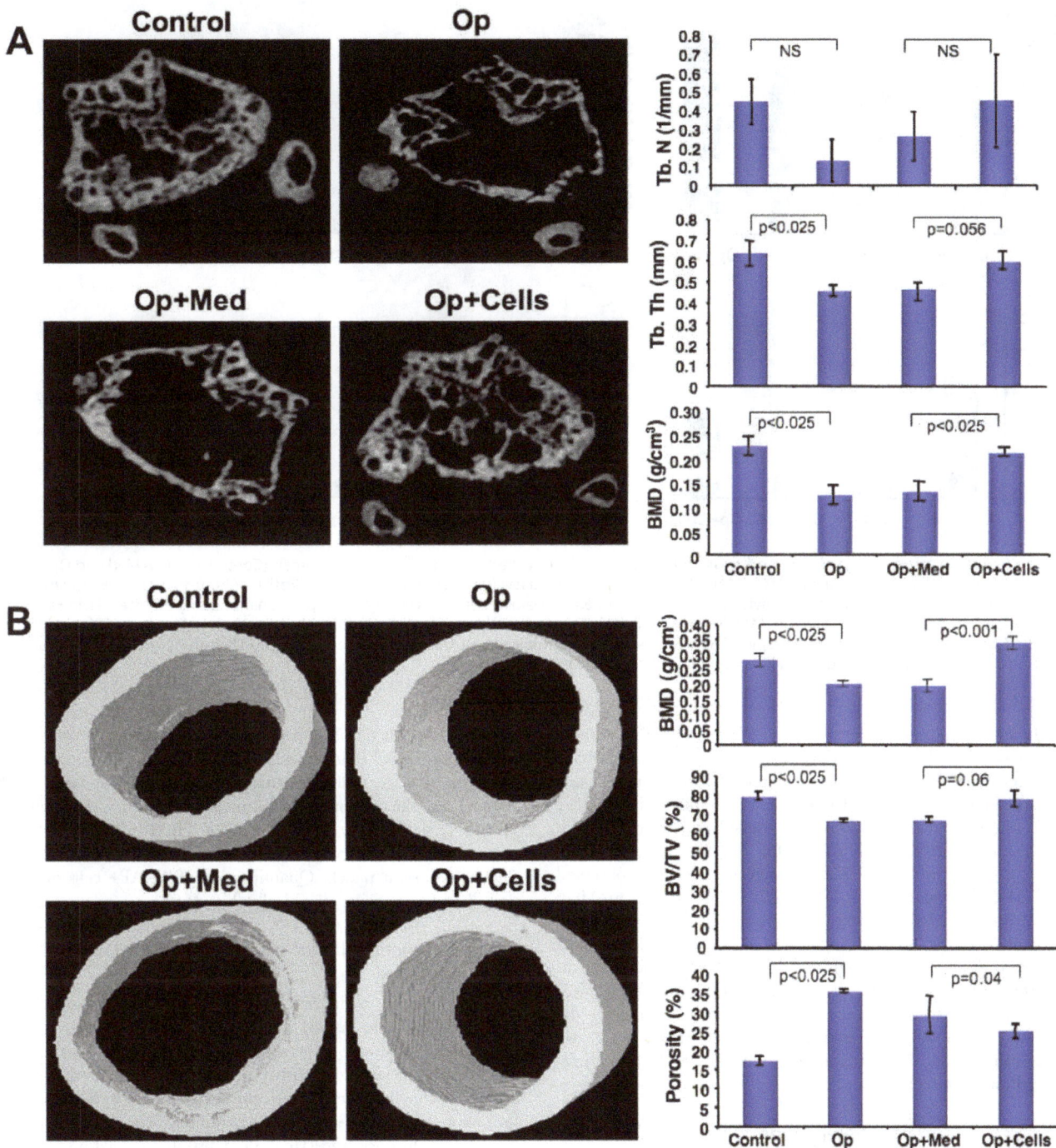

Figure 4. MicroCT images and analyses of bones. Formalin fixed femur bones were scanned using a high resolution MicroCT scanner (SkyScan 1172-D) established at 16 mm resolution and analyzed with the associated software (CTan). (**A**). Three dimensional image reconstruction of trabecular bones towards the distal side of the femur and, 0.1 mm away from the metaphyseal side of the growth plate is shown for each group (upper; left panel) and analysis is shown (upper; right panel) (n = 6/group). (**B**). MicroCT images (lower; left panel) and analyses of cortical bones (lower; right panel). Three dimensional (3D) image reconstruction of metaphyseal bones were generated at 2 mm away from growth plate and shown in the left panel. Analyzed data is presented in the lower; right panel (n = 6/group). NS = non-significant.

increase in the activation of osteoblasts and bone formation, as a consequence of CD34^{+}cell transplantation in Op mice.

Serum levels of cytokines and growth factors

It was reported that *in vitro* cultures of osteoblasts produce factors such as granulocyte-macrophage colony stimulating factor

(GM-CSF) and interleukin-1 (IL-1) [26]. Multiplex ELISA was performed to analyze the levels of serum cytokines and growth factors implicated to play significant role in bone homeostasis (from Quansys Biosciences, Logan Utah). Out of 20 markers tested (n = 4 mice/group) four (MCP-1, GM-CSF, and IL-10) showed marked changes in all groups (Figure 5). CD34^{+} cell transplan-

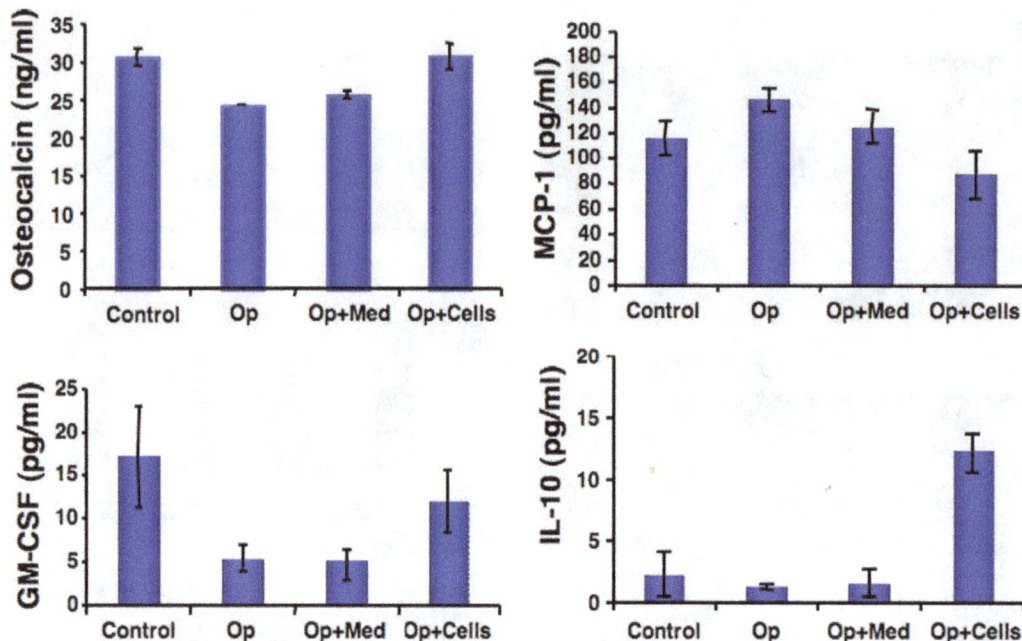

Figure 5. Serum levels of cytokines and growth factors. Blood was collected from all groups of animals (Control, Op, Op+Med and Op+Cells) before sacrifice and collected serum was stored at −80°C freezer. Increased levels of serum osteocalcin (indicative of bone formation) were observed in the mice that received CD34+ cell. Sandwich ELISA was performed to evaluate serum levels in all groups of animals using an osteoclacin ELISA kit (Biomedical Technologies, Inc, Staughton, MA), (n = 4 in triplicate). To assess the levels of various cytokines and growth factors (twenty factors) from collected serum (250 µl/animal) the multiplex ELISA was performed in triplicate by Quansys Biosciences, Logan Utah (n = 4/group). The values of MCP-1, GM-CSF and IL-10 were graphically reported as mean ± SEM.

tation appeared to direct normalization of the levels of markers of the osteoporosis. GM-CSF and MCP-1 levels were shown to have opposite effects on the osteoclast function [14]. Our data revealed a marked increase in MCP-1 levels in the Op mice while MCP-1 levels plummet after the CD34+ cell transplantation in Op mice (MCP-1 in control, 116.77±7.1; Op, 156.92±12.8; Op+Med, 125.57±7.8; Op+Cells, 87.95±9.3). Reverse trend was observed for GM-CSF levels (control, 17.95±2.7; Op, 5.6±1.3; Op+Med, 5.1±1.5; Op+Cells, 12.22±1.7). Interestingly, we observed that levels of IL-10 (pg/ml) were suppressed in Op and Op+Med mice but were dramatically upregulated in Op+Cells mice (IL-10 in control, 2.925±0.8; Op, 1.3± 0.1; Op+Med, 1.975±0.5; Op+Cells, 12.5±2.3). As there was a high variation among the animals and number of animals was small, results were not statistically significant when posthoc analysis was performed by using Bonferroni correction.

Impaired osteoclast differentiation following CD34+ cell transplantation

Our observations regarding altered levels of cytokines and growth factors and increased bone formation suggested possible effects of CD34+ cell transplantation on differentiation and/or function of bone resorbing osteoclasts. Thus, we investigated any changes in differentiation or function of osteoclasts in Op mice with or without CD34+ cell transplantation. Bone marrows harvested from mice from all groups were allowed to adhere to the plastic overnight in the presence of M-CSF. Non-adherent cells were then induced to osteoclastic differentiation in the presence of M-CSF and RANKL. During the course of differentiation, cells were harvested at various time points (day 3 and 6) and osteoclast specific tartrate resistant acid phosphatase (TRAP) staining was performed to detect cells differentiating into mature osteoclasts. Osteoclasts were defined multinucleated

TRAP+ cells. At day 3 and 6, significant numbers of cells were positive for TRAP staining in Op+Med mice. By day 6, extensive numbers of large multinucleated cells were positive for TRAP staining in the osteoporotic animals (Figure 6A, left panel). However, significantly less numbers of TRAP positive multinuclear cells were observed in animals that received CD34+ cells (Figure 6A, right panel). Quantification of TRAP+ cells at both days 3 and 6 is shown graphically (Figure 6A).

Reduced functionality of osteoclasts after CD34+ cell transplantation

Osteoclasts use actin rich, ring-shaped attachment structures called sealing zone instead of focal adhesions for adherence to mineralized substrate. Generation of the sealing zone is requirement for osteoclasts to resorb bone. Therefore, to evaluate the osteoclast function, cells were immunostained for F-actin ring formation using anti-F-actin specific antibody. The cells from bone marrow of Op mice (Op+Med), demonstrated formation of clear F-actin rings (Figure 6B, upper left panel). Contrarily, clear F-actin ring in the bone marrow cells from Op+Cells mice was not observed. We next assessed whether F-actin ring lacking bone marrow cells from Op+Cells mice could resorb bone, using ivory slices as substrate. As shown in Figure 6B, lower right panel, osteoclast-like cells from Op+Med mice resorbed bone as evidenced by the large pits formed in ivory slices. The number and size of resorbed pits were significantly reduced in cells from Op +Cells mice (Figure 6B, lower left panel), indicating that CD34+ cell therapy significantly reduced osteoclast differentiation and function (number of pits/ HPF: Op+Med, 15.5±2.1; Op+Cells, 4.5±0.7; and pit area (µm²)/ HPF: Op+Med, 1420.26±329.3; Op+Cells, 164.3±19.6).

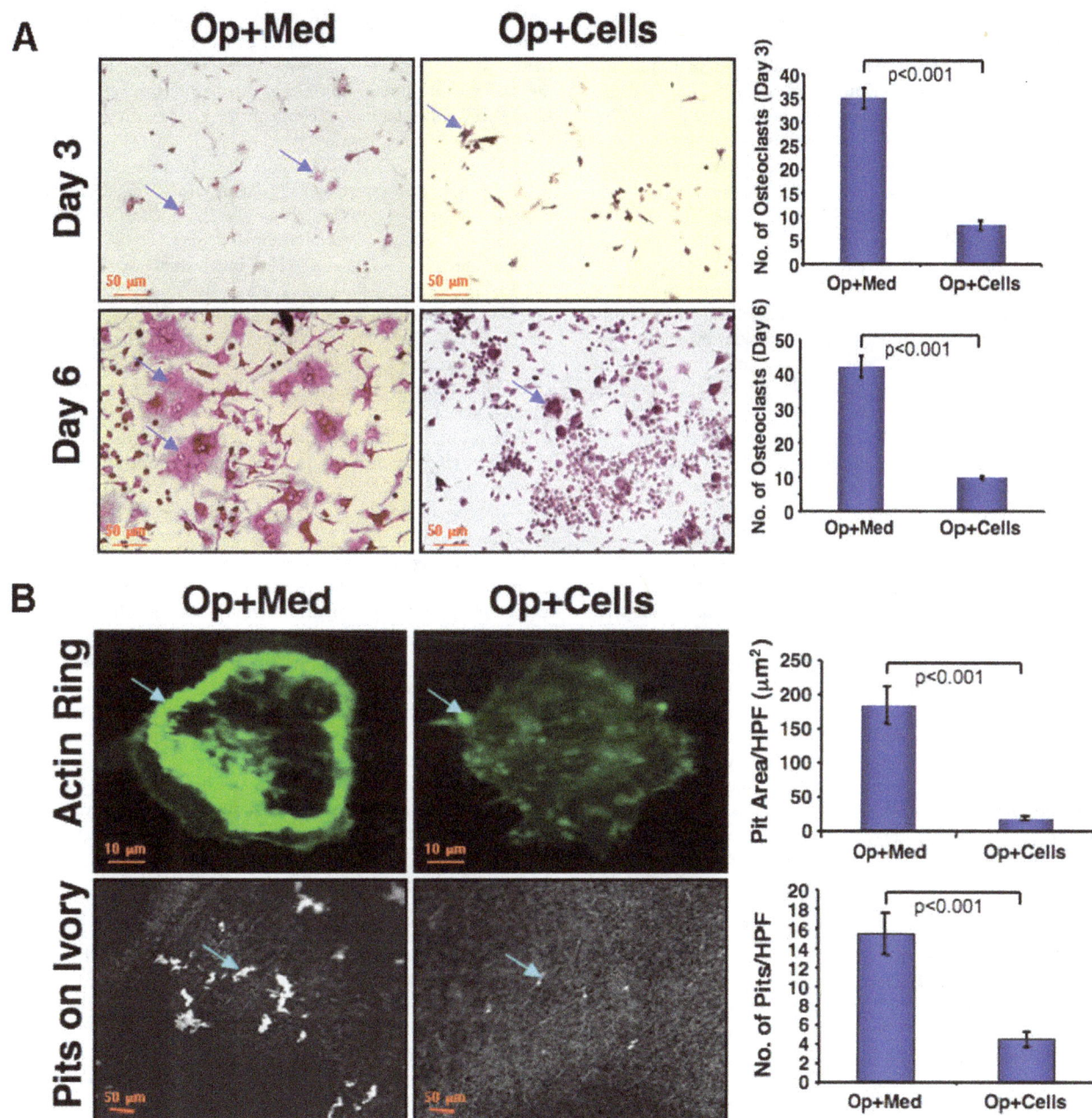

Figure 6. Impaired osteoclast differentiation, maturation and functionality in osteoporotic mice received CD34$^+$ cells. Harvested bone marrow was subjected to differentiation towards osteoclasts using M-CSF and sRANKL (n = 5). (**A**). During the course of differentiation at day 3 and 6, cells were stained with tartrate-resistant acid phosphatase (TRAP). The purple color was considered to indicate TRAP+ cells (arrows, left panel) and the yellow color as TRAP- cells. Nuclei were stained with DAPI for counting cell numbers. The Op+Med showed an increased number of TRAP+ cells at day 3 (upper, right panel) as well as day 6 compared to Op+Cells (lower, right panel). Evaluated values of differentiated osteoclasts are graphically presented. (**B**). To determine osteoclast functionality on day 4 of differentiation, osteoclasts were harvested and plated on thin ivory slices. Bone resorption assays were performed using osteoclasts from all four groups of animals and to analyze the formation of F-actin rings on ivory bone slices (arrow, upper; left panel). Ivory slices were stained with hematoxylin and analyzed for the resorbed pits on day 10 of differentiation. The formation of F-actin rings was assessed by F-actin specific antibody (green fluorescence). F-actin rings were prominent in osteoclasts derived from Op+Med animals (arrow, upper; left panel), however, osteoclasts derived from Op+Cells animals stained negative for F-actin ring (arrow, upper; right panel). Fewer and smaller resorption pits formed by osteoclasts from Op+Cells animals (arrow, lower; right panel) compared to those formed by animals from Op+Med (arrow, lower; left panel). Evaluated values of pit area/ high power field (HPF) and number of pits/ high power field (HPF) are shown graphical.

Discussion

Despite the hematopoietic origin of nanofiber expanded CD34$^+$ cells, herein we show that these cells could be differentiated towards osteogenic lineage. Both hematopoietic and osteogenic cells express similar families of transcription factors such as Cbfa/ Runx with some differences in expression levels of their sub family members [27,28]. These observations led us to believe that hUCB derived CD34$^+$ cells might also have potential to differentiate in the osteoblastic lineage. Indeed, we have observed that CD34$^+$ cells in response to osteogenic signals, ascorbic acid and b-glycerophosphate, expressed Runx2, osteocalcin, osteonectin, collagen1A1, alkaline phosphatase, and BMP, Smad and Wnt signaling molecules, which are characteristically expressed by osteoblasts [29]. Runx2 is required for osteogenic differentiation of mesenchymal cells, whereas osteocalcin, osteonectin and collagen type1A1 are integral to bone matrix [9,10,30]. BMPs expressed by osteoblasts, bind and transduce signals via receptors to activate Smad 1/5/8 signaling pathway, to induce gene expression for bone-associated proteins [10]. Wnt signaling associated proteins Dvl2 and Dvl3 are required to transmit signals during osteoblastic differentiation [31,32]. These findings provide evidence that hUCB derived CD34$^+$ cells are multipotent in nature and microenvironmental cues could drive their differentiation towards osteoblastic lineages.

Characteristic hallmark of osteoporosis is the loss of bone. We have observed that, following dexamethasone treatment mice exhibit significant decreases in trabecular and cortical BMDs compared to controls. Trabecular bone micro architectural parameters such as anisotropy and structure model index also provide strong evidences that dexamethasone was able to induce osteoporosis. This bone loss and changes in bone micro-architecture were almost restored within 28 days following application of a single bolus of hUCB derived CD34$^+$ cells. In osteoporosis, the balance of osteoblast and osteoclast cells is severely compromised. The number of osteoclasts is increased and they obliterate bone micro-architecture, which ultimately results in loss of bone mass [33,34]. This is further accompanied by the bone marrow stromal cells differentiation towards adipogenesis and inhibition of osteoblastogenesis [35]. In the current study, we found the loss of trabecular bone spicules and loss of cortical bones in the osteoporotic mice and concurrent increment of adipocytes. However, application of nanofiber-expanded CD34$^+$ cells induced significant reversion of osteoporosis, by increment of bone formation presumably by osteoblasts and concomitant decrease in number of adipocytes and osteoclasts. In fact, circulating CD34$^+$ cells have been shown to be recruited to the skeletal defect sites and heal non-union fractures in murine models [36,37]. The chemokine receptor, CXCR4 binds to stromal derived factor (SDF)-1 expressed highly in bone marrow stromal cells, and is required for efficient homing of cells to the bone marrow [38]. Since, nanofiber-expanded CD34$^+$ cells constitutively express high levels of CXCR4, this may be critical for homing of these cells to bone marrow. In a preclinical model of osteoporosis, adenoviral-mediated overexpression of CXCR4 gene was shown to be necessary for bone marrow derived mesenchymal cells, to home in the bone marrow [39]. However, advantages of using the nanofiber-expanded cells are that we do not need to induce CXCR4 expression using any viral methods, which has potential to integrate to the host genome [40]. Although nanofiber-expanded cells home to the other organs such as lung or spleen besides bone marrow, no bone formation was observed in other organs. Also, recently it was shown that CXCR4 expression on the precursor cells was important for bone formation [41]. Additionally, hUCB derived CD34$^+$ cells have greater advantage in that these cells have not been reported to induce oncogenic transformation in experimental model systems [20].

During osteoporosis, osteoblasts undergo apoptosis, thereby, altering the bone formation and lowering bone mineral density. This is paralleled by lower levels of serum osteoclacin, a marker for bone turnover [42]. Current findings show that CD34$^+$ cell transplantation decreased the numbers of adipocytes in bone marrow, increased trabecular numbers and thickness, and increased BMD, thereby indicating induction of osteoblast in bone. An increase in the osteocalcin levels coupled with an increase in vivo mineral apposition rate in the mice that received CD34$^+$ cell transplantation, confirms the regenerative potential of CD34$^+$ cells in bone formation.

Elevated levels of GM-CSF, and IL-10 and decreased level of MCP-1 in serum were also evident with the CD34$^+$ cell transplantation. Previous in vitro studies have shown that in the presence of CD34$^+$ cells, osteoblasts secrete GM-CSF and cytokines such as IL-6, IL-4 and IL-1 involved in bone homeostasis [15,43,44]. Current findings suggest that CD34$^+$ cells likely modulate cytokine secretions during induction of osteogenesis. In this respect, we have observed high level of IL-10 in serum of the mice that received CD34$^+$ cells. The importance of IL-10 in bone metabolism was demonstrated in IL-10 deficient mice, which develop osteopenia and decreased bone formation [45,46]. IL-10 exhibits anti-osteoclastic activity and may directly inhibit osteoclast precursor cell differentiation [47]. CD34$^+$ cell transplantation thus acts by upregulating the levels of IL-10 that may in turn regulate the bone remodeling by impairing osteoclastogenesis and restoring the bone formation [46,47].

Above findings thus demonstrate a novel therapeutic potential of nanofiber-expanded CD34$^+$ cells in resolving osteoporosis. These cells provide several advantages over other cell types as they are easily accessible, less immunogenic and maintain multi-potency. They can be available in unlimited numbers via expansion on nanofibers; constitutively express CXCR4 for efficient homing to the bone marrow; and differentiate into osteogenic lineage in vitro. These cells are biologically functional as they significantly improve bone mineral density, bone formation and bone micro-architecture in osteoporotic murine model. These characteristics make them an attractive choice of cells for bone induction in patients with severe bone loss due to osteoporosis.

Materials and Methods

Isolation of CD133$^+$ hematopoietic cells

Fresh human umbilical cord blood was obtained from The Ohio State University Medical Center with written consent from donors and prior approval from the internal review board. Briefly, heparinized cord blood was diluted with PBS (1:1) and carefully layered over 10 ml of Ficoll-Paque (GE Health Care-Biosciences, USA). After 30-min centrifugation in a swinging bucket rotor at 1400 rpm, the upper layer was aspirated and the mononuclear cell layer (buffy coat) was collected. Following labeling with magnetic bead conjugated anti-CD133 monoclonal antibody (Miltenyi Biotec Inc, Bergisch Gladbach, Germany), two cell separation cycles (with different columns) were performed using the AutoMACS cell sorter (Miltenyi Biotec) following manufacturer's protocol and reagents. After separation, purity of the cell product was determined by flow cytometry (more than 95% cells were CD133$^+$). Total 4–6 samples of cord blood were procured, isolated and used nanofiber mediated expansion and in vitro and in vivo experiments.

Expansion of CD133$^+$ hematopoietic cells

Electrospinning, surface grafting, and amination of PES nanofibers were carried out according to the procedure described earlier [48]. All chemicals were purchased from Sigma-Aldrich (USA) unless otherwise stated. PES granules were purchased from Goodfellow Cambridge Limited, UK. CD133$^+$ cells were expanded on nanofiber-coated plates using serum free expansion medium (SFEM) as previously described [19]. In brief, purified recombinant human stem cell factor (SCF), Flt-3 ligand (Flt3), thrombopoietin (TPO), and IL-3 were purchased from Peprotech Inc. (Rocky Hill, NJ). The StemSpan SFEM medium was purchased from StemCell Technologies (Vancouver, BC, Canada). Nanofiber meshes were securely glued to the bottoms of wells of a 24-well tissue culture plate. Eight hundred CD133$^+$ cells were seeded onto each scaffold in 0.6 ml StemSpanTM serum-free expansion medium, which consists of 1% BSA, 0.01 mg/ml recombinant human insulin, 0.2 mg/ml human transferrin, 0.1 mM 2-mercaptoethanol, and 2 mM L-glutamine in Iscove's MDM, supplemented with 0.04 mg/ml low-density lipoprotein (Athens Research and Technology Inc., USA), 100 ng/ml SCF, 100 ng/ml Flt3, 50 ng/ml TPO, and 20 ng/ml IL-3. Cells were cultured at 37°C in an atmosphere containing 5% CO$_2$ for 10 days without medium change. Cells were harvested after 10 days of expansion. All wells were washed once with non-enzymatic cell dissociation solution and twice with 2% FBS containing Hanks' buffer at 5 min intervals between each wash. The collected cells were then concentrated through centrifugation at 300× g for 5 min. Aliquots of the cells were then used for cell counting by a hemocytometer, flowcytometric analysis, as well as for further studies.

Flowcytometry

Flowcytometric analysis was performed by using standard two colors staining with a FACS Calibur flowcytometer (Becton Dickinson, Heidelberg, Germany) as described earlier [19]. Non-specific Fc-receptors were blocked with FcR-blocking reagent (Miltenyi Biotec Inc.) prior to adding primary antibodies. Primary antibody was incubated for 30 min at 4°C with the aliquots of expanded cells. Antibodies used were anti-CD34-PE, anti-CD133/2-FITC (all from Miltenyi Biotec Inc), PE labeled CXCR4, von Willebrand Factor, CD31, CD45, MHC class I, MHC class II, CD69, CD3, Mac-I, LFA-1, CD86, CD14 and isotype controls were purchased from BD Biosciences (USA) After incubation cells were washed with MACS buffer and resuspended in MACS buffer. Dead cells were excluded via propidium iodide staining. Data analysis was performed with BD Cell Quest software. The Milan-Mulhouse gating method was used for cell enumeration, where a double gating (CD133$^+$ and CD34$^+$) strategy was used to identify the primitive hematopoietic progenitor cell populations. At least 20,000 events were acquired.

Osteoblastic differentiation of nanofiber-expanded CD34$^+$ cells

After 10 days of CD133$^+$ cell expansion on nanofiber, cells were collected and reseeded in DMEM supplemented with 10% fetal bovine serum (FBS), penicillin, streptomycin, and glutamate (PSG) for three days in a 24-well plate or 4-chamber slides (Lab-Tek II Chamber slide System, Nalge Nunc International Corp., Naperville, IL, USA). The cultured cells were induced by specific osteoblast differentiating factors (60 μM ascorbic acid and 10 mM β-glycerophosphate) dissolved in fresh DMEM complete medium. The differentiation process was continued for 3 weeks with a change of fresh medium containing specific osteoblast inducing factors in every 3rd day. During the process of differentiation, some of the wells of differentiated cells were harvested at specific time points for further studies (n = 4).

Alizarin red S staining

To examine in vitro mineralization in osteoblastic differentiated cells, Alizarin Red S staining was performed in wells of a 24-well plate. Briefly, after 21 days of differentiation cells were fixed in

70% ethanol for one hour at room temperature followed by a wash with water (10 minutes, 2 times) and incubated with 1% Alizarin Red S solution for 30 minutes at room temperature (Chemicon International, USA). The red stain was washed with water three times and cells were mounted with mounting solution. Images were obtained by using a digital camera attached to the microscope (Axioplan2; Carl Zeiss) using Axio-vision software (Carl Zeiss, NY, USA). Nanofiber-expanded CD34$^+$ cells cultured in DMEM complete medium were used as a control.

Immunocytochemical staining

One quarter of a million nanofiber-expanded CD34$^+$ cells were induced to differentiate in each well of 4-chamber slides for three weeks. After three weeks of culture immunocytochemistry was performed following standard protocol to assess osteoblastic differentiation using osteoblast specific markers such as Smad 1/5/8, osteocalcin and IgG as an isotype control. Nuclear stain was performed with DAPI. Slides were observed under a fluorescence microscope (Axioplan2; Carl Zeiss) and images were captured with Zeiss Axiovision imaging software (Carl Zeiss, NY, USA).

RT-PCR and western blot analyses

Nanofiber-expanded CD34$^+$ cells were induced to osteoblastic differentiation in vitro. During the course of osteoblastic differentiation, total RNA and proteins were isolated at various time points using RNeasy Kit (Qiagen, USA) and RIPA, cell lysis buffer respectively. One microgram of RNA was used for cDNA synthesis using oligo dT (Invitrogen, USA) primer. Semi quantitative PCR was performed using one micro liter of cDNA for the gene specific primers such as Runx2, alkaline phosphatase, osteocalcin, osteonectin, collagen 1A1 and GAPDH. Fold increase for expression of each gene at mRNA level was analyzed using UN-SCAN-IT software (Silk Scientific, Inc.). Nanofiber-expanded cells were used as a control. Primers for RT-PCR reactions were designed using Primer Blast-NCBI software: Human Runx2 forward primer: 5' TAAGTACACGGGCTTCAGGG 3'; Human Runx2 reverse primer: 5' TTGTTGTCTTCTTGCCTCCA 3'; Human Alk Phos forward primer: 5' GGACATGCAGTAC-GAGCTGA 3'; Human Alk Phos reverse primer: 5' CAC-CAAATGTGAAGACGTGG 3'; Human osteocalcin forward primer:5' AAGCAAGTAGCGCCAATCT 3'; Human osteocalcin reverse primer: 5' GGAAGTAGGGTGCCATAACAC 3'; Human osteonectin forward primer:5' ACATCGGGCCTTG-CAAATACA 3'; Human osteonectin reverse primer: 5' GAAG-CAGCCGGCCCACTCATC 3'; Human collagen1A1 forward primer:5' CCTGGCCCCATTGGTAATGTT 3'; Human collagen1A1 reverse primer: 5' CCCCCTCACGTCCAGATTCAC 3'; Human GAPDH forward primer: 5' CTGATGCCCC-CATGTTCGTC 3'; Human GAPDH reverse primer: 5' CACCCTGTTGCTGTAGCCAAATTCG 3'.

Similarly, Western blot was performed for the level of BMP2, BMP4, Smad-1/5/8 (all from Santa Cruz Biotechnology, Inc., CA), Dvl2, Dvl3, and GAPDH (all from Cell Signaling Technology, Inc. MA) protein. Nanofiber-expanded cells were used as a control. Induced differentiated MC3T3 cells were also used as a positive control. Fold increase for expression of each gene at protein level was analyzed using UN-SCAN-IT software (Silk Scientific, Inc.).

Generation of osteoporosis

Seven month-old female NOD/SCID mice, retired breeder (body weight approximately 25 g) were obtained from Jackson Laboratory, Bar Harbor, ME and used for osteoporosis induction. The mice were housed in sterile IACUC-approved facilities at the

Biomedical Research Tower at The Ohio State University. After a week of acclimatization, mice were intraperitoneally (i.p.) injected with 5 mg/ kg body weight (b. wt.) of dexamethasone (American Regent, Inc. Shirley, NY) or with saline (as a control) for consecutive 21 days as described before [35]. Tapering doses of dexamethasone were given for 5 days for withdrawal. The mice were weighed every week during the injection to record any significant weight loss.

CD34+ cell transplantation

The mice, that received glucocorticoid injections were either sacrificed after 26 (21+5) days as an osteoporotic control or were used for CD34+ cell / medium injections (6 mice/group). The osteoporotic mice were anesthetized and injected with nanofiber-expanded CD34+ cells (0.5 million in 300 µl of serum free medium) via intra-cardio-ventricular injection or 300 µl of serum free medium (Op+Med) as a control for CD34+ cell therapy group. The osteoporotic mice of CD34+ cell therapy (Op+Cells) group received only one dose of CD34+ cells and were sacrificed after 28 days of injection. Osteoporotic mice receiving medium (Op+Med) were also sacrificed at the same time point.

CD34+ cell homing

To assess the homing of CD34+ cells, GFP overexpressed nanofiber-expanded CD34+ cells (0.5 million cells/mouse) were injected into the mice via intra-cardio-ventricular injection after induction of osteoporosis. Forty-eight hours and two weeks after cell injection, mice were sacrificed and various organs were harvested. Tissues were fixed in 10% formalin solution and subsequently embedded in paraffin block. Five-micron sections were cut and stained using anti-GFP primary antibody (Zymed Laboratories, Inc, CA, USA) and detected with 3,3'-Diamino-benzidine (DAB) and mounted. Slides were observed under a microscope (Axioplan2; Carl Zeiss) and images were captured with Zeiss, Axiovision imaging software (Carl Zeiss).

Mineral apposition rate (MAR)

A separate set of seven months old NOD/ SCID mice (3 mice / group) were subjected to generation of osteoporosis (21+5 days) and followed by CD34+ cell transplantation or medium (as a control) for 28 days as described above. Mice were intraperitone-ally (i.p.) injected with calcium binding dye, calcein (green flourescent dye; 10 mg/kg b.wt., Sigma); 10 days prior to sacrifice. Alizarin Red Dye (red fluorescent dye; 50 mg/kg b.wt., Sigma) was also injected to the same mice via i.p. route three days prior to sacrifice. Upon sacrifice, femurs were harvested and formalin fixed for 24 hours and then washed with 1x PBS, dehydrated with 70% ethanol, 95% ethanol, 100% ethanol, infiltrated and embedded in methylmethacrylate and polyester resin. Thirty-micrometer thick sections were cut with a diamond blade using Saw Microtome Leica SP1600 (Leica Microsystem, Wetzlar, Germany). The sections were mounted on the slides using Vecta Mount (Vector Labs, Inc. Burlingame, CA) and observed under a fluorescence microscope (Carl Zeiss, NY, USA) and images were captured with Zeiss Axiovision imaging software (Axioplan2). Images were analyzed to assess the mineral apposition rate (MAR) by using NIH Image J software. The mineral apposition rate (MAR, in µm per day) was determined by dividing the mean width of the double labels by the inter-label time as described previously [49].

Hematoxylin and eosin staining

All mice were euthanized after collecting blood and urine, and femurs were removed by surgical dissection and were preserved in 10% neutral buffered formalin. After decalcification, paraffin-blocked tissues were sectioned and stained with standard hematoxylin and eosin (H&E) staining protocol at the same depth from the growth plate.

Micro computed tomography (MicroCT)

Formalin fixed femur bones were encased in a tight fitted plastic tube to prevent any motion during scanning. Femurs were scanned using a high-resolution Micro CT scanner (SkyScan1172-D, Kontich, Belgium) at 16µm resolution. For measurements of bone mineral density (BMD; g/cm^3), phantoms of 25 and 75 g/cm^3 were scanned with the same settings as applied to the mice femur bones from all groups. The scanned images were reconstructed using Skyscan Nrecon software and analyzed with the CTan software (Kontich, Belgium). Analyses of trabecular bone were carried out in distal femur, 0.1 mm away from the growth plate. A threshold was established and the same threshold value was kept constant for all samples. Similarly, the metaphysial region, 2mm away from the growth plate, was selected for the cortical bone analysis. A separate threshold was established and kept constant for all cortical bone measurements. The analyses were performed for the bone volume, bone to tissue volume ratios, trabecular number (Tb.N; 1/mm), trabecular thickness (Tb.Th; mm), trabecular bone mineral density (BMD; g/cm^3), degree of anisotropy (DA), structure model index (SMI), cortical porosities (%), ratio of bone volume/ tissue volume (BV/TV) and cortical bone mineral density (BMD; g/cm^3) in animals from all groups using the Skyscan software and following manufacturer's protocol. The results were reported in mean ± SEM (n = 6/ per group). Three-dimensional (3D) models were reconstructed using CTvol software from SkyScan.

Serum osteocalcin assay

Sandwich ELISA was performed for the collected mouse serum using the osteocalcin ELISA kit (Biomedical Technologies, Inc, Staughton, MA). Briefly, the mouse was anesthetized and blood was collected from the descending aorta in an eppendorf tube and kept at room temperature for an hour to coagulate, then centrifuged at 14000 rpm for 20 minutes at 4°C. Serum was collected and stored at −80°C until further use. Standard curve was made and the serum samples were run in triplicates to assess the amount of osteocalcin in the serum. The samples from each group were diluted (5x) and incubated with the anti-serum osteocalcin overnight and detected using streptavidin-horseradish peroxidase (HRP) detecting system. The values were reported in mean ± SEM (n = 4/ per group, in triplicate).

Multiplex ELISA for cytokines and growth factors

To assess the levels of various cytokines and growth factors (twenty factors from 250 µl of serum) from collected serum (from all groups of animals before sacrifice and stored at −80°C), the multiplex ELISA was performed in triplicate by Quansys Biosciences, Logan Utah (n = 4/ per group). The values were reported in mean ± SEM.

Osteoclast differentiation

To assess the therapeutic effects of CD34+ cells on the bone resorbing cells; bone marrow cells were collected from femurs of animals of all the groups, after termination of experiments and were induced for osteoclastic differentiation in vitro. Cells were cultured overnight at 37°C incubator with 5% CO_2 in αMEM containing 10% heat inactivated fetal bovine serum in the presence of 20 ng/ml M-CSF (R & D Systems, Minneapolis,

MN). The next day, same number of non-adherent cells (1.5 million for all the groups) were collected and incubated for an additional 5–8 days in αMEM medium with 20 ng/ml M-CSF, and 50 ng/ml GST-RANKL [50]. The fresh medium was replaced every third day. At day 3 and 6 of differentiation, the cells were stained for TRAP staining using an acid phosphatase, leukocyte; TRAP staining kit (Sigma Aldrich, USA) and was viewed and imaged with a fluorescence microscope (Carl Zeiss, NY, USA). TRAP-positive cells (purple) containing at least three nuclei were counted as osteoclasts.

Osteoclast cytoskeleton structure and functionality

Osteoclasts were generated on plastic dishes as described above and on 3rd day of differentiation, osteoclasts cells were removed and equal number of osteoclasts cells were re-plated either on thinly cut ivory slices or glass cover slips. Cells were fixed at various time points of culture with 1% formaldehyde in pH 6.5 (30 minutes at room temp), stabilization buffer (127 mM NaCl, 5 mM KCl, 1.1 mM NaH$_2$PO$_4$, 0.4 mM KH$_2$PO$_4$, 2 mM MgCl$_2$, 5.5 mM glucose, 1 mM EGTA, 20 mM Pipes), and subsequently fixed and permeabilized with 2% formaldehyde, 0.2% Triton X-100, and 0.5% deoxycholate in the same stabilization buffer. Cells were stained with F-actin specific Ab and visualized using a Zeiss 510 META laser scanning confocal microscope (Campus Microscopy and Imaging Facility, The Ohio State University). Actin ring and podosome thicknesses were determined by generating Z-stack images of randomly selected cells and these structures were measured at their thickest points [50]. Bone resorption was assessed using ivory slices and

osteoclasts were gently removed with cotton swabs and washed with water. The ivory slices were then stained with hematoxylin stain for 5 minutes at room temperature and excess stain was removed by washing with water and pits were imaged with a confocal microscope mentioned above.

Statistical analysis

Values were expressed as mean ± SEM and statistical analysis was performed by using JMP software (version 9, SAS Institute Inc. NC). After checking equal variance two sample 't'-test was performed for assessment of significance. Posthoc analysis was performed by using Bonferroni correction and significance was determined when p values were obtained less than 0.025.

Acknowledgments

Authors are thankful to Drs. Jack F. Bukowski (Brigham and Women's Hospital, Harvard Medical School), Peter J. Mohler and Martin Lubow (The Ohio State University Medical Center) for their critical reading and suggestions for the manuscript. Authors would like to thank Dr. Haikady N. Nagaraja (COPH, Division of Biostatistics) for his help in statistical analyses.

Author Contributions

Conceived and designed the experiments: RA HD. Performed the experiments: RA JL SK MJ MD GN BM. Analyzed the data: RA JL SK MJ MD GN BM SA RH ZS BL TR RJ HD. Contributed reagents/materials/analysis tools: HM VP. Wrote the paper: RA HD.

References

1. Cooper C CG, Melton IJ 3rd (1992) Hip fractures in the elderly: a world-wide projection. Osteoporos International 2: 285–289.
2. Aguila HL, Rowe DW (2005) Skeletal development, bone remodeling, and hematopoiesis. Immunol Rev 208: 7–18.
3. Zaidi M (2007) Skeletal remodeling in health and disease. Nat Med 13: 791–801.
4. Weinstein RS, Jilka RL, Parfitt AM, Manolagas SC (1998) Inhibition of osteoblastogenesis and promotion of apoptosis of osteoblasts and osteocytes by glucocorticoids. Potential mechanisms of their deleterious effects on bone. J Clin Invest 102: 274–282.
5. Seeman E, Delmas PD (2006) Bone quality–the material and structural basis of bone strength and fragility. N Engl J Med 354: 2250–2261.
6. Lecka-Czernik B, Gubrij I, Moerman EJ, Kajkenova O, Lipschitz DA, et al. (1999) Inhibition of Osf2/Cbfa1 expression and terminal osteoblast differenti-ation by PPARgamma2. J Cell Biochem 74: 357–371.
7. Takada Y, Kouzmenko AP, Kato S (2009) Wnt and PPARgamma signaling in osteoblastogenesis and adipogenesis. Nat Rev Rheumatol 5: 442–447.
8. Pittenger MF, Mackay AM, Beck SC, Jaiswal RK, Douglas R, et al. (1999) Multilineage potential of adult human mesenchymal stem cells. Science 284: 143–147.
9. Ducy P, Karsenty G (1995) Two distinct osteoblast-specific cis-acting elements control expression of a mouse osteocalcin gene. Mol Cell Biol 15: 1858–1869.
10. Ducy P, Zhang R, Geoffroy V, Ridall AL, Karsenty G (1997) Osf2/Cbfa1: a transcriptional activator of osteoblast differentiation. Cell 89: 747–754.
11. Phimphilai M, Zhao Z, Boules H, Roca H, Franceschi RT (2006) BMP signaling is required for RUNX2-dependent induction of the osteoblast phenotype. J Bone Miner Res 21: 637–646.
12. Rawadi G, Vayssiere B, Dunn F, Baron R, Roman-Roman S (2003) BMP-2 controls alkaline phosphatase expression and osteoblast mineralization by a Wnt autocrine loop. J Bone Miner Res 18: 1842–1853.
13. Kobayashi H, Gao Y, Ueta C, Yamaguchi A, Komori T (2000) Multilineage differentiation of Cbfa1-deficient calvarial cells in vitro. Biochem Biophys Res Commun 273: 630–636.
14. Kim MS, Day CJ, Morrison NA (2005) MCP-1 is induced by receptor activator of nuclear factor-{kappa}B ligand, promotes human osteoclast fusion, and rescues granulocyte macrophage colony-stimulating factor suppression of osteoclast formation. J Biol Chem 280: 16163–16169.
15. Marie PJ, Hott M, Launay JM, Graulet AM, Gueris J (1993) In vitro production of cytokines by bone surface-derived osteoblastic cells in normal and osteoporotic postmenopausal women: relationship with cell proliferation. J Clin Endocrinol Metab 77: 824–830.
16. Vahle JL, Sato M, Long GG, Young JK, Francis PC, et al. (2002) Skeletal changes in rats given daily subcutaneous injections of recombinant human parathyroid hormone (1–34) for 2 years and relevance to human safety. Toxicol Pathol 30: 312–321.
17. Wilting I, de Vries F, Thio BM, Cooper C, Heerdink ER, et al. (2007) Lithium use and the risk of fractures. Bone 40: 1252–1258.
18. Khosla S, Westendorf JJ, Oursler MJ (2008) Building bone to reverse osteoporosis and repair fractures. J Clin Invest 118: 421–428.
19. Das H, Abdulhameed N, Joseph M, Sakthivel R, Mao HQ, et al. (2009) Ex vivo nanofiber expansion and genetic modification of human cord blood-derived progenitor/stem cells enhances vasculogenesis. Cell Transplant 18: 305–318.
20. Das H, George JC, Joseph M, Das M, Abdulhameed N, et al. (2009) Stem cell therapy with overexpressed VEGF and PDGF genes improves cardiac function in a rat infarct model. PLoS One 4: e7325.
21. Mifune Y, Matsumoto T, Kawamoto A, Kuroda R, Shoji T, et al. (2008) Local delivery of granulocyte colony stimulating factor-mobilized CD34-positive progenitor cells using bioscaffold for modality of unhealing bone fracture. Stem Cells 26: 1395–1405.
22. Chappard C, Brunet-Imbault B, Lemineur G, Giraudeau B, Basillais A, et al. (2005) Anisotropy changes in post-menopausal osteoporosis: characterization by a new index applied to trabecular bone radiographic images. Osteoporos Int 16: 1193–1202.
23. Ciarelli TE, Fyhrie DP, Schaffler MB, Goldstein SA (2000) Variations in three-dimensional cancellous bone architecture of the proximal femur in female hip fractures and in controls. J Bone Miner Res 15: 32–40.
24. Borah B, Dufresne TE, Cockman MD, Gross GJ, Sod EW, et al. (2000) Evaluation of changes in trabecular bone architecture and mechanical properties of minipig vertebrae by three-dimensional magnetic resonance microimaging and finite element modeling. J Bone Miner Res 15: 1786–1797.
25. Hildebrand T, Ruegsegger P (1997) Quantification of Bone Microarchitecture with the Structure Model Index. Comput Methods Biomech Biomed Engin 1: 15–23.
26. Taichman RS, Emerson SG (1996) Human osteosarcoma cell lines MG-63 and SaOS-2 produce G-CSF and GM-CSF: identification and partial characteriza-tion of cell-associated isoforms. Exp Hematol 24: 509–517.
27. Banerjee C, McCabe LR, Choi JY, Hiebert SW, Stein JL, et al. (1997) Runt homology domain proteins in osteoblast differentiation: AML3/CBFA1 is a major component of a bone-specific complex. J Cell Biochem 66: 1–8.
28. Zeng C, van Wijnen AJ, Stein JL, Meyers S, Sun W, et al. (1997) Identification of a nuclear matrix targeting signal in the leukemia and bone-related AML/CBF-alpha transcription factors. Proc Natl Acad Sci U S A 94: 6746–6751.
29. Beck GR, Jr., Zerler B, Moran E (2000) Phosphate is a specific signal for induction of osteopontin gene expression. Proc Natl Acad Sci U S A 97: 8352–8357.

30. Xiao G, Cui Y, Ducy P, Karsenty G, Franceschi RT (1997) Ascorbic acid-dependent activation of the osteocalcin promoter in MC3T3-E1 preosteoblasts: requirement for collagen matrix synthesis and the presence of an intact OSE2 sequence. Mol Endocrinol 11: 1103–1113.

31. Qiang YW, Hu B, Chen Y, Zhong Y, Shi B, et al. (2009) Bortezomib induces osteoblast differentiation via Wnt-independent activation of beta-catenin/TCF signaling. Blood 113: 4319–4330.

32. Day TF, Guo X, Garrett-Beal L, Yang Y (2005) Wnt/beta-catenin signaling in mesenchymal progenitors controls osteoblast and chondrocyte differentiation during vertebrate skeletogenesis. Dev Cell 8: 739–750.

33. Akune T, Ohba S, Kamekura S, Yamaguchi M, Chung UI, et al. (2004) PPARgamma insufficiency enhances osteogenesis through osteoblast formation from bone marrow progenitors. J Clin Invest 113: 846–855.

34. Hong JH, Hwang ES, McManus MT, Amsterdam A, Tian Y, et al. (2005) TAZ, a transcriptional modulator of mesenchymal stem cell differentiation. Science 309: 1074–1078.

35. McLaughlin F, Mackintosh J, Hayes BP, McLaren A, Uings IJ, et al. (2002) Glucocorticoid-induced osteopenia in the mouse as assessed by histomorphometry, microcomputed tomography, and biochemical markers. Bone 30: 924–930.

36. Matsumoto T, Kawamoto A, Kuroda R, Ishikawa M, Mifune Y, et al. (2006) Therapeutic potential of vasculogenesis and osteogenesis promoted by peripheral blood CD34-positive cells for functional bone healing. Am J Pathol 169: 1440–1457.

37. Matsumoto T, Mifune Y, Kawamoto A, Kuroda R, Shoji T, et al. (2008) Fracture induced mobilization and incorporation of bone marrow-derived endothelial progenitor cells for bone healing. J Cell Physiol 215: 234–242.

38. Yu X, Huang Y, Collin-Osdoby P, Osdoby P (2003) Stromal cell-derived factor-1 (SDF-1) recruits osteoclast precursors by inducing chemotaxis, matrix metalloproteinase-9 (MMP-9) activity, and collagen transmigration. J Bone Miner Res 18: 1404–1418.

39. Lien CY, Chih-Yuan Ho K, Lee OK, Blunn GW, Su Y (2009) Restoration of bone mass and strength in glucocorticoid-treated mice by systemic transplantation of CXCR4 and cbfa-1 co-expressing mesenchymal stem cells. J Bone Miner Res 24: 837–848.

40. Nakai H, Montini E, Fuess S, Storm TA, Grompe M, et al. (2003) AAV serotype 2 vectors preferentially integrate into active genes in mice. Nat Genet 34: 297–302.

41. Zhu W, Liang G, Huang Z, Doty SB, Boskey AL (2011) Conditional inactivation of the CXCR4 receptor in osteoprecursors reduces postnatal bone formation due to impaired osteoblast development. J Biol Chem 286: 26794–26805.

42. Godschalk MF, Downs RW (1988) Effect of short-term glucocorticoids on serum osteocalcin in healthy young men. J Bone Miner Res 3: 113–115.

43. Taichman RS, Emerson SG (1994) Human osteoblasts support hematopoiesis through the production of granulocyte colony-stimulating factor. J Exp Med 179: 1677–1682.

44. Taichman RS, Reilly MJ, Verma RS, Emerson SG (1997) Augmented production of interleukin-6 by normal human osteoblasts in response to CD34+ hematopoietic bone marrow cells in vitro. Blood 89: 1165–1172.

45. Al-Rasheed A, Scheerens H, Rennick DM, Fletcher HM, Tatakis DN (2003) Accelerated alveolar bone loss in mice lacking interleukin-10. J Dent Res 82: 632–635.

46. Dresner-Pollak R, Gelb N, Rachmilewitz D, Karmeli F, Weinreb M (2004) Interleukin 10-deficient mice develop osteopenia, decreased bone formation, and mechanical fragility of long bones. Gastroenterology 127: 792–801.

47. Evans KE, Fox SW (2007) Interleukin-10 inhibits osteoclastogenesis by reducing NFATc1 expression and preventing its translocation to the nucleus. BMC Cell Biol 8: 4.

48. Chua KN, Chai C, Lee PC, Tang YN, Ramakrishna S, et al. (2006) Surface-aminated electrospun nanofibers enhance adhesion and expansion of human umbilical cord blood hematopoietic stem/progenitor cells. Biomaterials 27: 6043–6051.

49. Sheng MH, Baylink DJ, Beamer WG, Donahue LR, Rosen CJ, et al. (1999) Histomorphometric studies show that bone formation and bone mineral apposition rates are greater in C3H/HeJ (high-density) than C57BL/6J (low-density) mice during growth. Bone 25: 421–429.

50. McMichael BK, Cheney RE, Lee BS (2010) Myosin X regulates sealing zone patterning in osteoclasts through linkage of podosomes and microtubules. J Biol Chem 285: 9506–9515.

6

The Effect of HIV-Hepatitis C Co-Infection on Bone Mineral Density and Fracture

Tyler J. O'Neill[1]*, Laura Rivera[1], Vladi Struchkov[1,3], Ahmad Zaheen[3], Hla-Hla Thein[1,2]

1 Dalla Lana School of Public Health, University of Toronto, Toronto, Ontario, Canada, **2** Ontario Institute for Cancer Research/Cancer Care Ontario, Toronto, Ontario, Canada, **3** Faculty of Medicine, University of Toronto, Toronto, Ontario, Canada

Abstract

Objective: There is a variable body of evidence on adverse bone outcomes in HIV patients co-infected with hepatitis C virus (HCV). We examined the association of HIV/HCV co-infection on osteoporosis or osteopenia (reduced bone mineral density; BMD) and fracture.

Design: Systematic review and random effects meta-analyses.

Methods: A systematic literature search was conducted for articles published in English up to 1 April 2013. All studies reporting either BMD (g/cm^2, or as a T-score) or incident fractures in HIV/HCV co-infected patients compared to either HIV mono-infected or HIV/HCV uninfected/seronegative controls were included. Random effects meta-analyses estimated the pooled odds ratio (OR) and the relative risk (RR) and associated 95% confidence intervals (CI).

Results: Thirteen eligible publications (BMD N = 6; Fracture = 7) of 2,064 identified were included with a total of 427,352 subjects. No publications reported data on HCV mono-infected controls. Meta-analysis of cross-sectional studies confirmed that low bone mineral density was increasingly prevalent among co-infected patients compared to HIV mono-infected controls (pooled OR 1.98, 95% CI 1.18, 3.31) but not those uninfected (pooled OR 1.47, 95% CI 0.78, 2.78). Significant association between co-infection and fracture was found compared to HIV mono-infected from cohort and case-control studies (pooled RR 1.57, 95% CI 1.33, 1.86) and compared to HIV/HCV uninfected from cohort (pooled RR 2.46, 95% CI 1.03, 3.88) and cross-sectional studies (pooled OR 2.30, 95% CI 2.09, 2.23).

Conclusions: The associations of co-infection with prevalent low BMD and risk of fracture are confirmed in this meta-analysis. Although the mechanisms of HIV/HCV co-infection's effect on BMD and fracture are not well understood, there is evidence to suggest that adverse outcomes among HIV/HCV co-infected patients are substantial.

Editor: Wenyu Lin, Harvard Medical School, United States of America

Funding: These authors have no support or funding to report.

Competing Interests: The authors have declared that no competing interests exist.

* Email: t.oneill@mail.utoronto.ca

Introduction

The success of antiretroviral therapy (ART) and other advanced therapeutics in reducing the mortality of human immunodeficiency virus (HIV)-infected patients has changed the clinical course of this disease. HIV infected patients are less likely to experience death as a result of 'AIDS-related' causes, but are susceptible to 'non-AIDS-related' conditions in the course of their treatment [1] including adverse metabolic outcomes of the skeletal system [2,3]. A common comorbid feature is co-infection with hepatitis C virus (HCV). Studies among HIV patients report hepatic-associated effects of chronic HCV infection, including hepatitis, fibrosis, cirrhosis, and carcinoma, are complicated by HIV co-infection [4]. The effect of non-hepatic outcomes, including mechanisms leading to low bone mineral density (BMD) and fractures associated with hepatic osteodystrophy, remains unclear due to limited evidence of the effects of co-infection [5,6,7].

Osteoporosis is a systemic skeletal disorder characterized by low bone mass. Osteopenia (BMD <1 standard deviations of the mean BMD of a sex-matched, young healthy population below normal BMD, i.e. T-score −1 to −2.5) often precedes osteoporosis (i.e. T-score <−2.5), predisposing affected patients to fracture [8,9,10]. Low BMD is prevalent in HIV patients [11]. Although the incidence of fractures among HIV patients is low, they can be debilitating and potentially life-threatening leading to lower quality of life [12,13,14,15,16,17,18,19,20]. Studies have found higher rates of osteoporotic-associated fractures in HIV patients compared to uninfected controls matched for age [21,22]. The use of ART by HIV mono-patients has also been implicated in exacerbating the severity of adverse skeletal outcomes [3,11,21]. However, it is unclear if it is HIV infection per se, ART, or both that lead to bone loss [10].

Multiple cross-sectional studies have reported an association between chronic HCV infections, reduced BMD [23,24,25,26], and increased risk of fracture [27]. HCV co-infection, compared to HIV mono-infected patients, significantly increases the risk of fractures at many sites [7,28,29]. Low BMD is a recognized complication of HIV infection [11], HIV/HCV co-infection [30], or use of ART [3]. Thus, the risk of fracture in co-infected patients may be greater than that of HIV or HCV mono-infected patients. Not only is co-infection globally prevalent [31], with osteoporotic fractures leading to $12–18 billion USD in direct health care costs annually. Loss of productivity from work because of continual pain, increased absenteeism, and psychological factors add significantly to the total cost of low BMD [32].

Conflicting evidence suggests that adverse bone outcomes are common amongst HIV [2] and HCV [29] mono-infected patients. For example, Lo Re et al. [7] did not find any significant difference in risk of hip fracture between HIV/HCV co-infected and HIV mono-infected patients. While in contrast, Lo Re et al. [30] reported a higher rate of hip fracture was found in co-infected patients compared to HCV mono-infected. However, the suspected synergistic effects of co-infection, including increased inflammation and higher risk of vitamin D deficiency [3], on these outcomes have not been reported as a primary outcome. Therefore, the objective of this systematic review and meta-analysis is to estimate the association of HIV/HCV co-infection on adverse skeletal outcomes (low BMD and risk of fracture). Furthermore, this study intends to generate an estimate for the associations of co-infection with both reduced BMD and bone fracture to stimulate investigation in this important area of growing understanding among HIV patients' comorbidities.

Methods

Search Strategy

Using MEDLINE, EMBASE, Cochrane Library (CENTRAL), and Scopus databases available to the University of Toronto, two investigators (VS and LR) performed a systematic search for relevant literature ever published up to 14 April 2013. The search strategy used MeSH terms ("human immunodeficiency virus" OR "human immunodeficiency virus infection" OR "HIV-1") and ("hepatitis co-infection" OR "hepatitis C" OR "HCV") and ("bone disease" OR "bone density" OR "bone mineral density" OR "osteoporosis" OR "osteopenia" OR "fracture" OR "bone fracture"). In addition, grey literature (e.g. government reports, theses) was searched in The NLM Gateway, The American Society for Bone and Mineral Research, and The Annual Conference on Retroviruses and Opportunistic Infections. The references of identified publications were crosschecked through review of references of relevant publications included in the review (Figure 1).

Study Selection

A Publication was considered eligible for inclusion if it: (1) evaluated the association between HIV-1/HCV co-infection and at least one skeletal outcome (BMD or fracture); (2) reported in English; (3) was a full-length, peer-reviewed observational or randomized control trial (RCTs); (4) reported controls that were either HIV or HCV mono-infected, or uninfected/seronegative; (5) had BMD measured by dual energy X-ray absorptiometry (DXA or DEXA); (6) reported the occurrence of osteoporosis or osteopenia as defined by The World Health Organization (WHO) [10]; and/or (7) reported incident pathologic fracture at any location was reported. Pathologic fractures were defined as fractures possibly due to low BMD (at least osteopenia), typically caused by low energy trauma [28]. Studies in non-human populations, individuals <18 years of age, review articles, case reports or studies that lacked relevant controls, studies on HIV-2 or other HIV strains, and those that did not clearly report the outcomes of interest were excluded from the review.

A two-step procedure was used to screen publications by title and abstract followed by full text review by two investigators (LR and AZ) independently. Any discrepancy concerning a publication's relevancy for inclusion was discussed until consensus was reached. If consensus was not reached, two investigators (HHT and TJO) adjudicated publications.

Data Abstraction

Using a standardized abstraction form, data were extracted by two reviewers (LR and TJO) applying inclusion and exclusion criteria. Information extracted from each study included: (1) study factors: publication status, year of publication, study design, duration of follow-up, inclusion and exclusion criteria, sample size; (2) host factors: age, gender, body mass index (BMI), baseline osteoporotic risk factors, fracture risk factors; (3) infection factors (HIV or HCV): HIV severity as measured by CD4 lymphocyte count and HIV RNA viral load, duration of HIV or HCV infection, clinical symptoms; (4) HCV treatment and ART duration and protocol(s); and (5) outcome factors, relating to BMD and/or fracture. The WHO (1994) criteria were used to define osteopenia (T-score −1.0 to −2.5) and osteoporosis (T-score <−2.5) at any anatomical site. Normal BMD was defined as a T-score greater than −1.0. Fracture could have occurred at any anatomical site. Ascertainments of fracture from radiological confirmation, reports of diagnosis from medical or insurance records, or by patient self-report were included.

Publications were included if they were population-based and reported co-infection as an independent variable and BMD (g/cm^2) or incident fracture as outcome measures. Furthermore, included publication were those in which summary estimates, such as odds ratio (OR) or risk ratio (RR) with 95% confidence interval (CI), were reported or if the publication allowed for the estimation of the summary estimates based on reported data.

Statistical analysis

For case-control and cross-sectional designs, if the adjusted OR of osteopenia or osteoporosis were reported, it was extracted along with covariates controlled for in the model. An unadjusted OR was extracted if an adjusted estimate was not reported. Where necessary, risk was estimated from reported odds according to King and Zeng [33]. The measure of association for cohort studies was summarized using the adjusted RR and 95% CI along with covariates.

Unadjusted measures were estimated where appropriate. For BMD, the mean and its standard deviation (SD) of BMD (g/cm^2) at any location for cases and controls were extracted. The T-score was then calculated comparing to a healthy 30-year old Caucasian female [10] and unadjusted odds were estimated. The odds of having a T-score consistent with osteopenia or osteoporosis were pooled to estimate a dichotomous outcome of low BMD. For publications reporting fracture data (e.g. number of fractures in each group), odds or risk and exact 95% CI were estimated using the reported number of individuals with incident fractures compared to controls.

Pooled analyses, comparing co-infected patients with mono- or uninfected controls, were estimated using random effects models to account for both within- and between-study variability [34]. An inverse variance method was used to weight each estimate. If BMD was measured with more than one control group (e.g. study reported both HIV negative and mono-infected controls) and an average was not reported, data were reported as separate studies within a single publication. If a study evaluated BMD at multiple time points, the value from the first measurement (most reflective of baseline) was selected to avoid dependence. Similarly, only

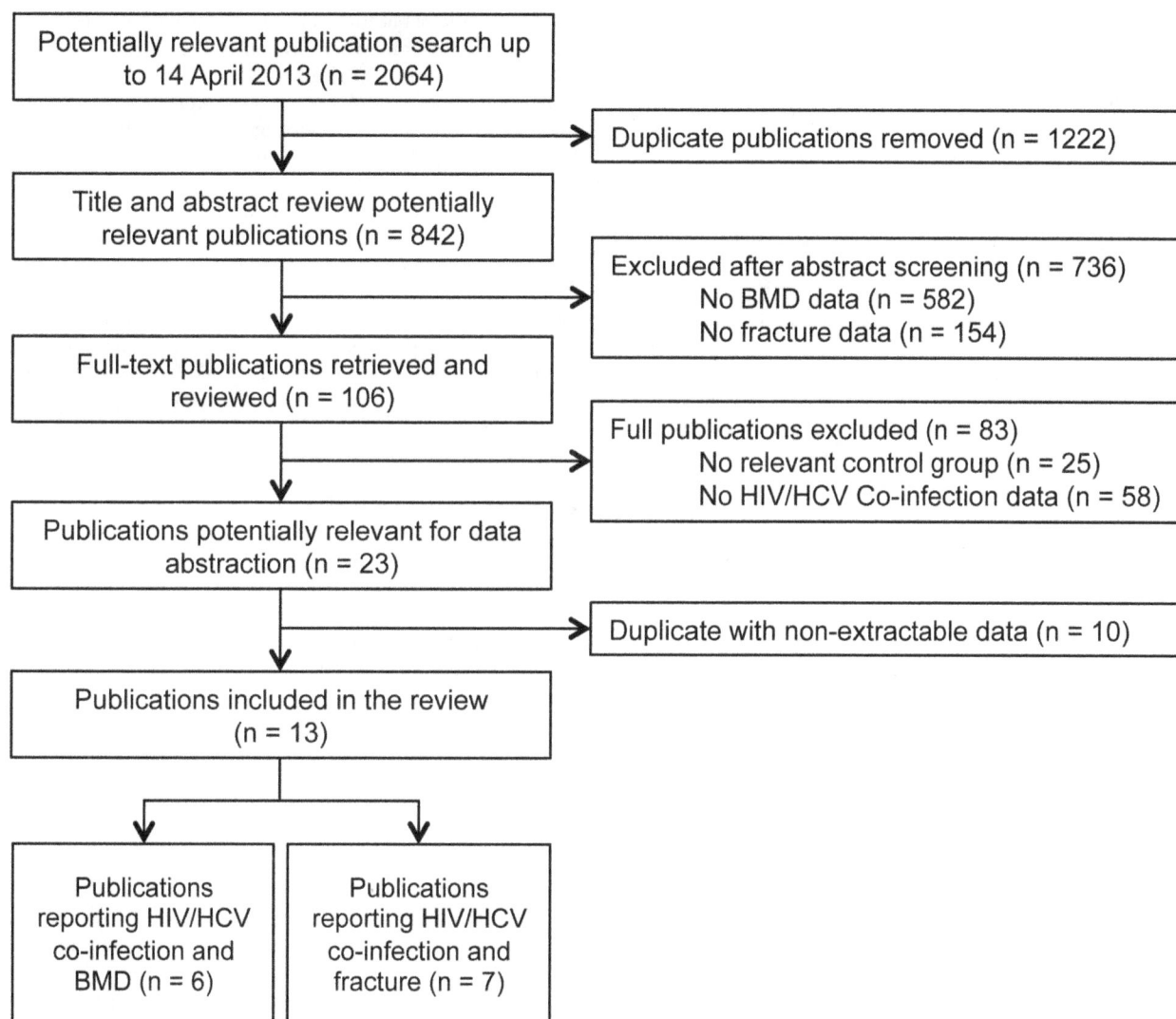

Figure 1. Identification of relevant literature on HIV/HCV co-infection and outcomes of (i) low bone mineral density (BMD) and (ii) fracture. BMD, bone mineral density; HCV, hepatitis C virus; HIV, human immunodeficiency virus.

incident fractures were considered. When sufficient information was provided to stratify data for multiple groups (e.g. gender, age), separate estimates were calculated for each group; again, treating the data as separate studies from a single publication.

The I^2 statistic was estimated as a measure of the total variation in point estimates attributable to between-study heterogeneity [35,36]. The magnitude was interpreted as low ($I^2 \leq 25\%$), medium ($I^2 = 50\%$) and high heterogeneity ($I^2 \geq 75\%$). A χ^2 test was used to assess statistical significance of heterogeneity within each analysis ($\alpha = 0.05$). Sensitivity analyses were employed to determine the causes of heterogeneity by evaluating whether BMD or fracture risk varied significantly based on demographic differences amongst publications. Furthermore, the included publications were selected for step-wise analysis of heterogeneity. Studies were systematically removed and replaced to estimate individual effects on pooled analyses. We evaluated publication bias using Egger regression asymmetry test and Begg's t. The analysis was conducted using Review Manager (RevMan, version 5.2, The Cochrane Collaboration, Copenhagen) and STATA (version 12, StataCorp, College Station, Tx). PRISMA reporting guidelines were adhered to in this publication (Checklist S1).

Results

Selection of Studies

The systematic search identified 2,064 potentially relevant publications (Figure 1). After exclusion of duplicates, and titles and abstracts were screened, 106 independent full-text publications were further evaluated. Studies were subsequently excluded due to lack of relevant control group (n = 25) or no co-infection data reported (n = 58), leaving 23 studies for data abstraction. Ten publications were excluded from abstraction because they did not report BMD or fractures in a co-infected population compared to controls. A total of 13 publications (n = 472,352 subjects) met all inclusion criteria and reported outcome(s) of interest. Manual review of included publication references did not yield any additional articles.

Only one publication required author contact [19] to clarify an adjusted OR point estimate and associated 95% CI due to a clerical error in the original publication. All reported adjusted measures of association were abstracted except one comparison of co- to mono-infected patients from Anastos et al. [19] that required unadjusted estimation of the OR based on reported data.

Demographic and Clinical Characteristics of Included Publications

Published between 2005 and 2012, all included publications reported observational study designs: 7 cohort, 5 cross-sectional, and a single matched case-control (Table 1). Publications were conducted in the United States (n = 7) [7,19,29,38,39,40,41] or Italy (n = 3) [30,37,42], with single publications reporting data from Iran [44], Denmark [28], and Australia [43]. Only effective sample sizes (those used to calculate the measure(s) of interest) were extracted, and ranged from 25 adults from a national multiyear, multicenter cohort [39] to 462,656 individuals in a retrospective cohort analysis of US Medicaid patients [7]. The majority of individuals included were male except for two publications [19,40] with an all-female population. Similar distribution of mean or median ages, BMI, and race was found across publications with no significant differences reported in included publications between cases and controls (Table 1). Lo Re et al. [30] stratified outcomes on gender; Lo Re et al. [7,30] stratified on both age and gender. In the analysis, these were treated as separate studies within each publication.

All studies reported control groups of either HIV mono- [7,19,29,30,39,41,42,43] or uninfected populations [7,19,28,40,44]. Lo Re et al. [7] did not find any significant difference in risk of hip fracture between HIV/HCV co-infected and HIV mono-infected patients. Thus, no data were reported in the publication and were not included in the analysis. In a single publication [30] evaluating rates of incident fracture among co-infected patients and HCV mono-infected controls, a higher rate of hip fracture was found in co-infected patients (HR 1.38, 95% CI 1.25, 1.53). In this study, there were insufficient data for pooled estimates using HCV mono-infection as a comparator.

Details of control selection were reported in all publications selected for pooled analyses. Five studies selected controls from within established cohorts: Lo Re et al. [7,30] used HIV mono- or uninfected controls from the US Medicaid recipients; the ANRS CO8 APROCOC-COPILOTE cohort [39] included HIV mono-infected controls on combination PI-ART; Bedimo et al. [29] used HIV mono-infected patients in the Veterans' Health Administration Clinical Case Registry data; and Anastos et al. [19] and Yin et al. [40] had HIV mono-infected (HAART naïve, non-PI HAART, PI HAART groups) and uninfected female controls, respectively, both from the Women's Interagency HIV Study. ART amongst co-infected patients was also reported in Lo Re et al. [7] compared to antiretroviral treated HIV mono-infected patients. Four publications used population-based controls. The NHANES III cohort in Fausto et al. [42] and Badie et al. [44], described hospital-based controls, matched on age, gender, HBV/HCV infection status, and injecting drug use. The NHAMCS-OPDs cohort in Young et al. [41] obtained controls matched on age and gender. Hansen et al. [28] linked the Danish HIV Cohort study to the Danish Civil Registration System and Danish National Hospital Registry. Hospital-based cohorts were included in three publications with age, gender, and duration of HIV infection individually matched by Yong et al. [43] to mono-infected controls, and HIV mono-infected controls at a single hospital included in Lo Re et al. [7,30].

Individuals on ART at the time of assessment were reported in all publications but one [38] (Table 2). Six publications had an outcome of BMD [19,30,37,38,42,44] whereas 8 reported fracture risk [7,28,29,30,39,40,41,43]. The wrist, hip, and lumbar spine were common locations for assessment of outcomes. All publications used DXA to evaluate BMD. T-scores and Z-scores equivalent to osteopenia or osteoporosis were reported by three [19,42,44] and one [30] publications, respectively. In contrast, less

than half of the publications identified incident fracture events by means of International Classification of Disease (ICD) version 9 (ICD-9) [29,43] or 10 (ICD-10) [28]. Diagnosis of fracture was included in the analysis of residents in multiple US states receiving Medicaid [7,30]. Cohort members from the HIV Outpatient Study (HOPS) [43] treated at non-HOPS sites self-reported incident fracture as did Yin et al. [40] and Young et al. [41], who abstracted incident fractures from patient charts similar to Collin et al. [39]. In the meta-analysis of 4 cross-sectional studies, low BMD was increasingly prevalent among co-infected patients compared to those HIV mono-infected (pooled OR 1.98, 95% CI 1.18, 3.31) despite substantial and significant heterogeneity ($I^2 = 83\%$, $p<0.001$) (Figure 2). In contrast, no significant changes in BMD odds or heterogeneity were found by pooling data from two cross-sectional that compared co-infected to uninfected individuals (pooled OR 1.47, 95% CI 0.78, 2.78) ($I^2 = 0\%$, $p = 0.54$). All publications reported adjusted measures.

In the meta-analysis of 5 cohort and 1 case-control study, significant associations between co-infected patients and fracture was estimated compared to HIV mono-infected patients (pooled RR 1.57, 95% CI 1.33, 1.86) with moderate, non-significant heterogeneity ($I^2 = 52\%$, $p = 0.06$) (Figure 3). An increased association with fracture among co-infected individuals compared to those uninfected with HIV or HCV was found from both cohorts (pooled RR 2.46, 95% CI 1.03, 3.88), despite substantial and significant heterogeneity ($I^2 = 94\%$, $p<0.001$), and cross-sectional studies (pooled OR 2.3, 95% CI 2.09, 2.53) with no heterogeneity identified ($I^2 = 1.0\%$, $p = 0.41$). All publications but one [28] reported adjusted measures. There was no evidence of publication bias as indicated by a non-significant Egger test (all $p > 0.05$) and Begg's test (all $p>0.05$) in all analyses.

Sensitivity analysis

Moderately attenuated heterogeneity and odds of low BMD (co-infected compared to HIV mono-infected) were found using step-wise publication of a single publication [19] (OR 1.58, 95% CI 1.02, 2.45; $I^2 = 44\%$, $p = 0.17$). Risk of fracture and heterogeneity were substantially attenuated using step-wise publication exclusion of Collin et al. [39] (co-infected compared to HIV mono-infected) (RR 1.51, 95% CI 1.22, 1.71; $I^2 = 31\%$, $p = 0.22$). No significant changes were observed when either analyses were repeated with omission of the total female populations reported in Yin et al. [40] or Anastos et al. [19], or by individual removal of publications from all comparisons.

Discussion

In this meta-analysis, low BMD and fracture was increasingly associated with HIV/HCV co-infection compared to HIV mono-infected and HIV/HCV uninfected or seronegative individuals, suggesting that HCV contributes to a burden a disease greater than HIV infection alone. Despite heterogeneity present in the analysis, the visual trends of the forest plots are suggestive of a positive clinical effect in the population. These findings confirm that co-infection is a risk factor for adverse bone health outcomes. This meta-analysis also confirmed the association between HIV mono-infection and low BMD or fracture as reported in previous studies [2,3]. This is the first attempt to synthesize data across publications to estimate the odds of low BMD or risk of fracture amongst HIV/HCV co-infected patients. Despite significant outcomes, the pooled associations of low BMD or risk of fracture among co-infected patients varied across publications, possibly due to differences in demographics of the study populations.

Table 1. Descriptive characteristics of studies meeting inclusion criteria for low BMD and fracture risk amongst HIV/HCV co-infected patients.

Author	Study Design	Country	N, Total	N, Co-infected (HIV+/HCV+)	Control group(s) — N, Monoinfected (HIV+)	Control group(s) — N, Uninfected	Sex (% Male)	Ethnicity (% HIV+)	Age (years)	Body Mass Index (kg/m², SD)
Anastos 2007	Cross-sectional	USA	387	112	152	123	0	Black (61.3) Caucasian (19.7) Hispanic (18.9)	36.7 (HIV−) 42.1 (HIV+ ART−) 40.5 (HIV+ non-PI ART+) 43.8 (HIV+ PI ART+) (median)	29.9, 6.72 (HIV−) 28.9, 6.24 (HIV+ ART−) 26.8, 5.81 (HIV+ non-PI ART+) 28.4, 6.87 (HIV+ PI ART+)
Badie 2011	Cross-sectional	Iran	101	61	40	-	79.2	Middle Eastern (100.0)	39.4, 7.7 (HIV+ ART+) 34.9, 7.3 (HIV+ ART−) 36.6, 10.5 (HIV−) (mean, SD)	22.7, 3.40 (HIV+ ART+) 22.7, 3.30 (HIV+ ART−) 22.8, 3.40 (HIV−)
Bedimo 2012	Cohort	USA	951	485	-	466	98.0	Black (56.0) Caucasian (18.0) Hispanic (23.0) Other (2.0)	46 (median)	Not reported
Collin 2009	Cohort	USA	25	13	-	12	77.2	Not reported	36.2 (median)	22.0 (Not reported) (HIV+)
El-Maouche 2011	Cross-sectional	USA	338	Not reported	Not reported	Not reported	55.0	Black (93.8)	42.5, 8 (mean, SD)	23.9, 2.90 (HIV+)*
Fausto 2006	Cross-sectional	Italy	161	55	-	106	64.0	Caucasian (100.0)	38.6, 4.18 (mean, SD)	22.9, 3.16 (HIV+ ART−) 23.1, 3.47 (HIV+ ART+)
Hansen 2012	Cohort	Denmark	5306	851	Not reported	-	76.0	Caucasian (80.0)	36.7, 30.5–44.5 (mean, 95% CI)	Not reported
Lo Re 2009	Cross-sectional	Italy	1237	625	-	612	62.0	Not reported	43, 10–18 (median, IQR)	23.5, 3.44 (HIV+)*
Lo Re 2012	Cohort	USA	462656	95827	366829		63.0	Black (43.1) Caucasian (27.4) Hispanic (8.3) Other (21.1)	39, 33–46 (mean, IQR)	23.1, 4.10 (HIV+ HCV+)* Not reported
Li Vecchi 2012	Cohort	Italy	188	41	76	71	55.9	Caucasian (100.0)	47, 9.7 (HIV+)	22.9, 3.62 (HIV+)*

Table 1. Cont.

Author	Study Design	Country	N, Total	N, Co-infected (HIV+/HCV+)	Control group(s)		Sex (% Male)	Ethnicity (% HIV+)	Age (years)	Body Mass Index (kg/m², SD)
					N, Monoinfected (HIV+)	N, Uninfected				
									49, 49, 11.3 (HIV−)* (mean, SD)	23.4, 3.81 (HIV−)*
Yin 2010	Cohort	USA	1101	438	663	-	0	Black (56.3) Caucasian (13.3) Hispanic (27.7) Other (3.2)	40.4, 8.8 (HIV+) 36.1, 9.9 (HIV−) (mean, SD)	28.5, 7.50 (HIV+) 30.0, 8.20 (HIV−)
Yong 2011	Case-control	Australia	46	16	-	30	88.5	Black (3.0) Caucasian (92.0) Asian (5.0)	49.8 (Case) 49.5 (Control) (mean)	24.2, 2.91 (Case)* 25.6, 3.47 (Control)*
Young 2011	Cohort	USA	193	51	-	142	79.0	Black (33.0) Caucasian (51.8) Hispanic (11.7) Other (3.5)	40, 34–46 (median, IQR)	26.7, 4.83 (HIV+)

HIV, Human Immunodeficiency Virus; HCV, Hepatitis C Virus; ART, antiretroviral therapy; CI, confidence interval; IQR, interquartile range; PI, protease inhibitor; SD, standard deviation.
*Mean (SD) estimated from descriptive categorical data reported in publication.

Table 2. Clinical characteristics and reported outcomes of publications included in the HIV/HCV co-infection review.

Author	ART exposure (%)	Reported outcome(s) (classification method)	Location	Co-variates adjusted
Anastos 2007	46.5	BMD (DXA)	Lumbar spine	White, Race, Nadir BMI, HIV+ ART naïve, HIV+ non-PI ART, HIV+ PI ART, post-menopausal
			Femoral neck	
Badie 2011	30.0	BMD (DXA)	Hip	Age, Gender, BMI, Smoking, Alcohol, Exercise, HBV infection, IV drug use, Prison
			Lumbar spine	
Bedimo 2012	69.4	Incident osteoporotic fracture (ICD-9 codes)	Wrist	ART+, CKD, Race, Age, Tobacco use, Diabetes, BMI
			Vertebra	
			Hip	
Collin 2009	100.0	Incident non-stress fracture (patient charts)	Any location	Age, HIV+, HIV-RNA, BMI, Location of birth, PI used first, Alcohol, CD4+ count,
El-Maouche 2011	Not reported	BMD (DXA)	Hip	Gender, Age, BMI, Race, Smoking, Alcohol, IV drug use, Hypogonadal/menopausal, HIV+, Methadone use, ART+, Hormone exposure, Vitamin D
			Femoral neck	
			Lumbar spine	
Fausto 2006	70.2	BMD (DXA)	Hip	Gender, Age, CDC Stage, IV drug use, Lypodistrophy, BMI, CD4+ count, HIV–RNA, HAART+, Length of HIV infection, Bone resorption, Bone formation, Vitamin D
			Lumbar spine	
Hansen 2012	78.0	Incident low energy fracture (ICD-10 codes)	Any location	
Lo Re 2009	79.0	BMD (DXA)	Lumbar spine	Age, Gender, BMI, Length of HIV infection, CD4+ count, ART+, Smoking, Alcohol, Exercise, Amenorrhea, eGFR
			Femoral neck	
Lo Re 2012	100	Incident low energy fracture (Medicaid claim codes)	Hip	Age, Gender, State (location), Propensity score
		BMD (DXA)		
Li Vecchi 2012	93.0	BMD (DXA)	Lumbar spine	Age, Yogurt intake, CD4+, Drug addiction
			Femoral neck	
Yin 2010	65.6	Incident low energy fracture (self-reported)	Hip	HIV+, Age, Race, BMI, Post-menopausal, Fracture before index, Serum creatinine
			Wrist	
			Spine	
Yong 2011	83.6	Incident non-stress fracture (ICD-9 codes)	Any location	HBV status, Previous opportunistic infection, CD4+ count, BMI, HIV-RNA, Duration of viral suppression, Type of DXA performed
Young 2011	72.7	Incident low energy fracture (patient charts; self-reported)	Wrist	Gender, Age, CD4+ count,
			Vertebra	
			Femoral neck	

ART, antiretroviral therapy; BMI, body mass index; CKD, chronic kidney disease; DXA, Dual energy x-ray absorbiometry; eGFR, estimated glomerular filtration rate; HAART, highly active antiretroviral therapy; HBV, hepatitis B virus; ICD, International Classification of Diseases; PI, protease inhibitor.

The inclusion of a co-infected state without regard for the estimated duration of HCV infection relative to HIV infection (and thus, the stage of dynamic fibrosis progression) limits our understanding of infection and its role on either outcome. Although a single study [7] reported significantly greater fracture risk among HCV patients compared to HIV mono-infected patients, we were unable to compare HCV alone to explore the relative contributions of either infection to fractures or BMD. Recent cross-sectional studies have suggested that HCV infected patients with hepatic decompensation have lower BMD than HCV-infected patients with healthy liver function [23,24,30]. The non-hepatic outcomes of HCV remain unclear, including mechanisms leading to low BMD and fractures associated with hepatic osteodystrophy [5,6,7].

Co-infection may have a compounded negative impact on bone strength due to reduced osteoclastic activity and hepatic osteodystrophy leading to increased fractures. This is consistent with findings in this analysis and Lo Re et al. [30], who reported both high odds of low BMD and risk of fracture compared to mono- and uninfected individuals. Unfortunately, no study in this analysis

[A]

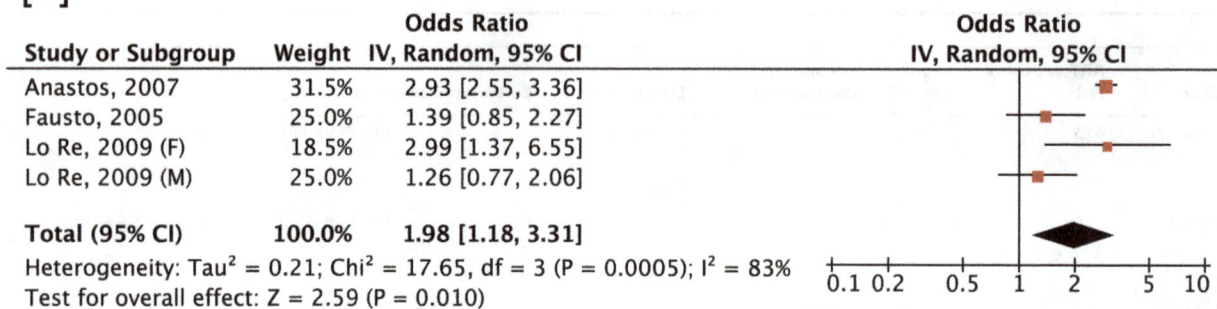

[B]

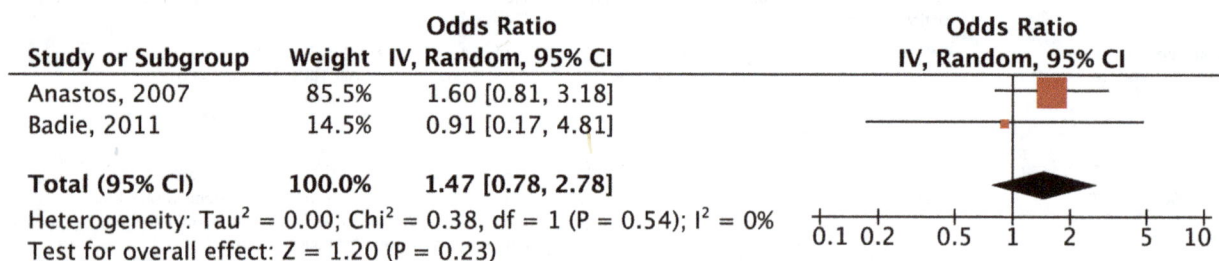

**Figure 2. Odds of low bone mineral density between individuals co-infected with HIV and hepatitis C virus compared to HIV mono-
(A) or uninfected (B) individuals.** HIV, human immunodeficiency virus; HCV, hepatitis C virus.

reported low BMD and risk of fracture as independent outcomes. Therefore, no association between low BMD and fracture risk could be estimated. The theories explaining the causal associations between co-infection and negative skeletal outcomes are reasonable, but require further research into clinical and pathological mechanisms for further clarification.

Risk factors and mechanisms that underlie the increased association between co-infection and low BMD or fracture have not been fully explained. It is likely to be multifactorial, representing complex interactions between infection, traditional osteoporotic risk factors, and ART. It is estimated that up to 9% of all HIV mono-infected patients have low BMD, irrespective of treatment modality [5,54,55] due to chronic inflammation leading to bone resorption [56]. HIV itself may also have direct effects on osteoclastic activity leading to osteoporosis, with the incidence greatly increased among those on ART [56]. Initiation of ART has been associated with 2–6% decrease in BMD over the first two years on therapy [11]. This magnitude in BMD reduction is similar to the first two years of a woman in early menopause. With increased duration of therapy, however, the BMD stabilizes or even improves thereafter. Large subsets of the HIV infected populations (both mono- and co-infected) were on ART of some variation. Insufficient data in the publications on ART duration precluded stratification or adjustment of this potential confounding variable. It is possible that ART patients may have biased the estimates towards a stronger association.

Comparisons between publications are only valid in so far as the groups were demographically similar in other respects. Several studies have reported the prevalence of low BMD in HIV infected patients compared to controls [3,16,50] but few have adjusted for potential confounding variables and heterogeneity of included study groups (e.g. including individuals who acquired HIV through different modes of transmission). No difference of low

BMD was estimated between co-infected patients and HIV/HCV uninfected individuals. This may be attributed to the small number of studies included in this analysis of co-infected individuals where the baseline risk of low BMD may have been greater in controls, which lead to conservative estimates.

No association was found when all female populations [19,40] were excluded. It is unlikely that the low BMD was entirely attributed to accelerated bone loss during the menopausal transition given that the reported mean ages were less than the average menopausal woman [52,53] in the United States, where the studies were conducted. Inflammation, leading to bone resorption, and higher risks of vitamin D deficiency have also been reported among mono- and co-infected patients [3,7,8]. Most publications reported a primarily middle-aged (40–55 years) male, Caucasian population. However, non-black race is a known risk factor for osteoporosis as noted in a recent meta-analysis by Shiau et al [2]. It was found that race modified the relationship between HIV infection and fracture, but co-infection was not reported. Although matching was reported in one case control study [43], some publications reported notable differences between HIV-infected individuals that may affect BMD, such as advancing age, menopausal status (estrogen deficiency), smoking history, and alcohol consumption. It is unclear if these potentially modifiable risk factors or other potentially important variables, such as dietary calcium intake, use of medications inducing bone loss (e.g. glucocorticoids), use of antidepressants (e.g. serotonin re-uptake inhibitors), or level of physical activity influenced the results [11,32]. Few publications adequately reported important potential confounding variables (e.g. gender; age; BMI; substance and alcohol consumption; sedentary lifestyle; digestive, renal, and endocrine disorders including diabetes; nadir CD4+ cell count; viral load) that could have potentially biased the measures

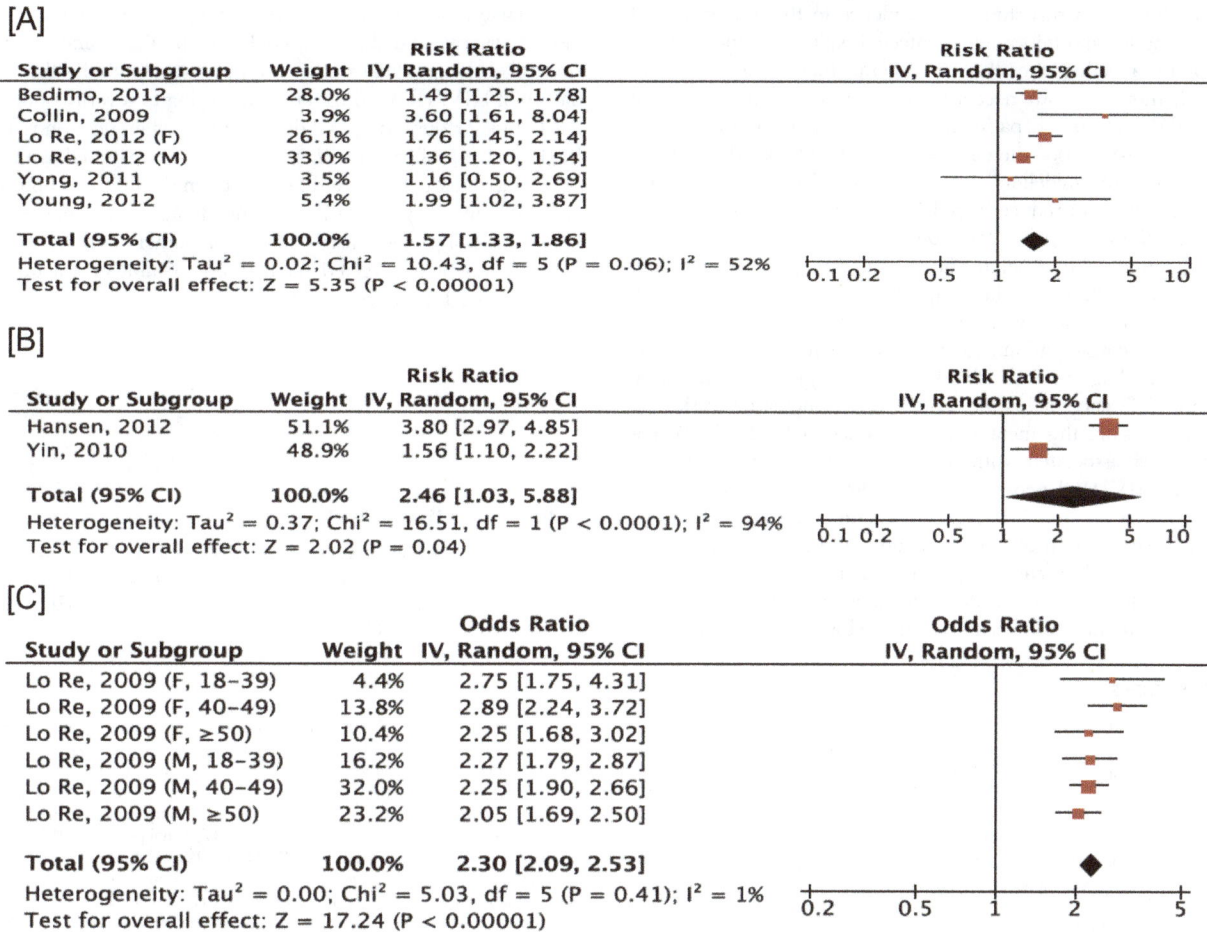

Figure 3. Risk of fracture between individuals co-infected with HIV and hepatitis C virus compared to HIV mono- (A) or uninfected individuals (B), with odds of fracture estimated from cross-sectional studies comparing HIV/HCV co-infected patients to HIV or HCV uninfected individuals (C). HIV, human immunodeficiency virus; HCV, hepatitis C virus.

estimated. Unfortunately, we were unable to adequately adjust in the analysis for this limitation due to inadequate reporting.

Osteopenia is not as sensitive as osteoporosis as a designation of reduced BMD [9]. Developed for post-menopausal women, the T-score has been applied to other adult populations despite controversy around its utility as a metric to quantify bone loss in men and pre-menopausal women [9,48,49]. Thus, age and T-scores are the key predictive factors in determining the BMD testing for screening purposes. The utility of estimating the association of low BMD in co-infected patients relates to the risk of future pathologic fracture. There is a continuous non-linear relationship between BMD and fracture risk [8,46], and measurement of BMD is regarded as the single best predictor of fractures [46,47]. The sensitivity of BMD for fracture prediction is low over most reasonable assumptions, but the specificity is high. Thus, many fractures will occur in individuals with BMD values in the normal range, but fracture risk is quite low. By contrast, fracture risk is very high in individuals with low BMD.

Reporting of fracture diagnosis varied among publications. Studies comparing results of questionnaires and information obtained by medical charts or ICD databases have been inconsistent with both over-reporting and underreporting [51]. The level of misclassification of incident fractures could not be estimated in the included publications and is a limitation of the present study. However, diagnosis of fractures from ICD

databases, insurance claims, and charted data for fractures has been reported to be highly valid [45].

This study had several limitations. First, the potential biases of the original studies, methodological issues, and different strategies for adjusting for confounders could affect the results of this meta-analysis. The cross-sectional association may have been confounded by other unadjusted factors or selection bias. Selection bias may also exist in studies using data from electronic records, claims-based, or primary care databases. Second, the number of cohort studies available was limited and the follow-up durations may not be sufficiently long to be able to detect associations. Third, different publications reported different definitions of incident fracture events that would affect the estimates of prevalence/incidence. However, all reported that pathologic fractures were likely due to low BMD [7,28,29,30,40,41,43] or lead to limited activity post-fracture possibly due to osteoporosis [39]. These differences could have also contributed to the observed high heterogeneity seen within some studies [57,58,59]. Last, publication bias may be of concern because studies that report statistically significant results are more likely to be published than studies reporting non-significant results, and this could have distorted the findings in this meta-analysis. Although the Egger's test and Begg's test indicated limited evidence of publication bias, the estimation may not be accurate enough as the number of studies may be insufficient.

The findings in this study add evidence to the importance of monitoring for and informing co-infected patients on the negative outcomes affecting the skeletal system. Increasing studies of multiple morbidities are necessary, as the incidence of co-infection with HIV and viral hepatitis increases and patients live longer. Outcomes will also directly benefit patient health through improved care guidelines (e.g. recommendations to improve physical activity to reduce bone loss once infected). Although the clinical validity of *a priori* chosen measures of association (relative effects) compared to absolute effects (important for interpretation) should be considered, the majority of publications reported adjusted odds or rates with insufficient data to estimate absolute risks. Thus, consideration should be made when interpreting the data as doubling of risk (i.e. 100% greater risk) may only mean an absolute difference of 1% (i.e. from 1 to 2% increase in risk).

In conclusion, this meta-analysis suggests that HIV/HCV co-infection is associated with significantly increased association between HIV/HCV co-infection and low BMD and fractures compared to an uninfected or HIV mono-infected population. The estimated significant cross-sectional and longitudinal associations in the analysis could suggest that there may be an increased risk for adverse bone health outcomes, including pathologic fractures, among co-infected patients. However, the impact of other factors on the estimated outcomes, such as HIV or HCV disease severity and duration, could not be determined. Further controlled, longitudinal studies are necessary to clarify the causal nature of HIV/HCV co-infection according to severity of disease, ART (type or duration), and demographic differences on reduced BMD and risk of fracture. This is especially warranted as the risk of skeletal disease is expected to increase in the future as both HIV and HCV-infected population continue to age. Better understanding of this will provide insight and improvement in screening and early treatment of targeted populations to mitigate fracture risk among aging HIV-infected patients.

Author Contributions

Conceived and designed the experiments: TJO LR HHT. Performed the experiments: TJO LR VS AZ HHT. Analyzed the data: TJO LR HHT. Contributed reagents/materials/analysis tools: TJO LR AZ HHT. Wrote the paper: TJO LR HHT.

References

1. Sackoff JE, Hanna DB, Pfeiffer MR, Torian LV (2006) Causes of death among persons with AIDS in the era of highly active antiretroviral therapy: New York City. Ann Intern Med 145: 397–406.
2. Shiau S, Broun EC, Arpadi SM, Yin MT (2013) Incident fractures in HIV-infected individuals. AIDS 27(12): 1949–57.
3. Brown TT, Qaqish RB (2006) Antiretroviral therapy and the prevalence of osteopenia and osteoporosis: a meta-analytic review. AIDS 20(17): 2165–74.
4. Seef LB (2002) Natural history of chronic hepatitis. Hepatology 36(S1): S35–46.
5. Tebas P, Powderly W, Yarasheski K (2000) Response to 'accelerate bone mineral loss in HIV-infected patients receiving potent antiretroviral therapy' by Drs Weil and Lenhard. AIDS 14(15): 2417.
6. Negredo E, Martinex E, Cinquegrana D, Estany C, Clotet B (2007) Therapeutic management of bone demineralization in the HIV-infected population. AIDS 21(6): 657–63.
7. Lo Re V, Volk J, Newcomb CW, Yang YX, Freeman CP, et al. (2012) Risk of hip fracture associated with hepatitis C virus infection and hepatitis C/human immunodeficiency virus coinfection. Hepatology 56(6): 1699–98.
8. Cummings SR, Nevitt MC, Haber RJ (1985) Prevention of osteoporosis and osteoporotic fractures. West J Med 143(5): 684–7.
9. Kanis JA (1994) Assessment of fracture risk and its application to screening for postmenopausal osteoporosis: synopsis of a WHO report. WHO Study Group. Osteoporosis Int 4(6): 368–81.
10. WHO (World Health Organization) (2000) Prevention and management of osteoporosis: report of the WHO scientific group. WHO Scientific Group on the Prevention and Management of Osteoporosis. Available: http://www.whqlibdoc.who.int/trs/WHO_TRS_921.pdf: Accessed 8 September 2013.
11. McComsey GA, Tebas P, Shane E, Yin MT, Turner Overton E, et al. (2010) Bone disease in HIV infection: a practical review and recommendations for HIV care providers. Clin Infect Dis 51(8): 937–46.
12. Tebas P (2001) Editorial comment: re-emerging infections – implicating the immune reconstitution syndrome. AIDS Read 11(12): 610.
13. Grinspoon SK, Bilesikian JP (1992) HIV disease and endocrine system. N Engl J Med 327(19): 1360–5.
14. Meyer D, Behrens G, Schmidt RE, Stoll M (1999) Osteonecrosis of the femoral head in patients receiving HIV protease inhibitors. AIDS 13(9): 1147–8.
15. Stephens EA, Das R, Madge S, Barter J, Johnson MA (1999) Symptomatic osteoporosis in two young HIV-positive African women. AIDS 13(18): 2605–6.
16. Moore AL, Vashisht A, Sabin CA, Mocroft A, Madge S, et al. (2001) Reduced bone mineral density in HIV-positive individuals. AIDS 15(13): 1731–3.
17. Knobel H, Guelar A, Vallecillo G, Nogues X, Diez A (2001) Osteopenia in HIV-infected patients: is it disease or is it treatment? AIDS 15: 807–8.
18. Thomas J, Doherty SM (2003) HIV infection – a risk factor for osteoporosis. JAIDS 33(3): 281–91.
19. Anastos K, Lu D, Shi O, Mulligan K, Tien PC, et al. (2007) The association of bone mineral density with HIV infection and antiretroviral treatment in women. Antiviral Therapy 12: 1049–58.
20. Paton NIJ, Macallan DC, Griffin GE, Pazianas M (1997) Bone mineral density in patients with Human Immunodeficiency Virus infection. Calcified Tissue Int 61(1): 30–2.
21. Triant VA, Brown TD, Lee H, Grinspoon SK (2008) Fracture prevalence among Human Immunodeficiency Virus (HIV)-infected versus non-HIV-infected patients in a large U.S. healthcare system. Endocrine Care 93(9): 3499.
22. Womack JA, Goulet JL, Gibert C, Brandt C, Chang CC, et al. (2011) Increased risk of fragility fractures among HIV infected compared to uninfected male vetrans. PLoS One 6(2): e17217, doi:10.1371/journal.pone.0017217.
23. Gallego-Rojo FJ, Gonzalez-Calvin JL, Munoz-Torres M, Mundi JL, Fernandez-Perez R, et al. (1998) Bone mineral density, serum insulin-like growth factor I, and bone turnover markers in viral cirrhosis. Hepatology 28(3): 695–9.
24. Gonzalez-Calvin JL, Gallego-Rojo F, Fernandez-Perez R, Casado-Caballero F, Ruiz-Escolano E, et al. (2004) Osteoporosis, mineral metabolism, and serum tumor necrosis factor receptor p55 in viral cirrhosis. J Clin Endocrinol Metab 89: 4325.
25. Leslie WD, Bernstein CN, Leboff MS (2003) AGA technical review on osteoporosis in hepatic disorders. Gastroenterology; 125: 941–66.
26. Rouillard S, Lane NE (2001) Hepatic osteodystrophy. Hepatology 33: 301–7.
27. Cummings SR, Black DM, Nevitt MC (1993) Bone density at various sites for prediction of hip fractures. Lancet 341: 72–5.
28. Hansen ABE, Gerstoft J, Kronborg G, Larsen CS, Pedersen G, et al. (2012) Incidence of low and high-energy fractures in persons with and without HIV infection: a Danish population-based cohort study. AIDS 26(3): 285–93.
29. Bedimo R, Maalouf NM, Zhang S, Drechsler H, Tebas P (2012) Osteoporotic fracture risk associated with cumulative exposure in tenofovir and other antiretroviral agents. AIDS 26(7): 825–31.
30. Lo Re V, Volk J, Newcomb CW, Yang YX, Freeman CP, et al. (2009) Viral hepatitis is associated with reduced bone mineral density in HIV-infected women but not men. AIDS 23: 2191–8.
31. Thein HH, Ti Q, Dore GJ, Krahn MD (2008) Estimation of stage-specific fibrosis progression rates in chronic hepatitis C virus infection: a meta-analysis and meta-regression. Hepatology 48(2): 418–31.
32. USPSTF (U.S. Preventive Services Task Force) (2011) Screening for osteoporosis: U.S. Preventive Services Task Force recommendation statement. Ann Intern Med 154: 356–64.
33. King G, Langche Z (2002) Estimating risk and rate levels, ratios, and difference in case-control studies. Stats Med 21: 1409–27.
34. Hedges LV, Pigott TD (2004) The power of statistical tests for moderators in meta-analysis. Psych Methods 9(4): 426–55.
35. Higgins JPT, Thompson SG (2002) Quantifying heterogeneity in meta-analysis. Stat Med 21(11): 1539–58.
36. Higgins JPT, Thompson SG, Deeks JJ, Altman DG (2003) Measuring inconsistency in meta-analyses. BMJ 327(7414): 557–60.
37. Li Vecchi V, Soresi M, Giannitrapani L, Mazzola G, La Sala S, et al. (2012) Dairy calcium intake and lifestyle risk factors for bone loss in HIV-infected and uninfected Mediterranean subjects. BMC Infect Dis 12: 192.
38. El-Maouche D, Mehta SH, Sutcliffe CG, Higgins Y, Torbenson MS, et al. (2013) Vitamin D deficiency and its relation to bone mineral density and liver fibrosis in HIV-HCV co-infection. Antivir Ther 18(2): 237–42.
39. Collin F, Duval X, Moing VL, Piroth L, Al Kaied F, et al. (2009) Ten year incidence and risk factors of bone fractures in a cohort of treated HIV1-infected adults. AIDS 23: 1021–6.

40. Yin MT, Shi Q, Hoover DR, Anastos K, Young M, et al. (2010) Fracture incidence in HIV-infected women: results from the Women's Interagency HIV Study. AIDS 24: 2678–86.

41. Young B, Dao CN, Baker R, Brooks JT (2011) Increased rates of bone fracture among HIV-infected persons in the HIV Outpatient Study (HOPS) compared with the US general population, 2000–2006. Clin Infect Dis 52: 1061–8.

42. Fausto A, Bongiovanni M, Cicconi P, Menicagli L, Ligabo EV, et al. (2006) Potential predictive factors of osteoporosis in HIV-positive subjects. Bone 38: 893–7.

43. Yong MK, Elliott JH, Woolley IJ, Hoy JF (2011). Low CD4 count is associated with an increased risk in fragility fracture in HIV fracture in HIV-infected patients. JAIDS 57: 205–10.

44. Badie BM, Soori T, Kheirandish P, Izadyar S (2011) Evaluation of bone mineral density in Iranian HIV/AIDS patients. Acta Medica Iranica 49(7): 460–7.

45. Ray WA, Griffin MR, Fought RL, Adams ML (1992) Identification of fractures from computerized medicare files. J Clin Epidemiol 45(7): 703–14.

46. Lofman O, Hallberg I, Berglund K, Wahsltrom O, Kartous L, et al. (2007) Women with low-energy fracture should be investigated for osteoporosis. Acta Orthop 78(6): 813–21.

47. Kanis JA, Melton LJ, Christiansen C, Johnston CC, Khaltaev N (1994) The diagnosis of osteoporosis. J Bone Miner Res 9: 1137–41.

48. Lewiecki EM (2004) Low bone mineral density in premenopausal women. South Med J 97(6): 544–50.

49. Lewiecki EM, Miller PD, Leib ES, Bilezikian JP (2005) Response to "The perspective of the International Osteoporosis Foundation on the Official Positions of the International Society for Clinical Densitometry," by John A. Kanis, et al. J Clin Densitom 8(2): 143–4.

50. Binkley N, Buehring B (2009) Beyond FRAX: It's time to consider "sarco-osteopenia". J Clin Densitom 12(4): 413–6.

51. Siggeirsdottir K, Aspelund T, Sigurdsson G, Mogensen B, Chang M, et al. (2007) Inaccuracy in self-report of fractures may underestimate association with health outcomes when compared with medical record based fracture registry. Eur J Epidemiol 22: 631–9.

52. Hernandez CJ, Beaupre GS, Carter DR (2003) A theoretical analysis of the relative influences of peak BMD age-related bone loss and menopause on the development of osteoporosis. Osteoporos Int 14: 843–47.

53. Palacios S, Henderson VW, Siseles N, Tan D, Villaseca P (2010) Age of menopause and impact of climacteric symptoms by geographical region. Climacentric 13(5): 419–28.

54. Amiel C, Ostertag A, Slama L, Baudoin C, N'Guyen T, et al. (2004). BMD is reduced in HIV-infected men irrespective of treatment. J Bone Min Res 19(3): 402–9.

55. Carr A, Miller J, Eisman J, Cooper D (2001) Osteopenia in HIV-infected men: association with asymptomatic lactic academia and lower weight preantire-troviral therapy. AIDS 15(6): 703.

56. Aukrust P, Haug C, Ueland T, Lien E, Muller F, et al. (1999) Decreased bone formative and enhanced resorptive markers in Human Immunodeficiency Virus infection: indication of normalization of the bone-remodeling process during highly active antiretroviral therapy. J Clinc Endocrin Metab 84(1): 145–50.

57. Egger M (1998) Meta-analysis bias in location and selection of studies. BMJ 316: 61.

58. Stroup DF, Berlin JA, Morton SC, Olkin I, Williamson GD, et al. (2000) Meta-analsysis of observational studies in epidemiology: a proposal for reporting. JAMA 283(15): 2008–12.

59. Huedo-Medina T, Sanchez-Meca J, Marin-Martinez F, Botella J (2006) Assessing heterogeneity in meta-analysis: Q statistic or I2 index? Psychol Methods 11(2): 193–206.

7

Clinical Disorders in a Post War British Cohort Reaching Retirement: Evidence from the First National Birth Cohort Study

Mary B. Pierce[1]*, Richard J. Silverwood[2], Dorothea Nitsch[2], Judith E. Adams[3], Alison M. Stephen[4], Wing Nip[4], Peter Macfarlane[5], Andrew Wong[1], Marcus Richards[1], Rebecca Hardy[1], Diana Kuh[1], on behalf of the NSHD Scientific and Data Collection Teams

1 MRC Unit for Lifelong Health & Ageing, London, England, 2 Department of Non-Communicable Disease Epidemiology, London School of Hygiene and Tropical Medicine, London, England, 3 Manchester Academic Health Science Centre, University of Manchester, Manchester, England, 4 MRC Human Nutrition Research, Elsie Widdowson Laboratory, Cambridge, England, 5 Electrocardiology Section, Royal Infirmary, University of Glasgow, Glasgow, Scotland

Abstract

Background: The medical needs of older people are growing because the proportion of the older population is increasing and disease boundaries are widening. This study describes the distribution and clustering of 15 common clinical disorders requiring medical treatment or supervision in a representative British cohort approaching retirement, and how health tracked across adulthood.

Methods and Findings: The data come from a cohort of 2661 men and women, 84% of the target sample, followed since birth in England, Scotland and Wales in 1946, and assessed at 60–64 years for: cardio and cerebro-vascular disease, hypertension, raised cholesterol, renal impairment, diabetes, obesity, hypothyroidism, hyperthyroidism, anaemia, respiratory disease, liver disease, psychiatric problems, cancers, atrial fibrillation on ECG and osteoporosis. We calculated the proportions disorder-free, with one or more disorders, and the level of undiagnosed disorders; and how these disorders cluster into latent classes and relate to health assessed at 36 years. Participants had, on average, two disorders (range 0–9); only 15% were disorder-free. The commonest disorders were hypertension (54.3%, 95% CI 51.8%–56.7%), obesity (31.1%, 28.8%–33.5%), raised cholesterol (25.6%, 23.1–28.26%), and diabetes or impaired fasting glucose (25.0%, 22.6–27.5%). A cluster of one in five individuals had a high probability of cardio-metabolic disorders and were twice as likely than others to have been in the poorest health at 36 years. The main limitations are that the native born sample is entirely white, and a combination of clinical assessments and self reports were used.

Conclusions: Most British people reaching retirement already have clinical disorders requiring medical supervision. Widening disease definitions and the move from a disease-based to a risk-based medical model will increase pressure on health services. The promotion of healthy ageing should start earlier in life and consider the individual's ability to adapt to and self manage changes in health.

Editor: Antony Bayer, Cardiff University, United Kingdom

Funding: This work was supported by the Medical Research Council grant numbers U1200632239 and U123092720. The funders had no role in study design, data collection and analysis, decision to publish, or preparation of the manuscript.

Competing Interests: The authors have declared that no competing interests exist.

* E-mail: m.pierce@nshd.mrc.ac.uk

Introduction

There is a longstanding and ongoing debate about the widening boundaries of disease and the costs and benefits of the medicalisation of health [1–5]. This debate is particularly relevant for the very old where multiple morbidity and polypharmacy are common and complicate treatment planning [6], and where medical problems may be overlooked or ignored [2]. It is also relevant for the early detection of disease at younger ages; for example, recent recommendations to screen everyone over 45 years for risk factors for cardiovascular disease [7] or prescribe statins or some form of 'polypill' for all those over 55 years old [8] would increase the proportion of the population with a disorder label and requiring regular medical supervision.

This debate needs to be informed about the current health status and treatment of older people. For the oldest old, in England, the Newcastle 85+ cohort [9] provides a description of their health status and treatment, and shows that nobody in this sample was disease free. National health surveys [10–12] also provide relevant information about the older population but they typically focus on different aspects of health in different years; and because they consist of a different population sample each year, it is impossible to estimate the extent of multiple morbidity. Moreover there is no way of defining in these surveys who is 'well' in the sense of being disease free.

In a national sample of the British population reaching retirement age, we investigate the extent of common clinical disorders, defined as an impairment of body system or structure for which there is evidence or a consensus for medical intervention, in terms of active monitoring or treatment. The data come from the Medical Research Council (MRC) National Survey of Health and Development (NSHD), a birth cohort study of men and women born in 1946 and followed ever since [13,14]. The generation that this cohort represents is important to study, being the first of the post World War II baby boom, and benefitting from increased longevity compared with earlier cohorts. This generation will contribute to the growing proportion of the population aged 65 years and over, which is expected to rise in the UK by 32% from 11.8 million in 2008 to reach 15.6 million by 2033 [15]. The health of the baby boomers as they age will dominate the work of the health and social care systems for the next three decades, not only in the UK but in all Western developed nations.

In this cohort aged 60–64 years, we describe: the proportions with, and sex differences in, fifteen common clinical disorders of later life; the extent to which these clinical disorders are already diagnosed and/or treated; how these disorders are distributed and relate to current self reported health; and how these disorders cluster into latent classes and relate to health status previously assessed at age 36 years.

Methods

Ethics statement

The study protocol received ethical approval from the Central Manchester Research Ethics Committee for data collection taking place in Manchester, Birmingham, Cardiff and London. Ethical permission was given by the Scotland A Research Ethics Committee for the data collection taking place in Edinburgh. Written informed consent was obtained from the study member at each stage of data collection.

Participants

The MRC NSHD is a socially stratified sample of 5362 singleton children born in one week in March 1946 in England, Scotland and Wales [14]. From an initial maternity survey in 1946 [16], the sample consisted of all single births to married women with husbands in non-manual and agricultural employment and one in four of all comparable births to women with husbands in manual employment. Of the 5362 original study members, the study team was still in contact with 3163 (59%) at age 60–64 years; 718 (13.4%) had died, 594 (11.1%) had previously withdrawn from the study, 567 (10.6%) lived abroad and 320 (5.9%) had been untraceable for more than ten years.

Study members received postal questionnaires between 2007 and 2008 and were invited for clinic visits between October 2007 and February 2011. If study members were unable or unwilling to come to one of the six Clinical Research Facilities (Edinburgh, Manchester, Cardiff, Birmingham, UCLH London or St Thomas' London) they were offered a slightly less comprehensive examination carried out in their own home by a trained nurse.

Of the 3163 people in the target sample, information was obtained from the postal questionnaire and/or visits from 2661 (84%). Of these, 2462 people completed the postal questionnaire and 2229 had a visit, of whom 1690 attended a clinic and 539 had a home visit.

Self-reported disorders

For stroke, diabetes, cancer, angina, myocardial infarction (MI) and thyroid disease we went back to the first occasion on which participants were asked if they had ever had a doctor diagnosis of these conditions. These reports were updated at subsequent data collections. In 1989, participants were first asked if they had ever been told by a doctor that they had had a stroke, diabetes or cancer; in 1999 a similar question referred to angina, MI and thyroid disease; and in the most recent data collection questions on coronary artery bypass graft, angioplasty or stent were included. Cancers were also picked up from registrations on the NHS Information Centre Registry.

Symptom scales

At age 60–64 years participants completed postal versions of the MRC Chronic Bronchitis [17] and the Rose Angina and Intermittent Claudication [18] questionnaires. The General Health Questionnaire (GHQ-28) [19] which asks about affective symptoms was self completed during the clinic or home visit.

Prescribed medications

As part of the postal questionnaire, participants were asked to list all their prescribed medications, and the reasons why these were prescribed. These were checked by the nurses and used to help define some disorders (see below).

Clinical assessments

Full details of the research protocol can be found elsewhere [14] but brief descriptions are given below. Those visited by a nurse at home received the same assessment except for the scans.

Cardiovascular assessment. Two measures of systolic and diastolic blood pressure were taken with an OMROM 705 with the participant seated, with the second reading used in this analysis. Participants visiting the clinic also had a 12 lead electrocardiogram recorded (Burdick Eclipse 850i). The output was sent by modem to the ECG Core Laboratory at the University of Glasgow for reporting.

DXA bone scans. Bone density scans were performed in the lumbar spine (L1–4) and proximal femur (femoral neck, total hip) using Hologic QDR 4500 Discovery scanners (Hologic Inc., Bedford MA, USA) according to standard protocols developed by Prof. J. Adams. Scans were sent to the central core laboratory in the University of Manchester for analysis.

Blood sample. Participants were asked to fast from 22.00 hours on the night before the visit, and the majority of blood samples were collected between 08.00 and 09.00 hours the following day. Samples were processed on site according to standardised protocols. Full blood counts were undertaken at the local hospital on the day of the visit. Aliquots were dispatched to Addenbrooke's Hospital Cambridge for HbA1c to be measured.

The remaining aliquots were stored at -80°C and couriered monthly, on dry ice, to the MRC Human Nutrition Research (HNR) laboratory in Cambridge. Serum lipids, fasting blood glucose, liver function tests, and serum creatinine were measured at HNR, and thyroid function tests at Addenbrooke's Hospital.

Serum total cholesterol, HDL cholesterol, triglycerides, glucose, and all liver function test parameters were measured colorimetrically on a Siemens Dimension Xpand analyser. LDL cholesterol was calculated from total cholesterol. HbA1c was analysed using the TOSOH G7 HPLC system. TSH and Free T4 were analysed using the Siemens Centaur Automated Immunoassay System. Free T3 was analysed using the Perkin Elmer AutoDELFIA Automated Immunoassay System until June 2009 and thereafter using the

Siemens Centaur. Serum creatinine measurements were carried out using the Jaffe method.

Defining the clinical disorders

We assessed 15 clinical disorders expected in people of this age group: cardio/cerebro-vascular disease, hypertension, raised cholesterol, renal impairment, diabetes, obesity, hypothyroidism, hyperthyroidism, anaemia, respiratory disease, liver disease, psychiatric problems, cancers, ECG abnormalities, and osteoporosis.

Clinical disorder status was derived from one or more of: a self-report of a doctor diagnosis of disease in response to a specific question; being positive on a validated scale for the disorder; a clinical assessment; currently receiving prescribed treatment for the disorder; or cancer registrations. The data sources and definitions for each clinical disorder are given in Table 1 [17–27]. For some conditions (hypertension, raised cholesterol, renal impairment, diabetes, obesity, hypothyroidism, and hyperthyroidism) two levels of disorder were defined, level 1 where intervention is required irrespective of other information and level 2 where the type of intervention may depend on other information. For example, whether or not to treat a person with a raised cholesterol level depends on the overall 10 year risk of a significant event.

Covariates

Health status at 36 years. Cohort members had previously been identified as being in the best of health (10%), intermediate (65%) or worst of health (25%) at age 36 years on the basis of measured blood pressure, lung function and body weight, self reported health problems and disability, and recent hospital admission [28].

Self-reported health status at 60–64 years. At age 60–64 years participants were asked to rate their current health on a 5 point scale from excellent to poor.

Statistical methods

The proportion with each clinical disorder was calculated as the number of participants meeting the relevant definition (see Table 1) divided by the number of participants with valid data for that measure. Where more than one measure was used in the definition of a disorder (for example total:HDL cholesterol ratio and reported statin/fibrate use for level 1 raised cholesterol), the sample was restricted to those with valid data for all relevant measures. The proportions were weighted to account for the social stratification in the original sample. Unweighted proportions were also calculated for comparison.

Undiagnosed disease. The number of participants who had diabetes, osteoporosis, hypertension, and thyroid disorders on examination, but who had not reported a doctor diagnosis of that condition or who were not on treatment for that specific disorder was divided by the total number of participants, to give the proportion of the total sample with undiagnosed disease. The proportion of those undiagnosed within the sample who had each of these disorders was also calculated. Social class-weighted results are presented, but unweighted results were produced for comparison.

Distribution and clustering of clinical disorders. For each participant for whom status on all the 15 disorders was defined, the number of identified clinical disorders was counted; this was initially restricted to level 1 disorders, then repeated to include those with level 2 disorders also. The number of disorders per participant was compared between sexes, and by self-rated health using a chi-squared test, grouping those with five or more clinical disorders together. This analysis was then repeated excluding the two disorders (osteoporosis and ECG abnormalities) that depended on the clinic visit for ascertainment. We assessed whether the number of disorders varied according to whether participants had a clinic or home visit, and by current self reported health status. Both weighted and unweighted analyses were again conducted.

To explore further the clustering of level 1 clinical disorders, latent class analysis (LCA) was performed on the level 1 clinical disorder variables. Latent class analysis is a multivariable regression model that describes the relationships between a set of observed dependent variables ('latent class indicators'), in this case the clinical disorders, and an unobserved categorical latent variable, each level of which is referred to as a 'latent class'. For dichotomous latent class indicators, as in the present application, the relationships are described by a set of logistic regression equations [29]. LCA assumes conditional independence of variables within each latent class. The objective is to identify the latent class indicators that best distinguish between classes and to categorise people into their most likely classes given their observed responses [30]. We used a variety of different tools to decide how many classes were required as no single approach is commonly accepted: the Lo-Mendell-Rubin adjusted likelihood ratio test (LRT), the bootstrap LRT, and three information criteria – Akaike's Information Criterion (AIC), Schwarz's Bayesian Information Criterion (BIC), and sample size-adjusted BIC (aBIC). The entropy, relative sizes, and meaningful interpretation of the latent classes were also considered. LCA was performed on complete cases only, then repeated using all study members who contributed data on at least one clinical disorder using full information maximum likelihood (FIML) under the assumption of missing at random for comparison [31]. LCA was conducted using Mplus version 6 [32].

The relationship between the latent classes and health status at 36 years was investigated using logistic regression of each latent variable on health status, weighted by the LCA posterior class membership probabilities.

Results

2657 survey members contributed to the analysis for one or more clinical disorders. Of these, 1104 (41.6%) belonged to the manual social class strata as defined at the initial sampling in 1946. This compares to 2370 (44.2%) of the 5362 study members originally in the cohort.

The commonest disorders were level 1 or level 2 hypertension (54%), obesity (31%), raised cholesterol (27%), and diabetes or impaired fasting glucose (26%). Other disorders affecting at least one in ten people were psychiatric disorders (19%), chronic respiratory disease (12%), cancers (11%), osteoporosis (11%), cardiovascular disease (11%) and renal impairment (10%); hypothyroidism (7%) and liver disease (5%) were less common. There was strong evidence for sex differences in many of the conditions examined. The others showed weak evidence (intermittent claudication, level 2 hyperthyroidism and cancers) or no evidence (anaemia, chronic respiratory disease, level 2 obesity and level 2 renal impairment); the number with level 1 renal impairment was too low to detect a sex difference. Hypertension, raised cholesterol, diabetes, cardiovascular problems, ECG abnormalities and abnormal liver function were more common in men, and psychiatric problems, thyroid disease, osteoporosis, and level 1 i.e. morbid obesity were more common in women (Table 2). The unweighted prevalences were similar for most clinical disorders, but slightly lower for several (results not shown).

Table 1. Clinical disorders, level 2 and level 1, with data sources and definitions.

Clinical disorder	Level 2/level 1	Constituent sub-disorders/definition
Level 1 CVD	Level 1	i) Angina (self-report of doctor diagnosed angina or self-reported by Rose chest pain questionnaire [18]; ii) CABG (self-report of CABG); iii) Angioplasty/stent (self-report of angioplasty or stent); iv) MI (self-report of doctor diagnosed MI); v) Stroke (self-report of doctor diagnosed stroke); or vi) Intermittent claudication (self-reported by Rose intermittent claudication questionnaire [18].
Hypertension	Level 1	Current SBP$\geq$160 mmHg or current DBP$\geq$100 mmHg, or reported being on anti-hypertensive medication.
	Level 2	Current SBP$\geq$140 mmHg or current DBP$\geq$90 mmHg but were not included in the 'level 1 hypertension' group.
Raised cholesterol	Level 1	Total:HDL cholesterol ratio $\geq$6.0 mmol/l or reported being on statins or fibrates.
	Level 2	Chance of developing a cardiovascular disease within the next 10 years$\geq$20% according to the Framingham risk score [20] but not included in the 'level 1 raised cholesterol' group. Risk score was calculated using current age, LDL and HDL cholesterol, current SBP and DBP, current smoking status (self-reported by direct questions), and 'level 1 diabetes' (see below).
Renal impairment	Level 1	eGFR<30 ml/min/1.73 m^2 [21]. eGFR calculated from serum creatinine using the MDRD formula [22].
	Level 2	30$\leq$eGFR<60 ml/min/1.73 m^2 or dipstick proteinuria$\geq$+ [22].
Diabetes	Level 1	FBG$\geq$7 mmol/l (restricted to study members who reported fasting appropriately), self-report of doctor diagnosed diabetes, or reported being on diabetes medication.
	Level 2	6.0>FBG<7 mmol/l (restricted to study members who reported fasting appropriately) [23].
Obesity	Level 1	BMI$\geq$40 kg/m^2 [20]. BMI calculated as weight (m)/height (kg)^2 [24].
	Level 2	30 kg/m^2$\leq$BMI]<40 kg/m^2 [24].
Hypothyroidism	Level 1	Self-report of doctor diagnosed hypothyroidism, TSH>5.5 mU/l and free T4<10.0 pmol/l (modified from Wilson 2006 [25]), or reported being on thyroxine.
	Level 2	TSH>5.5 mU/l and 10.0$\leq$free T4$\leq$19.8 pmol/l (modified from Wilson 2006 [25]).
Hyperthyroidism	Level 1	Self-report of doctor diagnosed hyperthyroidism, TSH<0.4 mU/l and free T3>7.5 pmol/l (modified from Wilson 2006 [25]), or reported being on medication.
	Level 2	TSH<0.4 mU/l and 3.0$\leq$free T3$\leq$7.5 pmol/l and 10.0$\leq$free T4$\leq$19.8 pmol/l (modified from Wilson 2006 [25]).
Anemia	Level 1	Haemoglobin <13 g/dl (males) or haemoglobin <12 g/dl (females) [26].
Respiratory disease	Level 1	Chronic bronchitis symptoms (MRC chronic bronchitis questionnaire [17]) or reported being on medication.
Liver disease	Level 1	Albumin <25 g/l, bilirubin >100 μmol/l, alkaline phosphatase >300 IU/l, alanine transaminase >300 IU/l, aspartate transaminase >300 IU/l, or gamma glutamyl transferase >100 IU/l.
Psychiatric problems	Level 1	GHQ 'caseness' ($\geq$5 items 'worse than usual' or 'much worse than usual') [19].
Cancers	Level 1	Self-report of doctor diagnosed cancer or cancer reported to the cancer registry.
ECG abnormalities	Level 1	Atrial fibrillation, atrial flutter or definite MI of any age.
Osteoporosis	Level 1	Bone density t-score by DXA scan $\leq$2.5 at spine, femoral neck, or hip [27].

CVD, cardiovascular disease; CABG, coronary artery bypass graft; MI, myocardial infarction; SBP, systolic blood pressure; DBP, diastolic blood pressure; HDL, high-density lipoprotein; LDL, low-density lipoprotein; eGFR, estimated glomerular filtration rate; MDRD, modification of diet in renal impairment; FBG, fasting blood glucose; TSH, thyrotrophin-stimulating hormone; T4, thyroxine; T3, triiodothyronine; MRC, Medical Research Council; GHQ, General Health Questionnaire; ECG, electrocardiogram; DXA, dual-emission X-ray absorptiometry.

This would be expected if the disorders were more prevalent in the manual social class, of which a smaller fraction were sampled.

Previously undiagnosed disorders

Table 3 shows the proportions with undiagnosed hypertension, diabetes, thyroid disease, and osteoporosis in the responding sample. Nine percent of the sample had undiagnosed untreated osteoporosis (79% of those with osteoporosis), 6% undiagnosed hypertension (15% of those with hypertension), 3% undiagnosed diabetes (39% of those with diabetes), and <1% undetected thyroid disease (8% of those with thyroid disease). Undiagnosed hypertension and diabetes were commoner in men. Undiagnosed osteoporosis was commoner in women in the full sample; however, within the group with osteoporosis, men were more likely to be undiagnosed (90%) than women (74%). There were no evidence of sex differences in undiagnosed thyroid disorders. The results from the unweighted analysis were very similar to those in the weighted analysis (results not shown).

Distribution of clinical disorders and relationship to current self reported health

Table 4 shows the distribution for the number of level 1 clinical disorders for those with information on all 15 or 13 clinical disorders. Thirty percent of the participants were free of all of the 15 level 1 disorders. The results on the larger sample, excluding the conditions only defined at the clinic visit (osteoporosis and ECG abnormalities), were similar, but slightly more participants (33%) were disorder free. In both cases the median number of level 1 disorders was 1 (range 0–8), and there was no evidence of sex difference in the number of disorders.

Table 5 shows the number of level 1 and level 2 clinical disorders in those with information on all 15 or 13 clinical disorders. Only 15% were free of either a level 1 or level 2

Table 2. Number and percent with level 1 and level 2 clinical disorders in men and women 60–64 years in the MRC National Survey of Health and Development.

Clinical disorder	Level 2/ level 1	Males		Females		Total		P for diff between sexes
		n/N	% (95% CI)[A]	n/N	% (95% CI)[A]	n/N	% (95% CI)[A]	
Level 1 CVD								
Angina	Level 1	97/1164	9.2 (7.3, 11.4)	60/1263	5.2 (3.9, 6.9)	157/2427	7.1 (5.9, 8.5)	0.002
CABG	Level 1	22/1136	2.3 (1.4, 3.6)	3/1209	0.3 (0.1, 1.2)	25/2345	1.3 (0.8, 2.0)	0.001
Angioplasty/stent	Level 1	40/1127	3.7 (2.6, 5.3)	13/1205	1.3 (0.7, 2.4)	53/2332	2.5 (1.8, 3.4)	0.002
MI	Level 1	59/1146	5.8 (4.3, 7.7)	15/1215	1.7 (0.9, 2.9)	74/2361	3.7 (2.8, 4.7)	<0.001
Stroke	Level 1	34/1181	3.1 (2.1, 4.6)	21/1268	2.1 (1.3, 3.4)	55/2449	2.6 (1.9, 3.5)	0.21
Intermittent claudication	Level 1	13/1152	1.4 (0.8, 2.6)	6/1235	0.4 (0.2, 1.1)	19/2387	0.9 (0.5, 1.5)	0.03
Any level 1 CVD	Level 1	133/1048	13.8 (11.5, 16.6)	71/1093	7.5 (5.8, 9.7)	204/2141	10.6 (9.1, 12.3)	<0.001
Hypertension	Level 1	407/1061	41.2 (37.6, 44.8)	348/1147	33.0 (29.8, 36.3)	755/2208	36.8 (34.4, 39.3)	0.001
	Level 2	225/1061	20.2 (17.5, 23.2)	188/1147	14.9 (12.6, 17.5)	413/2208	17.4 (15.6, 19.4)	0.005
Raised cholesterol	Level 1	269/960	28.0 (24.7, 31.5)	176/1024	18.2 (15.5, 21.3)	445/1984	22.9 (20.7, 25.2)	<0.001
	Level 2	63/785	8.9 (6.7, 11.6)	5/838	0.4 (0.1, 1.3)	68/1623	4.5 (3.4, 5.9)	<0.001
Renal impairment	Level 1	2/913	0.2 (0.0, 1.2)	0/942	0.0 (NA, NA)	2/1855	0.1 (0.0, 0.6)	NA
	Level 2	95/895	11.4 (9.1, 14.2)	78/932	9.4 (7.3, 12.0)	173/1827	10.4 (8.8, 12.3)	0.25
Diabetes	Level 1	101/834	12.8 (10.3, 15.9)	66/907	7.4 (5.6, 9.7)	167/1741	9.9 (8.4, 11.8)	0.002
	Level 2	180/917	20.5 (17.5, 23.9)	113/982	11.9 (9.7, 14.6)	293/1899	16.0 (14.1, 18.1)	<0.001
Obesity	Level 1	10/1061	0.7 (0.3, 1.5)	31/1158	3.0 (2.0, 4.5)	41/2219	1.9 (1.3, 2.7)	<0.001
	Level 2	290/1061	29.3 (26.1, 32.7)	320/1158	29.1 (26.0, 32.3)	610/2219	29.2 (26.9, 31.5)	0.93
Hypothyroidism	Level 1	20/903	1.8 (1.0, 3.0)	107/969	10.9 (8.7, 13.5)	127/1872	6.5 (5.3, 8.0)	<0.001
	Level 2	18/1000	1.5 (0.9, 2.7)	67/1063	6.4 (4.8,8.4)	85/2063	4.1 (3.2, 5.2)	<0.001
Hyperthyroidism	Level 1	6/903	0.6 (0.2, 1.6)	22/968	2.7 (1.7, 4.3)	28/1871	1.7 (1.1, 2.6)	0.003
	Level 2	7/1000	0.6 (0.2, 1.5)	17/1062	1.5 (0.8, 2.6)	24/2062	1.0 (0.6, 1.7)	0.09
Anemia	Level 1	45/999	3.8 (2.7, 5.5)	48/1063	5.1 (3.7, 7.0)	93/2062	4.5 (3.6, 5.7)	0.23
Respiratory disease	Level 1	140/1132	12.6 (10.4, 15.1)	140/1223	12.2 (10.2, 14.6)	280/2355	12.4 (10.9, 14.1)	0.84
Liver disease	Level 1	74/1002	7.3 (5.6, 9.5)	37/1059	3.3 (2.2, 4.8)	111/2061	5.2 (4.2, 6.5)	0.001
Psychiatric problems	Level 1	137/1047	13.5 (11.2, 16.2)	250/1136	23.3 (20.4, 26.4)	387/2183	18.7 (16.8, 20.7)	<0.001
Cancers	Level 1	108/1169	9.6 (7.8, 11.9)	164/1270	12.5 (10.5, 14.8)	272/2439	11.1 (9.7, 12.7)	0.06
ECG abnormalities	Level 1	47/785	6.2 (4.5, 8.6)	14/846	2.1 (1.1, 3.7)	61[B]/1631	4.1 (3.0, 5.4)	0.001
Osteoporosis	Level 1	50/780	7.3 (5.3, 10.0)	129/853	14.0 (11.5, 17.0)	179/1633	10.9 (9.2, 12.8)	<0.001

[A]Weighted according to original social class-stratified sampling. CVD, cardiovascular disease; CABG, coronary artery bypass graft; IC, intermittent claudication; MI, myocardial infarction; ECG, electrocardiogram.
[B]Of whom 31(2.3%) had atrial fibrillation.

disorders when 15 clinical disorders were considered, and 16% were disorder free when 13 clinical disorders were considered. In both cases the median number of level 2 or level 1 disorders was 2 (range 0 to 9). Women were somewhat more likely to be disorder free.

The distributions of the number of clinical disorders per study member were broadly similar in the unweighted analysis, though a slightly greater proportion of study members were disorder-free (results not shown). Again, this would be expected if disorders were more prevalent in the manual social class.

Those who had a home visit were less likely to be free from clinical disorders than those who had a clinic visit (23.3% v. 34.0%, p = 0.02 for level 1 clinical disorders).

In the total responding sample, 13% of participants described their health as excellent, 40% as very good, 32% as good, 13% as fair, and 2% as poor. These ratings were strongly associated with the number of level 1 and level 2 clinical disorders reported (p<0.001). For example, considering all 15 clinical disorders, 77% of those with no level 1 or 2 clinical disorders rated their health as excellent or very good and 2% rated it as fair or poor; but only 31% of those with 5 or more level 1 or 2 disorders rated their health as excellent or very good and 40% rated it as fair or poor. Around 50% of study members with cardiovascular disease or morbid obesity rated their health as fair or poor. These figures were essentially unchanged in the unweighted analysis.

Clustering of clinical disorders and relationship to health status at 36 years

Level 1 renal impairment was excluded from the LCA as the prevalence was too low. The remaining 14 clinical disorders meant that there were 16384 possible patterns of clinical disorders within

Table 3. Diagnosed and undiagnosed level 1 clinical disorders.

| | n/N (%[A]) | | | | | | |
| | Males | | Females | | Total | | |
Clinical disorder	Diagnosed	Undiagnosed	Diagnosed	Undiagnosed	Diagnosed	Undiagnosed	P for diff in undiagnosed between sexes
Hypertension	331/1061 (32.5)	76/1061 (8.7)	309/1147 (29.5)	39/1147 (3.5)	640/2208 (30.9)	115/2208 (5.9)	<0.001
Diabetes	58/834 (8.0)	43/834 (4.8)	43/907 (5.2)	23/907 (2.2)	101/1741 (6.5)	66/1741 (3.4)	0.01
Hypothyroidism	19/903 (1.6)	1/903 (0.2)	99/969 (10.2)	8/969 (0.6)	118/1872 (6.1)	9/1872 (0.4)	0.26
Hyperthyriodism	5/903 (0.6)	1/903 (0.1)	19/968 (2.4)	3/968 (0.3)	24/1871 (1.5)	4/1871 (0.2)	0.12
Osteoporosis	5/780 (0.5)	45/780 (6.8)	33/853 (3.7)	96/853 (10.3)	38/1633 (2.2)	141/1633 (8.6)	0.04

[A]Weighted according to original social class-stratified sampling.

the dataset. There was strong evidence that LCA models in which parameters were allowed to differ between males and females provided a better fit to the data than a model which combined both sexes. For both males and females a two class model provided the best fit to the data. Figures 1 and 2 show the latent classes of clinical disorders for males and females respectively using standardised probabilities, which are calculated by dividing the probability of each clinical disorder in each latent class by the observed proportion of study members with that disorder in the sample. For both males and females there was a smaller latent class (n = 77 for men and n = 112 for women) in which participants had a high probability of cardio-metabolic disorders (Figure 1a and 2a). The remaining larger latent class for men (n = 436) and women (n = 428) had a generally low probability of disorders (Figure 1b and 2b). As this larger cluster included participants with no disorders, the analysis was repeated excluding them. This gave essentially the same result, distinguishing those with a high probability of cardio-metabolic disorders from others. Repeating the LCA using all study members who contributed data on at least one clinical disorder using FIML increased the number of study members contributing to the analysis to 1283 men and 1374 women. Two latent classes were again required for both men and women, and the probabilities of each clinical disorder within each latent class were very similar to those in the complete case analysis

(results not shown). However, the classes were not as clearly separated (lower entropy) due to the inclusion of study members with reduced information.

In both males and females there was evidence of a trend in the relationship between the latent classes at 60–64 years and health status at age 36 years, with those in the worst health at age 36 more likely to be in the cardio-metabolic latent class almost thirty years later. Of those in the worst of health at 36 years, 25.5% of men and 30.9% of women were in the cardio-metabolic latent class at 60–4 years, whereas this was only true for only 13.2% of men and 14.6% of women in the best of health almost thirty years earlier (p = 0.02 and p = 0.003 respectively). When using the latent classes derived under FIML the magnitude of the associations was very similar (results not shown).

Discussion

Key findings

In this survey of common clinical disorders in the first wave of British baby boomers at 60–64 years, we found that most had clinical disorders even though the majority described their general health as good, or better. These disorders were widely spread across the population, with only one in six people being free of all the disorders considered i.e. not requiring any medical interven-

Table 4. Number (percent) of level 1 clinical disorders per study member.

| | n (%[A]) | | | | | |
| | All clinical disorders (max. 15)[B] | | | Excluding osteoporosis and ECG abnormalities (max. 13)[C] | | |
Number of clinical disorders	Males	Females	Total	Males	Females	Total
0	146 (26.3)	171 (32.4)	317 (29.5)	194 (30.8)	222 (34.2)	416 (32.6)
1	178 (34.4)	162 (29.6)	340 (31.8)	206 (32.0)	198 (31.6)	404 (31.8)
2	84 (18.2)	114 (19.6)	198 (18.9)	96 (16.1)	115 (17.6)	211 (16.9)
3	63 (12.8)	53 (10.5)	116 (11.6)	72 (12.5)	58 (10.0)	130 (11.2)
4	28 (5.2)	24 (4.4)	52 (4.8)	31 (5.5)	22 (3.8)	53 (4.6)
5+	14 (3.3)	15 (3.6)	29 (3.5)	16 (3.0)	13 (2.7)	29 (2.8)
Total	513	539	1052	615	628	1243

[A]Weighted according to original social class-stratified sampling.
[B]Range: 0–8; median: 1; P value for diff between sexes = 0.46.
[C]Range: 0–8; median: 1; P value for diff between sexes = 0.60.

Table 5. Number (percent) of level 1-level 2 clinical disorders per study member.

	n (%[A])					
	All clinical disorders (max. 15)[B]			Excluding osteoporosis and ECG abnormalities (max. 13)[C]		
Number of clinical disorders	Males	Females	Total	Males	Females	Total
0	69 (11.3)	92 (17.7)	161 (14.7)	91 (13.8)	117 (18.2)	208 (16.1)
1	116 (22.5)	128 (23.4)	244 (23.0)	148 (23.9)	160 (26.7)	308 (25.3)
2	108 (24.1)	128 (24.8)	236 (24.4)	119 (21.8)	150 (24.8)	269 (23.3)
3	89 (18.0)	83 (16.4)	172 (17.2)	103 (17.1)	90 (15.5)	193 (16.3)
4	61 (12.6)	50 (9.6)	111 (11.0)	64 (12.1)	52 (8.0)	116 (10.0)
5+	50 (11.5)	39 (8.1)	89 (9.7)	60 (11.3)	35 (6.8)	95 (9.0)
Total	493	520	1013	585	604	1199

[A]Weighted according to original social class-stratified sampling.
[B]Range: 0–9; median: 2; P value for diff between sexes = 0.13.
[C]Range: 0–9; median: 2; P value for diff between sexes = 0.03.

tion; this distribution was strongly related to self reported health. We identified a latent class of cardio-metabolic disorders, covering one in five of the population; this class was more likely to have had poor health as young adults.

Strengths and limitations of the study

As with all longitudinal studies NSHD has suffered from attrition. However, this is a large, national cohort that remains reasonably representative of the British born population. The NSHD study population is however all white, and therefore our findings cannot be extrapolated to the non-White British population. Non-White people make up 9% of the current population of England and Wales but they generally have a younger age profile, and only 5% of the population 60–64 years are non-White [33].

Some of our disorders are defined only on self–report of a doctor's diagnosis of disease. However, self-reports are generally

found to be reasonably accurate when compared with medical records in cases of definite diagnoses [34,35]. In the NSHD we sent questionnaires to GPs asking them to confirm self reports of chronic disease; for diabetes we found over 90% agreement [36]. We only measured blood pressure on one occasion so we may have overestimated the amount of previously undiagnosed hypertension, since in practice a diagnosis of hypertension is based on at least two readings taken at different times.

Rare disorders or common disorders in which confirmatory clinical assessments were not possible, and treatment is nonspecific e.g. arthritis, were not included. Hence this study estimated the extent of common clinical disorders rather than the full extent of health problems in this cohort at retirement age.

Although our analysis of the clustering of clinical disorders within study members was presented for complete cases only, obtaining very similar results using all study members who contributed data on at least one clinical disorder suggested that

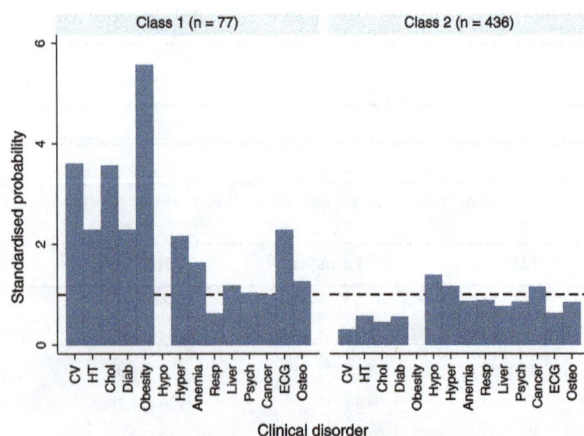

Figure 1. 1a and 1b. Latent classes of level 1 clinical disorders (excluding renalimpairment) in males (n = 513). Standardised probabilities are calculated by dividing the probability of each clinical disorder within each latent class by the observed proportion of study members with that disorder in the sample.

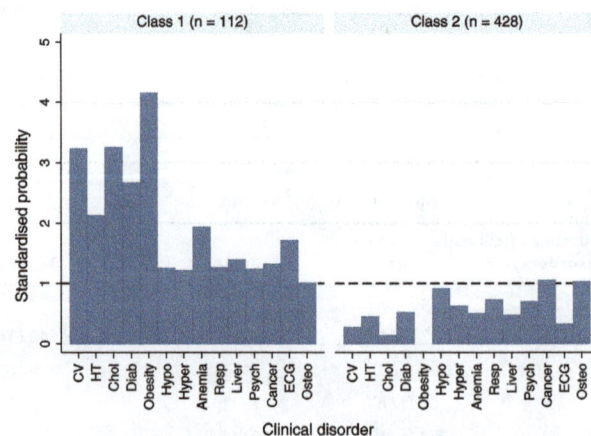

Figure 2. 2a and 2b. Latent classes of level 1 clinical disorders (excluding renal impairment) in females (n = 540). Standardised probabilities are calculated by dividing the probability of each clinical disorder within each latent class by the observed proportion of study members with that disorder in the sample.

significant bias was not introduced.

Comparison of our findings with other published studies

The proportions observed for cancers, diabetes, thyroid disease, obesity and psychiatric problems were similar to those in other studies, as were those for previously undiagnosed thyroid disorders and diabetes [20,22,36–44]. The major difference between our results and other reported studies was in relation to hypertension, the NSHD population had noticeably more people with hypertension than reported in HSE 2009 [37]. Our findings on renal impairment are not directly comparable with the other UK data [37,42] as these studies report CKD stages 3–5 (NICE 2008) [21] which exclude people with proteinuria but eGFR>60 ml/min/ 1.73 m^2 from being classified as having renal impairment. In NSHD the proportion with of CKD stages 3–5 is slightly lower than for the other studies [37,42]. However people with proteinuria alone do have a higher CVD and renal progression risk [22], and the NSHD identifies this group for the first time in a British general population. We found somewhat fewer MIs, strokes, and better respiratory function than has been reported in cross–sectional studies in people aged 64–69 in England [38], but this is probably accounted for by the age difference. NSHD women had somewhat less osteoporosis than estimated by WHO [27]; this may be an underestimation because participants who attended the clinics (where bone densitometry was available) had fewer clinical disorders than the people seen at home visits.

Undetected disorders. There was a high proportion of undetected osteoporosis in men and women. This is a condition that is not screened for as population screening is not cost effective [44]. National guidelines [44] do encourage case finding but this may not be widely applied and awareness of the problem in men is not high [45]. This may improve in the future with osteoporosis being introduced into the Quality Outcomes Framework in 2012. Undetected diabetes within the responding population was more frequent than found in the English Longitudinal Study of Ageing [39]; almost two fifths of those with diabetes had not been previously diagnosed. There was very little undetected thyroid disease, as found in the Birmingham Elderly Thyroid Study (BETS) [25]. This may be explained by GP awareness of thyroid disorders conditions and their success in case finding. The levels of undiagnosed hypertension and diabetes should reduce once the proposal for Vascular Screening system in the over 45 year-olds comes on-line in general practice [7].

Multiple disorders and clustering of disorders. In the Newcastle cohort study of those aged 85 years and older, nobody was disorder-free. This study also included heart failure, dementia and Parkinson's disease but we did not, as these conditions are rare in 65 years olds. Unlike our study, the authors found that women had more clinical disorders than men [9].

The picture we outline here is in many ways a best case scenario. It may be that that people born in the immediate post-war period are healthier than earlier or later born people because they have spent their whole lives within the post-war welfare state and only later experienced exposure to obesogenic lifestyles. There are a number of other conditions which we have not included, e.g. sarcopenia and osteopenia, that are as yet not monitored or treated but, given shifting boundaries, could easily become defined as clinical disorders [4]. We have not followed recent proposals for extending risk factors further back into the normal distribution identifying 'prehypertension' (SBP≥120 mmHg); impaired fasting glycaemia as beginning at 5.6 mmol/l ; and borderline risk of LDL as beginning at 3.6 mmol/l. In the US population Kaplan and Ong [46] estimate that such categorization of these

three risk factors alone would result in 97% of the population being under medical surveillance.

The study of patterns of multi-morbidity is relatively new field. There are few studies that have examined the way conditions cluster within groups of patients. One in the USA examined the records of 1.3 million primary care patients cared for by the Veterans Health Care System with two or more co morbidities and categorized 45 health conditions [47]. They reported that 83% of their sample fell into their metabolic cluster. An Australian study in working age adults [48] found that health conditions do not cluster neatly into organ or body systems as has been assumed by methods underpinning the Cumulative Index Rating Scale [49] and they identified 6 independent clusters of disorders.

Implications

Few people are without a clinical disorder on reaching retirement age. This highlights two sets of problems – the first is conceptual, related to our changing definition of disease and to current theories of ageing; and the second is pragmatic, and concerns the workload of health services going forward.

We have increasingly moved from a diseased-based model of medicine where doctors reacted to signs and symptoms presented by the patient, to a more proactive risk based model in which many clinical disorders are the end of a distribution of biological attributes, and are detected on the basis of case finding. This move has been driven by the success of epidemiological studies in identifying risk factors, and demonstrating effective interventions to reduce risk and to treat diseases early. Certainly this more proactive approach has coincided with a marked reduction in mortality rates for cardiovascular disease [50], although some would argue that the relationship between the two is not causal [51].

Individuals have different patterns of ageing. Such patterns have been postulated as; 'survivors' who live with extended morbidity due to age related disease diagnosed before old age; 'extenders' who live longer than expected without problems and have a shorter period of disability before death; and 'escapers' who attain very old age without disease [49,50]. As life expectancy increases there is a debate about whether we are facing a compression of morbidity, with people both living longer and having a longer period of healthy life (more extenders and escapers) or an expansion of morbidity with people living longer but having little or no increase in healthy life (more survivors). Alternatively, we may be facing some intermediate state involving more people living longer but with less severe morbidity (more survivors but with less disability). It has been proposed that ageing research should focus on extenders and escapers, to identify factors related to compression of morbidity and to avoid a pandemic of disability [52,53], and not just on age-related disease.

However, our research, and that emerging from the Netherlands [54], suggest that only a small minority of people in Western populations are 'escapers' or 'extenders', even by retirement age. Data from the Longitudinal Aging Study Amsterdam do not support the compression of morbidity scenario [54], and a study across OECD countries shows inconsistent results [55]. Thus ageing with clinical disorders may become the norm, and it might better to speak in terms of health relative to others of the same age. This situation is prompting new formulations of the meaning of health, especially in relation to older people, which focus on the individual's ability to adapt and self manage physically, psychologically and socially to their changing internal and external environment [56,57].

With our changing definitions of disease and the ageing population comes a significant load on the health services, especially general practice, in terms of monitoring and treatment. Not only is general practice delivering its traditional reactive role but it is increasingly expected to deliver the preventive care part of the public health agenda. The effect on workload is already being seen. Over the past decade patient consultation rates per patient in England and Wales have increased over 40% (from 3.9 in 1995/6 to 5.5 per patient per year 2008/9) [58], and this is also being seen in the other OECD countries [59].

The commonest conditions in this study are cardio-metabolic, cancers and osteoporosis which share common upstream causes in the nutritional deterioration of the nation's diet and sedentary behaviour. Unless we are able to tackle successfully these upstream causes on a societal level, we will be left with treating the effects in individuals, either monitoring and trying to change behaviour or prescribing medications. Our demonstration that health status at retirement is strongly associated with health status almost thirty years earlier suggests that a high risk group could be identified that may benefit from individual level interventions that start earlier than middle age. The current structure of the clinical care is still based on the disease model, and may be overwhelmed by the demands of proactive care. The purpose of this paper is not to give solutions to these problems, but to highlight the current position, and emphasize that the proportion of the population 'under the doctor' will only increase given an ageing population and diagnostic creep.

Acknowledgments

The authors are grateful to NSHD study members who took part in this latest data collection for their continuing support. We thank members of the NSHD scientific and data collection teams at the following centres: MRC Unit for Lifelong Health and Ageing, MRC Human Nutrition Research, Cambridge; MRC Epidemiology Unit, Cambridge; MRC Epidemiology Resource Centre, Southampton; Welcome Trust (WT) Clinical Research Facility (CRF) Manchester, the Manchester Heart Centre, and the Department of Clinical Radiology at the Central Manchester University Hospitals NHS Foundation Trust; WTCRF, Medical Physics and the Department of- Cardiology at the Western General Hospital in Edinburgh; WTCRF, Department of Nuclear Medicine and the Department of Cardiology at University Hospital Birmingham; WTCRF and the Department of Nuclear Medicine at University College London Hospital; CRF, the Department of Medical Physics and the Department of Cardiology at the University Hospital of Wales; CRF and Twin Research Unit at St Thomas' Hospital London; Vascular Physiology Unit, Institute of Child Health, London; National Heart and Lung Institute, Imperial College London; Divisional of Cardiovascular & Medical Sciences, Western Infirmary, Glasgow; Cardiovascular Institute, Sahlgrenska Academy, Gothenburg University.

We also thank Professor Jayne Franklyn from the University of Birmingham, Dr Joan Trowel (retired hepatologist) and Dr Ian Halsall who provided expert advice on blood analyte levels.

Author Contributions

Conceived and designed the experiments: DK MP JA PM DN MR RH. Performed the experiments: AW DK MR MP NSHD Data Collection Team. Analyzed the data: PM JA WN AS RS. Wrote the paper: MP DK. Revised the manuscript: MP RS DN JA AS WN PM AW MR RH DK.

References

1. Illich I (1975) Medical nemesis: the expropriation of health. London: Calder and Boyars.
2. Ebrahim S (2001) The medicalization of old age should be encouraged. BMJ 324:861–863.
3. Tinetti M and Fried T (2004) The end of the disease era. Am J. Med 116:179–185.
4. Moynihan R (2011) A new deal on disease definition. BMJ 342:1054–56.
5. Martin C (2010) Why medicine is overweight. BMJ 2010 340:c2800.
6. Ferrucci L, Studenski S (2012) Clinical problems of aging. In: Longo DL, Fauci AS, Kasper DL, Hauser SL, Jameson JL, Loscalzo J, editors. Harrison's Principles of Internal Medicine. 18th ed. New York, NY: McGraw-Hill. pp. 570–585.
7. Department of Health (2008) Putting prevention first—vascular checks: risk assessment and management. London: Department of Health Publications.
8. Wald NJ, Law MR (2003) A strategy to reduce cardiovascular disease by more than 80%. BMJ 326:1419–23.
9. Collerton J, Davies K, Jagger C, Kingston A, Bond J, et al. (2009) Health and disease in 85 year olds: baseline findings from the Newcastle 85+ cohort study. BMJ 339:b4904.
10. NHS Information centre (2012) The Health Survey for England. Available: http://www.ic.nhs.uk/hse. Accessed 20 April 2012.
11. The Scottish Government (2012) The Scottish Health Survey. Available http://www.scotland.gov.uk/Topics/Statistics/Browse/Health/scottish-health-survey. Accessed 20 April 2012.
12. Centres for Disease Control and prevention (2012) National Health and Nutrition Survey. Available: http://www.cdc.gov/nchs/nhanes.htm. Accessed 20 April 2012.
13. Wadsworth MEJ, Kuh D, Richards M, Hardy R (2006) Cohort profile: the 1946 birth cohort (MRC National Survey of Health and Development). Int J Epidemiol 35:49–54.
14. Kuh D, Pierce M, Adams J, Deanfield J, Ekelund U, et al. (2011) A Cohort profile: Updating the cohort profile for the MRC National Survey of Health and development: a new clinic based data collection for ageing research. Int J Epidemiol 40(1):e1–9.
15. Office for National Statistics (2009) National population projections-2008 based. Available:http://www.ons.gov.uk/ons/search/index.html?pageSize=50&newquery=age+sex+projections+2009. Accessed 10 January 2012.
16. Joint Committee of the Royal College of Obstetricians and Gynaecologists and the Population Investigation Committee (1948). Maternity in Great Britain. Oxford University Press, London.
17. Medical Research Council on the Aetiology of Chronic Bronchitis (1960) Standardised questionnaire on respiratory symptoms. BMJ 2:1665.
18. Rose G, McCartney P, Reid DD (1977) Self-administration of a questionnaire on chest pain and intermittent claudication. Br J Prev Soc Med 31: 42–8.
19. Goldberg DP, Hillier VF (1979) A scaled version of the General Health Questionnaire. Psychol Med 9:139–145.
20. Wilson PW, D'Agostino RB, Levy D, Belanger AM, Silbershatz H, et al. (1998) Prediction of coronary heart disease using risk factor categories. Circulation 97: 1837–47.
21. NHS. National Institute for Clinical Excellence (2008) Early identification and management of renal disease in adults in primary and secondary care. Clinical guidelines, CG73. Available: http://publications.nice.org.uk/chronic-kidney-disease-cg73. Accessed 17 April 2012.
22. Levey AS, de Jong PE, Coresh J, El Nahas M, Astor BC, et al. (2011) The definition, classification and prognosis of chronic kidney disease: a KDIGO Controversies Conference report. Kidney Int 80: 17–28.
23. World Health Organization (2006) Definition and diagnosis of diabetes mellitus and intermediate hyperglycaemia. Geneva: World Health Organization.
24. World Health Organization (2004) Obesity: preventing and managing the global epidemic. Geneva: World Health Organization.
25. Wilson S, Parle JV, Roberts LM, Roalfe AK, Hobbs FD, et al. (2006) Prevalence of subclinical thyroid dysfunction and its relation to socioeconomic deprivation in the elderly: a community-based cross-sectional survey. J Clin Endocrinol Metab 91: 4809–15.
26. World Health Organization (2008) Worldwide prevalence of anaemia 1993–2005: WHO global database on anaemia. Geneva: World Health Organization.
27. World Health Organization (1994) Assessment of fracture risk and its application to screening for postmenopausal osteoporosis. Geneva: World Health Organization.
28. Kuh D and Wadsworth MEJ (1993) Physical health at 36 years in a British national birth cohort. Soc Sci Med 37: 905–916.
29. Muthén LK, Muthén BO (1998–2007) Mplus User's Guide. Sixth Edition. Los Angeles, CA: Muthén & Muthén.
30. Nylund KL, Asparouhov T, Muthen BO (2007) Deciding on the Number of Classes in Latent Class Analysis and Growth Mixture Modeling: A Monte Carlo Simulation Study. Struct Equ Modeling 14(4): 535–69.
31. Little RJA, Rubin DB (2002). Statistical Analysis With Missing Data. Wiley: New York.
32. Muthén & Muthén (2010). Mplus statistical software, release 6. Muthén & Muthén: Los Angeles, CA.
33. Insightast (2001) Census table S101 Sex and Age by Ethnic Group (2001 Census). Available:http://insighteast.org.uk/viewResource.aspx?id=11003. Accessed 10 January 2012.
34. Tisnado DM, Adams JL, Liu H, Cen WP, Hu FA, et al. (2006) What is the concordance between the medical record and patient self-report as data sources for ambulatory care? Med Care 44:132–40.

35. Klungel OH, de Boer A, Paes AH, Seidell JC, Bakker A (1999) Cardiovascular diseases and risk factors in a population-based study in The Netherlands: agreement between questionnaire information and medical records. Neth J Med 55:177–83.

36. Pastorino S and Pierce M (2011) Validation of self-reported questionnaires for diagnosis of diabetes in a British birth cohort. Diabet Med 28:32–203.

37. NHS Information Centre (2009) Health Survey for England- 2009: Health and lifestyles. Available:http://www.ic.nhs.uk/pubs/hse09report. Accessed 10th January 2012.

38. NHS Information Centre (2005) Health Survey for England 2005. The health of older people. Available: http://www.ic.nhs.uk/webfiles/publications/hseolder/vol2.pdf .Accessed 10th January 2012.

39. Pierce MB, Zaninotto P, Steel N, Mindell J (2009) Undiagnosed diabetes-data from the English Longitudinal Study of Ageing. Diabet Med Jul;26(7):679–85.

40. Vanderpump MP, Tunbridge WM, French JM, Appleton D, Bates D, et al. (1995) The incidence of thyroid disorders in the community: a twenty-year follow-up of the Whickham Survey. Clin Endocrinol 43:55–68.

41. McManus S, Melter H, Bughra T, Bewbbington P, Jenkins R (2007). Adult psychiatric morbidity in England 2007. Results of a household survey. Available:http://www.ic.nhs.uk/pubs/psychiatricmorbidity07. Accessed 10th January 2012.

42. Stevens PE, O'Donoghue DJ, de Lusignan S, Van Vlymen J, Klebe B, et al. (2007) Chronic kidney disease management in the United Kingdom: NEOERICA project results. Kidney Int 72(1):92–9.

43. NHS Information Centre (2007) The Health Survey for England 2007, Vol 1. Healthy lifestyles, Knowledge and Behaviour. Available:http://www.ic.nhs.uk/webfiles/publications/HSE07/HSE%2007-Volume%201.pdf. Accessed 10 January 2012.

44. Royal College of Physicians (1999) Osteoporosis: guidelines for prevention and treatment. Royal College of Physicians, London, UK, pp 63–70.

45. Gielen E, Vanderschueren D, Callewaert F, Boonen S (2011) Osteoporosis in men. Best Pract Res Clin Endocrinol Metab 25:321–35.

46. Kaplan R M and Ong M (2007) Rationale and Public Health Implications of Changing CHD Risk Factor Definitions. Annual Review of Public Health 28; 321–44.

47. Cornell JE, Pugh JA, Williams JW, Kazis L, Lee AFS, et al. (2007) Multimorbidity clusters: Clustering binary data from multimorbidity clusters: Clustering binary data from a large administrative medical database. Applied Multivariate Research 2007, 12:163–182.

48. Holden l, Scuffham PA, Hilton MF, Muspratt A, Ng S, et al. (2011) Patterns of multi-morbidity in working Australians. Population Health Metrics 9:15.

49. Huddon C, Fotin M, Vanasse A (2005) Cumulative Illness Rating Scale was a valid and reliable index in a family practice context. J Clin Epidemiol 58:603–608.

50. O'Flaherty M, Ford E, Allender S, Scarborough P, Capewell S (2008) Coronary heart disease trends in England and Wales from 1984 to 2004: concealed levelling of mortality rates among young adults. Heart 94:178–81.

51. Kaplan GA, Baltrus PT, Raghunathan TE (2007) The shape of health to come: prospective study of the determinants of 30-year health trajectories in the Alameda County Study. Int J Epidemiol 36:542–48.

52. Fries JF, Bruce B, Chakravarty E (2011) Compression of morbidity 1980–2011: a focused review of paradigms and progress. J Aging Res 2011:261702.

53. Kivimaki M and Ferrie J (2011) Epidemiology of healthy ageing and the idea of more refined outcome measures. Int J Epidemiol 40:845–847.

54. Deeg D. New myths about ageing. About the growth of medical knowledge and its societal consequences. Chapter x in McDaniel SA, Zimmer Z, editors. Global Ageing in the Twenty-First Century: Challenges, Opportunities and Implications. Farnham, Surrey, UK: Ashgate Publishing. In press.

55. Lafortune G, Balestat G and the Disability Study Expert Group Members (2007) Trends in severe disability among elderly people: assessing the evidence in 12 OECD countries and the future implications. OECD Health working papers no. 26. Paris:OECD.

56. von faber M, Bootsma-vander Wiel A, van Excel E, Gussekloo J, Lagaay Am, et al. (2001) Successful ageing in the oldest old. Who can be characterized as successfully aged? Arc Int Medicine 161:2694–700.

57. Huber M, Knottnerus JA, Green L, van der Horst H, Jadad AR, Kromhout D, et al. (2011) How should we define health? BMJ 343:4163.

58. Hippsley-Cox J and Vinogardova Y (2009) Trends in consultation rates in general practice 1995/6 to 2005. Available:http://www.ic.nhs.uk/webfiles/publications/gp/Trends_in_Consultation_Rates_in_General_Practice_1995_96_to_2008_09.pdf. Accessed 11 January 2012.

59. OECD (2011) Consultations with doctors. In: OCED, health at a glance 2011:OECD indicators, OECD publishing. doi: 10.1787/health_glance-2011-29-en

8

A Modified Sagittal Spine Postural Classification and Its Relationship to Deformities and Spinal Mobility in a Chinese Osteoporotic Population

Hua-Jun Wang[1,2], Hugo Giambini[2], Wen-Jun Zhang[1], Gan-Hu Ye[3], Chunfeng Zhao[2], Kai-Nan An[2], Yi-Kai Li[1], Wen-Rui Lan[1], Jian-You Li[4], Xue-Sheng Jiang[4], Qiu-Lan Zou[5], Xiao-Ying Zhang[5], Chao Chen[1]*

1 Department of Orthopedics, School of Traditional Chinese Medicine, Southern Medical University, Guangzhou, China, 2 Biomechanics Laboratory, Division of Orthopedic Research, Mayo Clinic, Rochester, Minnesota, United States of America, 3 Chang Ping Hospital, Dongguan, China, 4 Orthopedic Department, Huzhou Central Hospital, Huzhou, China, 5 You-Hao Residential Care Home, Guangzhou, China

Abstract

Background: Abnormal posture and spinal mobility have been demonstrated to cause functional impairment in the quality of life, especially in the postmenopausal osteoporotic population. Most of the literature studies focus on either thoracic kyphosis or lumbar lordosis, but not on the change of the entire spinal alignment. Very few articles reported the spinal alignment of Chinese people. The purpose of this study was threefold: to classify the spinal curvature based on the classification system defined by Satoh consisting of the entire spine alignment; to identify the change of trunk mobility; and to relate spinal curvature to balance disorder in a Chinese population.

Methodology/Principal Findings: 450 osteoporotic volunteers were recruited for this study. Spinal range of motion and global curvature were evaluated noninvasively using the Spinal-Mouse® system and sagittal postural deformities were characterized.

Results: We found a new spine postural alignment consisting of an increased thoracic kyphosis and decreased lumbar lordosis which we classified as our modified round back. We did not find any of Satoh's type 5 classification in our population. Type 2 sagittal alignment was the most common spinal deformity (38.44%). In standing, thoracic kyphosis angles in types 2 (58.34°) and 3 (58.03°) were the largest and lumbar lordosis angles in types 4 (13.95°) and 5 (−8.61°) were the smallest. The range of flexion (ROF) and range of flexion-extension (ROFE) of types 2 and 3 were usually greater than types 4 and 5, with type 1 being the largest.

Conclusions/Significance: The present study classified and compared for the first time the mobility, curvature and balance in a Chinese population based on the entire spine alignment and found types 4 and 5 to present the worst balance and mobility. This study included a new spine postural alignment classification that should be considered in future population studies.

Editor: Dominique Heymann, Faculté de médecine de Nantes, France

Funding: This study is funded by the grant from National Natural Science Foundation of China (30700893 and 31171024), Huzhou Science and Technology R&D Fund (2009YS04 and 2010GS01) and the third phase of important subject construction programme of "211 Project" of Guangdong province. The funders had no role in study design, data collection and analysis, decision to publish, or preparation of the manuscript.

Competing Interests: The authors have declared that no competing interests exist.

* E-mail: chenchao@smu.edu.cn

Introduction

Osteoporosis, leading to an increased risk of fracture, poor posture and reduced functional ability is a significant global public health issue which has affected more than 200 million people and is expected to substantially increase by the year 2050 [1]. In the year 2005, approximately $19 billion was spent in osteoporosis related fractures, and by the year 2025, the cost is estimated to reach $25.3 billion (National Osteoporosis Foundation). The most common clinical manifestation of osteoporotic fractures are vertebral fractures. Older female patients are more severely affected due to the compromised resistance of bone as a consequence of decreased bone mineral, reduced bone quality

and destructive micro architecture resulting from post-menopause [2,3].

In addition to the above bone characteristic, more attention has been drawn into studies involving functional impairment including curvature deformity, balance disorder and the change of trunk mobility [3–19]. Such abnormal posture and spinal mobility is demonstrated to cause significant functional impairments in activities of daily living [3,11,15]. A series of studies by Miyakoshi et al. suggested lumbar kyphosis as a negative predictor of quality of life (QOL) and spinal mobility as a positive predictor and the most important factor relating QOL [15]. In addition, lumbar spinal mobility was proven to be the most important factor to QOL in patients with postmenopausal osteoporosis [13]. Conversely for middle-aged and elderly males, sagittal balance, lumbar lordosis angle, and spinal range of motion were also proved to be related to QOL [6]. On the other hand, studies have shown that thoracic hyperkyphosis is independently associated with decreased mobility and accompanied by a slower gait, poor balance, and greater body sway, which in turn is correlated with an increased tendency to falls [9,10,17]. Moreover it was reported that trunk deformities and spinal mobility also induce chronic back pain, increase vertebral fractures risk, reduce gait and stair-climbing function due to a decrease in lung function, and increase mortality rates, decreasing QOL and life satisfaction [5,7,16,19]. Therefore, rehabilitation intervention which has showed to influence a reduction in kyphosis may be an effective way to improve daily living functionality and QOL [4,18].

However an explanation to abnormal posture, spinal mobility and balance is multiplex and multifactorial. The proportion of older persons with the worst degrees of kyphosis who have vertebral fractures is only 36–37% [20]. Other causes impacting hyperkyphosis include postural changes, muscular weakness, degenerative disc disease and some genetic predisposition [20–23]. Consequently, there still exist some controversies which are not yet fully understood. Although lumbar lordosis tends to decrease with age in most research studies [22,24] other reports are inconsistent, reporting an increase [24] or no change in curvature [25], whereas Takahashi et al. showed that 11.9% of the participants had a decreased lumbar lordosis, and 4.7% exhibited an increased lumbar curvature [19]. While studies have demonstrated thoracic hyperkyphosis as an independent predictor of balance and QOL [6,9,17], lumbar kyphosis has been shown to affect spinal inclination and postural balance, presenting an additional risk factor for a tendency to falls [8,13,26]. Most notably, abnormal posture and spinal mobility should be studied as an overall alignment pattern including the thoracic and lumbar regions of the spine [15,27,28]. A same angular change in a similar segment of different persons may have a different effect on the global spine due to the compensatory and interactive relationship among separate segments of the spine in the process of senescence. Thus, it is important and meaningful to focus more attention on changes and relationships between different global spine curvature types [15,27,28]. Meanwhile a difference has been reported in the shape of the sagittal spinal curvature between Japan and the United States [29]. With one of the biggest populations in the world, a large elderly population and increasing longevity, osteoporosis has become a significant burden on society and healthcare systems in China [30]. An understanding of the changes of spinal deformity and functional impairment in the Chinese population would be useful in the planning of public health strategies in this region. However, there are very few articles reporting spinal functional impairment and alignment in Chinese people.

Thus, the objective of this study was to provide further evidence about the change of trunk mobility and the relationship between spinal curvature and balance disorder, especially for the different type of global spine deformity in a Chinese population.

Materials and Methods

Ethics Statement

Informed consent was obtained from all participants prior to examination, and ethical approval to undertake this study was obtained from Human Research Ethics Committee, Southern Medical University.

Participants

For this cross-sectional study, a total of 476 elderly women volunteers, over 60 years of age, with osteoporosis were recruited from local community centers. Diagnosis of osteoporosis was made according to the World Health Organization criteria defined by a bone mineral density (BMD) T-score of at least 2.5 standard deviations below the young normal sex-matched BMD of the reference database. In addition, participants were questioned about their medical history and were excluded if they had a history of neurologic and musculoskeletal disease such as acute or severe chronic back pain within the last 6 months that required medical attention or treatment, documented vertebral fractures within the last 6 months, previous surgery of the spine, dislocations of the spine, spondylolisthesis, spondylolysis, hip fractures, metastases, and rheumatologic disorder. Participants with any other possible disorder affecting bone metabolism were also excluded. Finally, 450 volunteers (mean 75 yrs., range 60–95) were eligible and joined our study.

Spine Range of Motion and Global Curvature Measurements

Using the Spinal-Mouse® we were able to evaluate spine range of motion (ROM) and global curvature (Idiag, Volkerswill, Switzerland). This is an electronic computer-aided device that measures sagittal spinal ROM and intersegmental angles noninvasively using a surface technique. The intra-class coefficients for curvature measurement with Spinal-Mouse® are 0.92–0.95 [31]. To avoid inter-measure variation, all the measurements were done by one examiner who was experienced in assessing spinal function using the Spinal-Mouse® system. Each measurement was conducted three times and the mean value obtained.

Spine curvature, spine inclination (angle of the plumb line bisecting the trochanter major and running through the middle of the supporting area of the feet) and sacral inclination angle (Sac/Hip: sacral slope defined as the angle between the horizontal and the sacral plate) were evaluated in the neutral upright position by sliding of the Spinal-Mouse® along the spine. All spine data were calculated and displayed on the computer automatically. Thoracic kyphosis was expressed as a positive value and lumbar lordosis expressed as a negative value. This process was repeated with the subject in a maximum bending position and a maximum extension position allowing for measurement of spinal mobility. Balance was related to spine inclination and the entire spine alignment measured by the angle of the whole trunk. A large angle indicated worst balance.

Postural Classification and Comparison

Classification of postures was made based on the visual curvature of the spine of the volunteers, palpation of the spine and curvature results from the spinal mouse®. Sagittal postural deformities were classified by two trained spine surgeons, and upon disagreement, a third spine surgeon was consulted before a final judgment was made. Sagittal postures were divided into the following five groups based on the entire spine alignment according to the classification proposed by *Satoh et al.* [27]: 1) Normal Posture (NP): without apparent change in spinal curve; 2) Round Back (RB): with increased thoracic kyphosis and normal lumbar lordosis; 3) Hollow Round Back (HRB): with increased thoracic kyphosis and lumbar lordosis; 4) Whole Kyphosis (WK): with extensive kyphosis from the thoracic to the lumbar spine and 5) Lower Acute Kyphosis (LAK): with localized lumbar kyphosis and a straight thoracic spine (*not found*) (Figure 1).

a)

Type 1:
Normal Posture

Type 2:
Round Back

Type 3:
Hollow Round Back

Type 4:
Whole Kyphosis

Type 5:
Modified Round Back

b)

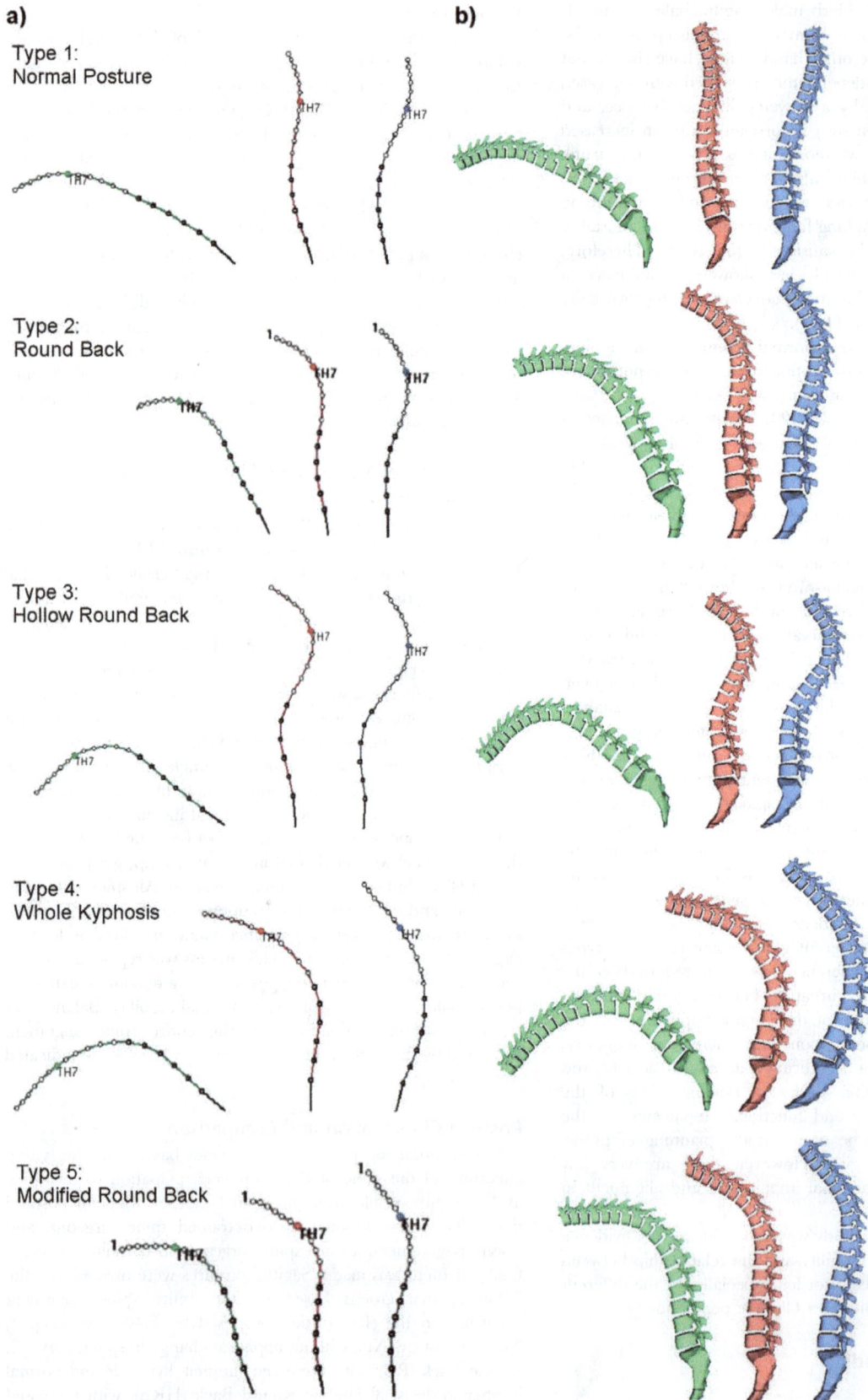

Figure 1. Sagittal spine alignments in flexed, standing and extended positions as acquired using the Spinal-Mouse® System. a) Type 1: Normal Posture; Type 2: Round Back; Type 3: Hollow Round Back; Type 4: Whole Kyphosis; Type 5: Modified Round Back. b) Representation of the different postural types in spine form.

Data Analysis and Statistics

All data are presented as mean and standard deviation (SD) and were analyzed using the Statistical Package for Social Sciences (SPSS, Chicago, IL; version 13.0). Descriptive statistics was used to describe the demographic and measurement variables of all the subjects. Categorical variables were expressed as frequencies and percentages for each variable. Continuous variables were presented as mean values±SD. The factorial design ANOVA and Student Newman Keuls was applied for a comparison between posture types. A *P-value* <0.05 was considered statistically significant.

Results

Volunteers were classified into five types according to Satoh's classification system. Notably, the type 5 (Lower Acute Kyphosis (LAK): localized lumbar kyphosis and a straight thoracic spine) was not found in our population but rather a new spine alignment was found consisting of an increased thoracic kyphosis and decreased lumbar lordosis which we classified as our modified type 5 and named Modified Round Back (MRB). Among the classified spines, types 2 (38.44%) and 5 (29.33%) sagittal alignment were the most common deformity with type 4 (4.44%) being the least common (Table 1).

In the standing position, thoracic kyphosis angles were significantly greater in types 2 (58.64°) and 3 (58.03°), and smaller in type 1 (39.24°) compared to those in types 4 (51.55°) and 5 (52.32°). In addition, lumbar lordosis and Sac/Hip angles were significantly greater in type 3 (−31.61° and 13.96°, respectively) compared with those in types 1 (−22.58° and 11.32°) and 2 (−21.49° and 8.16°), with type 4 (13.95° and −2.35°) and type 5 (−8.61° and 4.08°) being the smallest ones. Finally, the angle of the whole trunk was greater in types 4 (22.50°) and 5 (10.20°) compared with type 2 (6.10°), with types 1 (1.82°) and 3 (2.99°) being the smallest. Spine inclination, defined by the angle of the whole trunk, showed types 1 and 3 to have the worst balance followed by types 2, 4 and 5. Data is summarized in Table 1 as mean and standard deviation values.

The range of flexion (ROF) and range of flexion-extension (ROFE) of types 2 and 3 were usually greater than types 4 and 5, with type 1 being the largest. The range of extension (ROE) showed almost no difference in all posture types for the whole spine and individual segments, except on the Sac/Hip angles. These results are described in Table 1 and pictured in Figure 2.

Discussion

Abnormal posture and spinal mobility of the sagittal plane has been demonstrated to cause significant impairments in the elderly [3,11,15]. Prior studies have proven an existing, although conflicting, evidence linking different spinal postures to low back pain [27,32]. Recently, spinal posture and mobility have been established as important factors linked to quality of life (QOL) in the osteoporotic population [3,6,15]. Notably, most of the literature studies focus on either thoracic kyphosis or lumbar lordosis, but not on the change of the entire spinal alignment [3,11,13,15]. Also, there are still some controversies regarding whether the curvature and mobility of the lumbar region better relate to spinal function and balance compared to the thoracic spine, in both cases without fully understanding their progression [6,8,9,13,17,26]. Thus, it is meaningful to focus more attention on the global change of the spine and the relationship between the different spinal postural types.

Due to the large degree of variability in sagittal spinal alignment and relatively little work performed toward a classification of osteoporosis in sagittal spinal alignment, the comprehensive classification system and criteria are still ambiguous and equivocal. Roussouly et al. classified patients into four types mainly according to the reciprocal relationships between the sacral slope and the characteristics of the lumbar curvature [33]. Similarly, Lee et al. grouped 86 volunteers into three types based on the horizontal lumbar level [34]. Smith et al. established four subgroups by cluster analysis of three angular measurements of thoraco-lumbo-pelvic alignment [35]. Although those classifications are based on the overall sagittal pattern, the subjects are adolescent or middle-aged patients with or without low back pain who present different geometrical and physiological characteristics compared to an osteoporotic population. In the year 1889, Staffel arranged senile posture into five types: normal, round back, flat back, lordotic back and kypholordotic back, a classification still used at present [28]. Later, Wiles proposed five categories of the human posture based on a combination of the pelvic inclination and dorsolumbar kyphosis [36]. One of these types, round back, was then divided into two additional types according to the lower lumbar curve. Takemitsu et al. classified 105 patients into five types to study the relationship between posture and low back pain [32]. However, due to the complexity of the classification, they were barely used in mass examination studies. Furthermore, a classification system defined by Satoh et al. grouped 73 postmenopausal osteoporotic patients into five groups according to changes of the physiological thoracic and lumbar curvature [27]. Satoh's classification system was used in our study and proved to cover the whole range of our postmenopausal osteoporotic population.

In spite of the percentages of spinal types in our study differing from other literature results, there also exist substantial differences among previous published literature. In this study, type 2 (38.44%) was the most common spinal deformity, compared to the postural type 3 in Satoh's and Itoi's studies, 35.6% and 26% respectively [27,37]. Miyakoshi's study also presented a higher percentage (26.11%) of type 2 [15]. Moreover, Hongo et. al. suggested differences between a population from Minnesota, USA and a group from Japan, with the former presenting a typical type 2 (hollow round back) and the latter a single kyphotic or lower kyphosis apex [29]. However, until now, research has been done on small population cohorts, making it difficult to obtain decisive relations underlying postural deformity. For this reason, more studies from different ethnic groups, environments and populations are needed.

Most importantly, in addition to not finding Satoh's type 5 classification on our population, we found a new spine alignment. Having the second highest ratio of spinal deformity (29.33%) and consisting of an increased thoracic kyphosis and decreased lumbar lordosis, we classified this new spine posture as the *modified type 5 or Modified Round Back*. Reasons for the differences among populations of different geographic areas are multiple, but some of this variability may be related to lifestyle and genetic background.

There exists substantial disparity in the literature regarding the curvature of the thoracic and lumbar spines. Thoracic kyphosis has been reported to be in the 30–50 degrees range, while lumbar lordosis ranges from 20 to 60 degrees [3–7,9–11,13,15–19]. Comparatively, our study reports mean values of 54.21 and 17.95 degrees, respectively. Thus, compared to other geographical places, Chinese women seem to show more thoracic kyphosis with less lumbar lordosis, although many other reasons such as measurement technique, percentage of sex distribution and physical and anthropometric condition could also contribute to this difference.

Table 1. Summary of data for all curves types and conditions.

Table 1. Spinal Curvature and Mobility Comparison

	Type 1	Type 2	Type 3	Type 4	Type 5	Total
N (%)	50 (11.11%)	173 (38.44%)	75 (16.67%)	20 (4.44%)	132 (29.33%)	450 (100%)
Age	73.34 (6.98)	74.26 (7.80)	71.84 (7.17)	81.45 (7.10)[a, b, c]	78.36 (7.29)[a, b, c, d]	75.28 (7.87)
Thoracic spine						
Standing	39.24 (4.22)	58.64 (10.40)[a]	58.03 (8.63)[a]	51.55 (14.93)[a, b, c]	52.32 (11.61)[a, b, c]	54.21 (11.86)
ROF	16.90 (10.54)	8.30 (8.76)[a]	8.36 (9.25)[a]	3.65 (8.39)[a, b, c]	9.15 (11.06)[a, d]	9.31 (10.13)
ROE	−5.10 (10.76)	−5.14 (10.03)	−5.84 (7.55)	−8.55 (9.20)	−5.74 (8.24)	−5.58 (9.19)
ROFE	21.90 (14.07)	13.42 (12.90)[a]	14.16 (11.44)[a]	12.15 (10.45)[a]	14.86 (14.16)[a]	14.85 (13.29)
Lumbar spine						
Standing	−22.58 (4.82)	−21.49 (3.29)	−31.61 (3.45)[a, b]	13.95 (12.68)[a, b, c]	−8.61 (5.10)[a, b, c, d]	−17.95 (11.51)
ROF	42.54 (9.54)	37.60 (12.91)[a]	43.35 (13.52)[b]	17.80 (13.35)[a, b, c]	26.88 (11.64)[a, b, c, d]	35.08 (14.29)
ROE	−5.62 (5.70)	−5.43 (5.96)	−4.11 (5.46)	−6.40 (6.03)	−5.65 (5.72)	−5.34 (5.79)
ROFE	48.12 (10.16)	43.02 (15.44)	47.36 (15.46)	24.25 (14.08)[a, b, c]	32.41 (13.59)[a, b, c, d]	40.36 (15.88)
Whole trunk						
Standing	1.82 (3.21)	6.10 (6.71)[a]	2.99 (5.89) b	22.50 (15.84)[a, b, c]	10.20 (7.38)[a, b, c, d]	7.04 (8.38)
ROF	89.88 (19.17)	75.28 (22.52)[a]	85.92 (21.09)[b]	54.95 (29.35)[a, b, c]	63.58 (25.42)[a, b, c]	74.34 (25.16)
ROE	−18.20 (6.34)	−16.56 (5.82)	−16.63 (5.69)	−14.00 (8.07)	−15.63 (6.53)	−16.37 (6.22)
ROFE	108.00 (21.93)	91.73 (25.19)[a]	102.51 (23.16)[b]	68.95 (32.73)[a, b, c]	79.13 (28.07)[a, b, c, d]	90.63 (27.87)
Sac/Hip						
Standing	11.32 (5.20)	8.16 (5.93)[a]	13.96 (6.75)[a, b]	−2.35 (6.89)[a, b, c]	4.08 (6.68)[a, b, c, d]	7.81 (7.44)
ROF	49.96 (17.68)	42.38 (16.77)	47.92 (16.97)	39.60 (22.68)[a]	39.00 (20.46)[a]	43.03 (18.65)
ROE	−11.10 (7.75)	−9.47 (5.52)	−10.48 (5.17)	−6.05 (6.39)[a, b, c]	−8.82 (5.69)[d]	−9.48 (5.91)
ROFE	60.94 (20.99)	51.81 (18.20)	58.35 (17.42)	45.65 (24.18)[a, c]	47.77 (21.75)[a, c]	52.45 (20.25)

Type 1: Normal Posture; Type 2: Round Back; Type 3: Hollow Round Back; Type 4: Whole Kyphosis; Type 5: Modified Round Back.
Standing: Angle in standing position; **ROF**: Range of Flexion; **ROE**: Range of Extension; **ROFE**: Range of Flexion and Extension.
Whole trunk (Spinal Inclination): angle of the plumb line which bisects the trochanter major and runs through the middle of the supporting area of the feet.
Sac/Hip: Sacral slope defined as the angle between the horizontal and the sacral plate.
[a, b, c, d]Indicate significant differences (P<0.05) between: [a]Type 1, [b]Type 2, [c]Type 3, and [d]Type 4.

Spinal deformity has a significant impact on balance disorder and fall in the osteoporotic population [6,8,9,13,17,26]. The angle of the whole trunk in our study showed type 3, with a large thoracic kyphosis, to have the best balance, in contrast to type 4, presenting a mild thoracic kyphosis, and type 2, with a large thoracic kyphosis but normal lumbar lordosis, having the worst balance. This is due to the fact that the increased thoracic kyphosis (type 2- Round Back) is readily compensated by increasing lumbar lordosis, resulting in the formation of the type 3 (Hollow Round Back). If progressing round back cannot be compensated by either a reduced lumbar lordosis (type 5) or a kyphotic lumbar spine (type 4), then the spinal balance decreases progressively from worse (type 5) to worst (type 4). These results suggest that it is meaningful to focus more attention on the global change and relationship between different spinal types and balance, rather than "local" changes either thoracic or lumbar.

In this study we provided not only the mobility of individual regions of the spine but also of the whole trunk in both flexion and extension. In addition, the total mobility, from flexion to extension was also shown for individual regions and the whole spine. Our study showed an average range-of-flexion-to-extension (ROFE) of 90.63 degrees for all types, compared to previous studies which show a range of 68–116 degrees [6,8,13,15,16,31]. Our findings substantiate prior research showing that spinal mobility decreased in the elderly with postural deformities compared to normal (control) postures. However, we found that the change of spinal mobility was not directly accompanied with a change in thoracic or lumbar curvature, as previous studies have described [6,8,9,13]. For instance, type 3, with nearly most thoracic kyphosis and lumbar lordosis has the same mobility as type 1 without significant differences. On the other hand, as previously stated, those groups without compensation in curvature, either thoracic or lumbar, will have worse mobility. Because spinal mobility is best correlated with quality of life and function, prevention and therapy should be applied, especially for types 4 and 5 in Chinese elderly persons.

Spine curvature and balance is also affected by pelvic orientation and position in the sagittal plane [38–40]. When a spine deformity with sagittal imbalance occurs, compensatory mechanisms include not only the spinal column but also the pelvis expressed by sacral slope (SS), indicating the position of the pelvis

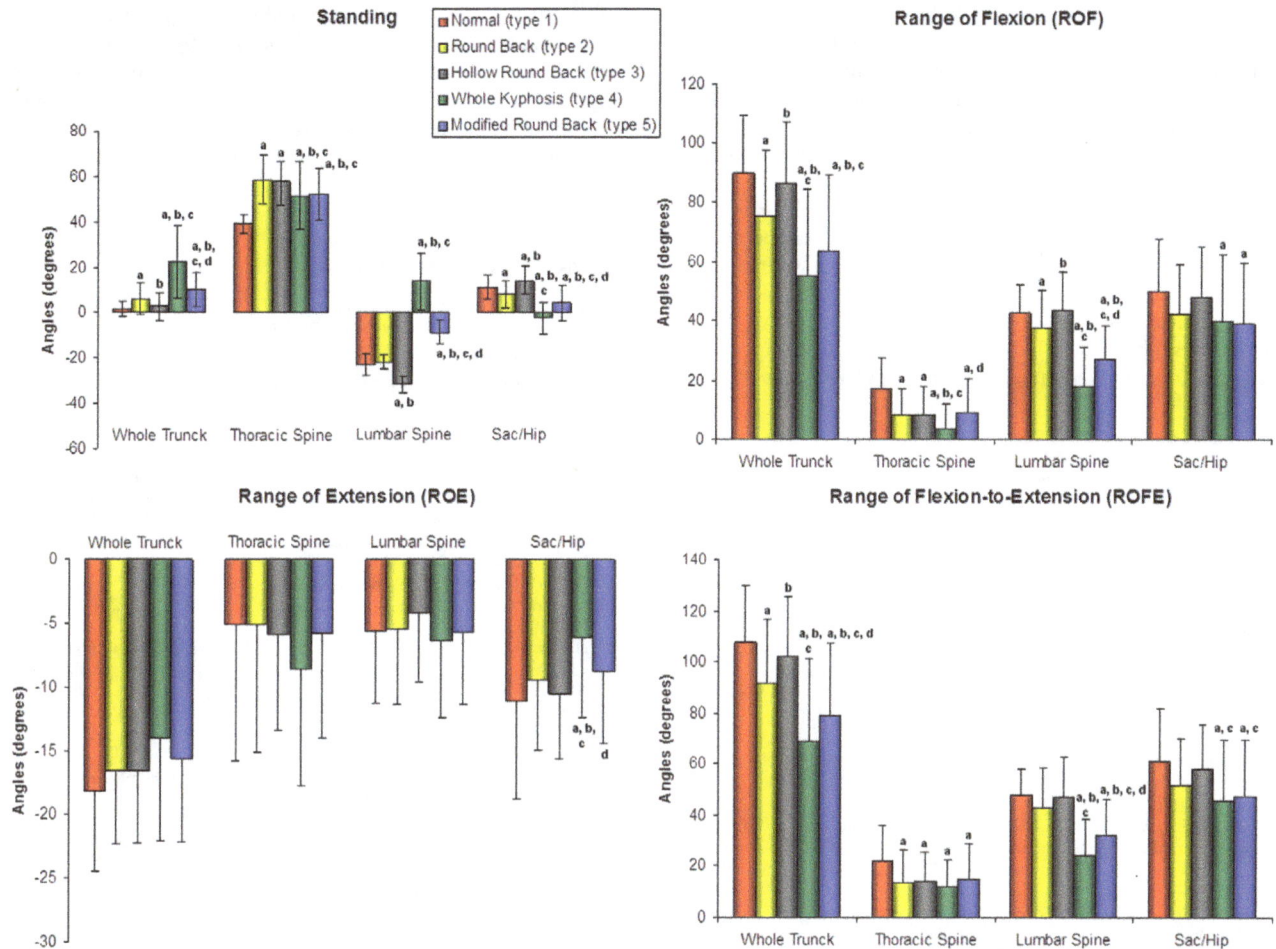

Figure 2. Angle data at different spine sections during standing, flexion and extension conditions. Standing: stand angle in standing; ROE: range of extension; ROF: range of flexion; ROFE: range of flexion-extension. [a, b, c, d] Indicate significant differences (P<0.05) between: [a]Type 1 (n = 50), [b]Type 2 (n = 173), [c]Type 3 (n = 75), and [d]Type 4 (n = 20). Modified type 5 (n = 132).

in the sagittal plane. Moreover, it is much easier to use the SS as an isolated parameter of pelvic orientation, since the measurement of the SS does not require the femoral heads to be visible on standing films [41]. It is commonly reported as a compensatory mechanism: "when the spine tilts forward due to age-related changes, sagittal imbalance, loss of lordosis or increase of kyphosis, the subject will try his/her best to maintain a minimum amount of energy posture and to keep the spine as vertical as possible" [40,41]. One way to maintain this spino-pelvic alignment is to retrovert the pelvis (decrease of SS) that may be seen as a backward rotation of the pelvis around the hips. In addition, correlations between the various parameters of lumbar and pelvic alignment indicate the sacral slope to be most associated with lumbar lordosis [42–44]. Our results are consistent with past observations, as the sacral slope decreases in types 4 and 5, accompanied with a reduction of lumbar lordosis. Also, in type 2, although there is no change in lumbar lordosis, as thoracic kyphosis increased, the sacral slope decreased in order to maintain sagittal balance. Type 3 is the only type with an increased lumbar lordosis and sacral slope. Sacral slope has been reported in only a few other studies using skin-surface devices, and the values obtained in the present study using the spinal mouse compare favorably with past research (all approx.. −13∼23°) [45,46]. However, these values are smaller than those measured in X-ray films (22∼56°) [39–44]. The main reason for this difference may be subject recruitment, as our study involved osteoporotic elderly women, while their research population consisted on young or asymptomatic adults. Furthermore, Barón had shown western population to have a significant lager SS than Asian population [47]. Therefore, in addition to instrumentation use, ethnicity also plays an important role in the differentiation of anthropometric values.

This study presents several limitations. First, there might have been some overlap between spinal types as spinal postural classification was based on changes in thoracic and lumbar curvatures, and there exist a wide range of curvatures. For this reason, the different curvatures types based on the angle change should be clearly and precisely defined to be useful. Second, since this is a cross-sectional study, we were not able to establish any cause-effect relationships and we are not able to verify the time point where the change in curvature occurred. Future longitudinal studies looking at different time point sequences should be undertaken to answer this question. Third, other factors such as body mass index, secondary effects of other fracture types (i.e. wrist and ribs), and exercise level were not recorded thus preventing their analysis on the effect of spinal postural deformities. Finally, position and anatomic pelvic parameters include not only the sacral slope (SS), but also pelvic tilt and pelvic incidence, which are proven to be associated with changes in pelvic spatial orientation and position [38,48]. However, our results only show SS as this was the only parameter that we could assess with the spinal mouse. All of these factors, as well as knee flexion during gait analysis, should be considered in future studies to confirm their influence in postural deformities, spinal mobility and QOL.

In conclusion, for the first time, the present study classified and compared the mobility and curvature in a Chinese population based on the entire spinal alignment. Types 4 and 5 were shown to have the worst balance in the Chinese elderly population, while type 3 demonstrated the best balance and mobility. We believe that future studies should look into the global spine change when trying to understand postural deformity and function. We also

believe that by doing so, it may serve as a convenient clinical marker signaling the falling risk and need for treatment strategies, including exercise and bracing which have shown to be useful for improving balance. Because spinal mobility was best correlated with quality of life and function, prevention and therapy should be especially applied to types 4 and 5 in the Chinese elderly population.

Author Contributions

Conceived and designed the experiments: HJW CC YKL. Performed the experiments: HJW WJZ WRL JYL XSJ QLZ XYZ GHY. Analyzed the data: HG HJW GHY. Wrote the paper: HG HJW CZ. Involved in the design of study analysis and revision of the manuscript: KNA.

References

1. Reginster JY, Burlet N (2006) Osteoporosis: a still increasing prevalence. Bone 38: S4–9. doi: 10.1016/j.bone.2005.11.024.
2. Briggs AM, Greig AM, Wark JD (2007) The vertebral fracture cascade in osteoporosis: a review of aetiopathogenesis. Osteoporosis International 18: 575–584. doi: 10.1007/s00198-006-0304-x.
3. Nevitt MC, Ettinger B, Black DM, Stone K, Jamal SA, et al. (1998) The association of radiographically detected vertebral fractures with back pain and function: a prospective study. Annals of Internal Medicine 128: 793–800.
4. Hongo M, Itoi E, Sinaki M, Miyakoshi N, Shimada Y, et al. (2007) Effect of low-intensity back exercise on quality of life and back extensor strength in patients with osteoporosis: a randomized controlled trial. Osteoporosis International 18: 1389–1395. doi: 10.1007/s00198-007-0398-9.
5. Huang MH, Barrett-Connor E, Greendale GA, Kado DM (2006) Hyperkyphotic posture and risk of future osteoporotic fractures: the Rancho Bernardo study. Journal of Bone & Mineral Research 21: 419–423. doi: 10.1359/JBMR.051201.
6. Imagama S, Matsuyama Y, Hasegawa Y, Sakai Y, Ito Z, et al. (2011) Back muscle strength and spinal mobility are predictors of quality of life in middle-aged and elderly males. European Spine Journal 20: 954–961. doi: 10.1007/s00586-010-1606-4.
7. Kado DM, Lui LY, Ensrud KE, Fink HA, Karlamangla AS, et al. (2009) Hyperkyphosis predicts mortality independent of vertebral osteoporosis in older women. Annals of Internal Medicine 150: 681–687.
8. Kasukawa Y, Miyakoshi N, Hongo M, Ishikawa Y, Noguchi H, et al. (2010) Relationships between falls, spinal curvature, spinal mobility and back extensor strength in elderly people. Journal of Bone & Mineral Metabolism 28: 82–87. doi: 10.1007/s00774-009-0107-1.
9. Katzman WB, Vittinghoff E, Kado DM (2011) Age-related hyperkyphosis, independent of spinal osteoporosis, is associated with impaired mobility in older community-dwelling women. Osteoporosis International 22: 85–90.
10. Lynn SG, Sinaki M, Westerlind KC (1997) Balance characteristics of persons with osteoporosis. Archives of Physical Medicine & Rehabilitation 78: 273–277. doi: 10.1016/S0003-9993(97)90033-2.
11. Martin AR, Sornay-Rendu E, Chandler JM, Duboeuf F, Girman CJ, et al. (2002) The impact of osteoporosis on quality-of-life: the OFELY cohort. Bone 31: 32–36. doi: 10.1016/S8756-3282(02)00787-1.
12. Mika A, Unnithan VB, Mika P (2005) Differences in thoracic kyphosis and in back muscle strength in women with bone loss due to osteoporosis. Spine 30: 241–246.
13. Miyakoshi N, Hongo M, Maekawa S, Ishikawa Y, Shimada Y, et al. (2007) Back extensor strength and lumbar spinal mobility are predictors of quality of life in patients with postmenopausal osteoporosis. Osteoporosis International 18: 1397–1403. doi: 10.1007/s00198-007-0383-3.
14. Miyakoshi N, Hongo M, Maekawa S, Ishikawa Y, Shimada Y, et al. (2005) Factors related to spinal mobility in patients with postmenopausal osteoporosis. Osteoporosis International 16: 1871–1874. doi: 10.1007/s00198-005-1953-x.
15. Miyakoshi N, Itoi E, Kobayashi M, Kodama H (2003) Impact of postural deformities and spinal mobility on quality of life in postmenopausal osteoporosis. Osteoporosis International doi: 14: 1007–1012. 10.1007/s00198-003-1510-4.
16. Ryan SD, Fried LP (1997) The impact of kyphosis on daily functioning. Journal of the American Geriatrics Society 45: 1479–1486.
17. Sinaki M, Brey RH, Hughes CA, Larson DR, Kaufman KR (2005) Balance disorder and increased risk of falls in osteoporosis and kyphosis: significance of kyphotic posture and muscle strength. Osteoporosis International 16: 1004–1010. doi: 10.1007/s00198-004-1791-2.
18. Sinaki M, Brey RH, Hughes CA, Larson DR, Kaufman KR (2005) Significant reduction in risk of falls and back pain in osteoporotic-kyphotic women through a Spinal Proprioceptive Extension Exercise Dynamic (SPEED) program. Mayo Clinic Proceedings 80: 849–855. doi: 10.4065/80.7.849.
19. Takahashi T, Ishida K, Hirose D, Nagano Y, Okumiya K, et al. (2005) Trunk deformity is associated with a reduction in outdoor activities of daily living and

life satisfaction in community-dwelling older people. Osteoporosis International 16: 273–279. doi: 10.1007/s00198-004-1669-3.
20. Schneider DL, von Muhlen D, Barrett-Connor E, Sartoris DJ (2004) Kyphosis does not equal vertebral fractures: the Rancho Bernardo study. Journal of Rheumatology 31: 747–752.
21. de Boer J, Andressoo JO, de Wit J, et al. (2002) Premature aging in mice deficient in DNA repair and transcription. Science 296: 1276–1279. doi: 10.1126/science.1070174.
22. Hinman MR (2004) Comparison of thoracic kyphosis and postural stiffness in younger and older women. Spine Journal: Official Journal of the North American Spine Society 4: 413–417. doi: 10.1016/j.spinee.2004.01.002.
23. Sinaki M, Wollan PC, Scott RW, Gelczer RK (1996) Can strong back extensors prevent vertebral fractures in women with osteoporosis? Mayo Clinic Proceedings 71: 951–956. doi: 10.4065/71.10.951.
24. Tuzun C, Yorulmaz I, Cindas A, Vatan S (1999) Low back pain and posture. Clinical Rheumatology 18: 308–312.
25. Jackson RP, McManus AC (1994) Radiographic analysis of sagittal plane alignment and balance in standing volunteers and patients with low back pain matched for age, sex, and size. A prospective controlled clinical study. Spine 19: 1611–1618.
26. Ishikawa Y, Miyakoshi N, Kasukawa Y, Hongo M, Shimada Y (2009) Spinal curvature and postural balance in patients with osteoporosis. Osteoporosis International 20: 2049–2053. doi: 10.1007/s00198-009-0919-9.
27. Satoh K, Kasama F, Itoi E, et al. (1988) Clinical features of spinal osteoporosis: spinal deformity and pertinent back pain. Contemp Orthop 16: 23–30.
28. Staffel F (1889) Die menschlichen Haltungstypen und ihre Beziehungen zu den Ruckgratverkrummungen. J. F. Bergman, Wiesbaden.
29. Hongo M, Miyakoshi N, Shimada Y, Sinaki M (2011) Association of spinal curve deformity and back extensor strength in elderly women with osteoporosis in Japan and the United States. Osteoporos Int doi: 10.1007/s00198-011-1624-z.
30. Cheung E, Tsang S, Bow C, Soong C, Yeung S, et al. (2011) Bone loss during menopausal transition among southern Chinese women. Maturitas 69: 50–56. doi: 10.1016/j.maturitas.2011.01.010.
31. Post RB, Leferink VJ (2004) Spinal mobility: sagittal range of motion measured with the SpinalMouse, a new non-invasive device. Archives of Orthopaedic & Trauma Surgery 124: 187–192. doi: 10.1007/s00402-004-0641-1.
32. Takemitsu Y, Harada Y, Iwahara T, Miyamoto M, Miyatake Y (1988) Lumbar degenerative kyphosis. Clinical, radiological and epidemiological studies. Spine 13: 1317–1326.
33. Roussouly P, Gollogly S, Berthonnaud E, Dimnet J (2005) Classification of the normal variation in the sagittal alignment of the human lumbar spine and pelvis in the standing position. Spine 30: 346–353.
34. Lee CS, Chung SS, Kang KC, Park SJ, Shin SK (2011) Normal patterns of Sagittal Alignment of the Spine in Young Adults Radiological analysis in a Korean population. Spine (Phila Pa 1976): 10.1097/BRS.0b013e318216b0fd.
35. Smith A, O'Sullivan P, Straker L (2008) Classification of sagittal thoraco-lumbo-pelvic alignment of the adolescent spine in standing and its relationship to low back pain. Spine 33: 2101–2107.
36. Wiles P (1937) Postural deformities of the anteroposterior curves of the spine. Lancet 17: 911–919. doi: 10.1016/S0140-6736(00)82825-1.
37. Itoi E (1991) Roentgenographic analysis of posture in spinal osteoporotics. Spine 16: 750–756.
38. Jean-Marc Mac-Thiong, P. Roussouly, Berthonnaud E (2011) Age-and sex-related variations in sagittal sacropelvic morphology and balance in asymptomatic adults. Eur Spine J 20 (Suppl 5): S572–S577.
39. Ibrahim Obeid, Olivier Hauger, Ste'phane Aunoble (2011) Global analysis of sagittal spinal alignment in major deformities: correlation between lack of lumbar lordosis and flexion of the knee. Eur Spine J 20 (Suppl 5): S681–S685.
40. Pierre Roussouly, Sohrab Gollogly, Eric Berthonnaud (2005) Classification of the Normal Variation in the Sagittal Alignment of the Human Lumbar Spine and Pelvis in the Standing Position. Spine (30) 3: 346 –353.

41. Sergio Mendoza-Lattes, Zachary Ries, Yubo Gao (2010) Natural History of Spinopelvic Alignment Differs From Symptomatic Deformity of the Spine. Spine (35) 16: E792–E798.

42. Stagnara P, De Mauroy JC, Dran G, Gonon G, Costanzo G, et al. (1982) Reciprocal angulation of vertebral bodies in a sagittal plane: approach to references for the evaluation of kyphosis and lordosis. Spine (Phila Pa 1976) 7(4): 335–342.

43. Barrey C, Jund J, Noseda O, Roussouly P (2007) Sagittal balance of the pelvis-spine complex and lumbar degenerative diseases. A comparative study of about 85 cases. Eur Spine J 16(9): 1459–1467.

44. Jang JS, Lee SH, Min JH, Maeng DH (2007) Changes in sagittal alignment after restoration of lower lumbar lordosis in patients with degenerative flat back syndrome. J Neurosurg Spine 7(4): 387–392.

45. A Mannion, K Knecht, G Balaban, J Dvorak, D Grob (2004) A new skin-surface device for measuring the curvature and global and segmental ranges of motion of the spine: reliability of measurements and comparison with data reviewed from the literature. Eur Spine J 13: 122–136. DOI 10.1007/s00586-003-0618-8.

46. Imagama S, Matsuyama Y, Hasegawa Y, Sakai Y, Ito Z, et al. (2011) Back muscle strength and spinal mobility are predictors of quality of life in middle-aged and elderly males. European Spine Journal 20: 954–961. doi: 10.1007/s00586-010-1606-4.

47. Barón Zárate-Kalfópulos, Samuel Romero-Vargas, Eduardo Otero-CáMara (2012) Differences in pelvic parameters among Mexican, Caucasian, and Asian populations. J Neurosurg: Spine 2: 1–4.

48. Legaye J, Duval-Beaup ère G, Hecquet J, et al. (1998) Pelvic incidence: a fundamental pelvic parameter for 3D regulation of spinal sagittal curves. Eur Spine J. 7: 99 –103.

9

Bone Turnover and Metabolism in Patients with Early Multiple Sclerosis and Prevalent Bone Mass Deficit

Stine Marit Moen[1]*, Elisabeth Gulowsen Celius[1], Leiv Sandvik[2], Magritt Brustad[3], Lars Nordsletten[4], Erik Fink Eriksen[5], Trygve Holmøy[6,7]

1 Department of Neurology, Oslo University Hospital Ullevål, Oslo, Norway, 2 Section of Epidemiology and Biostatistics, Oslo University Hospital Ullevål, Oslo, Norway, 3 Department of Community Medicine, University of Tromsø, Tromsø, Norway, 4 Orthopedic Department, Oslo University Hospital Ullevål, Oslo, Norway, 5 Department of Endocrinology, Oslo University Hospital, Oslo, Norway, 6 Department of Neurology, Akershus University Hospital, Lørenskog, Norway, 7 Institute of Clinical Medicine, University of Oslo, Oslo, Norway

Abstract

Background: Low bone mass is prevalent in ambulatory multiple sclerosis (MS) patients even shortly after clinical onset. The mechanism is not known, but could involve shared etiological risk factors between MS and low bone mass such as hypovitaminosis D operating before disease onset, or increased bone loss after disease onset. The aim of this study was to explore the mechanism of the low bone mass in early-stage MS patients.

Methodology/Principal Findings: We performed a population-based case-control study comparing bone turnover (cross-linked N-terminal telopeptide of type 1 collagen; NTX, bone alkaline phosphatase; bALP), metabolism (25-hydroxy- and 1, 25-dihydroxyvitamin D, calcium, phosphate, and parathyroid hormone), and relevant lifestyle factors in 99 patients newly diagnosed with clinically isolated syndrome (CIS) or MS, and in 159 age, sex, and ethnicity matched controls. After adjustment for possible confounders, there were no significant differences in NTX (mean 3.3; 95% CI −6.9, 13.5; p = 0.519), bALP (mean 1.6; 95% CI −0.2, 3.5; p = 0.081), or in any of the parameters related to bone metabolism in patients compared to controls. The markers of bone turnover and metabolism were not significantly correlated with bone mass density, or associated with the presence of osteoporosis or osteopenia within or between the patient and control groups. Intake of vitamin D and calcium, reported UV exposure, and physical activity did not differ significantly.

Conclusions/Significance: Bone turnover and metabolism did not differ significantly in CIS and MS patients with prevalent low bone mass compared to controls. These findings indicate that the bone deficit in patients newly diagnosed with MS and CIS is not caused by recent acceleration of bone loss, and are compatible with shared etiological factors between MS and low bone mass.

Editor: Celia Oreja-Guevara, University Hospital La Paz, Spain

Funding: Study funding: Supported by research grants from the South-Eastern Norway Regional Health Authority, Ulleval University Hospital, Odd Fellow Research Foundation for Multiple Sclerosis, the Endowment of K. and K. H. Hemsen, and the Endowment of Fritz and Ingrid Nilsen. The funders had no role in study design, data collection and analysis, decision to publish, or preparation of the manuscript.

Competing Interests: I have read the journal's policy and have the following conflicts. Stine Marit Moen has received funding for travel from Biogen Idec and European Charcot Foundation and has received research support from the South-Eastern Norway Regional Health Authority, Ullevål University Hospital, Biogen Idec, Odd Fellow Research Foundation for Multiple Sclerosis, the Endowment of K. and K.H. Hemsen, and the Endowment of Fritz and Ingrid Nilsen. Elisabeth Gulowsen Celius has received funding for travel and speaker honoraria from Sanofi-Aventis, Merck Serono, Biogen Idec, Bayer Schering Pharma, Teva, and Novartis; and receives research support from Biogen Idec and Novartis. Lars Nordsletten serves on scientific advisory boards for Novartis and DePuy Mitek, Inc.; has received funding for travel and speaker honoraria from Novartis, DePuy Mitek, Inc., Biomet Inc., Amgen, and Stryker, and serves on the editorial board of Acta Orthopaedica. Erik Fink Eriksen has served as a consultant for Eli Lilly and Company, Amgen, and Novartis; and serves on speakers' bureaus for Novartis and Eli Lilly and Company. Trygve Holmøy has received funding for travel and speaker honoraria from Sanofi-Aventis, Merck Serono, Biogen Idec, Bayer Schering Pharma, and Novartis. This does not alter our adherence to all the PLoS ONE policies on sharing data and materials. The authors Magritt Brustad and Leiv Sandvik have declared that no competing interests exist.

* E-mail: s.m.moen@medisin.uio.no

Introduction

Multiple sclerosis (MS) is a demyelinating inflammatory disease of the central nervous system [1]. Patients with long-standing MS have an increased risk of osteoporosis and fractures due to reduced bone mass and falls [2–5]. As in many other chronic diseases, disability leading to disuse and reduced mechanical loading of bone is likely an important risk factor for osteoporosis in patients

with long-standing MS [6,7]. The roles of other possible factors contributing to reduced bone mass or bone mineral density (BMD), such as low levels of vitamin D, medications in the course of disease, and the inflammatory process itself, are less clear [8].

MS results from an interplay between genetic susceptibility and environment, and growing evidence suggests that hypovitaminosis D is a risk factor [9]. Vitamin D is essential for bone growth, preservation, and mineral homeostasis, and has also immunomodulatory effects [10]. Environmental factors such as hypovitaminosis D acting from conception to early adult life might be of importance for the risk of MS [11–13]. During the same period the skeleton acquires a peak bone mass influenced by genetic and environmental factors, including vitamin D status [14]. If hypovitaminosis D is a risk factor for MS, it is conceivable that MS patients have low bone mass already at the time of diagnosis. We have earlier found that low bone mass was more prevalent in newly diagnosed patients with MS and clinically isolated syndrome (CIS) suggestive of demyelinating disease than in controls [15]. This finding is compatible with the hypothesis that MS and osteoporosis share etiological factors, and that the bone deficit in the newly diagnosed patients could be explained by low bone mass before disease onset. An alternative explanation could be increased bone loss after disease onset, which would be reflected by increased bone turnover or perturbated bone metabolism at the time of BMD assessment.

The bone tissue is continually adapting to various inputs, and coupled bone formation and bone resorption is a dynamic process that occurs throughout life [16]. While BMD reflects the sum of peak bone mass and the amount of subsequent bone loss, changes in bone turnover markers occur more rapidly and provide a dynamic view into the current bone metabolism. The bone resorption marker cross-linked N-terminal telopeptide of type 1 collagen (NTX) is a breakdown product of type 1 collagen and reflects degradation of bone matrix, whereas bone alkaline phosphatase (bALP) secreted from osteoblasts reflects bone formation [17]. The overall aim of this study was to explore the mechanism of the low bone mass previously recorded in patients newly diagnosed with CIS and MS compared to controls [15]. We therefore assessed NTX, bALP, vitamin D metabolites, and other biochemical and lifestyle factors related to bone metabolism in patients newly diagnosed with MS or CIS and controls.

Methods

Ethics Statement

The study was approved by the Regional Ethics Committee for Medical Research in South-Eastern Norway Regional Health Authority, the Review Board of Oslo University Hospital Ullevål, and the National Population Registry, Norway and carried out in accordance with the Helsinki Declaration. Written informed consent was obtained from all participants.

Study Design and Participants

The design of this population-based case-control study has been described previously [15]. Briefly, all 107 patients living in Oslo and diagnosed with CIS or MS according to the McDonald criteria [18] between January 2005 and January 2008 were invited to participate. Ninety-nine (92.5%) patients participated in the study. The mean duration from first symptom of demyelinating disease to study examination was 1.6±1.3 years, and mean expanded disability status scale (EDSS) score was 1.4±1.1. Age-, sex-, and ethnicity-matched controls were randomly selected from the National Population Registry, and 275 (45.8%) of the subjects selected responded, of whom 219 (79.6%) were willing to participate. Of these, one control was randomly selected for each patient. In addition, the patients recruited 60 unrelated controls of the same sex, age (±5 years), ethnicity, and for women the same menopausal phase.

Data Collection

Blood and urine samples from paired patients and controls were preferentially collected at the same date or during a restricted time period (±2 weeks) from May 2007 to September 2008. Serum 25-hydroxyvitamin D (25(OH)D) and 1,25-dihydroxyvitamin D (1,25(OH)$_2$D) were measured by competitive radioimmunoassay (RIA) (DiaSorin, Stillwater, MN, USA), vitamin D binding protein (DBP) was measured with RIA using human Gc-globulin (Sigma, St.Louis, USA) and rabbit polyclonal anti-Gc-globulin antibody (DakoCytomation, Glostrup, Denmark), and parathyroid hormone (PTH) was measured with non-competitive immunoluminometric assay (ILMA, Immulite 2500 Diagnostic Products Corporation, Los Angeles, Ca, USA) at the Hormone Laboratory at Oslo University Hospital Aker. The RIA detected both the D$_2$ and D$_3$ forms of 25(OH)D and 1,25(OH)$_2$D. The coefficients of variation (CV) were 6% intra-assay and 13–16% inter-assay for 25-(OH)D, 8–12% intra-assay and 14–20% inter-assay for 1,25(OH)$_2$ D, 5% intra-assay and 12–14% inter-assay for DBP, 3–5% intra-assay and 8–9% inter-assay for PTH. Serum bALP was measured by an enzyme immunoassay kit (Metra Biosystems Inc., Mountain View, CA, USA), and the enzyme activity was measured in U/l where one unit of bALP activity was defined as 1 µmol of p-nitrophenyl phosphate hydrolyzed per minute at 25°C in 2-amino-2 methyl-1-propanol. The intra-assay and inter-assay CV values were 2–6% and 12–13%, respectively. Serum ionized calcium (Ca), creatinine, and phosphate were measured according to standard laboratory techniques. NTX in the second morning void urine was measured by competitive enzyme immunoassay (12–20% intra-assay and 12–19% inter-assay CV).

A questionnaire including medication, comorbidity, menstrual status, smoking, alcohol, diet (food frequency), physical activity, and sun exposure was mailed to the participants and collected at the time of study examination. Comorbidity was assessed by asking the participants if they had any chronic diseases with the answer categories "yes" or "no", with further specification if "yes". Relevant medications with possible skeletal effects were noted to determine possible confounding [15]. A validated self-administered food frequency questionnaire [19] was used to assess average intake of vitamin D (µg per day) and calcium (mg per day) the preceding year. The nutrients were computed using nutrient values from the Norwegian Food Composition Table (2006) and analyzed with Statistical Analysis System (SAS) software package, version 9.1 (SAS Institute Inc, Cary, NC) at the Department of Community Medicine, University of Tromsø, Norway. Current physical activity was recorded on a scale ranging from 1 to 10 and categorized as "low" (1–3), "moderate" (4–7), and "high" (8–10) [20]. The questionnaire also covered ultraviolet (UV)/sun exposure including solarium use, sun holidays in southern latitudes (Mediterranean and near equator), and sun tanning in Norway and in northern latitudes the two months prior to blood and urine sampling [19]. The level of disability (EDSS) [21] and other details related to past medical history, including recent childbirth and breastfeeding (last 12 months), were recorded by a neurologist.

Missing Data

Four PTH, three Ca, one bALP, one phosphate, and three NTX values from controls, and one phosphate value from a patient were missing due to technical errors. One patient and six controls did not answer the question about current physical activity. One patient and one control did not answer the question about solarium use, and one patient did not answer the question about sun tanning in Norway the preceding two months.

Statistical Analysis

Statistical analyses included independent-samples two-tailed t tests for continuous variables, Mann-Whitney U test for not normally distributed data, and Chi-square test for dichotomous variables for comparison of groups. Unpaired analyzes were used because the parity of the matching was incomplete. Results are expressed as mean ± SD or as number (percentages) unless otherwise stated. Pearson's or Spearman's rank correlation coefficients (r) were calculated for bivariate correlations between variables depending on their distribution. Possible confounders were identified by checking whether the variable in question was associated with the measure, or whether it differed significantly between patients and controls. Adjustments for the possible confounders were performed using multivariate linear regression for numerical outcomes. The possible confounders were analyzed as independent variables separately and simultaneously in the regression models. The following outcome variables were analyzed as dependent: NTX, phosphate, left femoral neck BMD, total body BMD, and nondominant radius BMD. Multiple linear regression was also used to analyze the interactions between bone mass status (osteoporosis/osteopenia or normal) and participant status (patient or control) in the association analyses of biochemical parameters. The interaction term was a combination of bone mass status (osteoporosis or osteopenia/normal bone mass) and participant status (patient/control). A variance inflation factor >5 was used as criterion for multicollinearity. Missing values were not replaced. Statistical significance was defined as $p < 0.05$. All analyses were conducted using SPSS (version 18, SPSS, Chicago, IL).

Results

The blood and urine samples from paired patients and controls were obtained within mean 4.4±8.7 days (median 0, range 0–64.0). Patients exhibited higher urine NTX and serum phosphate levels compared to controls (Table 1). The other biochemical parameters of bone turnover and metabolism, including vitamin D status–serum levels of 25(OH)D, 1, 25(OH)$_2$D, DBP, bALP, Ca, and PTH–did not differ between patients and controls. Two (2.0%) patients and 3 (1.9%) controls had vitamin D deficiency defined as 25(OH)D <25 nmol/l, and 21 (21.2%) patients and 31 (19.5%) controls were below 50 nmol/l. Thirty-eight (38.4%) patients and 60 (37.7%) controls had 25(OH)D ≥75 nmol/l.

In order to identify possible confounders we assessed factors that may influence bone metabolism. Use of systemic glucocorticoids, current smoking, use of alcohol, recent childbirth, and breastfeed-

ing differed significantly between patients and controls (Table 2). There was no significant difference in estimated daily intake of vitamin D and calcium between patients and controls, or in current physical activity, use of solarium, or sun tanning in Norway or at lower latitudes in the preceding two months. Participants who had recently given birth, were breastfeeding, had begun menopausal transition, or reported no sun exposure in northern latitudes the preceding 2 months revealed higher NTX levels than those not being exposed to these factors ($p < 0.001$, $p < 0.001$, $p = 0.043$, and $p = 0.001$, respectively). NTX did not differ significantly between those who had or had not been exposed to the other variables that could affect bone metabolism or remodeling listed in Table 2.

The impact on NTX of potential confounders (variables that either differed significantly between patients and controls or were significantly associated with NTX) were analyzed both separately and simultaneously with multiple linear regression. NTX was analyzed as a dependent variable and the following as independent variables: use of systemic glucocorticoids, current smoking, use of alcohol, recent childbirth, breastfeeding, begun menopausal transition, sun tanning in northern latitudes preceding two months, and phosphate. After adjusting for these factors, the difference in NTX between patients and controls was no longer significant (Table 3).

As patients exhibited higher serum levels of phosphate than controls, the impact of possible confounders on phosphate was investigated. Phosphate was higher in participants who had recently given birth ($p < 0.001$), were breastfeeding ($p < 0.001$), or had used systemic glucocorticoids ($p = 0.017$) compared to those who had not been exposed to these factors. Phosphate was included as a dependent variable and use of systemic glucocorticoids, recent childbirth, and breastfeeding as independent variables in the regression model (again recent childbirth and breastfeeding were not included simultaneously in the regression analysis due to the high correlation).The difference in phosphate between patients and controls did not remain significant when adjusting for recent childbirth and use of systemic glucocorticoids ($\beta = 0.026$; 95% CI -0.019, 0.071; $p = 0.262$), or breastfeeding and use of systemic glucocorticoids ($\beta = 0.025$; 95% CI -0.020, 0.070; $p = 0.273$).

In order to further examine whether there were perturbations in bone metabolism in the CIS and MS patients, we compared the

Table 1. Biochemical markers (mean ± SD) of vitamin D status, bone turnover and metabolism in patients and controls.

	Patients (n = 99)	Controls (n = 159)	95% CI	p value
25(OH)D (nmol/l)	68.4±24.5	68.5±22.9	−6.0, 5.9	0.992
1,25(OH)$_2$D (pmol/l)	119.9±43.7	127.0±44.9	−18.4, 4.1	0.211
PTH (pmol/l)	3.55±1.89	3.68±1.83	−0.60, 0.34	0.585
Ionized calcium (mmol/l)	1.27±0.03	1.27±0.04	−0.01, 0.01	0.986
Phosphate (mmol/l)	1.14±0.15	1.09±0.16	0.01, 0.09	0.012
DBP (μmol/l)	4.28±0.72	4.18±0.73	−0.08, 0.29	0.255
Creatinine (μmol/l)	66.2±11.1	69.0±11.8	−5.7, 0.1	0.060
bALP (U^a/l)	24.2±7.6	22.6±7.2	−0.2, 3.5	0.081
NTX (nmol/l BCE^b/mmol/l Cr^c)	54.7±42.2	44.6±23.0	2.1, 18.2	0.030

25(OH)D: 25-hydroxyvitamin D, 1,25(OH)$_2$D: 1,25-dihydroxyvitamin D, PTH: parathyroid hormone, DBP: vitamin D binding protein, bALP: bone alkaline phosphatase, NTX: cross-linked N-terminal telopeptide of type 1 collagen (all measured in serum, except NTX that was measured in urine).
^{a}Enzyme activity measured in U/l, 1U: one unit of bALP activity was defined as 1 μmol of p-nitrophenyl phosphate hydrolyzed per minute at 25°C,
^{b}BCE: Bone Collagen Equivalents,
^{c}Cr: Creatinine. Comparison of groups was calculated using independent two-tailed t test. CI: mean difference confidence interval.

Table 2. Distribution of factors that may influence current bone metabolism.

	Patients (n=99)	Controls (n=159)	p value
Vitamin D intake (µg per day), **preceding year**, (mean ± SD)	8.1±8.1	8.0±6.4	0.899
Calcium intake intake (mg per day), **preceding year**, (mean ± SD)	648±293	633±268	0.667
UV/sun exposure preceding 2 months, n (%)			
Solarium >1 per month	15 (15.3)	23 (14.6)	0.870
Sun tanning in northern latitudes ≥1 week	17 (17.3)	35 (22.0)	0.366
Sun tanning in southern latitudes[a] ≥1 week	10 (10.1)	21 (13.2)	0.455
Current physical activity, n (%)			0.057
Low	23 (23.5)	19 (12.4)	n/a
Moderate	61 (62.2)	114 (74.5)	n/a
High	14 (14.3)	20 (13.1)	n/a
Ever used iv or po glucocorticoids, n (%)	38 (38.4)	1 (0.6)	<0.001
Ever used inhalation glucocorticoids, n (%)	3 (3.0)	7 (4.4)	0.579
Have other relevant diseases, n (%)	8 (8.1)	11 (6.9)	0.728
Use other relevant medication, n (%)	8 (8.1)	10 (6.3)	0.583
Current smokers, n (%)	31 (31.3)	27 (17.0)	0.007
Alcohol more often than 1/week, n (%)	33 (33.3)	76 (47.8)	0.022
Begun menopausal transition[b], n (%)	8 (11.3)	10 (8.5)	0.539
Absent menstruation[b], n (%)	15 (21.1)	15 (12.8)	0.132
Hormonal treatment[b], n (%)	11 (15.5)	15 (12.8)	0.607
Recently given birth[b], n (%)	7 (9.9)	2 (1.7)	0.011
Breastfeeding[b], n (%)	6 (8.5)	1 (0.9)	0.008

iv: intravenous, po: per oral.
[a]Mediterranean or other destinations nearer equator than Norway.
[b]percentages of female participants (female patients, n=71; female controls, n=117). Comparison of groups was calculated using Chi-square test and independent-samples two-tailed t test.

Table 3. Differences in urine NTX between patients and controls, without and with adjustment for possible confounders.

	β (95% CI)	p value
Unadjusted	10.2 (2.1, 18.2)	0.014
Adjusted for:		
Recent childbirth	6.9 (−0.8, 14.7)	0.079
Breastfeeding	6.0 (−1.5, 13.6)	0.117
Ever used iv or po glucocorticoids	8.1 (−1.3, 17.5)	0.090
Current smoking	10.6 (2.4, 18.8)	0.011
Alcohol use	9.7 (1.6, 17.9)	0.020
Begun menopausal transition	9.6 (0.3, 18.9)	0.044
Sun tanning in northern latitudes preceding 2 months	9.6 (1.6, 17.7)	0.019
Phosphate	8.9 (0.7, 17.0)	0.033
Recent childbirth, systemic glucocorticoids, current smoking, alcohol use, begun menopausal transition, sun tanning in northern latitudes preceding 2 months, and phosphate.	3.6 (−6.9, 14.1)	0.497
Breastfeeding, systemic glucocorticoids, current smoking, alcohol use, begun menopausal transition, sun tanning in northern latitudes preceding 2 months, and phosphate.	3.3 (−6.9, 13.5)	0.519

β: unstandardized β coefficient, CI: β confidence interval. NTX (cross-linked N-terminal telopeptide of type 1 collagen) was analyzed as dependent and the following as independent variables (separately and simultaneously): recent childbirth, breastfeeding, systemic glucocorticoids, current smoking, alcohol use, began menopausal transition, sun tanning in northern latitudes, and phosphate. Recent childbirth and breastfeeding were not included simultaneously in the regression analysis due to their high correlation (r=0.921; p<0.001).

correlations between markers of bone turnover and metabolism between patients and controls. Both bALP and NTX showed positive correlations in both patients (r = 0.553; p<0.0001) and controls (r = 0.405; p<0.0001). Serum 25(OH)D and 1,25(OH)$_2$D also exhibited positive correlations in patients (r = 0.342; p = 0.001) and in controls (r = 0.255; p = 0.001). There was a significant inverse correlation between 25(OH)D and PTH in the controls (r = −0.218; p = 0.007), but this inverse correlation was not significant among the patients (r = −0.123; p = 0.226). There was a significant inverse correlation between PTH and Ca in both patients (r = −0.280; p = 0.005) and controls (r = −0.402; p<0.001). The strength of these correlations did not differ between patients and controls.

There were no significant differences in the levels of 25(OH)D, 1,25(OH)$_2$D, bALP, NTX, PTH, or Ca among patients or controls with either osteoporosis or osteopenia compared to those with normal bone mass (Table 4). Applying multiple linear regression with a combination of bone mass status (osteoporosis or osteopenia/normal bone mass) and participant status (patient/control) as interaction term, we found that the associations between the biochemical parameters and bone status were unaffected by participant status (data not shown).

There was no significant correlation between 25(OH)D and BMD at any of the skeletal sites in patients or controls (Table 5). There was, however, a significant inverse correlation between 1,25(OH)$_2$D and BMD in the left femoral neck, total body, and nondominant ultradistal radius among the patients, but not among the controls (Table 5). The correlations between BMD and 1,25(OH)$_2$D did not remain significant after adjusting for variables associated with BMD at each skeletal site (i.e. use of inhalation glucocorticoids) or variables which differed significantly between patients and controls (i.e. use of systemic glucocorticoids, current smoking, use of alcohol, recent childbirth, breastfeeding, NTX, and phosphate) in multivariate linear regression analyses (left femoral neck; p = 0.518, total body; p = 0.586, and nondominant ultradistal radius; p = 0.071), using BMD at each skeletal site as dependent variables and use of inhalation glucocorticoids, use of systemic glucocorticoids, current smoking, use of alcohol, recent childbirth, breastfeeding, NTX, and phosphate as independent variables. Finally, there were no significant associations (analyzed with linear regression) between EDSS and any of the markers of

bone turnover or metabolism in the patient group (data not shown).

Table 5. Correlations between bone mineral density (BMD) and vitamin D metabolites and PTH.

	Patients (n = 99)		Controls (n = 159)	
	Pearson's r	p value	Pearson's r	p value
Correlation between 25(OH)D and BMD				
Lumbar spine	0.008	0.939	0.108	0.176
Total hip	0.130	0.198	0.046	0.570
Left femoral neck	0.107	0.291	0.046	0.565
Right femoral neck	0.094	0.354	0.048	0.547
Total body	0.083	0.414	−0.024	0.767
Nondominant ultradistal radius	−0.063	0.536	−0.027	0.741
Correlation between 1,25(OH)$_2$D and BMD				
Lumbar spine	−0.078	0.444	0.057	0.475
Total hip	−0.190	0.060	0.029	0.715
Left femoral neck	−0.221	0.028	0.026	0.749
Right femoral neck	−0.160	0.114	0.002	0.980
Total body	−0.218	0.030	0.055	0.492
Nondominant ultradistal radius	−0.306	0.002	−0.013	0.872
Correlation between PTH and BMD				
Lumbar spine	−0.023	0.822	−0.022	0.788
Total hip	−0.011	0.911	−0.117	0.149
Left femoral neck	−0.087	0.391	−0.134	0.097
Right femoral neck	−0.077	0.449	−0.127	0.117
Total body	−0.023	0.825	−0.078	0.336
Nondominant ultradistal radius	0.114	0.259	−0.129	0.112

BMD: bone mineral density, 25(OH)D: 25-hydroxyvitamin D, 1,25(OH)$_2$D: 1,25-dihydroxyvitamin D, PTH: parathyroid hormone, r: correlation coefficient.

Table 4. Biochemical measures (mean ± SD) of vitamin D status, bone turnover and metabolism in patients and controls with different bone status.

	Patients				Controls			
	Low BM (n = 50)	Normal BM (n = 49)	Mean diff (95% CI)	p value	Low BM (n = 59)	Normal BM (n = 100)	Mean diff (95% CI)	p value
25(OH)D	67.1±23.7	69.8±25.5	−2.6 (−12.4, 7.2)	0.598	66.9±22.3	69.4±23.2	−2.5 (−9.9, 4.9)	0.513
1,25(OH)$_2$D	123.2±46.0	116.5±41.4	6.6 (−10.8, 24.1)	0.452	127.9±39.9	126.5±47.8	1.4 (−13.3, 16.0)	0.855
PTH	3.64±1.91	3.46±1.89	0.18 (−0.58, 0.95)	0.637	3.90±1.92	3.54±1.78	0.36 (−0.24, 0.96)	0.238
ionCa	1.27±0.04	1.27±0.03	0.003 (−0.01, 0.02)	0.648	1.27±0.04	1.28±0.04	−0.009 (−0.02, 0.003)	0.135
bALP	24.6±8.9	23.9±6.1	0.7 (−3.8, 2.4)	0.648	22.3±6.7	22.7±7.5	−0.4 (−2.0, 2.7)	0.764
NTX	60.9±52.8	48.5±26.6	12.5 (−29.2, 4.3)	0.142	48.8±25.0	42.1±21.6	6.7 (−14.2, 0.8)	0.080

Low BM: low bone mass; osteoporosis or osteopenia, mean diff: mean difference, 25(OH)D: 25-hydroxyvitamin D, 1,25(OH)$_2$D: 1,25-dihydroxyvitamin D, PTH: parathyroid hormone, ionCa: ionized calcium, bALP: bone alkaline phosphatase, NTX: cross-linked N-terminal telopeptide of type 1 collagen. Comparison of groups was calculated using independent two-tailed t test. CI: confidence interval.

Discussion

The main findings in this study were that biochemical markers of bone turnover and metabolism, including vitamin D status, did not differ significantly between newly diagnosed CIS and MS patients with prevalent low bone mass and controls after adjusting for relevant confounders. There were no significant associations of biochemical parameters with bone status within or between the patient and control groups.

The lack of association between markers of bone turnover and BMD is in line with previous findings in ambulatory premenopausal female patients [22] and also in physically active patients of both sexes [23], both with more long-standing MS and higher EDSS than in our patients. Several studies of young MS patients (<55 years) with longer disease duration than our patients have found that vitamin D levels were not associated with reduced BMD [24–27]. Our findings are at odds with a study showing negative correlation between bALP and trochanter BMD [24]. Notably, these patients had much longer disease duration and more pronounced disability than our patients, and no other associations between biochemical bone markers and BMD were found. Nevertheless, one of these studies reported lower levels of the bone formation marker osteocalcin, higher bone resorption markers (pyridinoline and deoxypyridinoline), and higher PTH in premenopausal women with relapsing remitting MS compared to controls [22]. However, only PTH was inversely correlated with lumbar BMD [22]. Differences in disability levels, disease duration, biochemical parameters of bone metabolism, and measured BMD sites may contribute to the conflicting results.

Vitamin D deficiency may cause reduced acquisition of bone during growth and enhanced bone loss in adults [10,14]. At latitudes ≥42° North (e.g. Oslo, Norway, 59° North) the solar UV-B radiation in winter is insufficient for cutaneous production of vitamin D [28]. The major circulating vitamin D metabolite, 25(OH)D, is sensitive to both recent UV exposure and vitamin D intake [10,19]. Hydroxylation of 25(OH)D to bioactive 1,25(OH)$_2$D by 25-hydroxyvitamin D-1α-hydroxylase (CYP27B1) in the kidneys is tightly regulated by Ca, phosphate, PTH, and by negative feedback from 1,25(OH)$_2$D [10]. Both the genes encoding CYP27B1 and 25-hydroxyvitamin D-24-hydroxylase (CYP24A1) that catalyzes breakdown of 1,25(OH)$_2$D may be associated with MS risk [29,30]. PTH enhances the renal reabsorption of calcium and stimulates production of 1,25(OH)$_2$D and bone resorption. 1,25(OH)$_2$D increases intestinal absorption of Ca and phosphate. Vitamin D deficiency leads to decreased intestinal Ca absorption and secondary increased PTH [10]. Given the high prevalence of low BMD among the patients in our study, one might have expected to find perturbations in bone turnover and metabolism. However, the relationship between markers of bone formation (bALP) and resorption (NTX) and the correlations between biochemical indices of bone metabolism (25(OH)D and PTH, PTH and Ca) were consistent and not significantly different between patients and controls. Thus, the bone deficit found in these newly diagnosed patients seems less likely to be a result of a recent acceleration of bone turnover.

We did not find significant differences in measured 25(OH)D or 1,25(OH)$_2$D, estimated vitamin D intake, or reported sun/UV exposure in patients compared to controls. This is at variance with studies that have reported lower 25(OH)D [25,31–36] or 1,25(OH)$_2$D [33] levels in MS patients than in controls, but concur with other studies showing no significant differences in 25(OH)D [37–40] or 1,25(OH)$_2$D [37,39], including patients with low disability [32] and short disease duration [31]. These differences might be due to small sample sizes and different

selection of participants between studies (e.g. exclusion of subjects with possible negative bone-influential factors and controls chosen from hospital staff rather than general population). Higher EDSS has been found to be associated with reduced sun exposure [32]. As expected from the vitamin D measurements, our patients did not report different recent sun/UV exposure compared to controls. We confirm the positive association between serum 25(OH)D and 1,25(OH)$_2$D previously reported in MS patients [37,41], indicating dependency on the availability of 25(OH)D for 1,25(OH)$_2$D synthesis, although the renal activity of CYP27B1 is strictly regulated.

Smoking is another potential risk factor for both MS and osteoporosis [14,42] and was more common among patients than controls in our study. However, the proportion of current smokers was relatively low, and smoking did not influence the levels of NTX. Short-term glucocorticoid treatment of MS relapses can trigger immediate changes in bone metabolism and turnover [43,44], but has not been consistently related to markers of bone turnover in MS [22]. The use of systemic glucocorticoids did not significantly influence the levels of NTX or bALP in our participants. Our findings cohere with observations in non MS-populations [45]. As the use of systemic glucocorticoids was mainly in the patient group, it could be argued that such treatment was approaching a status as an intermediary variable/mediator (in the causal path between MS and bone status) and should consequently not be adjusted for. When excluding the use of systemic glucocorticoids from the analyses of NTX, the difference in mean NTX between MS patients and controls remained non-significant (data not shown). However, both patients and controls could have and had used systemic glucocorticoids, and therefore this use was adjusted for.

The major strength of this study is the population-based design with rigorous recruitment of newly diagnosed incident cases. The public health care system in Norway provides equal free-of-charge access to medical services for all Norwegian citizens. It is therefore likely that almost all incident cases of MS and CIS in Oslo were invited to participate, and that the included patients were representative of the source population. The case-control design allowed comprehensive collection of relevant lifestyle factors as well as biological data, making it possible to adjust for potential confounders. Biochemical measures and BMD obviously complement each other, as do markers of bone turnover and metabolism, because turnover markers reflect but do not regulate bone metabolism. In addition, neither self-reported recent UV exposures, assessed intake of vitamin D, nor measured serum 25(OH)D differed significantly between patients and controls. Because serum 25(OH)D is a marker of recent sun exposure and vitamin D intake, this consistency is reassuring.

There are also several limitations to this study. Markers of bone turnover are affected by a number of factors [17], and even if we have taken many of these into account, we lacked data on genetics, gonadal steroids, and inflammatory cytokines. Because of the case-control design, there could be potential recall bias for lifestyle factors that were assessed by questionnaire. In order to minimize recall bias, the participants did not know their vitamin D or bone status when completing the questionnaire, which contained a wide range of questions regarding the diet, health, and lifestyle without giving prime focus to any section. Notably, at the time of examination there was not yet general awareness among patients or controls in Norway about of the possible role of vitamin D and bone health in MS. Although we aimed to minimize the impact of self-selection by randomly recruiting controls from the general population and by letting the patients recruit additional controls, we cannot rule out the possibility that persons with an unhealthy lifestyle participated to a lesser extent than persons with a healthier lifestyle. Smoking habits could be an indicator of such bias. Data from Statistics Norway (www.ssb.no\english) show that 17% of the Norwegian population aged 16–74 years and even fewer under 25 years were daily smokers in 2011. Thus, the smoking habits of our controls seem to be in line with the general population and do not suggest a bias towards particularly health-conscious controls. Moreover, body mass index (BMI), which is an indicator of general health and also associated with BMD and vitamin D status [46], did not differ between patients and controls [15]. BMI was also consistent with previous Oslo health surveys [47–49]. One of these evaluated the impact of self-selection and non-attendance on BMI and smoking and found that prevalence estimates were robust and that self-selection had little impact [50]. Importantly, most of the source population and the participating controls were likely too young to be concerned about osteoporosis, and low bone mass is asymptomatic. Knowledge of risk factors for osteoporosis is not evident, and in order to minimize differential selection bias we did not inform about such risk factors in the invitation letter.

Our previous study showed low bone mass at isolated skeletal sites but no significant difference in the total body bone mass in patients compared to controls [15]. Biochemical markers reflect the metabolism of the entire skeleton and not specific skeletal sites. We can therefore not completely exclude the possibility of a minor increase in bone turnover contributing over time, as increased turnover at some sites may have been insufficient to induce a difference in the systemic levels of the measured markers.

The low bone mass in these newly diagnosed patients with CIS and MS compared to controls was not mirrored by significant differences in bone turnover or metabolism. In addition, the lack of association between biochemical indices of bone metabolism and bone status might indicate a longstanding BMD deficit rather than a recent bone loss. Shared etiological factors between MS and osteoporosis such as vitamin D deficiency could cause low peak bone mass and low BMD at disease onset. The lack of difference in vitamin D status between patients and controls in our study does not rule out the possible role of low vitamin D in the

pathogenesis of MS, as vitamin D measures after disease onset are not considered representative of vitamin D status prior to disease onset [51]. Alterations in behavior, medication, and the disease process itself may affect vitamin D status after disease onset. Risk factors may also normalize from susceptibility periods in early life or youth until the time in adult life when symptoms appear. Thus, obese female adolescents were found to have increased MS risk, but there was no association between adult body size and MS risk [52]. The findings presented here and previously [15] are therefore in line with the hypothesis that if vitamin D status exerts a major effect on MS risk, skeletal consequences of hypovitaminosis D should be apparent from the onset of disease. This suggestion does not exclude other possible links not related to vitamin D between MS and osteoporosis, including shared genetic risk factors, and genetic variation in the interleukin-6 gene is one example that has been associated with both diseases [53,54].

We know that low bone mass may occur early in MS and that patients with MS are at high risk of osteoporosis and fractures. Newly diagnosed patients have many years of disease ahead. Osteoporosis, fractures, and their sequelae may therefore have important impact on the patients' quality of life. Bone health in the early stage of MS deserves awareness and is far from fully explored. This lack of knowledge should trigger prospective studies on the mechanisms involved as well as prophylaxis and treatment.

Acknowledgments

The authors thank all the participants, Guri Skei at the Department of Community Medicine, University of Tromsø, for technical assistance, and Jan A. Falch for participation in study design.

Author Contributions

Conceived and designed the experiments: SMM EGC LS MB LN TH. Performed the experiments: SMM. Analyzed the data: SMM LS MB. Contributed reagents/materials/analysis tools: MB LN EFE. Wrote the paper: SMM EGC TH. Revised the manuscript: SMM EGC LS MB LN EFE TH.

References

1. Compston A, Coles A (2002) Multiple sclerosis. Lancet 359: 1221–1231.
2. Nieves J, Cosman F, Herbert J, Shen V, Lindsay R (1994) High prevalence of vitamin D deficiency and reduced bone mass in multiple sclerosis. Neurology 44: 1687–1692.
3. Cosman F, Nieves J, Komar L, Ferrer G, Herbert J, et al. (1998) Fracture history and bone loss in patients with MS. Neurology 51: 1161–1165.
4. Bazelier MT, van Staa TP, Uitdehaag BM, Cooper C, Leufkens HG, et al. (2011) The risk of fracture in patients with multiple sclerosis: the UK general practice research database. J Bone Miner Res 26: 2271–2279.
5. Bazelier MT, de Vries F, Bentzen J, Vestergaard P, Leufkens HG, et al. (2012) Incidence of fractures in patients with multiple sclerosis: the Danish National Health Registers. Mult Scler 18: 622–627.
6. Gibson JC, Summers GD (2011) Bone health in multiple sclerosis. Osteoporos Int 22: 2935–2949.
7. Zikan V (2011) Bone health in patients with multiple sclerosis. J Osteoporos 2011: 596294. 10.4061/2011/596294 [doi].
8. Hearn AP, Silber E (2010) Osteoporosis in multiple sclerosis. Mult Scler 16: 1031–1043.
9. Ascherio A, Munger KL, Simon KC (2010) Vitamin D and multiple sclerosis. Lancet Neurol 9: 599–612.
10. Holick MF (2007) Vitamin D deficiency. N Engl J Med 357: 266–281.
11. Willer CJ, Dyment DA, Sadovnick AD, Rothwell PM, Murray TJ, et al. (2005) Timing of birth and risk of multiple sclerosis: population based study. BMJ 330: 120. bmj.38301.686030.63 [pii];10.1136/bmj.38301.686030.63 [doi].
12. Smestad C, Sandvik L, Holmoy T, Harbo HF, Celius EG (2008) Marked differences in prevalence of multiple sclerosis between ethnic groups in Oslo, Norway. J Neurol 255: 49–55.
13. Mirzaei F, Michels KB, Munger K, O'Reilly E, Chitnis T, et al. (2011) Gestational vitamin D and the risk of multiple sclerosis in offspring. Ann Neurol 70: 30–40.
14. Heaney RP, Abrams S, Dawson-Hughes B, Looker A, Marcus R, et al. (2000) Peak bone mass. Osteoporos Int 11: 985–1009.

15. Moen SM, Celius EG, Sandvik L, Nordsletten L, Eriksen EF, et al. (2011) Low bone mass in newly diagnosed multiple sclerosis and clinically isolated syndrome. Neurology 77: 151–157.
16. Clarke B (2008) Normal bone anatomy and physiology. Clin J Am Soc Nephrol 3 Suppl 3: S131–S139.
17. Seibel MJ (2003) Biochemical markers of bone remodeling. Endocrinol Metab Clin North Am 32: 83–113.
18. McDonald WI, Compston A, Edan G, Goodkin D, Hartung HP, et al. (2001) Recommended diagnostic criteria for multiple sclerosis: guidelines from the International Panel on the diagnosis of multiple sclerosis. Ann Neurol 50: 121–127.
19. Brustad M, Alsaker E, Engelsen O, Aksnes L, Lund E (2004) Vitamin D status of middle-aged women at 65–71 degrees N in relation to dietary intake and exposure to ultraviolet radiation. Public Health Nutr 7: 327–335.
20. Brustad M, Braaten T, Lund E (2004) Predictors for cod-liver oil supplement use–the Norwegian Women and Cancer Study. Eur J Clin Nutr 58: 128–136.
21. Kurtzke JF (1983) Rating neurologic impairment in multiple sclerosis: an expanded disability status scale (EDSS). Neurology 33: 1444–1452.
22. Terzi T, Terzi M, Tander B, Canturk F, Onar M (2010) Changes in bone mineral density and bone metabolism markers in premenopausal women with multiple sclerosis and the relationship to clinical variables. J Clin Neurosci 17: 1260–1264.
23. Stepan JJ, Havrdova E, Tyblova M, Horakova D, Ticha V, et al. (2004) Markers of bone remodeling predict rate of bone loss in multiple sclerosis patients treated with low dose glucocorticoids. Clin Chim Acta 348: 147–154.
24. Tuzun S, Altintas A, Karacan I, Tangurek S, Saip S, et al. (2003) Bone status in multiple sclerosis: beyond corticosteroids. Mult Scler 9: 600–604.
25. Ozgocmen S, Bulut S, Ilhan N, Gulkesen A, Ardicoglu O, et al. (2005) Vitamin D deficiency and reduced bone mineral density in multiple sclerosis: effect of ambulatory status and functional capacity. J Bone Miner Metab 23: 309–313.

26. Steffensen LH, Mellgren SI, Kampman MT (2010) Predictors and prevalence of low bone mineral density in fully ambulatory persons with multiple sclerosis. J Neurol 257: 410–418.
27. Triantafyllou N, Lambrinoudaki I, Thoda P, Andreadou E, Kararizou E, et al. (2012) Lack of association between vitamin D levels and bone mineral density in patients with multiple sclerosis. J Neurol Sci 313: 137–141.
28. Edvardsen K, Engelsen O, Brustad M (2009) Duration of vitamin D synthesis from weather model data for use in prospective epidemiological studies. Int J Biometeorol 53: 451–459.
29. Sundqvist E, Baarnhielm M, Alfredsson L, Hillert J, Olsson T, et al. (2010) Confirmation of association between multiple sclerosis and CYP27B1. Eur J Hum Genet 18: 1349–1352.
30. Sawcer S, Hellenthal G, Pirinen M, Spencer CC, Patsopoulos NA, et al. (2011) Genetic risk and a primary role for cell-mediated immune mechanisms in multiple sclerosis. Nature 476: 214–219.
31. Soilu-Hanninen M, Airas L, Mononen I, Heikkila A, Viljanen M, et al. (2005) 25-Hydroxyvitamin D levels in serum at the onset of multiple sclerosis. Mult Scler 11: 266–271.
32. van der Mei IA, Ponsonby AL, Dwyer T, Blizzard L, Taylor BV, et al. (2007) Vitamin D levels in people with multiple sclerosis and community controls in Tasmania, Australia. J Neurol 254: 581–590.
33. Correale J, Ysrraelit MC, Gaitan MI (2009) Immunomodulatory effects of Vitamin D in multiple sclerosis. Brain 132: 1146–1160.
34. Shaygannejad V, Golabchi K, Haghighi S, Dehghan H, Moshayedi A (2010) A Comparative Study of 25 (OH) Vitamin D Serum Levels in Patients with Multiple Sclerosis and Control Group in Isfahan, Iran. Int J Prev Med 1: 195–201.
35. Gelfand JM, Cree BA, McElroy J, Oksenberg J, Green R, et al. (2011) Vitamin D in African Americans with multiple sclerosis. Neurology 76: 1824–1830.
36. Lucas RM, Ponsonby AL, Dear K, Valery PC, Pender MP, et al. (2011) Sun exposure and vitamin D are independent risk factors for CNS demyelination. Neurology 76: 540–548.
37. Barnes MS, Bonham MP, Robson PJ, Strain JJ, Lowe-Strong AS, et al. (2007) Assessment of 25-hydroxyvitamin D and 1,25-dihydroxyvitamin D3 concentrations in male and female multiple sclerosis patients and control volunteers. Mult Scler 13: 670–672.
38. Soilu-Hanninen M, Laaksonen M, Laitinen I, Eralinna JP, Lilius EM, et al. (2008) A longitudinal study of serum 25-hydroxyvitamin D and intact parathyroid hormone levels indicate the importance of vitamin D and calcium homeostasis regulation in multiple sclerosis. J Neurol Neurosurg Psychiatry 79: 152–157.
39. Kragt J, van Amerongen B, Killestein J, Dijkstra C, Uitdehaag B, et al. (2009) Higher levels of 25-hydroxyvitamin D are associated with a lower incidence of multiple sclerosis only in women. Mult Scler 15: 9–15.
40. Lonergan R, Kinsella K, Fitzpatrick P, Brady J, Murray B, et al. (2011) Multiple sclerosis prevalence in Ireland: relationship to vitamin D status and HLA genotype. J Neurol Neurosurg Psychiatry 82: 317–322.
41. Smolders J, Menheere P, Kessels A, Damoiseaux J, Hupperts R (2008) Association of vitamin D metabolite levels with relapse rate and disability in multiple sclerosis. Mult Scler 14: 1220–1224.
42. Hawkes CH (2007) Smoking is a risk factor for multiple sclerosis: a metanalysis. Mult Scler 13: 610–615.
43. Cosman F, Nieves J, Herbert J, Shen V, Lindsay R (1994) High-dose glucocorticoids in multiple sclerosis patients exert direct effects on the kidney and skeleton. J Bone Miner Res 9: 1097–1105.
44. Dovio A, Perazzolo L, Osella G, Ventura M, Termine A, et al. (2004) Immediate fall of bone formation and transient increase of bone resorption in the course of high-dose, short-term glucocorticoid therapy in young patients with multiple sclerosis. J Clin Endocrinol Metab 89: 4923–4928.
45. Minisola S, Del Fiacco R, Piemonte S, Iorio M, Mascia ML, et al. (2008) Biochemical markers in glucocorticoid-induced osteoporosis. J Endocrinol Invest 31: 28–32.
46. Lagunova Z, Porojnicu AC, Lindberg F, Hexeberg S, Moan J (2009) The dependency of vitamin D status on body mass index, gender, age and season. Anticancer Res 29: 3713–3720.
47. Gilboe IM, Kvien TK, Haugeberg G, Husby G (2000) Bone mineral density in systemic lupus erythematosus: comparison with rheumatoid arthritis and healthy controls. Ann Rheum Dis 59: 110–115.
48. Lilleby V, Lien G, Frey FK, Haugen M, Flato B, et al. (2005) Frequency of osteopenia in children and young adults with childhood-onset systemic lupus erythematosus. Arthritis Rheum 52: 2051–2059.
49. Alver K, Meyer HE, Falch JA, Søgaard J (2005) Bone mineral density in ethnic Norwegians and Pakistani immigrants living in Oslo–The Oslo Health Study. Osteoporos Int 16: 623–630.
50. Sogaard AJ, Selmer R, Bjertness E, Thelle D (2004) The Oslo Health Study: The impact of self-selection in a large, population-based survey. Int J Equity Health 3: 3. 10.1186/1475-9276-3-3 [doi];1475-9276-3-3 [pii].
51. Munger KL, Levin LI, Hollis BW, Howard NS, Ascherio A (2006) Serum 25-hydroxyvitamin D levels and risk of multiple sclerosis. JAMA 296: 2832–2838.
52. Munger KL, Chitnis T, Ascherio A (2009) Body size and risk of MS in two cohorts of US women. Neurology 73: 1543–1550.
53. Mirowska-Guzel D, Gromadzka G, Mach A, Czlonkowski A, Czlonkowska A (2011) Association of IL1A, IL1B, ILRN, IL6, IL10 and TNF-alpha polymorphisms with risk and clinical course of multiple sclerosis in a Polish population. J Neuroimmunol 236: 87–92.
54. Czerny B, Kaminski A, Kurzawski M, Kotrych D, Safranow K, et al. (2010) The association of IL-1beta, IL-2, and IL-6 gene polymorphisms with bone mineral density and osteoporosis in postmenopausal women. Eur J Obstet Gynecol Reprod Biol 149: 82–85.

10

Impact of Generic Alendronate Cost on the Cost-Effectiveness of Osteoporosis Screening and Treatment

Smita Nayak[1]*, Mark S. Roberts[1,2], Susan L. Greenspan[3]

1 Section of Decision Sciences and Clinical Systems Modeling, Division of General Internal Medicine, Department of Medicine, University of Pittsburgh School of Medicine, Pittsburgh, Pennsylvania, United States of America, 2 Department of Health Policy and Management, University of Pittsburgh Graduate School of Public Health, Pittsburgh, Pennsylvania, United States of America, 3 Division of Endocrinology and Metabolism and Division of Geriatric Medicine, Department of Medicine, University of Pittsburgh School of Medicine, Pittsburgh, Pennsylvania, United States of America

Abstract

Introduction: Since alendronate became available in generic form in the Unites States in 2008, its price has been decreasing. The objective of this study was to investigate the impact of alendronate cost on the cost-effectiveness of osteoporosis screening and treatment in postmenopausal women.

Methods: Microsimulation cost-effectiveness model of osteoporosis screening and treatment for U.S. women age 65 and older. We assumed screening initiation at age 65 with central dual-energy x-ray absorptiometry (DXA), and alendronate treatment for individuals with osteoporosis; with a comparator of "no screening" and treatment only after fracture occurrence. We evaluated annual alendronate costs of $20 through $800; outcome measures included fractures; nursing home admission; medication adverse events; death; costs; quality-adjusted life-years (QALYs); and incremental cost-effectiveness ratios (ICERs) in 2010 U.S. dollars per QALY gained. A lifetime time horizon was used, and direct costs were included. Base-case and sensitivity analyses were performed.

Results: Base-case analysis results showed that at annual alendronate costs of $200 or less, osteoporosis screening followed by treatment was cost-saving, resulting in lower total costs than no screening as well as more QALYs (10.6 additional quality-adjusted life-days). When assuming alendronate costs of $400 through $800, screening and treatment resulted in greater lifetime costs than no screening but was highly cost-effective, with ICERs ranging from $714 per QALY gained through $13,902 per QALY gained. Probabilistic sensitivity analyses revealed that the cost-effectiveness of osteoporosis screening followed by alendronate treatment was robust to joint input parameter estimate variation at a willingness-to-pay threshold of $50,000/QALY at all alendronate costs evaluated.

Conclusions: Osteoporosis screening followed by alendronate treatment is effective and highly cost-effective for postmenopausal women across a range of alendronate costs, and may be cost-saving at annual alendronate costs of $200 or less.

Editor: Joseph S. Ross, Yale University School of Medicine, United States of America

Funding: This study was supported by grant 1R01AR060809-01 from the National Institute of Arthritis and Musculoskeletal and Skin Diseases (Dr. Nayak); grant KL2 RR024154 from the National Center for Research Resources (a component of the National Institutes of Health) and National Institutes of Health Roadmap for Medical Research (Dr. Nayak); and grant K24 DK062895 from the National Institute of Diabetes and Digestive and Kidney Diseases (Dr. Greenspan). The funders had no role in study design, data collection and analysis, decision to publish, or preparation of the manuscript.

Competing Interests: The authors have read the journal's policy and have the following conflicts: Dr. Greenspan has consulted for and received research funding from Merck & Co. The funding from Merck & Co. was not for this specific study. This does not alter the authors' adherence to all the PLoS ONE policies on sharing data and materials..

* E-mail: nayaks@upmc.edu

Introduction

Osteoporosis affects approximately 10 million individuals in the United States, most of whom are postmenopausal women [1,2]. It is estimated that half of women over the age of 50 will sustain an osteoporotic fracture during their lifetime [2], with potentially severe consequences including mortality, chronic pain, mobility limitation, and nursing home placement. Osteoporosis-related costs in the U.S. were nearly $17 billion in 2005 [3], and are projected to double or triple by 2040 [4]. The US Preventive Services Task Force (USPSTF) recommends osteoporosis screening for women aged 65 and older, to identify individuals who may be candidates for treatment [5].

Medical treatment of osteoporosis reduces fracture risk, and multiple studies have demonstrated the cost-effectiveness of osteoporosis treatment [6,7,8] and osteoporosis screening followed by treatment [9,10]. Alendronate is a first-line medication for osteoporosis treatment, and is among the most cost-effective treatments for osteoporosis [6,10,11]. In 2008, alendronate became available in generic form in the U.S., with a resulting drop in its cost and widening of the gap in price between alendronate and other treatment options. Most published studies of the cost-effectiveness of alendronate therapy have assumed pre-2008 costs; the cost of alendronate has continued to drop since 2008; with prices currently as low as approximately $84 annually at discount pharmacies [12].

The aim of this study was to evaluate the effect of various alendronate costs on the cost-effectiveness of osteoporosis screening and treatment.

Methods

We constructed a Monte Carlo microsimulation model of osteoporosis screening followed by alendronate treatment compared to no screening with treatment only if fracture occurs for US women age 65 and older. The model estimates direct costs in 2010 US dollars, quality-adjusted life-years (QALYs), and incremental cost-effectiveness ratios (ICERs) in units of cost per QALY gained for osteoporosis screening followed by alendronate treatment. A lifetime time horizon was used. We followed guidelines of the Panel on Cost-Effectiveness in Health and Medicine [13], and ran our analyses using TreeAge Pro Suite 2009 (TreeAge Software, Williamstown, MA). Our methods are summarized briefly here – more details can be found in a related paper in the Annals of Internal Medicine on the cost-effectiveness of different screening strategies for osteoporosis in postmenopausal women [14].

Model Development

General Structure. Figure 1 is a simplified schematic of the model, in which cohorts of 65 year old community-dwelling women are either screened with dual-energy x-ray absorptiometry (DXA) of the femoral neck and lumbar spine, or not screened and offered treatment only if an osteoporotic fracture occurs. Each woman who tests positive for osteoporosis by DXA criteria (T-score≤−2.5 at either the femoral neck or lumbar spine) is offered alendronate treatment, and each who tests negative (i.e. T-score>−2.5) receives usual care only (calcium and vitamin D). During each 3-month time period (cycle) in the model, the woman may sustain a fracture of the hip, vertebra, or wrist; may survive or die; may remain community-dwelling or enter a nursing home; and may develop an alendronate adverse event. Prior fracture history affects future fracture risk. Occurrence of a hip fractures

increases the probability of nursing home placement and short-term death. Osteoporotic fractures, nursing home residence, and alendronate-related adverse events incur direct costs and "disutility" (decrease in health-related quality of life). Individuals continue cycling through the model until death. Table S1 shows model parameter assumptions.

Screening. We modeled initiation of screening at age 65 with DXA, with repeat screening every 5 years for individuals who test negative. With repeat screening, individuals who did not have osteoporosis at age 65 but who subsequently developed osteoporosis as their BMD declined with age would be offered treatment at the older age at which they are diagnosed. We used 65 as the screening initiation age for women in the absence of additional risk factors in accordance with current guidelines from the U.S. Preventive Services Task Force [5]. Initial DXA T-scores for each simulated individual were assigned by sampling from National Health and Nutrition Examination Survey (NHANES III) femoral neck data for non-Hispanic white women [15], and lumbar spine reference data for white women from a DXA manufacturer (Hologic, Inc., Bedford, MA). We incorporated correlations between sampled femoral neck and lumbar spine values based on published data(R = 0.603); and modeled the average annual change in T-scores at the lumbar spine and femoral neck [15,16]. Constant, linear decrement in T-scores over time was assumed.

Treatment. We assumed that women with positive DXA results (T-scores≤−2.5) or who experienced a fracture of the hip, vertebra (clinically detected), or wrist were offered treatment with 70 mg of alendronate once weekly. We assumed 5 years of treatment [17,18] and medication compliance of 50% [19,20] in base case analysis. We assumed that the 50% of individuals who were initially compliant remained compliant with treatment for the entire duration of recommended therapy unless they sustained side effects requiring discontinuation. We assumed that 50% of individuals were entirely noncompliant with treatment recommendations, and that these individuals remained noncompliant for the entire period or recommended therapy unless they experienced an osteoporotic fracture. We assumed that previously noncompliant individuals who sustained an osteoporotic fracture had a 50% probability of becoming newly compliant. We assumed that noncompliant individuals did not

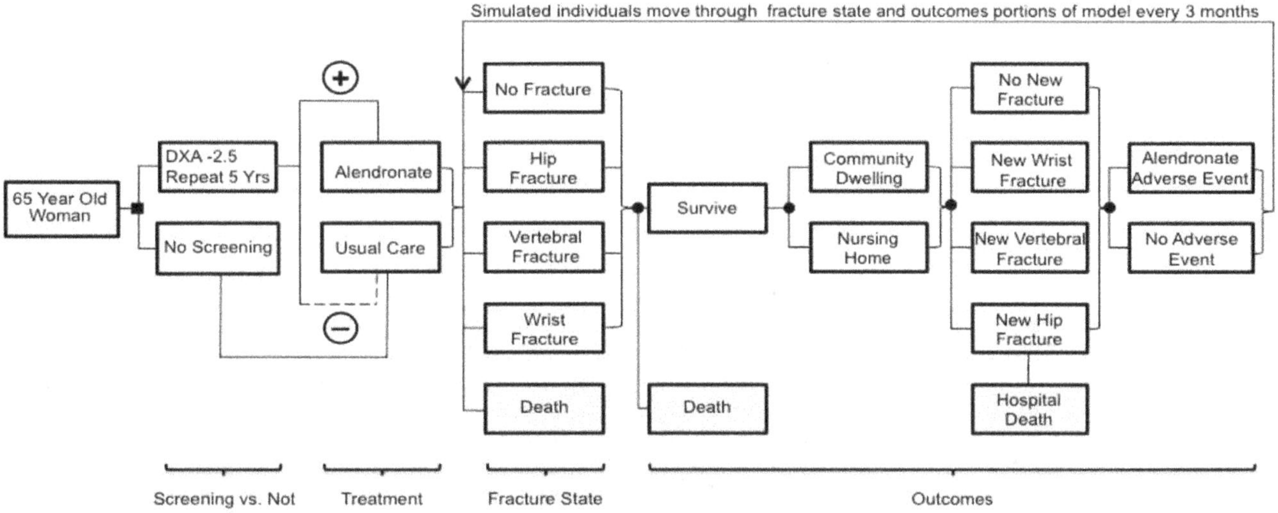

Figure 1. Model Schematic. A simplified and partial representation of the full model.

incur the fracture reduction benefits or costs of alendronate therapy. All individuals, whether receiving alendronate or not, were assumed to be taking vitamin D and calcium, without additional protection against fracture.

Fracture Rates. Fracture rates for women not on alendronate treatment were based on Study of Osteoporotic Fractures (SOF) data, with future fracture probability predicted as a function of age, femoral neck or lumbar spine BMD, and history of fracture [14,21]. We assumed that 35% of vertebral fractures were clinically detected [22]. For women taking alendronate, fracture relative risk was based on data from several published clinical trials and a meta-analysis [23,24,25,26,27]. For individuals who incurred a fracture, future fracture relative risk was predicted using data for women with previous fractures [27]. For women receiving alendronate treatment without a history of osteoporotic fracture, we based future fracture relative risk on data for women without previous fractures [23–26], using the fracture risk estimates corresponding to the lower of the T-scores from the lumbar spine or femoral neck.

We assumed a constant, linear decline in fracture risk reduction benefit over 5 years after completion of alendronate treatment [28].

Mortality Rates. We used US national vital statistics data for baseline mortality rates [29]; and data on hip fracture-related mortality from several published sources [30,31].

Nursing Home Characteristics. Nursing home admission rates, length of stay, and mortality data were obtained from several published sources [31,32,33,34].

Costs. We included direct costs of DXA screening ($97.71) [35], alendronate therapy, fracture treatment, physician visits, nursing home residence, and alendronate-related adverse events. In separate base-case analyses, we evaluated annual alendronate costs of $20, $40, $60, $80, $100, $200, $400, $600, and $800. These costs were chosen to represent a spectrum of possible alendronate annual costs, including a cost higher than the 2010 CMS Federal Upper Limit price for alendronate (approximately $738) and costs lower than the current annual cost of alendronate at discount pharmacies (approximately $84) [12]. Costs for fracture-related treatment, other relevant medical services, and nursing home stay were obtained from several sources [35–37]. We inflated costs to 2010 U.S. dollars using the US Consumer Price Index for Medical Care [38]. We discounted future costs by 3% annually.

Utilities. We used data from a sample of older women in the U.S. for baseline health state utilites [39]. We modeled disutility from osteoporotic fractures, nursing home placement, and alendronate adverse events using data from multiple published sources [40,41,42,43,44,45,46]. We discounted future utility values by 3% annually.

Adverse Events. We modeled medication adverse events of esophagitis and esophageal ulceration with rates obtained from clinical trials data [27].

Analyses

We performed base-case and sensitivity analyses separately for each alendronate cost evaluated. Key parameter values used for base-case analyses and the range of values used for sensitivity analyses are shown in Table S1. Sensitivity analyses included evaluation of different assumptions for key model parameters of costs (higher than base-case); discount rate (5% annually instead of 3%); fracture risks (50% lower than base-case); and probability of admission to a nursing home after hip fracture (30% instead of 60%). Additionally, probabilistic sensitivity analyses were performed to evaluate the impact of joint input parameter uncertainty

on the model findings. For each base-case analysis and for the sensitivity analyses of costs, discount rate, fracture risks, and probability of nursing home admission, we ran the model with 1 million trials. For each probabilistic sensitivity analysis, we ran 500 simulations with 2,000 trials per simulation.

Model Validation

We compared the model's fracture and life expectancy predictions with published U.S. outcomes data.

Results

Model Validation

Our model predicted a mean life expectancy of 19.3 years for 65-year-old women who were not screened for osteoporosis. This is similar to the U.S. National Vital Statistics figure of 19.8 years reported for 65-year-old women in 2006 [47]. The model predicted that 49% of 65-year-old women who were not screened would experience at least one osteoporotic fracture during their lifetime. Our model predicted that 28% of women would experience a vertebral fracture; this figure matches that reported in a prior study of older US women [48]. Our model predicted that 24% of women would sustain a hip fracture during their lifetime, and 17% would sustain a wrist fracture; these estimates are higher than those reported in a study of Medicare beneficiaries who sustained a fracture by age 90, which used data from 1986–1990 [49]. However, women's life expectancies have increased by 1.3 years since 1988, and 29% of women lived to be at least 90 years old in our modeling analysis; 17% of women in our analysis experienced a hip fracture before age 90, close to the figure reported by Barrett et al. [49].

Base-Case Analyses

Osteoporosis screening initiated at age 65 followed by alendronate treatment was more effective than no screening with treatment only if fracture occurs, resulting in 10.6 additional quality-adjusted life-days. When assuming alendronate costs of $200 or less, osteoporosis screening and treatment was cost-saving, resulting in lower total costs than no screening as well as more QALYs (Table 1). Lifetime direct cost savings ranged from $171 to $343 when assuming alendronate annual costs of $200 or $20, respectively. When assuming alendronate costs of $400, $600, or $800, screening and treatment resulted in greater lifetime costs than no screening but was highly cost-effective, with ICERs ranging from $714 per QALY gained to $13,902 per QALY gained when assuming annual alendronate costs of $400 or $800, respectively (Table 1).

Sensitivity Analyses

Table 2 shows results (ICERs and cost savings) from sensitivity analyses of assumptions for costs, discount rate, fracture risks, and probability of nursing home admission after hip fracture. In general, these results were similar to base-case analysis findings in demonstrating the value of osteoporosis screening followed by alendronate treatment across a range of alendronate annual costs. However, ICERs or cost savings associated with different alendronate costs varied. When assuming 50% lower fracture risks, screening and treatment remained cost-effective across the range of costs evaluated, but with higher ICERs than in base-case analysis; additionally, none of the alendronate costs evaluated were associated with cost savings. When assuming nursing home admission probability of 30% after hip fracture instead of 60%, screening and treatment remained highly cost-effective, but with ICERs higher than in base-case analysis; additionally, the annual

Table 1. Base-Case Analysis Results, Various Alendronate Costs.

Alendronate Cost ($)	Incremental Cost-Effectiveness Ratio ($/QALY)[a]
20	Cost-saving: $343[b]
40	Cost-saving: $324[b]
60	Cost-saving: $305[b]
80	Cost-saving: $286[b]
100	Cost-saving: $266[b]
200	Cost-saving: $171[b]
400	$712
600	$7307
800	$13,902

[a]Incremental cost-effectiveness of osteoporosis screening followed by alendronate treatment, compared to no screening with treatment only if fracture occurs; in 2010 US dollars per quality-adjusted life-year (QALY).
[b]Lifetime direct costs saved.

cost at which alendronate became cost-saving was $40 instead of $200. When assuming high costs for fracture-related treatment, nursing home care, and DXA, screening and treatment remained highly cost-effective, but with ICERs higher than in base-case analysis; additionally, the cost at which alendronate became cost-saving was $100 instead of $200. When assuming a discount rate of 5% instead of 3%, results were similar to base-case analysis, with screening and treatment becoming cost-saving at annual alendronate costs of $200 or lower.

Probabilistic sensitivity analyses revealed that the cost-effectiveness of osteoporosis screening followed by alendronate treatment was relatively robust to variations in input parameter estimates at a willingness-to-pay threshold of $50,000/QALY for all alendronate costs evaluated (Figure 2). When assuming annual alendronate costs of $100 or less, the probability that osteoporosis screening followed by alendronate treatment was cost-effective was 95%. The probability that screening followed by alendronate treatment was cost effective remained high at 84% when assuming an annual alendronate cost of $800.

Discussion

Our analyses demonstrated that osteoporosis screening followed by alendronate treatment is effective and highly cost-effective for women aged 65 and older across a wide range of alendronate costs; and potentially cost-saving at annual alendronate costs of $200 or less, depending on assumptions about fracture risk, nursing home admission probability after hip fracture, and health care costs. Sensitivity analyses showed that the value (cost-effectiveness) of alendronate treatment for all alendronate costs evaluated was relatively robust to key model parameter uncertainty; but the price at which alendronate becomes cost-saving is sensitive to the parameters specified above. These results indicate that osteoporosis screening followed by alendronate treatment is an advantageous use of healthcare resources for women age 65 and older, that can be expected to improve health outcomes and may result in potential cost savings when alendronate annual costs are $200 or less, as is currently the case at discount pharmacies. As the cost of alendronate continues to fall, the value and potential for cost savings for the U.S. healthcare system resulting from osteoporosis screening of older women followed by alendronate treatment can be expected to increase, assuming appropriate selection of candidates for treatment. This is a significant finding, given how few preventive services can result in cost savings [50,51].

Our model has several limitations. First, our analyses did not incorporate the costs of added life days from osteoporosis screening. However, the costs of added life days would likely be small as the age of death was very similar in the screening followed by treatment and no screening model arms. Second, our analysis assumed that only women with DXA T-scores in the osteoporotic range would be offered treatment, in accordance with evidence that treatment of women with osteopenia (low bone mass) is not

Table 2. Sensitivity Analysis Results; Costs, Discount Rate, Fracture Risk, Nursing Home Probability.

Alendronate Cost ($)	Incremental Cost-Effectiveness Ratio ($/QALY)[a]			
	High Costs Scenario[b]	High Discount Rate Scenario[c]	Low Fracture Risk Scenario[d]	Low Nursing Home Probability Scenario[e]
20	Cost-saving: $116[f]	Cost-saving: $275[f]	$5483	Cost-saving: $28[f]
40	Cost-saving: $97[f]	Cost-saving: $258[f]	$6728	Cost-saving: $9[f]
60	Cost-saving: $77[f]	Cost-saving: $241[f]	$7973	$362
80	Cost-saving: $58[f]	Cost-saving: $223[f]	$9218	$1047
100	Cost-saving: $39[f]	Cost-saving: $206[f]	$10463	$1733
200	$1948	Cost-saving: $119[f]	$16688	$5161
400	$8543	$2561	$29138	$12018
600	$15138	$10638	$41588	$18874
800	$21733	$18715	$54037	$25731

[a]Incremental cost-effectiveness of osteoporosis screening followed by alendronate treatment, compared to no screening with treatment only if fracture occurs; in 2010 US dollars per quality-adjusted life-year (QALY).
[b]High fracture-related, nursing home, and dual-energy x-ray absorptiometry costs (high values of the sensitivity analysis range for costs shown in Table S1).
[c]Discount rate for future costs and health state utilities of 5% annually.
[d]Fracture risks (hip, vertebral, and wrist) 50% lower than in base-case analysis.
[e]Probability of nursing home admission after hip fracture of 30%.
[f]Lifetime direct costs saved.

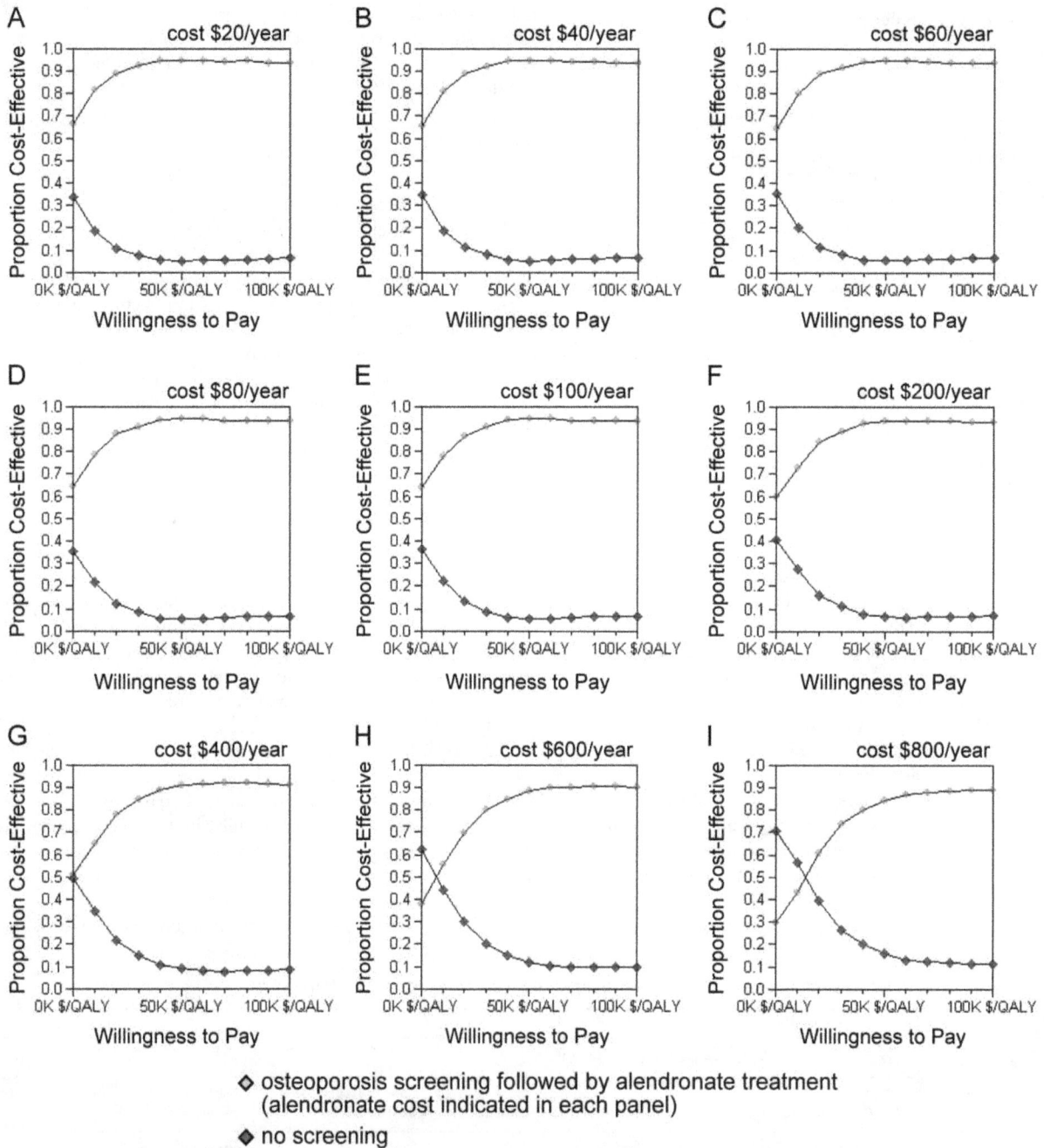

Figure 2. Probabilistic Sensitivity Analysis Cost-Effectiveness Acceptability Curves.

cost-effective [52]. However, if screening leads to inappropriate treatment of individuals at lower risk for osteoporotic fracture, it's cost-effectiveness and potential cost savings would be lessened. Additionally, we did not model all potential adverse events of alendronate treatment, including arthalgias, myalgias, osteonecrosis of the jaw, or atypical femoral neck fractures; such adverse events may require additional physician visits, labwork, or discontinuation of medication. However, osteonecrosis of the jaw and atypical femoral neck fractures are rare reported adverse events, and their association with alendronate treatment is still under investigation. Moreover, the effectiveness and adherence with generic bisphosphonate therapy may be lower than with proprietary formulations [53]. If this is the case, and adherence or

fracture risk reduction with generic alendronate is lower than our model assumptions, generic alendronate therapy would be less cost-effective than our findings suggest. Finally, our model parameter inputs were primarily based on data from white women, and thus our results may be less applicable to women of other races.

In conclusion, our analyses indicate that osteoporosis screening followed by alendronate treatment is highly cost-effective for women aged 65 and older when assuming annual alendronate costs of $400 through $800, and potentially cost-saving when assuming annual alendronate costs of $200 or less, depending on key parameter assumptions. Thus, osteoporosis screening followed by alendronate treatment in appropriately selected patients represents an excellent healthcare value, and this important preventive health service should be promoted. Although our analyses were limited to alendronate, other osteoporosis treatments with similar effectiveness and costs may be expected to be similarly cost-effective. For example, other available oral bisphosphonates (e.g. risedronate) may be similarly cost-effective if costs of the medication were to decrease. However intravenous bisphosphonates, which have additional costs for the infusions, different adverse event profiles, as well as different fracture reduction outcomes would not be expected to have similar cost-effectiveness to alendronate. This would apply to other osteoporosis medications that have different costs, adverse event profiles, adherence patterns, and routes of administration.

Future research should evaluate the cost-effectiveness of "real-world" osteoporosis screening and treatment practices, in which some patients will be inappropriately selected for treatment. Furthermore the effects of assuming treatment duration longer than 5 years or a drug holiday should be examined. However, assuming appropriate selection of individuals for treatment, osteoporosis screening followed by alendronate treatment in women aged 65 and old represents a superb healthcare value across the variety of alendronate costs evaluated.

Acknowledgments

The authors thank Hau Liu, MD, MPH, MBA and Kaleb Michaud, PhD for assistance with development of the cost-effectiveness model.

Author Contributions

Conceived and designed the experiments: SN MSR SLG. Performed the experiments: SN. Analyzed the data: SN. Contributed reagents/materials/analysis tools: SN. Wrote the paper: SN SLG. Review of the manuscript: MSR.

References

1. National Osteoporosis Foundation (2005) About Osteoporosis: Fast Facts. Washington, DC: National Osteoporosis Foundation.
2. Nelson HD, Helfand M, Woolf SH, Allan JD (2002) Screening for postmenopausal osteoporosis: a review of the evidence for the U.S. Preventive Services Task Force. Ann Intern Med 137: 529–541.
3. Burge R, Dawson-Hughes B, Solomon DH, Wong JB, King A, et al. (2007) Incidence and economic burden of osteoporosis-related fractures in the United States, 2005–2025. J Bone Miner Res 22: 465–475.
4. US Department of Health and Human Service, Office of the Surgeon General (2004) Bone Health and Osteoporosis: A Report of the Surgeon General. Rockville, MD.
5. US Preventive Services Task Force (2011) Screening for osteoporosis: U.S. preventive services task force recommendation statement. Ann Intern Med 154(5): 356–64.
6. Liu H, Michaud K, Nayak S, Karpf DB, Owens DK, et al. (2006) The cost-effectiveness of therapy with teriparatide and alendronate in women with severe osteoporosis. Arch Intern Med 166: 1209–1217.
7. Tosteson AN, Burge RT, Marshall DA, Lindsay R (2008) Therapies for treatment of osteoporosis in US women: cost-effectiveness and budget impact considerations. Am J Manag Care 14: 605–615.
8. Schousboe JT (2007) Cost-effectiveness modeling research of pharmacologic therapy to prevent osteoporosis-related fractures. Curr Rheumatol Rep 9: 50–56.
9. Schousboe JT, Ensrud KE, Nyman JA, Melton LJ, 3rd, Kane RL (2005) Universal bone densitometry screening combined with alendronate therapy for those diagnosed with osteoporosis is highly cost-effective for elderly women. J Am Geriatr Soc 53: 1697–1704.
10. Mobley LR, Hoerger TJ, Wittenborn JS, Galuska DA, Rao JK (2006) Cost-effectiveness of osteoporosis screening and treatment with hormone replacement therapy, raloxifene, or alendronate. Med Decis Making 26: 194–206.
11. Fleurence RL, Iglesias CP, Johnson JM (2007) The cost effectiveness of bisphosphonates for the prevention and treatment of osteoporosis: a structured review of the literature. Pharmacoeconomics 25: 913–933.
12. Drug Topics Red Book.: Physician's Desk Reference.
13. Weinstein MC, Siegel JE, Gold MR, Kamlet MS, Russell LB (1996) Recommendations of the Panel on Cost-effectiveness in Health and Medicine. JAMA 276: 1253–1258.
14. Nayak S, Roberts MS, Greenspan SL (2011) Cost-effectiveness of different screening strategies for osteoporosis in postmenopausal women. Ann Intern Med 155(11): 751–61.
15. Looker AC, Wahner HW, Dunn WL, Calvo MS, Harris TB, et al. (1998) Updated data on proximal femur bone mineral levels of US adults. Osteoporos Int 8: 468–489.
16. Lu Y, Genant HK, Shepherd J, Zhao S, Mathur A, et al. (2001) Classification of osteoporosis based on bone mineral densities. J Bone Miner Res 16: 901–910.
17. Black DM, Schwartz AV, Ensrud KE, Cauley JA, Levis S, et al. (2006) Effects of continuing or stopping alendronate after 5 years of treatment: the Fracture Intervention Trial Long-term Extension (FLEX): a randomized trial. JAMA 296: 2927–2938.
18. Schwartz AV, Bauer DC, Cummings SR, Cauley JA, Ensrud KE, et al. (2010) Efficacy of continued alendronate for fractures in women with and without prevalent vertebral fracture: the FLEX trial. J Bone Miner Res 25(5): 976–982.
19. Solomon DH, Avorn J, Katz JN, Finkelstein JS, Arnold M, et al. (2005) Compliance with osteoporosis medications. Arch Intern Med 165: 2414–2419.
20. Recker RR, Gallagher R, MacCosbe PE (2005) Effect of dosing frequency on bisphosphonate medication adherence in a large longitudinal cohort of women. Mayo Clin Proc 80: 856–861.
21. Cummings SR, Nevitt MC, Browner WS, Stone K, Fox KM, et al. (1995) Risk factors for hip fracture in white women. Study of Osteoporotic Fractures Research Group. N Engl J Med 332: 767–773.
22. Melton LJ, 3rd, Lane AW, Cooper C, Eastell R, O'Fallon WM, et al. (1993) Prevalence and incidence of vertebral deformities. Osteoporos Int 3: 113–119.
23. Liberman UA, Weiss SR, Broll J, Minne HW, Quan H, et al. (1995) Effect of oral alendronate on bone mineral density and the incidence of fractures in postmenopausal osteoporosis. The Alendronate Phase III Osteoporosis Treatment Study Group. N Engl J Med 333: 1437–1443.
24. Karpf DB, Shapiro DR, Seeman E, Ensrud KE, Johnston CC, Jr., et al. (1997) Prevention of nonvertebral fractures by alendronate. A meta-analysis. Alendronate Osteoporosis Treatment Study Groups. JAMA 277: 1159–1164.
25. Cummings SR, Black DM, Thompson DE, Applegate WB, Barrett-Connor E, et al. (1998) Effect of alendronate on risk of fracture in women with low bone density but without vertebral fractures: results from the Fracture Intervention Trial. JAMA 280: 2077–2082.
26. Black DM, Thompson DE, Bauer DC, Ensrud K, Musliner T, et al. (2000) Fracture risk reduction with alendronate in women with osteoporosis: the Fracture Intervention Trial. FIT Research Group. J Clin Endocrinol Metab 85: 4118–4124.
27. Black DM, Cummings SR, Karpf DB, Cauley JA, Thompson DE, et al. (1996) Randomised trial of effect of alendronate on risk of fracture in women with existing vertebral fractures. Fracture Intervention Trial Research Group. Lancet 348: 1535–1541.
28. Tosteson AN, Jonsson B, Grima DT, O'Brien BJ, Black DM, et al. (2001) Challenges for model-based economic evaluations of postmenopausal osteoporosis interventions. Osteoporos Int 12: 849–857.
29. Arias E (2007) United states life tables, 2004. Natl Vital Stat Rep 56: 1–39.
30. Johnell O, Kanis JA, Oden A, Sernbo I, Redlund-Johnell I, et al. (2004) Mortality after osteoporotic fractures. Osteoporos Int 15: 38–42.
31. US Congress, Office of Technology Assessment (1994) Hip Fracture Outcomes in People Age 50 and Over - Background Paper. OTA-BP-H-120. Washington, DC: U.S. Government Printing Office.
32. Corliss GR, Lucas R, Newton M, Tillman K (2004) Long-Term Care Experience Committee Intercompany Study 1984–2001. Society of Actuaries.
33. Braithwaite RS, Col NF, Wong JB (2003) Estimating hip fracture morbidity, mortality and costs. J Am Geriatr Soc 51: 364–370.
34. Fitzgerald JF, Moore PS, Dittus RS (1988) The care of elderly patients with hip fracture. Changes since implementation of the prospective payment system. N Engl J Med 319: 1392–1397.
35. Centers for Medicare and Medicaid Services national physician fee schedule website. Available: http://www.cms.hhs.gov/PFSlookup/. Accessed 2010 Dec 16.
36. Gabriel SE, Tosteson AN, Leibson CL, Crowson CS, Pond GR, et al. (2002) Direct medical costs attributable to osteoporotic fractures. Osteoporos Int 13: 323–330.
37. GE Financial Nursing Home Cost of Care Survey. Richmond, VA: GE Financial Assurance Holdings Inc.
38. U.S. Consumer Price Index for Medical Care for All Urban Consumers U.S. Department of Labor Bureau of Labor Statistics.
39. Hanmer J, Lawrence WF, Anderson JP, Kaplan RM, Fryback DG (2006) Report of nationally representative values for the noninstitutionalized US adult

population for 7 health-related quality-of-life scores. Med Decis Making 26: 391–400.

40. Brazier JE, Green C, Kanis JA (2002) A systematic review of health state utility values for osteoporosis-related conditions. Osteoporos Int 13: 768–776.

41. Oleksik A, Lips P, Dawson A, Minshall ME, Shen W, et al. (2000) Health-related quality of life in postmenopausal women with low BMD with or without prevalent vertebral fractures. J Bone Miner Res 15: 1384–1392.

42. Dolan P, Torgerson D, Kakarlapudi TK (1999) Health-related quality of life of Colles' fracture patients. Osteoporos Int 9: 196–199.

43. Fryback DG, Dasbach EJ, Klein R, Klein BE, Dorn N, et al. (1993) The Beaver Dam Health Outcomes Study: initial catalog of health-state quality factors. Med Decis Making 13: 89–102.

44. Brazier J, Kohler B, Walters S (2000) A prospective study of the health related quality of life impact of hip fractures University of Sheffield.

45. Kanis JA, Johnell O, Oden A, Borgstrom F, Zethraeus N, et al. (2004) The risk and burden of vertebral fractures in Sweden. Osteoporos Int 15: 20–26.

46. Tosteson AN, Gabriel SE, Grove MR, Moncur MM, Kneeland TS, et al. (2001) Impact of hip and vertebral fractures on quality-adjusted life years. Osteoporos Int 12: 1042–1049.

47. Heron M, Hoyert DL, Murphy SL, Xu J, Kochanek KD, et al. (2009) Deaths: final data for 2006. Natl Vital Stat Rep 57: 1–134.

48. Cummings SR, Black DM, Rubin SM (1989) Lifetime risks of hip, Colles', or vertebral fracture and coronary heart disease among white postmenopausal women. Arch Intern Med 149: 2445–2448.

49. Barrett JA, Baron JA, Karagas MR, Beach ML (1999) Fracture risk in the U.S. Medicare population. J Clin Epidemiol 52: 243–249.

50. Russell LB (2009) Preventing chronic disease: an important investment, but don't count on cost savings. Health Aff (Millwood) 28: 42–45.

51. Woolf SH (2009) A closer look at the economic argument for disease prevention. JAMA 301: 536–538.

52. Schousboe JT, Nyman JA, Kane RL, Ensrud KE (2005) Cost-effectiveness of alendronate therapy for osteopenic postmenopausal women. Ann Intern Med 142: 734–741.

53. Kanis JA, Reginster JY, Kaufman JM, Ringe JD, Adachi JD, et al. (2012) A reappraisal of generic bisphosphonates in osteoporosis. Osteoporos Int 23: 213–21.

11

Mechanical Behaviour of Umbrella-Shaped, Ni-Ti Memory Alloy Femoral Head Support Device during Implant Operation: A Finite Element Analysis Study

Wei Yi[1], Qing Tian[2], Zhipeng Dai[3], Xiaohu Liu[4]*

1 Department of Mechanics, Huazhong University of Science and Technology, Wuhan, Hubei, China, 2 Tongji Medical College, Huazhong University of Science and Technology, Wuhan, Hubei, China, 3 Tongji Medical College, Huazhong University of Science and Technology, Wuhan, Hubei, China, 4 Department of Mechanics, Huazhong University of Science and Technology, Wuhan, Hubei, China

Abstract

A new instrument used for treating femoral head osteonecrosis was recently proposed: the umbrella-shaped, Ni-Ti memory femoral head support device. The device has an efficacy rate of 82.35%. Traditional radiographic study provides limited information about the mechanical behaviour of the support device during an implant operation. Thus, this study proposes a finite element analysis method, which includes a 3-step formal head model construction scheme and a unique material assignment strategy for evaluating mechanical behaviour during an implant operation. Four different scenarios with different constraints, initial positions and bone qualities are analyzed using the simulation method. The max radium of the implanted device was consistent with observation data, which confirms the accuracy of the proposed method. To ensure that the device does not unexpectedly open and puncture the femoral head, the constraint on the impact device should be strong. The initial position of sleeve should be in the middle to reduce the damage to the decompression channel. The operation may fail because of poor bone quality caused by severe osteoporosis. The proposed finite element analysis method has proven to be an accurate tool for studying the mechanical behaviour of umbrella-shaped, Ni-Ti memory alloy femoral head support device during an implant operation. The 3-step construct scheme can be implemented with any kind of bone structure meshed with multiple element types.

Editor: Mikko Lammi, University of Eastern Finland, Finland

Funding: This work was supported by the National Natural Science Foundation of China through the project No. 11172110. The funders had no role in study design, data collection and analysis, decision to publish, or preparation of the manuscript.

Competing Interests: The authors have declared that no competing interests exist.

* Email: xhliu@mail.hust.edu.cn

Introduction

Osteonecrosis of the femoral head is a devastating disease that typically presents in young patients between the ages of thirty and forty [1]. If osteonecrosis is not effectively treated, many patients will experience femoral head collapse [2]. Hip replacement is not an optimal choice for the younger patients because of the validity of the artificial joint. Therefore, several minimally invasive surgery modalities [3] have been used to prevent the collapse of the femoral head. The following treatments, in the order they've been introduced, have been used in therapy: transtrochanteric osteotomy [4], core compression [5], Nonvascularized bone graft [6], vascularized bone graft [7], porous tantalum implant [8], Ni-Ti superelastic cage implant [3]. Of these treatments, those that used implant techniques were much more effective than the others [3]. This is because the structural stiffness of the implanted device provides a high level of support. However, all of these devices come with certain limitations, including a support area that is too small. Recently, an umbrella-shaped, Ni-Ti alloy femoral head support device [9] was proposed to treat the early stage osteonecrosis of the femoral head. Based on 17 devices implanted in 10 patients, the device showed an 82.35% efficacy rate. As reported, the support area was much larger than the traditional implant treatment. Note, however, that there are also risks

associated with this operation. The biomechanical mechanism was not entirely clear, and the operation process has not yet been perfected.

Ni-Ti shape memory alloy, as a functional metal material, has many advantages including a remarkable resistance to wear and corrosion, good biocompatibility, and other special mechanical characters: SME (shape memory effect) [10], PE (pseudo elastic) and pseudo plastic [11]. These distinct characteristics make the shape memory alloy very useful in bone surgery instrument design [12]. The many studies on the biomechanical characteristics of the Ni-Ti SMA (shape memory alloy) have increased its used in orthopedics. From the work of Auricchio [13], Lsdyna provides a linearized macroscopic phenomenological model for SMA spans, which is widely used for SMA simulation. Although this model did not include permanent strain, PE was still in effect.

The major focus on Ni-Ti surgery instruments has been in clinical practice, with few computational studies conducted on the instruments. This is particularly true for the umbrella-shaped formal head support device, which has yet to be computationally researched. The FEA (finite element analysis) can serve as the deformation field, strain field and stress field of the femoral head and support device, which is almost impossible to determine in a radiological imaging study. More importantly, the computational simulation study can predict the whole process without actually performing the surgery. Because the bone is damaged inside the femoral head, and a traditional static analysis is unable to address issues related to element failure, the explicit integration method is used.

The aim of present study is to propose a finite element analysis method based on Lsdyna to simulate the mechanical behaviour of the Ni-Ti umbrella-shaped femoral head support device during the implant process. This method includes 1) a 3-step model construction and particular material assignment strategy for the femoral head in FEA pre-processing and 2) a dynamic relaxation analysis (the normal step) in which the stress initialization file is derived from a pre-analysis (the pre-step) of the support device.

We attempted to illustrate the expanding process within the femoral head during surgery, and review the accuracy of the simulation method by comparing the literature data with the simulation. Two different cases of sleeve initial positions were simulated. The results suggested that the open shape might be similar, but different kinds of damage were found inside the femoral neck. Finally, we conducted a simulation of the same patient with moderate osteoporosis. The results show that moderate osteoporosis might lead to surgery failure because the femoral head was not strong enough to resist the expending of the implant device. Since the finite element simulation method was effective and accurate, it might also be used as a rehearsal for selecting both the best implant location and implant device size for patients with varying bone qualities. Equation Chapter 1 Section 1.

Materials and Methods

The FEA study is based on a 3-step model construction scheme, outlined below. Initially, the model is digitized based on a CT (Computed Tomography) scan experiment. Then, the geometric model is created with Mimics and Geomagic Studio. The finite element is then discretized and a special material assignment strategy is carried out. Finally, an analyses is conducted during which the pre-step simulates the reshape phase under $0°C$ in vitro and the normal step simulates the opening phase under $50°C$ in vivo. The Boundary conditions and loading are explained in a following subsection.

CT Scan Experiment

The first step of the 3-step construction scheme was to digitize the geometric and bone quality information of the femoral head. An anonymous 45-year-old male patient with Stage I femoral head osteonecrosis was CT scanned every two millimeters from the femoral head to the lesser trochanter and then at five millimeter intervals along the femur bone. A Brilliance 128 iCT scanner (Philips) was used to scan the patient. The CT slice image data were saved and exported in DICOM (Digital Imaging and Communications in Medicine) format.

The second step was to reconstruct a high quality 3D geometric model based on the digitized slice image data. The slice images were imported into Mimics software (Materialise, Leuven, Belgium) for the model reconstruction. Then, using Geomagic Studio V13.0 (Raindrop Geomagic, TrianglePark, NC) with a reverse modeling process, a fine geometric model was made (Fig. 1(a)).

FEA Analysis

Mesh and material assignment of femoral head and femur. After the Geometric model was constructed from the CT images, an operation channel with a 9 mm outer diameter at the greater tuberosity to a 5 mm diameter under the subchondral bone along the femur neck was cut in the formal head. The last step of the construction scheme was element discrete.

In HyperMesh, we used the geometric model created during the pre-step to carry out the mesh process. The whole bone structure was divided into 3 parts: the femoral head, the femur, and part in-between. The first 2 parts were meshed with 8-node 1st order hexahedron elements. Because the femoral head part was the main area of focus, the mesh with the element edge in the range of 0.28 ~0.62 mm was much finer then the femur part. The 3rd part was meshed with 4-node 1st order tetrahedron. The element numbers, element types, and support device are shown in Table 1.

The low quality (2 mm resolution) of the CT scan data prevented a clear view of the internal femoral bone microstructure and distribution of the internal trabecular bone, but it provided enough information to establish a high quality 3D geometric model of the femur. The quality of the mesh depends only on the meshing skill when the geometric model is adequate. In other words, the low quality of the CT scan has no effect on the element quality when a high quality 3D geometric model can be made.

After the 3-step model construction, we assigned a material property for each element. Because of the limitations of the Mimics auto-assignment function (it is only available when the mesh is created with 4-node elements), an assignment strategy was used.

Unable to use the Mimics auto-assignment function for the mixed-type mesh (mesh II), we generated a 4-node tetrahedron element mesh, named mesh I, and auto-assigned material in Mimics. The problem then presented is how to link Mesh I and II to each other. The detailed process for solving this problem is as follows:

Step 1: Generate an auto-assigned density for Mesh I in Mimics as N sets of elements. All of the sets are created based on the range of the apparent density which was evenly distributed and shown as the left side of each sub-graph in Fig. 2.

Step 2: Correspond Mesh II to Mesh I using the mass centroid coordination of each element. Since Mesh I is divided into N sets, Mesh II is also divided into N sets with the same apparent density as Mesh I. This can be seen in the right side of each sub-graph in Fig. 2.

Table 1. Mesh Information.

Parts	femoral head	femur	connector	umbrella	sleeve	total
Number	113680	59080	139366	11904	5412	329442
Element nodes	8	8	4	8	8	4 & 8
Element type	hexahedron	hexahedron	tetrahedron	hexahedron	hexahedron	h & t

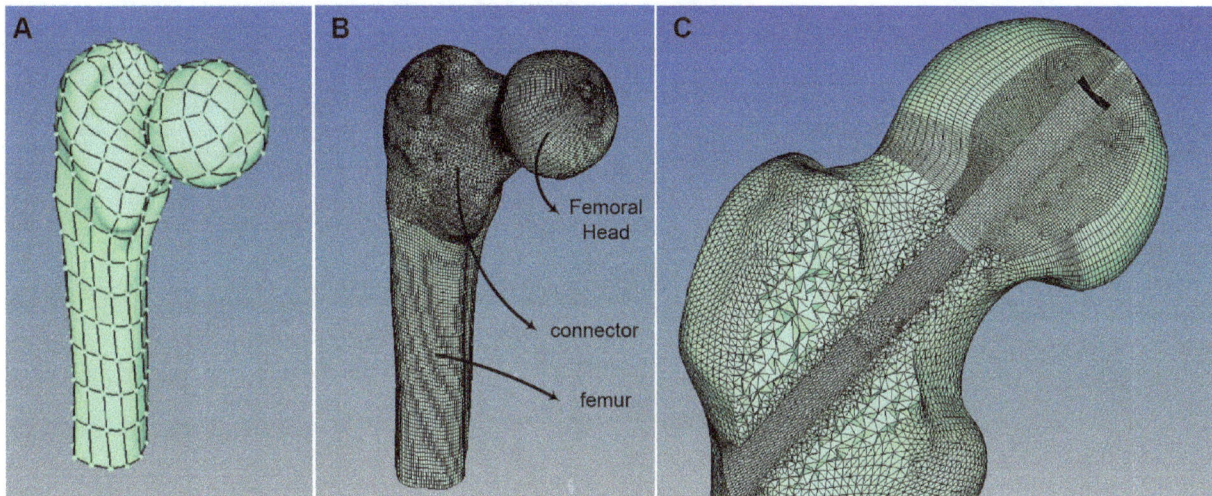

Figure 1. Digitized femur. (A) Geometric Model; (B) FE mesh model; (C) FE mesh model (local view).

Step 3: Based on the porosity-elastic module squared relation [14], E_N for set N is determined along with the failure strain for all the bone elements [15].

It's important to note that Mesh II is much finer than Mesh I. Hence, a cubic search bucket with a width 20 times the longest side of the current element E_i^{I} is created. In this bucket, we searched the corresponded element E_j^{II} that the mass centroid of E_i^{I} belonged to.

The N is set to 10, and the density, elastic module, failure strain and Poisson's ratio of each set are shown in Table 2. The corresponding elements of each set in Mesh I and II are shown with the same color, side by side. (Mesh I is show on the left side, and mesh II on the right).

In Mimics, a linear formula is used to translate the Hounsfield into the bone mass density field by the linear formula:

$$\rho = \rho_{\max} \frac{HU_j}{HU_{\max}} \qquad (1)$$

Where, j is the material property number. It is important to note that material property number and element set number are not necessarily the same, as shown in Table 2. HU_j represents the HU value of the material property j, and can be calculated with formula (2):

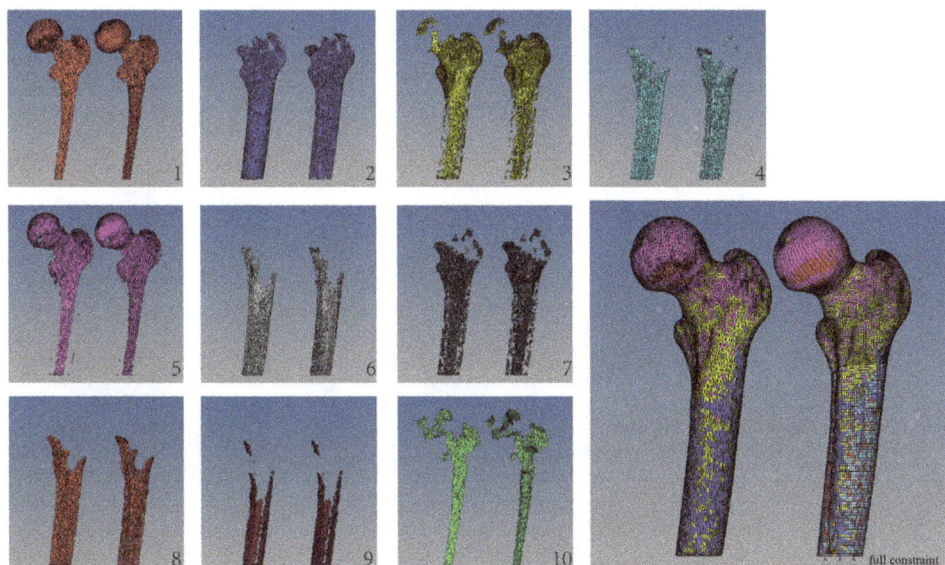

Figure 2. Bone material assignment results of 10 individual groups and the overall model. Constraint on the bone structure: In the normal step, a full constraint was applied at the bottom to eliminate rigid displacement of the whole structure.

Table 2. Material parameters for 10 different sets of bone elements.

Set | Material Property	Density (mg/mm³)	Elastic module (Gpa)	Failure strain	Poisson's ratio
1 | 2	0.63(0.53)	0.80(0.56)	0.009	0.3
2 | 5	1.57(0.31)	5.00(3.5)		
3 | 4	1.26(1.05)	3.20(2.24)		
4 | 7	2.19(1.83)	9.80(6.68)		
5 | 3	0.94(0.79)	1.80(1.26)		
6 | 9	2.83(2.37)	16.20(11.34)		
7 | 6	1.88(1.57)	7.20(5.04)		
8 | 8	2.51(2.10)	12.80(8.96)		
9 | 10	3.14(2.63)	20.00(14.00)		
10 | 1	0.32(0.27)	0.20(0.14)		

$$HU_j = \begin{cases} 168 & HU \leq 252 \quad and \quad j=1 \\ j \times 168 & j*168-84 < HU \leq j*168+84 \quad and \quad j=2,9 \\ 1680 & 1596 < HU \leq 1680 \quad and \quad j=10 \end{cases} \quad (2)$$

The HU value range 168~1680 was used to separate the muscle and soft tissue, while maintaining the best shape of the femur and formal head.

With $\rho_{max} = 3.14 \times 10^{-6}$ Kg/mm³, the bone mass density field is calculated. Then, the squared relation [14] is used to calculate the elastic module:

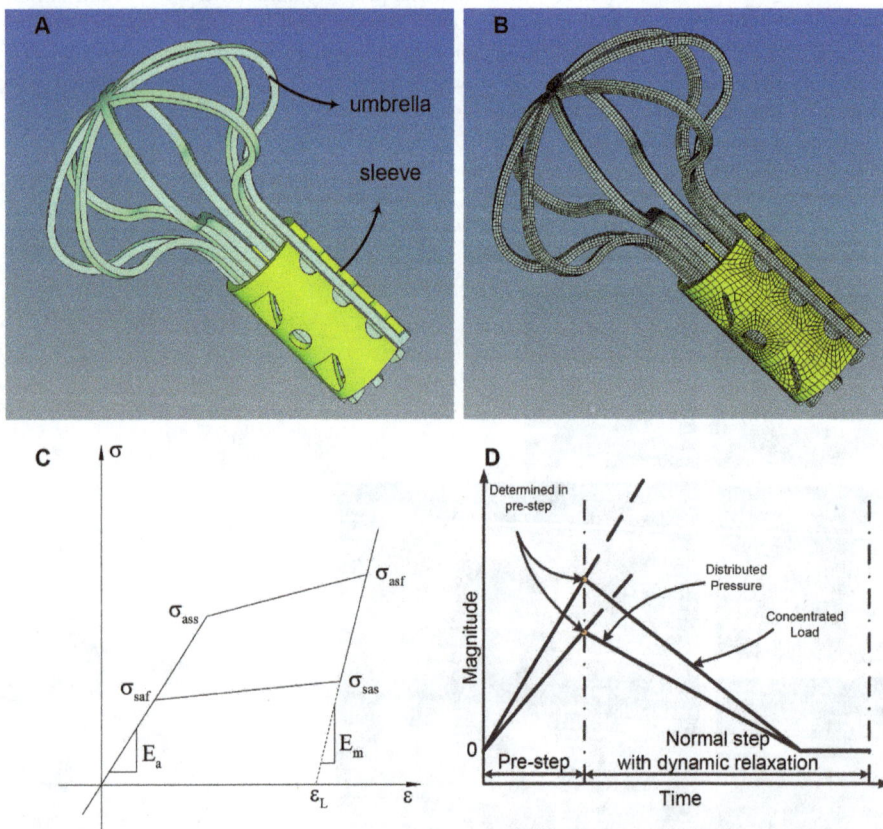

Figure 3. Implant devices and analysis setting in Lsdyna. (A) Umbrella-shaped femoral head support device geometric model; (B) Umbrella-shaped femoral head support device FE mesh model; (C) Material model in Lsdyna; (D) User-defined load curve in pre-step and normal step in: Lsdyna.

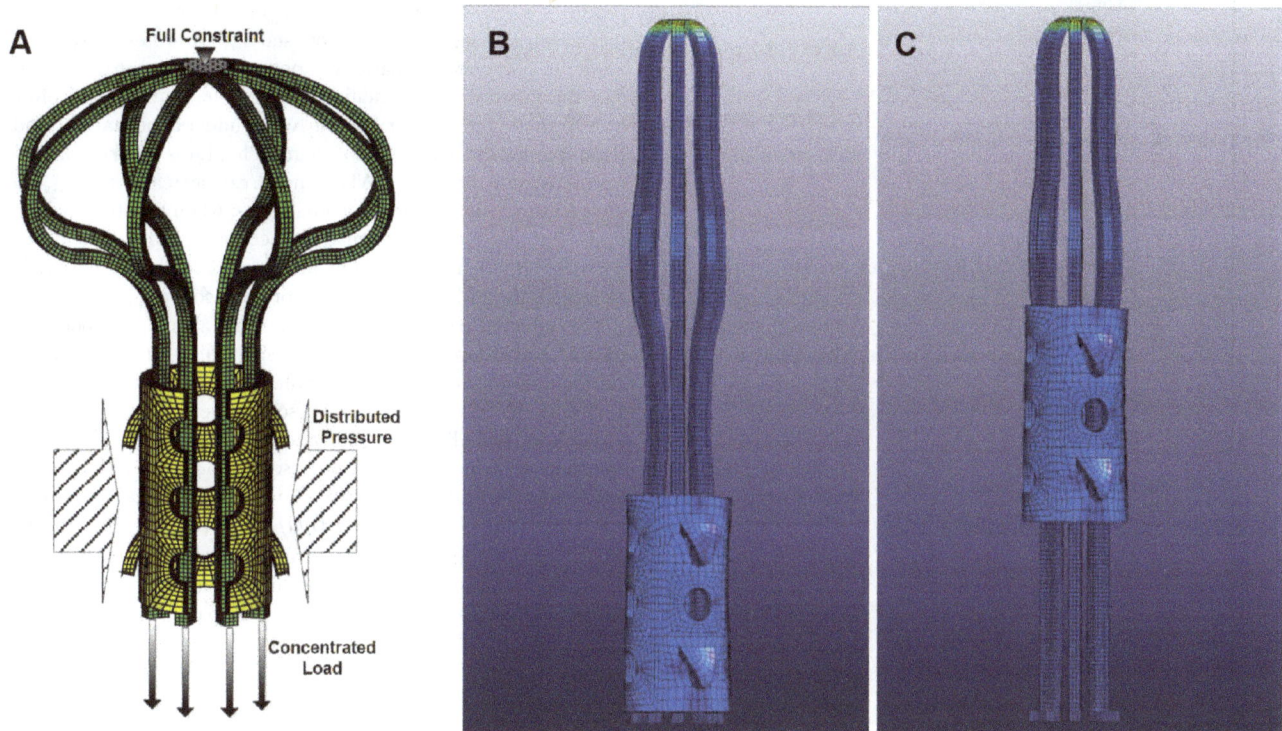

Figure 4. Constraint and load on implant devices and two different positions of the sleeve. (A) constraint and load on implant devices in pre-step and normal step:a full constraint at the top of the umbrella, concentrated load on the bottom of the umbrella, distributed pressure on the sleeve, the loads increase with time in the pre-step and decrease with time in the normal step; (B) Position I: sleeve at the bottom; (C) Position II: sleeve in the middle.

$$E = E_0 (\frac{\rho}{\rho_0})^2 \qquad (3)$$

Where $\rho_0 = 3.14 \times 10^{-6}$ Kg/mm^3, $E_0 = 20.0$ Gpa. Because of a lack of previous experiments conducted on actual femoral head bone material, the approximate squared relationship is a good and relatively simple choice. Moreover, it is often used for bone structure simulations [21].

The equivalent strain failure criterion was used to judge the failure of the bone element. When the equivalent strain reached 0.009, the bone element was damaged and removed from the calculation. This element deletion will damage the original contact surface area, which forms on the bone element's surface. Thus, all the contacts involving bone are set to an eroding-type contact, in which the contact surface can be updated whenever the original contact surface was damaged.

When the patient suffered from severe osteoporosis, a 16.34% bone mass loss was assumed and the elastic module was 30% less than normal (Table 2). The values in and out of the brackets correspond respectively to the osteoporosis bone and normal bone.

Umbrella-shaped Femoral Head Support Device

The geometric model of the Ni-Ti umbrella-shaped femoral head support device at 50°C is shown in Fig. 3(a). The implant device contains two parts: the umbrella and the sleeve, marked in green and yellow, respectively. The outer diameter of the sleeve is 12 mm. The umbrella height is 50 mm; the outer diameter is 36.25 mm; and the width of the umbrella arm is 1.2 mm. The thickness is 1 mm in both parts. The umbrella and sleeve are all meshed with 8-node hexahedron elements. There are at least 3 layers of elements width-wise. The element numbers of the umbrella and sleeve are shown in Table 1.

Ni-Ti SMA Constitutive Relation

There are three kinds of constitutive relations that can be used to describe the shape of the memory alloy: a microscopic thermodynamic model, macroscopic phenomenological model [16], and multivariant micromechanical model [17]. The microscopic thermodynamic model is useful for determining the nucleation, interfacial movement, growth of martensite, and other microscopic mechanisms of a material. Using the microscopic thermodynamic model, the macroscopic constitutive relation in the Multi-scale model is determined. Although the physical meaning of these two methods is clear, they remain difficult to use in practical engineering. The macroscopic phenomenological model [18,19,20] has developed rapidly in concert with the enrichment of experimental results. However the phenomenological constitutive model equation and the phase transition thermodynamics equations are nonlinear. In other words, it's easy to not use these equations as they require a many resources and demand a great deal of time to solve.

As previously mentioned, Lsdyna provides a simplified macroscopic phenomenological model through which the phase-changing process is made linear (Fig. 4(a)). Where σ_{ass} and σ_{asf} are the start and final stress values for the forward phase transformation, respectively. σ_{sas} and σ_{saf} are the start and final stress value for the reverse phase transformation, respectively. When the ambient temperature of 50°C was higher than A_f, which is the Austenite Finish temperature (material parameter which is 37 °C), the stress-strain curve of the SMA under an isothermal environment is determined (Fig. 3(c)). The mechanical load placed upon the alloy

Table 3. SMA material parameters setting.

Density (mg/mm³)	E_m (Gpa)	E_a (Gpa)	Poisson's Ratio	σ_{ass} (Gpa)	σ_{asf} (Gpa)	σ_{sas} (Gpa)	σ_{saf} (Gpa)	EPSL	ALPHA
6.3×10^{-6}	63.0	26.3	0.3	0.3528	0.4228	0.2856	0.1794	0.067	0.0

produces a stress on the martensite phase transformation; when the stress reaches σ_{ass} the alloy starts to transform from the austenite phase to the martensite phase. When the stress reaches σ_{asf} the forward transformation is complete. This type of phase transformation remains stable only when under a mechanical load. Even if unheated, when the mechanical load was lifted the inverse transformation occurred. When the stress decreases to σ_{sas}, the inverse transformation to austenite begins; when the stress reaches σ_{saf}, the inverse transformation occurred. When the stress decreased to 0, i.e. when the mechanical load was essentially cancelled, the SMA recovers to its original shape.

The material parameters are shown in Table 3. Temperatures M_f, M_s, A_s, A_f (representing Martensite Finish, Martensite Start, Austenite Start, and Austenite Finish, respectively) are set to 9°C, 18.4°C, 29.3°C, and 37°C. These temperatures are set in accordance with Brinskon [20] and Yu [9]. The transformation constants C_m and C_A, used to describe the relationship of the temperature and the critical stress to the induced transformation, are 0.008 $Gpa/°C$ and 0.0138 $Gpa/°C$, respectively. σ_s^{cr} and σ_f^{cr} which represent the critical stress value below M_s are 0.1 Gpa and 0.17 Gpa, respectively. Equations for evaluating the four stress values used in Lsdyan from the material parameters mentioned above are:

$$\sigma_{ass} = \sigma_s^{cr} + C_m(T - M_s) \tag{4}$$

$$\sigma_{asf} = \sigma_f^{cr} + C_m(T - M_s) \tag{5}$$

$$\sigma_{sas} = C_A(T - A_f) \tag{6}$$

$$\sigma_{saf} = C_A(T - A_s) \tag{7}$$

When the temperature was set to 50°C, the material parameters used in Lsdyna are obtained and shown in Table 3.

The EPSL refers to the maximum residual strain; and the ALPHA refers to the parameter measuring the differences between the material responses in for both the tension and compression.

Constraint and Load

The simplified linearized pseudo elastic model does not include permanent strain. In other words, after unloading, there is no stable deformation. This remains true even if the deformation is larger than the maximum strain set to .067, as described in more detail above. To properly maintain the shape below 0°C, the constrained boundary and a tension load are applied on the umbrella. A pressure is also applied on the sleeve in the normal step, as seen in Fig. 4(a). Note that the constrain and load shown above are the same values used to calculate the shape of the support device under 0°C in the pre-step. The magnitudes of these loads, i.e. the inflection points in Fig. 3(d), are chosen so that the device matches the shape presented in previous study [9]. More specifically, the outer diameter of the umbrella is 8 mm and the outer diameter of the sleeve is 9 mm.

After the reshape phase under 0°C (the pre-step), the bone structure with a full constraint at the bottom was added to the simulation (the normal step). When the distributed pressure and concentrated load began decreasing, the umbrella and sleeve began to recover to their original shape, leading to bone element

Table 4. Information of four different scenarios.

Scenario	Initial Position		Bone Quality		Constraint and Load	
	I	II	Normal	Osteoporosis	Yes	No
1	√		√			√
2	√		√		√	
3	√			√	√	
4		√	√		√	

failure. By the end of the simulation, the artificial load on the device has decreased to zero, and the final shape is obtained. The user-defined load curves of the distributed pressure and concentrated load are shown in Fig. 3(d). Two different phases–the reshape phase (pre-step phase) and open phase (normal step phase)–are included. The inflection points are determined in the pre-step phase with multiple computations.

Although the surgery process has been comprehensively described, the optimized initial position of the support device has not been determined. Likewise, there are problems remaining that relate to the damage inside the femoral head as well as variability of bone quality as seen in different patients. Thus, in the normal step phase, 4 different scenarios are simulated (Table 4).

Scenario 1 is the only one scenario without a constraint: the umbrella and sleeve can move freely, no load has been applied the umbrella and the sleeve, and the initial position I is used (Fig. 4(b)). In Scenario 2, we constrain the umbrella at the top; the concentrated load and distributed pressure are slowly released. Scenario 3 is almost the same as scenario 2, except that the bone material is different. Scenario 4 is the only scenario that uses the initial position II (Fig. 4(c)); otherwise, the conditions are identical to Scenario 2.

In all 4 scenarios, the contacts are set for the umbrella, the sleeve and formal head with each other. Two self-contacts are set for the umbrella and sleeve. More specifically, eroding-type contacts are implemented when formal bone is involved. When bone elements are deleted because of failure, a new contact surface is generated in the eroding-type contact.

Results

After reshaping under 0°C, the Ni-Ti alloy umbrella-shaped support device is implanted in the formal head. Hot saline (50°C) is poured into the formal head, and the support device begins to recover to its original shape. The primary focus of this research is to evaluate how the final shape of the support device functions in the human body. However, because of the resistance of the cancellous bone inside the formal head, the final shape is not the same as original shape, (Fig. 5(a)). In other words, the support device cannot totally recover its shape. Likewise, there is a compression deformation with respect to the original shape. Thus, the support device contains a potential energy expansion, and plays an active role in allowing the formal head to resist the pressure caused by normal bodily activities.

After the simulation, several conclusions were reached:

1) The top of the umbrella should be fully constrained to avoid the umbrella opening in an unexpected location (Fig. 5(c)). When the umbrella penetrates the formal head, the head suffers severe bone damage.

2) In Scenario 2, the final shape of the support device is similar to the original shape but with a decreased outer diameter. The outer diameter of the sleeve decreased, on average, from 12 mm to 11.26 mm (Fig. 5(b)). The maximum outer diameter of the umbrella decreased on average from 36.225 mm to 31.62 mm, which is quite close to previously observed data (32 mm) [9]. A typical pair of 4 opposite umbrella arm pairs for each scenario is shown in Fig. 5(a).

3) In Scenario 3, the operation failed, penetrating the femoral heads of the patients with severe osteoporosis. The failure position was near the bottom of the femoral head (marked in black circle in Fig. 5(e)). This failure was caused by the low elastic module, which itself was the result of severe osteoporosis (Table 2). The osteoporosis bone elements are much more vulnerable than normal bone elements.

4) The final shape of the umbrella is almost identical in Scenario 2 and 4, which means that the initial position of the sleeve does not affect the final shape of umbrella. However, the traces left by the sleeve are much different. In Scenario 2, when the sleeve is placed at the bottom and the temperature is rising, the sleeve expanded and dragged by the umbrella-shaped support device. A columnar hole of 20 mm diameter and 22.5 mm depth is formed along the decompression channel (Fig. 5(d)). However, in Scenario 4, the sleeve was placed in the middle and there was no additional damage done to the decompression channel (Fig. 5(f)).

5) There are stresses placed upon the support device and formal head because of the shape taken during the recovery process (Fig. 5(g) and (h)). These stresses correspond to the strains caused by the deformation of the umbrella-shaped device. The cancellous bone inside the femoral bone partially prevents the device from recovering to its original shape; thus the device squeezes the femoral head from inside to outside. The stresses and strain are helpful for the formal head to support the pressure brought upon the femoral head during daily activities. This means the umbrella-shaped support device is much more effective than other devices. The usefulness of this feature can be seen in the porous tantalum rod implant [21]: when there is almost no deformation in the implant device, additional enforcement of the femur head is only created by the implant device's stiffness.

Discussion

The implant surgery process includes opening the umbrella-shaped device. This device cuts through the cancellous bone and soft tissue inside the femoral head, thus causing element failure. The explicit integration method in Lsdyna is used to simulate the implant process.

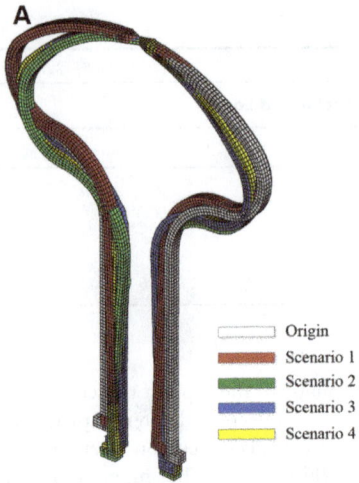

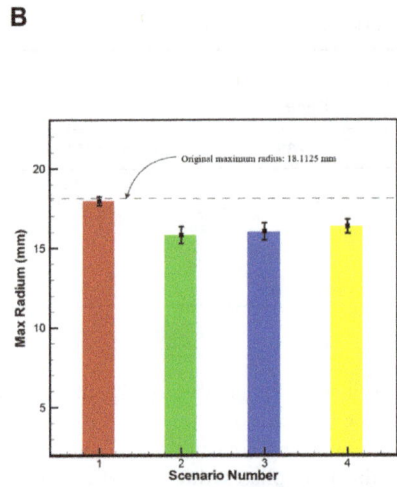

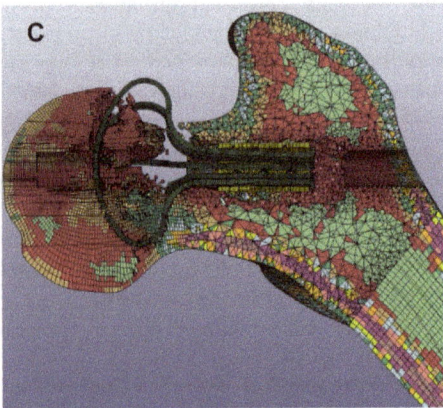

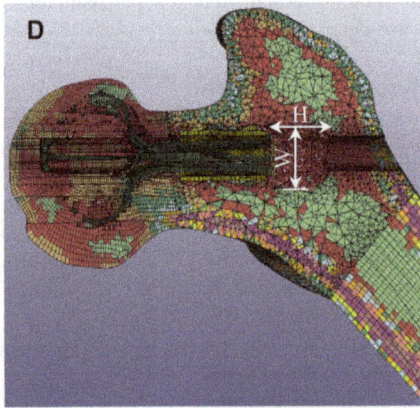

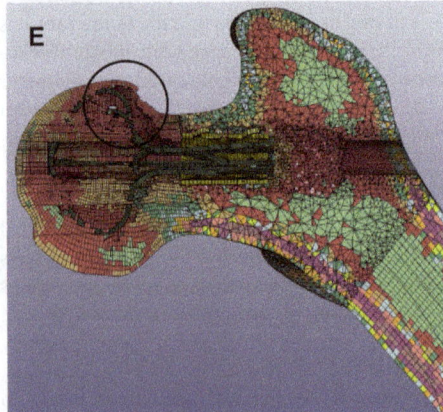

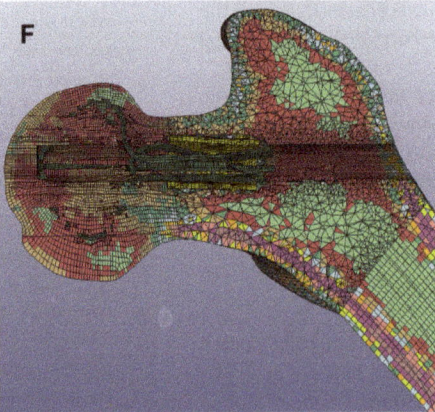

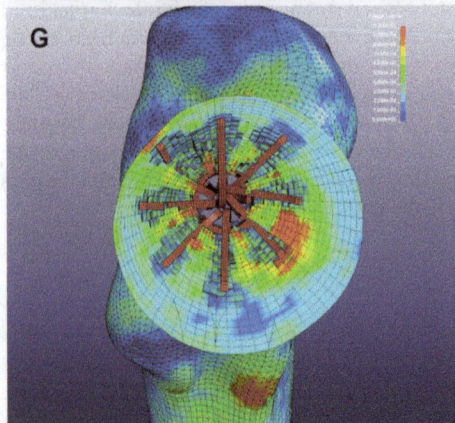

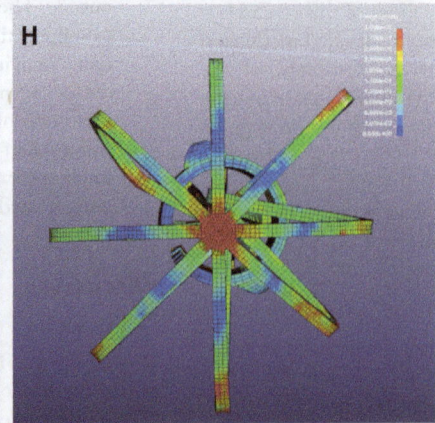

Figure 5. Analysis results. (A) Final shape of one typical pair of 4 opposite umbrella arm pairs in each scenario; (B) Statistical figure of maximum radius of each scenario; (C) scenario 1, without constraint; (D) scenario 2, initial position 1, Normal bone quality. H = 22.5 mm, W = 20 mm; (E) scenario 3, with osteoporosis, failure location marked with black circle line; (F) scenario 4, initial position 2; (G) Stress field distrubution inside femoral head in secnario 4; (H) Stress field distrubution of umberalle-shape device in secnario 4.

In this study, a 3-step scheme is used to construct the formal head FEA mesh model. The Correspond Method is used for assigning material to the mixed-element type mesh which is not suitable for auto-assigning material in Mimics. Finally, based on Lsdyna, an analysis is conducted with a dynamic relaxation for the stress initialization wherein the prescribed geometry is obtained from the pre-step.

The simulation revealed that inside the formal head the final shape of the umbrella-shaped device is not the same as the original shape. An outward expansion strain is formed inside the formal head because of the resistance created during the recovery process of the device. Penetration traces corresponding to the umbrella arms were formed inside the formal head. The traces were not strictly made along the radial direction, with some deflection caused by the uneven bone density.

The results of the analysis indicate that the simulation method is suitable and accurate. More specifically, the maximum radius of the simulation's umbrella-shaped device was almost identical to the observation data. Placing the sleeve in the middle (position II) is a better choice than the bottom of the umbrella (position I), because there is no additional damage caused in this position to the decompression channel.

Interestingly, during the simulation we noted that if the patient suffered from severe osteoporosis, and then the operation would

fail. More specifically, the failure occurred when the umbrella arm punctured the formal head. In other words, a bone mineral density test will help a doctor determine if a patient is suitable for the implant surgery.

The proposed FEA method for a computational study on the surgery simulation is proven to be reasonable and effective. For an individual patient, different sizes of support devices, initial positions and other conditions can be simulated. In other words, an individual treatment for different patients is possible with pre-FEA for specialized treatment. Our later study will focus on the evaluation of the effect of the Ni-Ti implant treatment by comparing the bearing capacity of the formal head before and after surgery through FEA.

Acknowledgments

The authors would like to thank Kangyu Jia for his contribution to syntax correction.

Author Contributions

Conceived and designed the experiments: ZD. Performed the experiments: QT. Analyzed the data: WY XL. Contributed reagents/materials/analysis tools: WY XL. Wrote the paper: WY XL.

References

1. Zhao G, Yamamoto T, Ikemura S, Motomura G, Mawatari T, et al. (2010) Radiological outcome analysis of transtrochanteric curved varus osteotomy for osteonecrosis of the femoral head at a mean follow-up of 12.4 years. J Bone Joint Surg Br 92B: 781–786.
2. Marker DR, Seyler TM, McGrath MS, Delanois RE, Ulrich SD, et al. (2008) Treatment of early stage osteonecrosis of the femoral head. J Bone Joint Surg Am 90 (Supplement 4): 175–187.
3. Wang Y, Chai W, Wang Z, Zhou Y, Zhang G, et al. (2009) Superelastic cage implantation: a new technique for treating osteonecrosis of the femoral head with mid-term follow-ups. J Arthroplasty 24: 1006–1014.
4. Sugioka Y, HOTOKEBUCHI T, TSUTSUI H (1992) Transtrochanteric anterior rotational osteotomy for idiopathic and steroid-induced necrosis of the femoral head: indications and long-term results. Clin Orthop Relat Res 277: 111–120.
5. Koo KH, Kim R, Ko GH, Song HR, Jeong ST, et al. (1995) Preventing collapse in early osteonecrosis of the femoral head. A randomised clinical trial of core decompression. J Bone Joint Surg Br 77: 870–874.
6. Plakseychuk AY, Kim S, Park B, Varitimidis SE, Rubash HE, et al. (2003) Vascularized compared with nonvascularized fibular grafting for the treatment of osteonecrosis of the femoral head. J Bone Joint Surg Am 85: 589–596.
7. AldridgeIII JM, Berend KR, Gunneson EE, Urbaniak JR (2004) Free Vascularized Fibular Grafting for the Treatment of Postcollapse Osteonecrosis of the Femoral HeadSurgical Technique. J Bone Joint Surg Am 86: 87–101.
8. Shuler MS, Rooks MD, Roberson JR (2007) Porous tantalum implant in early osteonecrosis of the hip: preliminary report on operative, survival, and outcomes results. J Arthroplasty 22: 26–31.
9. Yu X, Jiang W, Pan Q, Wu T, Zhang Y, et al. (2013) Umbrella-shaped, memory alloy femoral head support device for treatment of avascular osteonecrosis of the femoral head. Int Orthop: 1–8.
10. Kainuma R, Matsumoto M, Honma T. The mechanism of the all-round shape memory effect in a Ni-rich TiNi alloy; 1986. 717–722.

11. Christ D, Reese S (2009) A finite element model for shape memory alloys considering thermomechanical couplings at large strains. Int J Solids Struct 46: 3694–3709.
12. Necchi S, Taschieri S, Petrini L, Migliavacca F (2008) Mechanical behaviour of nickel-titanium rotary endodontic instruments in simulated clinical conditions: a computational study. Int Endod J 41: 939–949.
13. Auricchio F, Taylor RL (1997) Shape-memory alloys: modelling and numerical simulations of the finite-strain superelastic behavior. Comput Method Appl Mech Eng 143: 175–194.
14. Gibson LJ, Ashby MF (1999) Cellular solids: structure and properties. Cambridge university press. 449 p.
15. Burgers TA, Mason J, Niebur G, Ploeg HL (2008) Compressive properties of trabecular bone in the distal femur. J Biomech 41: 1077–1085.
16. Tanaka K (1986) A thermomechanical sketch of shape memory effect: one-dimensional tensile behavior. Res Mechanica 18: 251–263.
17. Gao X, Huang M, Brinson LC (2000) A multivariant micromechanical model for SMAs Part 1. Crystallographic issues for single crystal model. Int J Plasticity 16: 1345–1369.
18. Müller I (1979) A model for a body with shape-memory. Arch Ration Mech Anal 70: 61–77.
19. Sun QP, Hwang KC (1993) Micromechanics modelling for the constitutive behavior of polycrystalline shape memory alloys-I. Derivation of general relations. J Mech Phys Solids 41: 1–17.
20. Brinson LC (1993) One-dimensional constitutive behavior of shape memory alloys: thermomechanical derivation with non-constant material functions and redefined martensite internal variable. J Intell Mater Syst Struct 4: 229–242.
21. Lutz AE, Nackenhorst U, von Lewinski G, Windhagen H, Floerkemeier T (2011) Numerical studies on alternative therapies for femoral head necrosis. Biomech Model Mechanobiol 10: 627–640.

12

Use of Alendronate Sodium (Fosamax) to Ameliorate Osteoporosis in Renal Transplant Patients

Wen-Hung Huang[1,2], Shen-Yang Lee[1,2], Cheng-Hao Weng[1,2], Ping-Chin Lai[1,2]*

1 Department of Nephrology, Chang Gung Memorial Hospital, Linkou, Taiwan, Republic of China, 2 Chang Gung University College of Medicine, Taoyuan, Taiwan, Republic of China

Abstract

Background: Renal transplant patients often have severe bone and mineral deficiencies. While the clinical effects of immunosuppressive agents like calcineurin inhibitors (CIs) and sirolimus on bone turnover are unclear, bisphosphonates are effective in bone recovery in these patients. Gender is significantly associated with osteoporosis and affects bone turnover, which is different in women and men. The effective gender-related site of action of bisphosphonates is unknown.

Methods: Initially, we enrolled 84 kidney recipients who had received their transplants at least 5 months ago; of these, 8 were excluded and 76 were finally included in the study. First bone mineral density (BMD) at the lumbar spine, hip, and femoral neck was determined using dual-energy X-ray absorptiometry (DXA) between September 2008 and March 2009. These 76 patients underwent a repeat procedure after a mean period 14 months. Immunosuppressive agents, bisphosphonates, patients' characteristics, and biochemical factors were analyzed on the basis of the BMD determined using DXA.

Results: After the 14-month period, the BMD of lumbar spine increased significantly (from 0.9 g/cm^2 to 0.92 g/cm^2, p<0.001), whereas that of the hip and femoral neck did not. Ordinal logistic regression analysis was used to show that Fosamax improved bone condition, as defined by WHO (p = 0.007). The use of immunosuppressive agents did not affect bone turnover (p>0.05). Moreover, in subgroup analysis, Fosamax increased the BMD at the lumbar spine and the hipbone in males (p = 0.028 and 0.03, respectively) but only at the lumbar spine in females (p = 0.022).

Conclusion: After a long periods after renal transplantation, the detrimental effects of steroid and immunosuppressive agents on bone condition diminished. Short-term Fosamax administration effectively improves BMD in these patients. The efficacy of Fosamax differed between male and female renal transplant patients.

Editor: Bin He, Baylor College of Medicine, United States of America

Funding: The authors have no support or funding to report.

Competing Interests: The authors have declared that no competing interests exist.

* E-mail: williammaxima@gmail.com

Introduction

Patients maintained on dialysis for end-stage renal disease exhibit severe mineral and bone deficiencies. While renal transplantation restores defective kidney function in patients with chronic renal disease, the associated steroid and other immuno-suppressive therapies continuously damage the bones [1,2]; the expected correction of established bone lesions does not occur. Although transplantation can resolve many biochemical imbalances, such as hyperparathyroidism, associated with chronic renal failure, progressive loss of BMD in the trabecular bone often occurs early after renal transplantation [3]. Investigators have not agreed on the risk factors that are most strongly associated with reduced BMD [4,5] after renal transplantation, except on an accumulated dose of steroid. At present, the use of biochemical markers of bone turnover in the serum or urine is not recommended for diagnosis [6]. The World Health Organization (WHO) defines osteoporosis as a condition in which the difference between the mean BMDs for the lumbar spine (LS), femoral neck (FN), or hip (H) of the patients and healthy young adults is more than 2.5 standard deviations (SDs), as measured by dual energy X-ray absorptiometry (DXA). Further, osteopenia is defined as a condition in which the difference between the mean BMDs of the patients and healthy young adults is between 1 and 2.5 SDs [6]. Several studies have shown the beneficial effects of bisphospho-nates on post-transplantation osteoporosis [7–9]. Other studies have shown that calcineurin inhibitors (CIs) have deleterious effects on bone mineral metabolism in rats [10–12], and that at least one cyclosporine has a protective effect on bone [13]. Other immune-modifying drugs, such as azathioprine, mycophenolate mofetil, and sirolimus, which are used in conjunction with glucocorticoids and CIs, have not been shown to promote bone loss, neither experimentally nor clinically [14,15]. Osteoporosis caused by portosystemic shunting [16], or by steroid or CIs through receptor activator of nuclear factor kappa-B ligand

(RANKL)-dependent pathways, may be partially ameliorated using sirolimus [17]. Moreover, the physiology of bone turnover differs according to gender, particularly in menopausal women [18–21], and the efficacy of alendronate in the treatment of postmenopausal osteoporosis has been well established [22]. To our knowledge, the gender-related efficacy of alendronate in renal transplant subjects has rarely been reported. The aim of this randomized case-control study was to assess the impact of immunosuppressive agents and alendronate on BMD, as estimated by DXA, and to determine whether the response to alendronate in renal transplant subjects is gender-dependent.

Materials and Methods

This case-control study complied with the guidelines of the Declaration of Helsinki and approved by the Medical Ethics Committee of Chang Gung Memorial Hospital, a tertiary referral center located in the northern part of Taiwan. Since this study involved retrospective review of existing data, the Institutional Review Board approval was obtained, but without specific informed consent from patients. In addition, all individual information was securely protected (by delinking identifying information from main data set) and available to investigators only. Furthermore, all the data were analyzed anonymously. On the other hand, if this study involved retrospective review of existing data plus retrospective analysis of remaining biological samples, both Institutional Review Board approval and specific informed consent must be obtained from all patients. The Institutional Review Board of Chang Gung Memorial Hospital has specifically waived the need for consent. Finally, all primary data were collected according to strengthening the reporting of observational studies in epidemiology guidelines. The form described above was referenced from the Liu et al.'s publication [23].

Study population

We randomly enrolled 84 kidney recipients (40 men and 44 women) who had undergone transplantation at least 5 months ago. We used DXA to obtain BMD measurements of the lumbar spine (LS), left hip (H), and femoral neck (FN) between September 2008 and March 2009 [24]. Bone condition was defined on the basis of the WHO criteria: a BMD value >2.5 standard deviations (SD, T score) below the young adult mean indicated osteoporosis and that between 1.0 and 2.5 SDs below the mean indicated osteopenia. The immunosuppressive agents that the patients had received included prednisolone (5 mg/tablet), cyclosporine (25 mg/tablet and 100 mg/tablet), tacrolimus (0.5 mg/tablet and 1 mg/tablet), sirolimus (1 mg/tablet), and mycophenolate (250 mg/tablet). Fosamax (alendronate sodium; 70 mg/tablet, 70 mg per week) was administered to the patients who were initially diagnosed with osteoporosis. Fasting blood levels of serum creatinine (Cr), blood urea nitrogen (BUN), calcium, inorganic phosphate, and uric acid were obtained. The patients' medical records were studied for the history of diabetes mellitus (DM), smoking frequency, alcohol intake, and hepatitis B (HBV), hepatitis C (HCV), and cytomegalovirus (CMV) infections. All the doses of immunosuppressive agents administered between the 2 BMD measurements were considered as the accumulated dose. After 14 ± 1.6 months of follow-up, the 76 remaining patients (8 of the 84 patients were excluded—2 subjects had died, 2 had graft failure, and the initial BMD measurements of 4 patients was lost) received a second measurement of BMD and fasting blood tests.

Precautions and contraindications for the use of Fosamax

The first DXA report was obtained between September 2008 and March 2009. Fosamax (70 mg per week) was administered to the patients diagnosed with osteoporosis based on this DXA report unless 1 or more of the following conditions was present: bisphosphonate allergy; blood calcium levels <8 mg/dL; active stomach problems (e.g., esophagitis, gastritis, or ulcers); renal insufficiency (estimated glomerular filtration rate [eGFR] <30 mL/[min·1.73 m^2] or serum Cr level >3 mg/dL); difficulty swallowing or the inability to stand/sit upright for at least 30 min, and pregnancy and breastfeeding. The patients did not receive Fosamax prior to obtainment of the first DXA data. Furthermore, the patients were informed that they should take the drug only upon rising for the day with 3 to 4 swallows of water and that they should stand, walk, or sit and fast for 30–45 min afterwards, and then eat breakfast. Lying down or reclining after taking the drug is prohibited. At least 30 min should pass after the intake of alendronate before taking supplements or other drugs.

Immunosuppressive protocol

In our hospital, we mainly use a CI-based immunosuppressive regimen in the initial months of transplantation. Most of our patients also receive mycophenolic acid plus prednisolone during this stage. Immediately after transplantation, the targeted cyclosporine concentration at 2 h post-dose (C$_2$) is approximately 1300–1100 ng/mL and the tacrolimus trough level is maintained at approximately 12–10 ng/mL. These concentrations are tapered gradually in the first year. In patients that have been transplanted for more than 12 months, the cyclosporine C$_2$ level is maintained at approximately 500–600 ng/mL and tacrolimus level at 3–4 ng/mL. Prednisolone is maintained at 1.25–10 mg per day, according to patient's condition. An mTOR inhibitor is added to the regimen if the patient's condition is suitable (proteinuria <800 mg/day and eGFR >40 mL/[min·1.73 m^2]). The trough level of the mTOR inhibitor is maintained at approximately 3–8 ng/mL. Once the mTOR inhibitor has been added, the CI and mycophenolic acid dose are cut by 50% overnight, while prednisolone is maintained at the same dosage. Subsequently, the CI dose is tapered as much as possible. Most of the patients in this study received only 25 mg cyclosporine or 0.5 mg tacrolimus per day if an mTOR inhibitor was used.

Statistical analysis

The data, given as median and interquartile ranges in nonnormal distribution variables, are expressed as mean $\pm$ SD in normal distribution variables. The paired t test and the Wilcoxon signed-rank test were used to compare data of the patients at presentation and follow-up. The Kruskal–Wallis test and one-way analysis of variance (ANOVA) were performed to compare data of the different bone conditions defined by the WHO criteria. Comparisons among groups were performed using the Mann–Whitney test and Student's t test. We used multivariate ordinal logistic regression to test the expected value between clinical variables and the change of bone condition (grade 1: change to better, grade 2: no change, and grade 3: deterioration; change to better: from osteoporosis to osteopenia or normal, or from osteopenia to normal; no change: no change in bone condition at start and follow-up; deterioration: from normal to osteopenia or osteoporosis, or from osteopenia to osteoporosis), as defined by WHO. The Chi-square test was used to determine the correlation between the 2 binary variables; a p value <0.05 was considered statistically significant. All statistical analyses were performed using the Statistical Package for the Social Sciences (SPSS) Version 12.0 for Windows (SPSS Inc., Chicago, IL, USA).

Results

Characteristics of the study population

After a follow-up period of 14±1.6 months, 76 subjects received a second BMD measurement. Among these patients, 12 had a medical history of DM; 10 were infected with HBV, 15 with HCV, and 13 with CMV; 10 men were habitual tobacco users, and 8 men and 1 woman regularly consumed alcohol. Thirty-four patients received Fosamax, 57, prednisolone; 55, mycohenolate; 30, tacrolimus; 26, cyclosporine; and 34, sirolimus. Eight patients (11%) received a single immunosuppressive agent, 21 patients (28%) received 2 immunosuppressive agents, 36 (47%) received 3, and 11 (14%) received 4.

Bone mineral density (BMD) at baseline and at follow-up

Table 1 shows the changes in BMD and blood biochemistry after 14±1.6 months of follow-up. In the 76 patients, calcium level decreased from 9.45±0.51 mg/dL to 9.29±0.52 mg/dL ($p<0.001$) and albumin from 4.42±0.29 g/L to 4.34±0.4 g/L ($p = 0.009$), both levels were still within the normal range. However, BMD of the lumbar spine increased from 0.9 to 0.92 g/cm^2, ($p<0.001$). No correlation between the use of Fosamax and that of the immunosuppressive agents could be demonstrated, as determined by the Chi-square test ($p>0.05$). No patient who received Fosamax exhibited a deterioration in the condition of his bone structure, as defined by WHO criteria. Thirty patients showed no change in their bone condition, but 4 showed improvement. In patients who had not received Fosamax, 6 (14%) showed deterioration and 1 (2%) showed improvement.

BMD in patients with osteoporosis and without

In 41 patients with and 35 without osteoporosis at baseline, the lumbar spine bone density increased (from 0.83 to 0.86 g/cm^2 [$p<0.001$] and from 0.99 to 1.0 g/cm^2 [$p = 0.02$]; respectively) after the mean 14-month follow-up period, but hip and femoral neck densities did not (Table 2). In order to detect any difference in BMD due to the use of immunosuppressive agents in different conditions of the bone, the patients were divided into 3 groups: normal, osteopenia, and osteoporosis, on the basis of the initial DXA findings. The osteoporosis group received a greater cumulative steroid dose than the osteopenia group (1326.5 mg vs. 724.5 mg; $p = 0.005$; Figure 1A), and the increase in the lumbar spine BMD was greater in the osteoporosis group (0.033 g/cm^2 vs. 0.009 g/cm^2; $p = 0.028$; Figure 1B). Otherwise, the cumulative dose of immunosuppressive agents among the 3 groups did not differ significantly ($p>0.05$; Figure 1A). Interestingly, of our 41 osteoporosis patients, 7 did not receive Fosamax due to their intolerance of the side effects. Among those 41 patients, those administered Fosamax showed a greater increase in BMD (0.035 g/cm^2 vs. 0.003 g/cm^2) but not significant ($p>0.05$).

Factors associated with bone turnover

To deepen our investigation of the influence of clinical features on bone condition, we used a univariate binary logistic regression to evaluate the association between bone condition (osteoporotic and not osteoporotic at follow-up) and the clinical variables in 76 patients. The use of both prednisolone (odds ratio [OR], 5.18; 95% confidence interval [CI], 1.6–16.4; $p = 0.005$) and Fosamax (OR, 18.75; 95% CI, 5.42–64.76; $p<0.001$) showed an association in patients with osteoporosis (Figure 2A). In an ordinal logistic regression with multivariate analysis of the change in bone condition (grade 1, improvement; grade 2, no change; and grade 3, deterioration; as defined by WHO criteria) and the clinical variables, after adjusting for age, sex, status of diabetes, smoking,

Table 1. Data reported at baseline and at follow-up, n = 76.

	Baseline	follow-up	P value
LS-BMD (g/cm²)	0.90±0.14	0.92±0.14	<0.001
H-BMD (g/cm²)	0.81±0.14	0.81±0.14	NS
FN-BMD (g/cm²)	0.68±0.12	0.69±0.13	NS
LS T	−1.53±1.24	−1.32±1.26	<0.001
H T	−1.76±0.97	−1.68±1.07	NS
FN T	−2.45±0.96	−2.42±1.02	NS
Smoking	10/76		
Alcohol	9/76		
DM	12/76		
HBV	10/76		
HCV	15/76		
CMV	13/76		
BUN (mg/dL)	19.7±10.0	19.8±10.9	NS
Cr (mg/dL)	1.18±0.54	1.20±0.54	NS
Ca (mg/dL)	9.45±0.51	9.29±0.52	<0.001
P (mg/dL)	3.21±0.54	3.23±0.59	NS
Uric acid (mg/dL)	6.24±1.68	6.45±1.70	NS
Albumin (g/L)	4.42±0.29	4.34±0.40	0.009
TC (mg/dL)	201±44	190±46	NS
TG (mg/dL)	147±82	148±113	NS
Normal	5/76	5/76	
Osteopenia	30/76	29/76	
Osteoporosis	41/76	42/76	

At follow-up, LS-BMD was significantly greater than its initial value. The albumin and calcium levels also had decreased significantly, but they remained within normal range.
Abbreviations: LS-BMD, lumbar spine bone mineral density; H-BMD, hip bone mineral density; FN-BMD, femoral neck bone mineral density; T, number of standard deviations (SD) above or below the mean value of a sex-matched, young adult mean of BMD. DM, diabetes mellitus; BUN, blood urea nitrogen; Cr, blood creatinine; Ca, serum calcium; P, serum inorganic phosphate; TC, serum total cholesterol; TG, serum triglyceride; HBV, hepatitis B virus infection; HCV, hepatitis C virus infection; CMV, cytomegalovirus infection; NS, no significance, $p>0.05$.

alcohol consumption, time since transplantation, age at transplant, and use of prednisolone, the use of Fosamax (OR, −3.115; 95% CI, −5.364; −0.866; $p = 0.007$) was found to be associated with a positive prognosis (Figure 2B).

Gender differences in the effect of Fosamax on bones

In our study, we found no gender-related differences in bone turnover of renal transplant patients during the mean 14-month follow-up period. Seeking a gender-related difference in the physiology of bone turnover, we examined the bone response to Fosamax in the 2 sexes. We found no differences in bone turnover with respect to age, time since transplant, or the changes in blood values for creatinine, albumin, or calcium, and neither was the change in BMD or the cumulative immunosuppressive agents different in the 2 sexes. However, when we compared BMD before and after Fosamax treatment within the male and female groups, we found Fosamax to be more effective in men than in women. Among the patients who received Fosamax, BMD in the lumbar spine and the hip ($p = 0.028$ and $p = 0.03$, respectively) increased in 14 men; however, the increase in the BMD was observed only

A

B

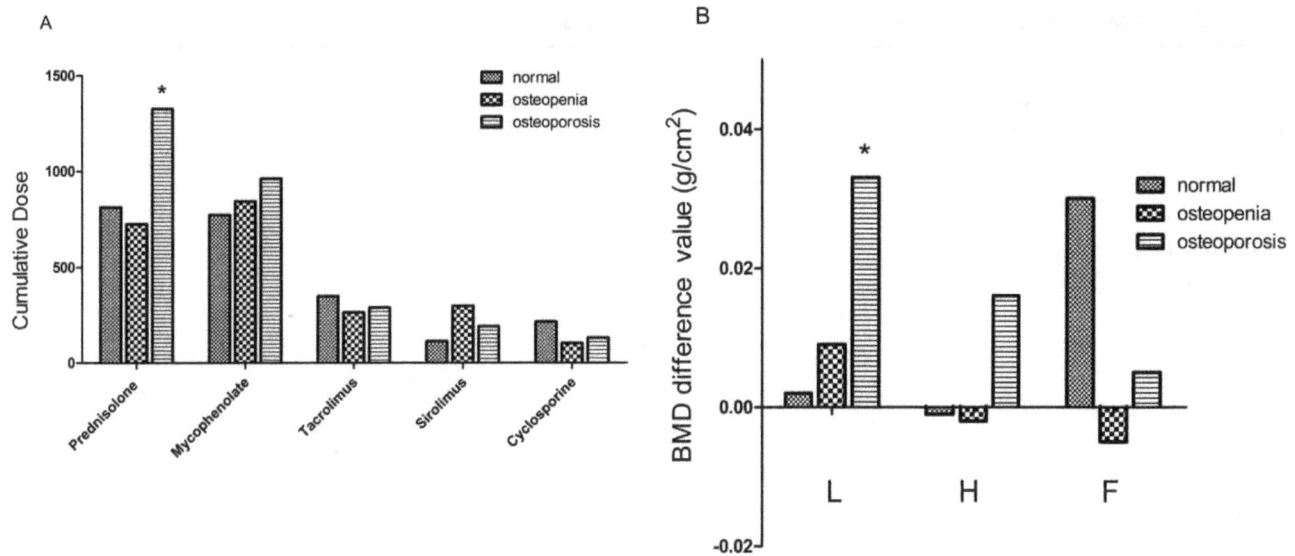

Figure 1. Cumulative dose of immunosuppressive agents and bone mineral density change between three bone conditions by WHO. The patients were divided, according to their baseline DXA, into normal (n = 5), osteopenia (n = 30), and osteoporosis (n = 41) groups. The osteoporosis group received a significantly greater cumulative prednisolone dose than did the osteopenia group (1326.5 mg vs. 724.5 mg; p = 0.005; Figure 1A), and the increase in lumbar spine bone mineral density was also significantly greater in the osteoporosis group (0.033 g/cm² vs. 0.009 g/cm²; p = 0.028; Figure 1B). The drugs included in the analysis of cummulative immunosuppresive therapy were prednisolone, 5 mg; mycophenolate, 250 mg; tacrolimus, 0.5 mg; sirolimus, 1 mg; and cyclosporine, 100 mg. Abbreviations: L, lumbar spine; H, hipbone; F, femoral neck. *Statistical significance at p<0.05.

in the lumbar spine (p = 0.022; Table 3) in 20 women. Among the above-mentioned men and women who used Fosamax, the BMD difference values were not different (p>0.05). Thus, we find that the sites of action of Fosamax differ across the 2 sexes.

Discussion

In this study, we have shown that short-term weekly use of Fosamax can improve both BMD and bone condition, in accordance with the WHO criteria, regardless of effect of immunosuppressive agents after a long period after renal transplantation. In renal transplant subjects with osteoporosis, Fosamax improved the BMD of the lumbar spine. Although the bone condition after renal transplantation did not vary according to gender, the bone regions in which Fosamax was effective did vary.

An increase in bone mass loss is multifactorial and is affected by age [21], sex [19–21], renal function, and duration of time for which the patient was on dialysis before transplantation [20]. A major influencing and well-known factor causing increased loss of bone mass is high-dose steroid therapy during the early period after transplantation and continuous long-term steroid administration [2]. CIs such as cyclosporine and tacrolimus also are known to have serious effects and cause rapid and severe bone losses in both animal models and humans. The role of T-lymphocyte action via RANKL seems to be of essence in triggering bone loss [14]. Other immune-modifying drugs such as azathioprine, mycophenolate mofetil, and sirolimus, which are used in conjunction with glucocorticoids and CIs, have—neither experimentally nor clinically—been shown to promote bone loss. Recent studies [17,25] suggest that sirolimus could promote an osteoclastic balance between the effects of steroid and of calcineurine inhibitors. Moreover, under sirolimus-based maintenance immunosuppression [26] after bone surgery, no radiologic advantage or disadvantage to bone healing was noted. Therefore, in our clinical

estimation, a bias may exist between the biochemical markers and DXA–WHO criteria in osteoporosis to evaluate bone condition.

Interestingly, the lumbar spine BMD in our 35 non-osteoporotic patients increased slightly. As was true with the steroids, the cumulative dose of immunosuppressive agents in the non-osteoporosis and osteoporosis groups did not differ. In the past decade, the use of corticosteroids in the peritransplantation period has been dramatically reduced and replaced by CIs and other adjunctive agents. To our knowledge, the first 3 to 6 months after transplantation is the critical period for the loss in bone mass [4,27,28]. In a long-term study, the ongoing accelerated lumbar bone mass loss was 1.7±2.8% per year [29], but in the 12 months following cardiac transplantation, the LS BMD value was restored to that at the time of transplant [30]. Twenty-four months after transplantation, the yearly loss of absolute BMD was parallel to the age-dependent physiological decline in absolute BMD [5]. In our study, the time since transplant of non-osteoporotic subjects was 78±60 months. From the studies cited above and from our observations during the long post-transplantation period, we can explain the slightly increased BMD of lumbar spine in our patients who did not receive Fosamax. Otherwise, as the use of immunosuppressive agents changes in the long period of renal transplantation, the effective power of steroid on bone turnover may be increasingly minor.

In this study, when we analyzed the subgroups of the subjects with osteoporosis, we observed that Fosamax was not equally effective in men and women in the different bone regions. Several previous studies have shown that bisphosphonates continued to improved bone mineral density after renal transplantation [7–9,31,32] and most of them showed the effect on both lumbar spine and femoral neck BMD. In a meta-analysis review of 1209 patients [33], treatment with bisphosphonates increased BMD in lumbar spine and femoral neck. No measurable change in the BMD of the hip area was observed. In another population-based longitudinal study [18], both the bone turnover and the sites of bone loss

Table 2. Comparison of patients with (41) and without (35) osteoporosis at presentation and follow-up.

	Non-osteoporosis patients (35)			Osteoporosis patients (41)			P value
	Baseline	1st follow up	P value	Baseline	1st follow up	P value	
LS-BMD(g/cm^2)	0.99±0.12	1.00±0.13	0.02	0.83±0.11	0.86±0.12	<0.001	
H-BMD(g/cm^2)	0.91±0.12	0.90±0.13	NS	0.72±0.11	0.73±0.10	NS	
FN-BMD (g/cm^2)	0.78±0.09	0.78±0.11	NS	0.605±0.058	0.607±0.066	NS	
LS T score	−1.0 [−1.6,−0.2]	−0.9 [−1.5,0.3]	0.047	−2.15±1.02	−1.9±1.07	<0.001	
H T score	−1.06±0.65	−1.01±0.89	NS	−2.35±0.79	−2.25±0.86	NS	
FN T score	−1.59±0.68	−1.68±0.78	NS	−3.14±0.47	−3.09±0.54	NS	
Gender (F/M)	16/19			24/17			
Smoking	5/35			5/41			
Alcohol	5/35			4/41			
DM	7/35			5/41			
BUN (mg/dL)	17.7±7.6	17.7±6.3	NS	21.27±11.77	21.55±13.46	NS	NS*
Cr (mg/dL)	1.09±0.45	1.15±0.41	0.043	1.24±0.6	1.28±0.62	NS	NS*
Ca (mg/dL)	9.52±0.49	9.33±0.56	0.002	9.4±0.53	9.24±0.49	0.007	NS*
P (mg/dL)	3.22±0.58	3.22±0.57	NS	3.2±0.52	3.25±0.62	NS	NS*
Uric acid (mg/dL)	6.0±1.7	6.6±1.9	NS	6.44±1.73	6.26±1.59	NS	NS*
Albumin (g/L)	4.48±0.31	4.39±0.43	0.035	4.38±0.27	4.31±0.41	NS	NS*
TC (mg/dL)	198.1±40.2	190.5±44.3	NS	203.67±47.5	187.78±49.4	NS	NS*
TG (mg/dL)	159.9±85.5	152.5±106.3	NS	137.77±79.35	146.03±129.37	NS	NS*
Normal	5	5		0	0		
Osteopenia	30	25		0	4		
Osteoporosis	0	5		41	37		
Cumulative dose of immunosuppressant agent							
Prednisolone (mg)	872±730			1326.5±961			p=0.003
Mycophenolate (tablets)	833.6±823.8			962.2±812.5			NS*
Tacrolimus (tablets/1 mg)	275.0±393.6			288.1±447.1			NS*
Sirolimus (tablets)	270.8±302.0			191.5±301.1			NS*
Cyclosporine (100 mg tablets)	119.20±210.85			131.12±177.79			NS*
Increase in BMD							
LS-BMD (g/cm^2)	0.011±0.027			0.030±0.028			p=0.005
H-BMD (g/cm^2)	−0.005±0.03			0.007±0.036			NS*
FN-BMD (g/cm^2)	0.003 ±0.052			0.002±0.031			NS*

The mean follow-up period was 14 months. In both the non-osteoporosis and the osteoporosis group, the LS-BMD significantly increased. At the end of the period, the cumulative dose of prednisolone and the LS-BMD differential were greater in the osteoporosis group.

NS*: p>0.05 between the osteoporosis and non-osteoporosis group.

Abbreviations: LS-BMD, lumbar spine bone mineral density; H-BMD, hip bone mineral density; FN-BMD, femoral neck bone mineral density; T score, number of standard deviations (SD) different from the mean value of the corresponding gender-matched young adult mean BMD. DM, diabetes mellitus; BUN, blood urea nitrogen; Cr, blood creatinine; Ca, serum calcium concentration; P, serum inorganic phosphate level; TC, serum total cholesterol level; TG, serum triglyceride level; NS: not significant, p>0.05.

differed according to gender. In a 2-year double-blind trial of men with osteoporosis (mean age, 63 years), alendronate significantly increased bone mass of spine and hipbone and helped prevent vertebral fractures [34]. Iwamoto et al. [35] have suggested that although alendronate treatment in men effectively increased lumbar BMD from baseline, its efficacy appeared to be no greater than that in postmenopausal women with osteoporosis. Studies on the comparative effects in a renal transplant population of bisphosphonates according to gender and bone site are limited. In our study on men and women who presented no significant differences in the increase in their BMD with Fosamax, the 14

osteoporotic men showed improved BMD at the hip and lumbar spine and the 20 osteoporotic females responded well only at the lumbar spine.

Fosamax is absorbed and partitioned rapidly, with approximately 50% binding to the exposed bone surface and the remainder being excreted unchanged by the kidneys [36]. Therefore, Fosamax should be used carefully in patients with renal insufficiency or in anuric patients because of concerns regarding drug accumulation. The major side effect of Fosamax is ulceration of the esophagus, which may require hospitalization and intensive treatment. Gastric and duodenal ulceration may also

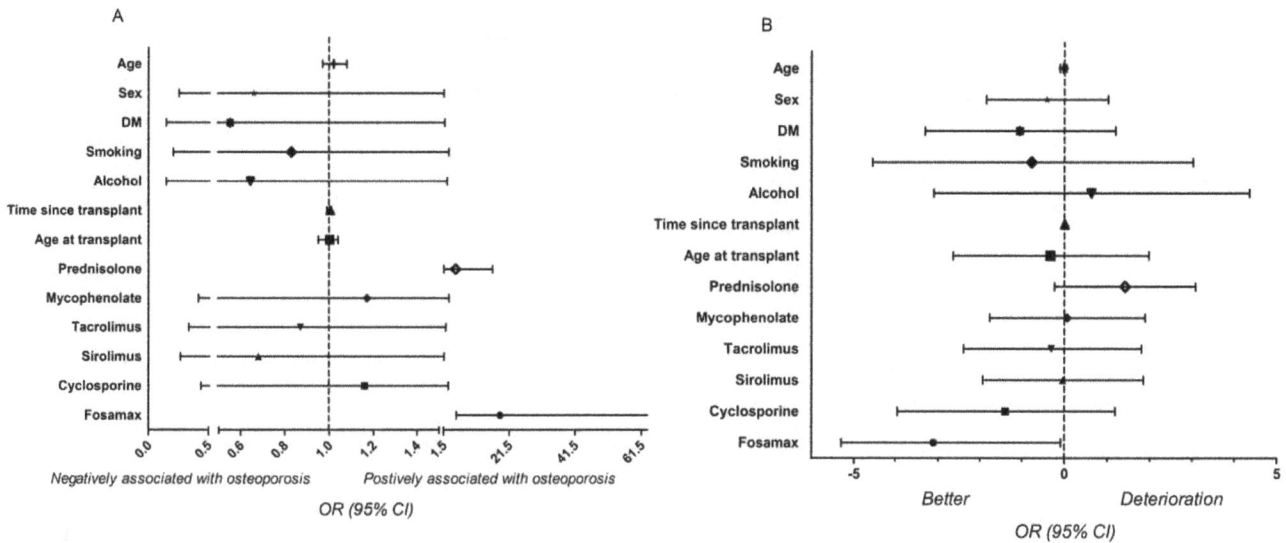

Figure 2. Clinical variables associated with bone condition change. A binary (non-osteoporosis and osteoporosis in follow-up) logistic regression analysis was performed to identify the variables associated with osteoporosis. The dependent variable was non-osteoporosis or osteoporosis. The independent variables were age, sex, DM, smoking, alcohol consumption, age at transplantation, time since transplant, use of immunosuppressive agents and use of Fosamax. Both the use of prednisolone (odds ratio [OR], 5.18; 95% confidence interval [CI], 1.6–16.4; p = 0.005) and the use of Fosamax (OR, 18.75; 95% CI, 5.42–64.76; p<0.001) were associated with the symptoms of osteoporosis (Figure 2A). In an ordinal logistic regression with multivariate analysis of the change of bone condition (grade 1, changed to the better; grade 2, no change; and grade 3, deterioration, as defined by WHO criteria and clinical variables), after adjusting for age, sex, status of diabetes (DM), smoking, alcohol consumption, time since transplant, age at transplant, and use of prednisolone, the use of Fosamax (OR, −3.115; 95% CI, −5.364 to −0.866; p = 0.007) was found to be associated with a positive prognosis (Figure 2B).

Table 3. Comparison of the use and non-use of Fosamax in men and women.

	Male patients (36)			Female patients (40)			P value
	Non-Fosamax (22)	Fosamax (14)	P value	Non-Fosamax (20)	Fosamax (20)	P value	
Age (years)	48±10.4	51.9±9.0	NS	49.7±7.6	53.3±8.8	NS	NS*
Time since transplant (months)	92±68.1	103.7±59.4	NS	61.4±39.6	97.6±72.9	NS	NS*
Creatinine difference value (mg/dL)	0 (−0.072, 0.122)	0.04 (−0.09, 0.21)	NS	0.05 (−0.035, 0.225)	0.01 (−0.075, 0.16)	NS	NS*
Albumin difference value (g/L)	−0.06 (−0.21, 0.08)	0.01 (−0.33, 0.18)	NS	−0.02 (−0.26, 0.047)	−0.1 (−0.21, 0.15)	NS	NS*
Calcium difference value (mg/dL)	−0.3 (−0.4, 0)	−0.2 (−0.4, 0.025)	NS	−0.15 (−0.27, 0)	−0.1 (−0.5, 0.17)	NS	NS*
BMD difference value							
LS-BMD difference value (g/cm^2)	0.018 (−0.002, 0.036)	0.039 (0.02, 0.056)	0.028	0.004 (−0.004, 0.033)	0.032 (0.01, 0.051)	0.022	NS*
H-BMD difference value (g/cm^2)	−0.0085 (−0.025, 0.015)	0.015 (−0.0035, 0.029)	0.03	0.003 (−0.015, 0.019)	0.023 (−0.043, 0.039)	NS	NS*
FN-BMD difference value (g/cm^2)	0.004 (−0.021, 0.030)	0.0095 (−0.0065, 0.03)	NS	−0.0015 (−0.024, 0.017)	−0.0035 (−0.024, 0.016)	NS	NS*
Cumulative dose of Immunosuppressive agents							
Prednisolone (mg)	1054±700	1477±1072	NS	434 (0, 616)	1295 (751, 2151)	<0.001	NS*
Mycophenolate (tablets)	971±933	1079±902	NS	613±487	994±856	NS	NS*
Tacrolimus (tablets/1 mg)	0 (0, 178)	0 (0, 677)	NS	0 (0,705)	147 (0, 770)	NS	NS*
Sirolimus (tablets)	350 (0, 556)	0 (0, 425)	NS	0 (0, 383)	0 (0, 385)	NS	NS*
Cyclosporine (tablets/100 mg)	0 (0,402)	0 (0, 404)	NS	0 (0, 192)	0 (0, 253)	NS	NS*

Under similar conditions (characteristics, BMD differences, and cumulative use of immunosuppressive agents) the use of Fosamax in male patients increased the BMD of both lumbar spine and hip bone, but in female patients it increased the BMD only of lumbar spine.
NS*: p>0.05 between male and female patients.
Abbreviations: LS-BMD, lumbar spine bone mineral density; H-BMD, hip bone mineral density; FN-BMD, femoral neck bone mineral density; NS, no significance, p>0.05.

occur [37,38]. The co-administration of Fosamax and calcium, antacids, or oral medications containing multivalent cations interferes with the absorption of alendronate [38]. The short-term use of a low dose of Fosamax (40 mg per week) was safe in hemodialysis patients [39]. Alendronate treatment safely and effectively increased BMD and decreased fractures in women with normal to severely impaired renal function [40], and no differences in adverse events were observed in these women according to their renal function. The use of Fosamax for a mean of 14 months did not deteriorate renal function in male and female renal transplant patients (Table 3). To our knowledge, studies on the interaction between Fosamax and immunosuppressant agents are limited. The studies cited above and our own observations suggest that the interaction between these agents is subtle.

Although the limitations of our study with regard to its retrospective design and small sample size are evident, to our knowledge, these are the first data reporting the differences between men and women with regard to the sites at which Fosamax is effective in renal transplant patients; these findings refer to short-term treatment after a long post-renal transplantation period.

Conclusions

In conclusion, this randomized case-control study has shown that short-term use of Fosamax increased BMD and that the effect of concomitant steroid was not significantly correlated with bone turnover. Moreover, Fosamax increased the BMD of the lumbar spine and hip significantly in men, but only in the lumbar spine in women. Immunosuppressive agents such as CIs, sirolimus, and mycohenolate were not correlated with any change in BMD.

Acknowledgments

We thank the members of the Immune Transplant Center in Chang Gung Memorial Hospital for their invaluable and dedicated assistance.

Author Contributions

Conceived and designed the experiments: WHH PCL. Performed the experiments: WHH SYL CHW. Analyzed the data: WHH SYL PCL. Contributed reagents/materials/analysis tools: WHH CHW. Wrote the paper: WHH.

References

1. Parker CR, Freemont AJ, Blackwell PJ, Grainge MJ, Hosking DJ (1999)Cross-sectional analysis of renal transplantation osteoporosis. J Bone Miner Res 14(11):1943–1951.
2. Kodras K, Haas M (2006) Effect of kidney transplantation on bone. Eur J Clin Invest 36:Suppl-75.
3. Rodino MA, Shane E (1998) Osteoporosis after organ transplantation. Am J Med 104(5):459–469.
4. Julian BA, Laskow DA, Dubovsky J, Dubovsky EV, Curtis JJ, et al. (1991) Rapid loss of vertebral mineral density after renal transplantation. N Engl J Med 325(8):544–550.
5. Grotz WH, Mundinger FA, Rasenack J, Speidel L, Olschewski M, et al. (1995) Bone loss after kidney transplantation: a longitudinal study in 115 graft recipients. Nephrol Dial Transplant 10(11):2096–2100.
6. Sweet MG, Sweet JM, Jeremiah MP, Galazka SS (2009) Diagnosis and treatment of osteoporosis. Am Fam Physician 79(3):193–200.
7. Nayak B, Guleria S, Varma M, Tandon N, Aggarwal S, et al. (2007)Effect of bisphosphonates on bone mineral density after renal transplantation as assessed by bone mineral densitometry. Transplant Proc 39(3):750–752.
8. Palmer SC, McGregor DO, Strippoli GF (2007) Interventions for preventing bone disease in kidney transplant recipients. Update of Cochrane Database Syst Rev (3):CD005015
9. El-Agroudy AE, El-Husseini AA, El-Sayed M, Mohsen T, Ghoneim MA (2005) A prospective randomized study for prevention of postrenal transplantation bone loss. Kidney Int 67(5):2039–2045.
10. Buchinsky FJ, Ma Y, Mann GN, Rucinski B, Bryer HP, et al. (1996)T lymphocytes play a critical role in the development of cyclosporin A-induced osteopenia. Endocrinology 137(6):2278–2285.
11. Movsowitz C, Epstein S, Fallon M, Ismail F, Thomas S (1988) Cyclosporin-A in vivo produces severe osteopenia in the rat: effect of dose and duration of administration. Endocrinology 123(5):2571–2577.
12. Schlosberg M, Movsowitz C, Epstein S, Ismail F, Fallon MD, et al. (1989)The effect of cyclosporin A administration and its withdrawal on bone mineral metabolism in the rat. Endocrinology 124(5):2179–2184.
13. Carlini RG, Rojas E, Weisinger JR, Lopez M, Martinis R, et al. (2000) Bone disease in patients with long-term renal transplantation and normal renal function. Am J Kidney Dis 36(1):160–166.
14. Tamler R, Epstein S (2006) Nonsteroid immune modulators and bone disease. Ann N Y Acad Sci 1068:284–296.
15. Abdelhadi M, Ericzon BG, Hultenby K, Sjoden G, Reinholt FP, et al. (2002) Structural skeletal impairment induced by immunosuppressive therapy in rats: cyclosporine A vs tacrolimus. Transpl Int 15(4):180–187.
16. van der Merwe SW, Conradie MM, Bond R, Olivier BJ, Fritz E, et al. (2006) Effect of rapamycin on hepatic osteodystrophy in rats with portasystemic shunting. World J Gastroenterol 12(28):4504–4510.
17. Westenfeld R, Schlieper G, Woltje M, Gawlik A, Brandenburg V, et al. (2011) Impact of sirolimus, tacrolimus and mycophenolate mofetil on osteoclastogen-esis-implications for post-transplantation bone disease. Nephrol Dial Transplant 26(12):4115–4123.
18. Dennison E, Eastell R, Fall CH, Kellingray S, Wood PJ, et al. (1999) Determinants of bone loss in elderly men and women: a prospective population-based study. Osteoporos Int 10(5):384–391.
19. Kokado Y, Takahara S, Ichimaru N, Toki K, Kyo M, et al. (2000) Factors influencing vertebral bone density after renal transplantation. Transpl Int 13:Suppl-5.
20. Aroldi A, Tarantino A, Montagnino G, Cesana B, Cocucci C, et al. (1997) Effects of three immunosuppressive regimens on vertebral bone density in renal transplant recipients: a prospective study. Transplantation 63(3):380–386.
21. Hung CJ, Lee PC, Song CM, Chang YT, Tsai MT, et al. (1996) Clinical implication of hormone treatment in postmenopausal kidney transplants. Transplant Proc 28(3):1548–1550.
22. Cranney A, Guyatt G, Griffith L, Wells G, Tugwell P, et al. (2002) Meta-analyses of therapies for postmenopausal osteoporosis. IX: Summary of meta-analyses of therapies for postmenopausal osteoporosis. Endocr Rev 23(4):570–578.
23. Liu SH, Lin JL, Weng CH, Yang HY, Hsu CW, et al.(2012) Heart rate-corrected QT interval helps predict mortality after intentional organophosphate poisoning. PLoS One 7(5):e36576.
24. Huang WH, Lai PC (2011)Age at transplant–one of the factors affecting bone mineral density in kidney recipients–a single-center retrospective study. Ren Fail 33(8):776–80.
25. Campistol JM, Holt DW, Epstein S, Gioud-Paquet M, Rutault K, et al. (2005) Bone metabolism in renal transplant patients treated with cyclosporine or sirolimus. Transpl Int 18(9):1028–1035.
26. Cavadas PC, Hernan I, Landin L, Thione A (2011) Bone healing after secondary surgery on hand allografts under sirolimus-based maintenance immunosuppression. Ann Plast Surg 66(6):667–669.
27. Horber FF, Casez JP, Steiger U, Czerniak A, Montandon A, et al. (1994) Changes in bone mass early after kidney transplantation. J Bone Miner Res 9(1):1–9.
28. Ezaitouni F, Westeel PF, Fardellone P, Mazouz H, Brazier M, et al. (1998) Long-term stability of bone mineral density in patients with renal transplant treated with cyclosporine and low doses of corticoids. Protective role of cyclosporine?. Presse Med 27(15):705–712.
29. Pichette V, Bonnardeaux A, Prudhomme L, Gagne M, Cardinal J, et al. (1996) Long-term bone loss in kidney transplant recipients: a cross-sectional and longitudinal study. Am J Kidney Dis 28(1):105–114.
30. Leidig-Bruckner G, Hosch S, Dodidou P, Ritschel D, Conradt C, et al. (2001) Frequency and predictors of osteoporotic fractures after cardiac or liver transplantation: a follow-up study. Lancet 357(9253):342–347.
31. Torregrosa JV, Fuster D, Pedroso S, Diekmann F, Campistol JM, et al. (2007)Weekly risedronate in kidney transplant patients with osteopenia. Transpl Int 20(8):708–711.
32. Giannini S, D'Angelo A, Carraro G, Nobile M, Rigotti P, et al. (2001) Alendronate prevents further bone loss in renal transplant recipients. J Bone Miner Res 16(11):2111–2117.
33. Palmer SC, Strippoli GF, McGregor DO (2005) Interventions for preventing bone disease in kidney transplant recipients: a systematic review of randomized controlled trials. Am J Kidney Dis 45(4):638–649.
34. Orwoll E, Ettinger M, Weiss S, Miller P, Kendler D, et al. (2000) Alendronate for the treatment of osteoporosis in men. N Engl J Med 343(9):604–610.
35. Iwamoto J, Takeda T, Sato Y, Uzawa M (2007) Comparison of the effect of alendronate on lumbar bone mineral density and bone turnover in men and postmenopausal women with osteoporosis. Clin Rheumatol 26(2):161–167

36. Shinkai I, Ohta Y (1996) New drugs–reports of new drugs recently approved by the FDA. Alendronate. Bioorg Med Chem 4(1):3–4.

37. de Groen PC, Lubbe DF, Hirsch LJ, Daifotis A, Stephenson W, et al. (1996) Esophagitis associated with the use of alendronate. N Engl J Med 335(14):1016–1021

38. Full prescribing information for FOSAMAX (2012) Merck Sharp & Dohme, June 2012.

39. Wetmore JB, Benet LZ, Kleinstuck D, Frassetto L (2005) Effects of short-term alendronate on bone mineral density in haemodialysis patients. Nephrology 10(4):393–399.

40. Jamal SA, Bauer DC, Ensrud KE, Cauley JA, Hochberg M, et al. (2007) Alendronate treatment in women with normal to severely impaired renal function: an analysis of the fracture intervention trial. J Bone Miner Res 22(4):503–508.

13

Comorbidity and Sex-Related Differences in Mortality in Oxygen-Dependent Chronic Obstructive Pulmonary Disease

Magnus P. Ekström[1]*, Claes Jogréus[2], Kerstin E. Ström[3]

1 Department of Respiratory Medicine & Allergology, Institution for Clinical Sciences, University of Lund, Lund, Sweden, 2 Department of Mathematics and Science, School of Engineering, Blekinge Institute of Technology, Karlskrona, Sweden, 3 Department of Respiratory Medicine & Allergology, Institution for Clinical Sciences, University of Lund, Lund, Sweden

Abstract

Background: It is not known why survival differs between men and women in oxygen-dependent chronic obstructive pulmonary disease (COPD). The present study evaluates differences in comorbidity between men and women, and tests the hypothesis that comorbidity contributes to sex-related differences in mortality in oxygen-dependent COPD.

Methods: National prospective study of patients aged 50 years or older, starting long-term oxygen therapy (LTOT) for COPD in Sweden between 1992 and 2008. Comorbidities were obtained from the Swedish Hospital Discharge Register. Sex-related differences in comorbidity were estimated using logistic regression, adjusting for age, smoking status and year of inclusion. The effect of comorbidity on overall mortality and the interaction between comorbidity and sex were evaluated using Cox regression, adjusting for age, sex, Pa_{O_2} breathing air, FEV_1, smoking history and year of inclusion.

Results: In total, 8,712 patients (55% women) were included and 6,729 patients died during the study period. No patient was lost to follow-up. Compared with women, men had significantly more arrhythmia, cancer, ischemic heart disease and renal failure, and less hypertension, mental disorders, osteoporosis and rheumatoid arthritis ($P < 0.05$ for all odds ratios). Comorbidity was an independent predictor of mortality, and the effect was similar for the sexes. Women had lower mortality, which remained unchanged even after adjusting for comorbidity; hazard ratio 0.73 (95% confidence interval, 0.68–0.77; $P < 0.001$).

Conclusions: Comorbidity is different in men and women, but does not explain the sex-related difference in mortality in oxygen-dependent COPD.

Editor: Christian Taube, Leiden University Medical Center, The Netherlands

Funding: The study was supported by grants from the Swedish Heart and Lung Foundation (URL: http://www.hjart-lungfonden.se), the Swedish National Board of Health and Welfare (URL: http://www.socialstyrelsen.se), and the Research Council of Blekinge (http://www.ltblekinge.se/omlandstinget/blekingekompetenscentrum). The funders had no role in study design, data collection and analysis, decision to publish, or preparation of the manuscript.

Competing Interests: The authors have declared that no competing interests exist.

* E-mail: pmekstrom@gmail.com

Introduction

Severe Chronic Obstructive Pulmonary Disease (COPD) can be a devastating illness with high morbidity and mortality. [1] Long-term oxygen therapy (LTOT) is an established treatment in hypoxic (oxygen-dependent) COPD, as it was shown to approximately double survival in two randomized trials. [2,3] The incidence of LTOT has increased markedly in women; in fact, the majority of patients starting LTOT in Sweden are now women. [4] Studies of sex-related differences in survival on LTOT for COPD have shown conflicting results. Women had better survival than men after starting LTOT in most studies, [4,5,6,7] but in a study of Machado et al., survival was worse in women than men. [8] These inconsistent findings could be related to the heterogeneity of research settings, patient selection and covariates included in the analyses. Co-existing diseases, or comorbidity, was only evaluated in two of the studies, which both found a high overall

prevalence of comorbidity but did not report any significant differences in comorbidity between men and women. [7,8] Interestingly, one study found that comorbidity predicted mortality, but only in women. [7] It remains unknown whether the effect of comorbidity on mortality differs between men and women, as this has only been evaluated in one previous, relatively small, study, which found no effect measure interaction between comorbidity and sex. [8]

The prevalence of comorbidity in COPD is high, [9] and increases with age and COPD severity. [10,11] Comorbidity has been shown to predict mortality in COPD, [11,12] and may be more prevalent in men than in women. [11,13] An analysis from the TORCH study, in which patients with significant comorbidity were excluded, found no significant difference in mortality between men and women. [14] In a study of patients matched in terms of COPD severity, [13] mortality was found to be higher in men than in women, and comorbidity to predict mortality in men only. This study formulated the hypothesis that the higher mortality in men was attributable to sex-dependent differences in comorbidity, especially in severe COPD. [14]

The present national prospective study evaluates whether there are differences in comorbidity between men and women in oxygen-dependent COPD, and tests the hypothesis that comorbidity contributes to sex-related differences in mortality.

Materials and Methods

Patients aged 50 years or older, starting LTOT for physician diagnosed COPD between 1 January 1992 and 31 December 2008 in the Swedish National Oxygen Register were included prospectively. The indications for LTOT and details of the register have been reported previously, [4] and part of the database was used in recently published studies. [15,16] For patients who had started LTOT more than once (n = 99), only the latest treatment episode was included in the analysis. At baseline, defined as the date of starting LTOT, data were collected on arterial gas tension of oxygen (Pa_{O2}) and carbon dioxide (Pa_{CO2}) when breathing air and during oxygen therapy, forced expiratory volume in one second (FEV_1), forced vital capacity (FVC), concomitant home mechanical ventilator use, smoking history (never, past or current smoking), the prescribed oxygen dose, and the prescribed duration of oxygen therapy per day.

Discharge diagnoses, the number of hospitalizations and in-hospital days within five years prior to starting LTOT were collected for all patients from the Swedish Hospital Discharge Register, which covers more than 98% of all hospitalizations in Sweden after 1 January 1987. [17] In addition, data on all lung transplantations and lung volume reduction procedures before starting LTOT and during follow up was collected.

Patients were followed until withdrawal of LTOT, death or 31 December 2008, whichever came first. Vital status and underlying cause of death was obtained from the Swedish Causes of Death Register. All diagnoses, procedure codes, and causes of death were coded according to the ninth (before 1997) and tenth revisions of the International Classification of Disease (ICD). [18,19] Definitions of all diagnosis entities and procedures are found in a supporting information table (Table S1).

Ethics statement

All patients gave their informed written consent to participate. The study was approved by the Lund University Research Ethics Committee (157/2007 and 350/2008), the Swedish National Board of Health and Welfare, and the Data Inspection Board.

Statistical methods

Differences in baseline data were tested using chi square-test, Student's t-test, and Wilcoxon's rank-sum test for categorical, normally and non-normally distributed variables. Comorbidities were defined as relevant registered discharge diagnoses, primary or secondary, within five years prior to starting LTOT. In the analyses, comorbidity was categorized into the Charlson comorbidity score, [20] with COPD removed from the list of weighted diagnoses, in order to only include comorbidities of COPD. Age was not incorporated in the Charlson score and was included as an independent variable in all analyses.

Odds ratios for women as compared to men for individual comorbidities and for the Charlson score, adjusted for age, smoking history and start year, were analyzed using logistic regression and a generalized ordered logit model. [21] The ordered odds ratio for Charlson score was interpreted as the odds ratio of having a higher score than the present category. [21] The

Hosmer-Lemeshow test was used to test the fit of the logistic models. [22]

The effect of comorbidity, categorized as Charlson score and individual diagnoses not included in the score, on overall mortality was evaluated using Cox regression, [23] adjusted for age, sex, Pa_{O2} breathing air, FEV_1 (included as absolute values or percent of predicted, [24] respectively), start year and smoking history. The effect of adding body mass index (BMI) to the model was evaluated in the cohort starting LTOT 1995–2008, as BMI was registered during this time period only. Interactions between comorbidity and sex, age and start year, respectively, and between age and sex were analyzed on the multiplicative scale by entering interaction terms into the fully adjusted model. Biological interaction between sex and comorbidity (defined as a Charlson score of one or higher) on the additive scale was explored by calculating the adjusted attributable proportion, which is the proportion of the relative risk among exposed that is attributable to the interaction, [25] adjusted for all covariates in the Cox regression. The attributable risk among all men was calculated as: [the attributable proportion] × [the prevalence of Charlson score one or more among men].

The proportional hazards assumption of the Cox model was assessed graphically with log-log plots and by testing for interaction with analysis time for all covariates. The overall fit of the model was assured using Cox-Snell residuals.

All statistical tests were two-sided and P-values below the standard value of 0.05 were considered statistically significant. All confidence intervals were 95% intervals. All statistical analyses were performed with Stata version 11.1 (StataCorp LP; College Station, TX).

Results

A total of 8,712 patients, 3,929 men and 4,783 (54.9%) women were included in the study after exclusion of 15 patients (0.2%) because of data irregularities. Concomitant home mechanical ventilator was used at baseline by 2% of both women and men. Lung transplantation was performed in only 7 patients before starting LTOT, and in 45 (0.5%) patients, 29 women and 16 men, during follow up. Only 60 patients (27 women) had had lung volume reduction surgery before starting LTOT, and during follow up, it was performed in 17 patients (8 women). The cohort was followed for a total of 20718.7 person-years with a median follow-up of 1.65 years (range 0–16.85 years). LTOT was withdrawn before death in 415 patients (4.8%), mainly owing to improved oxygenation. No patient was lost to follow up. In total, 6,729 patients, 3,199 men and 3,530 women, died under observation. Nonrespiratory causes of deaths were slightly more common in men than women (31.1% vs 27.4%; P = 0.001). Baseline characteristics are shown in Table 1. Compared with men, women were younger, had a lower mean absolute FEV_1 but similar FEV_1% of predicted, higher Pa_{CO2}, and more in-hospital days, although the median number of hospitalizations were the same as for men. In the subset of patients starting LTOT 1995 or later (n = 7593), the mean BMI [± SD] was 23.0±5.1 and 23.5±6.7 kg/m^2 in men and women, respectively.

Of all patients, 98.3% had been hospitalized at least once within five years prior to starting LTOT and 75% three or more times. The patients who had no hospitalization (1.7%) were evenly distributed between men (N = 77) and women (n = 73).

Sex-related differences in comorbidity

As shown in Table 2, women had more hypertension, mental disorders, osteoporosis and rheumatoid arthritis, but less arrhyth-

Table 1. Baseline characteristics of patients starting long-term oxygen therapy for chronic obstrucitve pulmonary disease, 1992–2008.

Characteristic	Women, n = 4,783 (55%)	Men, n = 3,929	P-value
Age, years	71.8 ± 8.4	73.7 ± 7.8	<0.001
Pa$_{O2}$ air, kPa	6.5 ± 0.9	6.7 ± 0.9	<0.001
Pa$_{CO2}$ air, kPa	6.5 ± 1.2	6.1 ± 1.2	<0.001
Pa$_{O2}$ oxygen, kPa	8.8 ± 1.1	8.9 ± 1.1	<0.001
Pa$_{CO2}$ oxygen, kPa	6.8 ± 1.2	6.3 ± 1.2	<0.001
FEV$_1$, L	0.7 ± 0.3	1.0 ± 0.5	<0.001
FEV$_1$ of predicted, %	34.0 ± 17.0	35.5 ± 19.6	0.005
FVC, L	1.5 ± 0.5	2.2 ± 0.9	<0.001
Smoking history, %			
Never	6	4	<0.001
Past	91	94	<0.001
Current	3	2	0.129
All Hospitalizations, n*	5 (3–9)	5 (3–9)	0.013
Hospitalizations for COPD, n*	2 (1–4)	2 (1–4)	<0.001
In-hospital days*	48 (25–87)	41 (21–77)	<0.001

Data presented as mean ± SD unless otherwise specified.
Definition of abbreviations: FEV$_1$ = forced expiratory volume in one second; FVC = forced vital capacity; Pa$_{CO2}$ air = arterial blood gas tension of carbon dioxide while breathing ambient air; Pa$_{CO2}$ oxygen = arterial blood gas tension of carbon dioxide while breathing oxygen; Pa$_{O2}$ air = arterial blood gas tension of oxygen while breathing ambient air; Pa$_{O2}$ oxygen = arterial blood gas tension of oxygen while breathing oxygen.
*Hospitalizations and in-hospital days within 5 years prior to starting LTOT, presented as median (first quartile – third quartile).

mias, cancer, ischemic heart disease and renal failure, as compared to men. There were no significant sex-related differences for anemia, cerebrovascular disease, diabetes mellitus, digestive organ disease, heart failure, lung cancer or pulmonary embolism. Men were more likely to have high Charlson scores than women, and this sex-related difference increased with each additional category in the Charlson score (Table 3).

Comorbidity and mortality

Comorbidity was an independent predictor of adjusted mortality, with increasing mortality for each additional category in the Charlson score (Table 4). In addition, anemia, arrhythmia, mental disorders and osteoporosis, which are not included in the Charlson score, independently predicted mortality. When individual diagnoses were entered in the model instead of the Charlson score, the comorbidities which were statistically significant and increased mortality with 10% or more were anemia, arrhythmia, cancer, ischemic heart disease, heart failure, mental disorder, and osteoporosis (Table 5).

The crude overall mortality was lower for women than for men, hazard ratio (HR) 0.76 (95% confidence interval (CI), 0.73–0.80; P<0.001). As shown in Table 4 and 5, this survival benefit for women was not explained by comorbidity, since it remained relatively unchanged in multiple regression models which adjusted for Charlson score and individual comorbidities, as well as the other covariates. The sex-related difference remained unchanged even after adjusting, in addition to the covariates above, for the number of hospitalizations in the preceding five years or when excluding patients with no prior hospitalization, HR 0.73 (95% CI, 0.68–0.77; P<0.001) and HR 0,73 (95% CI, 0.68–0.78; P<0.001), respectively. In addition, the model estimates remained unchanged when including BMI and FEV$_1$ in percent of predicted instead of the absolute values, as shown in the supplemental Table S2. There were no signs of multiplicative interaction between

comorbidity and sex; P-values for interaction terms ranging 0.669–0.842, or comorbidity and age (P ranging 0.108–0.924), comorbidity and start year (P ranging 0.100–0.862), or age and sex (P ranging, 0.436–0.892). Although not statistically significant, data indicated a small biological interaction between comorbidity and sex on the additive scale, attributable proportion 0.073 (95% CI; −0.01, 0.16). Thus, interaction may have attributed to 7.3% of the relative risk in men with comorbidity, and 3.7% of the relative risk among all men.

Discussion

The main findings in the present study are that in oxygen-dependent COPD 1) comorbidity differs between men and women, 2) comorbidity is an independent predictor of mortality with similar effects for both sexes, and 3) comorbidity does not explain the survival difference between men and women.

To the authors' knowledge, this is the first study to evaluate sex-related differences in the prevalence of individual diagnosis entities in a large cohort of patients with oxygen-dependent COPD. The only two previous studies of sex-stratified comorbidity in the field included relatively few patients and found no significant difference in the mean number of comorbidities [7] or Charlson score, [8] respectively.

The higher prevalence of cardiovascular disease among men is consistent with previous studies of patients with a broader range of COPD-severity. [11,26] The finding of more hypertension among women than men is consistent with some previous studies, [26,27] but not all. [11] The lack of sex-related difference in heart failure in the present study, in spite of a previous report of a higher prevalence among men, [11] might be due to the differences in patient selection and the particular difficulty of detecting heart failure in severe COPD. For this reason, the heart failure estimates should be interpreted with caution. Interestingly, mental disorders

Table 2. Prevalence and sex-related odds of comorbidity in patients starting long-term oxygen therapy for chronic obstructive pulmonary disease, 1992–2008.

Diagnosis	Prevalence in Women, n (%)	Prevalence in Men, n (%)	Adjusted Odds Ratio for Women Compared to Men*	95% Confidence Interval	P-value
All cancers[†]	460 (10)	503 (13)	0.74	0.64–0.84	<0.001
Lung cancer	76 (2)	79 (2)	0.74	0.53–1.02	0.065
Anaemia	245 (5)	183 (5)	1.11	0.90–1.36	0.329
Arrhythmia[†]	578 (12)	662 (17)	0.72	0.63–0.81	<0.001
Cerebrovascular disease	236 (5)	214 (5)	0.88	0.73–1.08	0.224
Diabetes mellitus	414 (9)	369 (9)	0.87	0.74–1.01	0.062
Digestive organ disease	922 (19)	831 (21)	0.90	0.81–1.01	0.062
Heart failure	1543 (32)	1254 (32)	1.09	0.99–1.20	0.072
Hypertension[†]	673 (14)	429 (11)	1.26	1.10–1.1.45	0.001
Ischemic heart disease[†]	864 (18)	880 (22)	0.77	0.69–0.86	<0.001
Mental disorder[†]	482 (10)	291 (7)	1.27	1.09–1.49	0.003
Osteoporosis[†]	485 (10)	131 (3)	3.42	2.80–4.19	<0.001
Pulmonary embolism	114 (2)	89 (2)	0.99	0.74–1.32	0.931
Renal failure[†]	72 (2)	101 (3)	0.58	0.42–0.79	0.001
Rheumatoid arthritis[†]	103 (2)	52 (1)	1.56	1.10–2.20	0.012

Percentages may not add up to 100 due to rounding.
*Odds ratio adjusted for age, smoking history and year of starting long-term oxygen therapy.
[†]Entities with significant sex-related difference in odds.

were more common among women than men, supporting recent findings that female sex is a determinant of depression in COPD. [28]

In the present study, comorbidity predicted mortality, independent of age, sex, degree of hypoxia, FEV_1, year of starting LTOT, and smoking status. Previous studies of whether Charlson score predicts mortality in COPD have shown conflicting results, [7,8,10,11,12,13,29,30,31] which may be due to relatively small study populations, [7,29] inclusion of few women, [12,29,30] or inclusion of covariates that captured part of the effect of comorbidity in the multiple regression models, such as dyspnea, measures of physical capacity and quality of life, [8,13] which may have biased the estimates for comorbidity toward less effect. Although often used, the Charlson score has not been validated in COPD. In the present study, several comorbidities predicted mortality independent of the Charlson score, which was also found

in another recent study. [31] This highlights the need for an updated comorbidity score validated specifically for COPD.

A previous study of our group showed that women had a better adjusted survival than men in oxygen-dependent COPD, but that this unexplained survival advantage for women also exists in the Swedish general population. [16] In fact, women had higher relative mortality than men, when the mortality was compared with the expected mortality in the general population for women and men respectively. [16] The driving hypothesis behind the present study was that differences in comorbidity, which was not evaluated in the previous study, explain part of the survival advantage for women compared with men after starting LTOT for COPD. [4,5,6,7] Surprisingly, the present findings strongly argue against any such effect on the sex-related difference in survival. Furthermore, the effect of comorbidity on the mortality rate-ratio was not modified by sex, and any biological interaction was small. Thus, the longer survival for women as compared with men is not

Table 3. Prevalence and sex-related odds of Charlson score in patients starting long-term oxygen therapy for chronic obstructive pulmonary disease, 1992–2008.

Charlson score	Prevalence in Women, n (%)	Prevalence in Men, n (%)	Adjusted Odds Ratio for Women Compared to Men*	95% Confidence Interval	P-value
0	2440 (51)	1962 (50)	1.00	0.91–1.09	0.921
1	1371 (29)	1012 (26)	0.79	0.71–0.88	<0.001
2	616 (13)	517 (13)	0.62	0.53–0.72	<0.001
3	224 (5)	235 (6)	0.49	0.39–0.62	<0.001
>3	132 (3)	203 (5)	-	-	-

Percentages may not add up to 100 due to rounding.
*Generalized ordered odds ratio adjusted for age, smoking history and year of inclusion. It is interpreted as the odds ratio of having a higher score than the present category.

Table 4. Cox regression of overall mortality in patients starting long-term oxygen therapy, 1992–2008.

Characteristic	Hazard ratio	95% confidence interval	P-value
Age	1.04	1.04–1.04	<0.001
Female	0.73	0.68–0.77	<0.001
Pa$_{O2}$ air	0.88	0.86–0.91	<0.001
FEV$_1$	0.82	0.76–0.88	<0.001
Past smoking*	1.05	0.94–1.20	0.356
Current smoking*	1.33	1.07–1.64	0.010
Start year	1.00	1.00–1.01	0.391
Charlson score†			
1	1.14	1.07–1.22	<0.001
2	1.39	1.26–1.52	<0.001
3	1.52	1.32–1.75	<0.001
>3	1.69	1.42–2.02	<0.001
Anemia	1.28	1.10–1.48	0.001
Arrhythmia	1.23	1.13–1.34	<0.001
Mental disorder	1.18	1.06–1.32	0.003
Osteoporosis	1.31	1.17–1.48	<0.001

Definition of abbreviations: FEV$_1$ = forced expiratory volume in one second; Pa$_{O2}$ air = arterial blood gas tension of oxygen while breathing ambient air.
*Never smoking is used as reference category.
†Charlson score 0 is used as reference category.

Table 5. Cox regression of the effects of individual comorbidities on overall mortality.

Characteristic	Hazard ratio	95% confidence interval	P-value
Age	1.04	1.04–1.04	<0.001
Female	0.72	0.68–0.77	<0.001
Pa$_{O2}$ air	0.88	0.85–0.91	<0.001
FEV$_1$	0.81	0.75–0.87	<0.001
Past smoking*	1.08	0.95–1.23	0.228
Current smoking*	1.36	1.10–1.69	0.005
Start year	1.00	1.00–1.01	0.300
All cancers	1.28	1.17–1.41	<0.001
Anemia	1.31	1.12–1.52	<0.001
Arrhythmia	1.24	1.14–1.36	<0.001
Cerebrovascular disease	1.01	0.88–1.16	0.914
Diabetes mellitus	1.11	1.00–1.24	0.060
Heart failure	1.10	1.03–1.17	0.006
Hypertension	1.03	0.93–1.14	0.591
Ischemic heart disease	1.12	1.04–1.21	0.004
Mental disorder	1.17	1.05–1.31	0.005
Osteoporosis	1.30	1.15–1.47	<0.001
Pulmonary embolism	1.20	0.96–1.50	0.101
Renal failure	1.11	0.87–1.43	0.394
Rheumatoid arthritis	1.15	0.93–1.42	0.197

*Never smoking is used as reference category.

explained by differences in comorbidity or differences in the effect of comorbidity on mortality.

The strength of the present study is the prospective inclusion of a large national cohort of patients starting LTOT for COPD with complete follow-up. The National Oxygen Register covers some 85% of all patients who have started LTOT since 1987 in Sweden, with loss of data from whole counties mainly due to temporary shortages of staff. [32]

Several potential weaknesses in the present study need to be mentioned. This study included patients starting LTOT and the distribution of comorbidities and their effects on mortality may not be representative for the whole population of patients with very severe COPD. Although diagnoses in the Swedish Hospital Discharge Register have been recently validated as having high specificity throughout as well as good sensitivity to certain conditions, such as cardiovascular disease, the register's sensitivity is lower for less acute or less serious conditions, such as hypertension and diabetes mellitus. [33] The sensitivity for cardiovascular disease might be lower in these patients with severe COPD than indicated by the validation studies, as cardiac disease may remain undiagnosed. [34] The misclassification from low sensitivity would likely tend to underestimate the association between these comorbidities and mortality, as unregistered comorbidity in the "healthy" group will make their mortality more similar to that of patients with registered comorbidity. [35] On the other hand, the estimates for comorbidities may be biased towards a higher effect, as patients with more severe illness may be more likely to be hospitalized and to get comorbidities registered. However, a too high effect of comorbidity is not a threat to the validity of the present finding that comorbidity does not explain the sex-related difference in mortality. We lacked data on prognostic predictors such as the level of dyspnea and exercise capacity, but inclusion of these factors, which are likely directly related to comorbidity, would have biased the associations between comorbid-

ity and mortality. There were also insufficient data on duration and severity of comorbidities, but the sensitivity of the Discharge Register has been shown to be high for serious and more severe forms of comorbidity, [33] known to have prognostic impact in COPD. Thus, the present finding that comorbidity cannot explain sex-related differences in mortality is likely to have a high validity. In the authors' opinion, the mentioned potential weaknesses do not substantially alter the main finding of the present study.

What could be the mechanisms behind the survival difference between men and women in oxygen-dependent COPD, [4,5,6,7] since it does not seem to be explained by comorbidity? The present data do not suggest that women started LTOT earlier in the course of their disease, or had less severe respiratory insufficiency, since FEV$_1$% of predicted were similar and women in fact had a lower mean Pa$_{O2}$ and a higher mean Pa$_{CO2}$ on ambient air than men when starting LTOT. Whether the effect of LTOT or the compliance to the therapy differs between the sexes has not been evaluated because few women were included in the randomized trials and compliance has generally not been assessed. [2,3] One hypothesis is that women, as compared to men, might develop COPD at lower smoking exposure [36] and report more dyspnea and lower quality of life independent of COPD severity. [27,37] It is possible that women, due to less total smoking and different exposure to other biological factors (such as sex hormones) as well as environmental factors (such as alcohol, social and nutritional factors), might have lower frailty with the same degree of respiratory insufficiency than men after starting LTOT. There may also be phenotypical differences between men and women in COPD. Men have been found to have more emphysema than women at all levels of COPD severity and smoking, [38] which could contribute to the survival difference since the extent of emphysema predicts mortality.

[39] Clearly, the sex-related survival difference in COPD with LTOT warrants further research.

For the clinician, this study shows that comorbidity has a major impact on mortality even in the most severe stages of COPD and highlights the importance of improved preventive treatments for conditions such as osteoporosis, as well as of optimized diagnosis and treatment of manifest comorbidity in order to improve the high morbidity and mortality in severe COPD.

In conclusion, this study shows that comorbidity differs between men and women, but differences in prevalence or effect of comorbidity do not explain the sex-related difference in mortality in oxygen-dependent COPD.

Supporting Information

Table S1 Definitions of diagnosis entities and surgical procedures according to ICD9 (used before 1997) and ICD-10.

Table S2 Cox regression of overall mortality in patients (n = 7,593) who started LTOT 1995–2008. The analysis includes FEV_1 in percent of predicted instead of absolute values, as well as BMI, which was available for this time period only.

Acknowledgments

The authors thank Philippe Wagner at the National Competence Centre for Musculoskeletal Disorders for valuable advice regarding statistical methodology, Anders Behrens at Blekinge Hospital for help with data formatting, and above all, the nurses and physicians who included and cared for the patients.

Author Contributions

Conceived and designed the experiments: ME KS. Performed the experiments: ME KS. Analyzed the data: ME CJ KS. Contributed reagents/materials/analysis tools: ME KS. Wrote the paper: ME CJ KS.

References

1. Global Strategy for the Diagnosis, Management and Prevention of COPD, Global Initiative for Chronic Obstructive Lung Disease (GOLD) (2011) Available from http://www.goldcopd.org/.
2. Nocturnal Oxygen Therapy Trial Group (1980) Continuous or nocturnal oxygen therapy in hypoxemic chronic obstructive lung disease: a clinical trial. Ann Intern Med 93: 391–398.
3. Report of the Medical Research Council Working Party (1981) Long term domiciliary oxygen therapy in chronic hypoxic cor pulmonale complicating chronic bronchitis and emphysema. Lancet 1: 681–686.
4. Franklin KA, Gustafson T, Ranstam J, Strom K (2007) Survival and future need of long-term oxygen therapy for chronic obstructive pulmonary disease–gender differences. Respir Med 101: 1506–1511.
5. Miyamoto K, Aida A, Nishimura M, Aiba M, Kira S, et al. (1995) Gender effect on prognosis of patients receiving long-term home oxygen therapy. The Respiratory Failure Research Group in Japan. Am J Respir Crit Care Med 152: 972–976.
6. Chailleux E, Fauroux B, Binet F, Dautzenberg B, Polu JM (1996) Predictors of survival in patients receiving domiciliary oxygen therapy or mechanical ventilation. A 10-year analysis of ANTADIR Observatory. Chest 109: 741–749.
7. Crockett AJ, Cranston JM, Moss JR, Alpers JH (2001) Survival on long-term oxygen therapy in chronic airflow limitation: from evidence to outcomes in the routine clinical setting. Intern Med J 31: 448–454.
8. Machado M-CL, Krishnan JA, Buist SA, Bilderback AL, Fazolo GP, et al. (2006) Sex differences in survival of oxygen-dependent patients with chronic obstructive pulmonary disease. American Journal of Respiratory And Critical Care Medicine 174: 524–529.
9. Soriano JB, Visick GT, Muellerova H, Payvandi N, Hansell AL (2005) Patterns of comorbidities in newly diagnosed COPD and asthma in primary care. Chest 128: 2099–2107.
10. Curkendall SM, Lanes S, de Luise C, Stang MR, Jones JK, et al. (2006) Chronic obstructive pulmonary disease severity and cardiovascular outcomes. Eur J Epidemiol 21: 803–813.
11. Mannino DM, Thorn D, Swensen A, Holguin F (2008) Prevalence and outcomes of diabetes, hypertension and cardiovascular disease in COPD. Eur Respir J 32: 962–969.
12. Antonelli Incalzi R, Fuso L, De Rosa M, Forastiere F, Rapiti E, et al. (1997) Comorbidity contributes to predict mortality of patients with chronic obstructive pulmonary disease. Eur Respir J 10: 2794–2800.
13. de Torres JP, Cote CG, Lopez MV, Casanova C, Diaz O, et al. (2009) Sex differences in mortality in patients with COPD. Eur Respir J 33: 528–535.
14. Celli B, Vestbo J, Jenkins CR, Jones PW, Ferguson GT, et al. (2011) Sex differences in mortality and clinical expressions of patients with chronic obstructive pulmonary disease: the TORCH experience. Am J Respir Crit Care Med 183: 317–322.
15. Ekstrom MP, Wagner P, Strom KE (2011) Trends in Cause-Specific Mortality in Oxygen-dependent Chronic Obstructive Pulmonary Disease. American Journal of Respiratory and Critical Care Medicine 183: 1032–1036.
16. Ekstrom M, Franklin KA, Strom KE (2010) Increased relative mortality in women with severe oxygen-dependent COPD. Chest 137: 31–36.
17. Swedish National Board of Health and Welfare (2008) Quality and Contents of the Swedish Hospital Discharge Register. Stockholm: Swedish National Board of Health and Welfare. The Center for Epidemiology.
18. WHO (1978) Manual of the International Classification of Diseases, Injuries and Causes of Death. 9th revision. Geneva, Switzerland: World Health Organization.
19. WHO (1992) Manual of the International Statistical Classification of Diseases and Health Related Problems. 10th revision. Geneva, Switzerland: World Health Organization.
20. Charlson ME, Pompei P, Ales KL, MacKenzie CR (1987) A new method of classifying prognostic comorbidity in longitudinal studies: development and validation. J Chronic Dis 40: 373–383.
21. Williams R (2006) Generalized ordered logit/partial proportional odds models for ordinal dependent variables. Stata Journal 6: 58–82.
22. Hosmer D, Lemeshow S (2000) Applied Logistic Regression. New York: John Wiley & Sons.
23. Cox DR (1972) Regression Models and Life-Tables. Journal of the American Statistical Association 34: 187–220.
24. Berglund E, Birath G, Bjure J, Grimby G, Kjellmer I, et al. (1963) Spirometric studies in normal subjects. I. Forced expirograms in subjects between 7 and 70 years of age. Acta medica Scandinavica 173: 185–192.
25. Andersson T, Alfredsson L, Källberg H, Zdravkovic S, Ahlbom A (2005) Calculating measures of biological interaction. European Journal of Epidemiology 20: 575–579.
26. Almagro P, Lopez Garcia F, Cabrera F, Montero L, Morchon D, et al. (2010) Comorbidity and gender-related differences in patients hospitalized for COPD. The ECCO study. Respiratory Medicine 104: 253–259.
27. de Torres JP, Casanova C, Hernández C, Abreu J, Aguirre-Jaime A, et al. (2005) Gender and COPD in Patients Attending a Pulmonary Clinic*. Chest 128: 2012–2016.
28. Hanania NA, Mullerova H, Locantore NW, Vestbo J, Watkins ML, et al. (2011) Determinants of Depression in the ECLIPSE Chronic Obstructive Pulmonary Disease Cohort. Am J Respir Crit Care Med 183: 604–611.
29. Marti S, Munoz X, Rios J, Morell F, Ferrer J (2006) Body weight and comorbidity predict mortality in COPD patients treated with oxygen therapy. Eur Respir J 27: 689–696.
30. Almagro P, Calbo E, Ochoa de E, x00Fc, en A, et al. (2002) Mortality after hospitalization for COPD. Chest 121: 1441–1448.
31. Lash T, Johansen M, Christensen S, Baron J, Rothman K, et al. (2011) Hospitalization Rates and Survival Associated with COPD: A Nationwide Danish Cohort Study. Lung 189: 27–35.
32. Strom K, Boe J (1988) A national register for long-term oxygen therapy in chronic hypoxia: preliminary results. Eur Respir J 1: 952–958.
33. Ludvigsson J, Andersson E, Ekbom A, Feychting M, Kim J-L, et al. (2011) External review and validation of the Swedish national inpatient register. BMC Public Health 11: 450.
34. Rutten FH, Cramer M-JM, Lammers J-WJ, Grobbee DE, Hoes AW (2006) Heart failure and chronic obstructive pulmonary disease: An ignored combination? European Journal of Heart Failure 8: 706–711.
35. Rothman KJ, Greenland S, Lash TL (2008) Validity in Epidemiologic Studies. In: Greenland S, Lash TL, Rothman KJ, eds. Modern Epidemiology. Third Edition ed. Philadelphia: Lippincott Williams & Wilkins. pp 128–147.
36. Xu X, Weiss ST, Rijcken B, Schouten JP (1994) Smoking, changes in smoking habits, and rate of decline in FEV1: new insight into gender differences. Eur Respir J 7: 1056–1061.
37. de Torres JP, Casanova C, Hernandez C, Abreu J, Montejo de Garcini A, et al. (2006) Gender associated differences in determinants of quality of life in patients with COPD: a case series study. Health and Quality of Life Outcomes 4: 72.
38. Dransfield MT, Washko GR, Foreman MG, Estepar RSJ, Reilly J, et al. (2007) Gender differences in the severity of CT emphysema in COPD. Chest 132: 464–470.
39. Haruna A, Muro S, Nakano Y, Ohara T, Hoshino Y, et al. (2010) CT Scan Findings of Emphysema Predict Mortality in COPD. Chest 138: 635–640.

14

Common Genetic Variants Are Associated with Accelerated Bone Mineral Density Loss after Hematopoietic Cell Transplantation

Song Yao[1], Lara E. Sucheston[1], Shannon L. Smiley[2], Warren Davis[1], Jeffrey M. Conroy[3], Norma J. Nowak[3,4], Christine B. Ambrosone[1], Philip L. McCarthy Jr.[2◦], Theresa Hahn[2*◦]

1 Department of Cancer Prevention and Control, Roswell Park Cancer Institute, Buffalo, New York, United States of America, 2 Department of Medicine, Roswell Park Cancer Institute, Buffalo, New York, United States of America, 3 Department of Cancer Genetics, Roswell Park Cancer Institute, Buffalo, New York, United States of America, 4 Department of Biochemistry, University at Buffalo, Buffalo, New York, United States of America

Abstract

Background: Bone mineral density (BMD) loss commonly occurs after hematopoietic cell transplantation (HCT). Hypothesizing that genetic variants may influence post-HCT BMD loss, we conducted a prospective study to examine the associations of single nucleotide polymorphisms (SNP) in bone metabolism pathways and acute BMD loss after HCT.

Methods and Findings: We genotyped 122 SNPs in 45 genes in bone metabolism pathways among 121 autologous and allogeneic HCT patients. BMD changes from pre-HCT to day +100 post-HCT were analyzed in relation to these SNPs in linear regression models. After controlling for clinical risk factors, we identified 16 SNPs associated with spinal or femoral BMD loss following HCT, three of which have been previously implicated in genome-wide association studies of bone phenotypes, including rs2075555 in *COL1A1*, rs9594738 in *RANKL*, and rs4870044 in *ESR1*. When multiple SNPs were considered simultaneously, they explained 5–35% of the variance in post-HCT BMD loss. There was a significant trend between the number of risk alleles and the magnitude of BMD loss, with patients carrying the most risk alleles having the greatest loss.

Conclusion: Our data provide the first evidence that common genetic variants play an important role in BMD loss among HCT patients similar to age-related BMD loss in the general population. This infers that the mechanism for post-HCT bone loss is a normal aging process that is accelerated during HCT. A limitation of our study comes from its small patient population; hence future larger studies are warranted to validate our findings.

Editor: Michael Hendricks, Harvard University, United States of America

Funding: This work was supported, in part, by a Cancer and Leukemia Group B (CALGB) Investigator Award for junior oncology faculty (S.L.S). The DataBank and BioRepository and the Genomics Shared Resource at Roswell Park Cancer Institute are Cancer Center Support Grant (CCSG) Shared Resources (NIH 5P30CA016056-34). The funding organizations played no roles during the conduct of the study or the preparation of the manuscript. The funders had no role in study design, data collection and analysis, decision to publish, or preparation of the manuscript.

Competing Interests: The authors have declared that no competing interests exist.

* E-mail: Theresa.hahn@roswellpark.org

◦ These authors contributed equally to this work.

Introduction

After the second decade of life, bone mineral density (BMD) gradually declines as a result of normal aging [1]. This process is accelerated in patients undergoing hematopoietic cell transplantation (HCT) [2,3]. Rapid bone loss weakens bone strength and may permanently impair bone remodeling capability [4,5], putting HCT survivors at high risk of premature fracture. We previously demonstrated that BMD loss within 4 months after HCT is equivalent to 7 to 17 years of normal bone aging [6]. Moreover, this loss occurs following autologous and allogeneic HCT with a similar incidence and severity.

In the general population, the inherited genetic background accounts for a large proportion of phenotypic variation in BMD loss and fracture risk [7,8]. In numerous candidate gene association studies, a variety of genetic variants, mostly in the form of single nucleotide polymorphisms (SNP), have been associated with regulation of BMD and risk of fracture [9], with less than a handful of them confirmed in a recent large-scale meta-analysis performed by the Genetic Factors for Osteoporosis (GEFOS) Consortium [10]. A genome-wide association (GWA) approach has also been used to search for loci associated with various bone phenotypes, which identified a number of novel SNPs [11,12,13,14,15]. These genetic markers may have clinical significance in predicting risk of BMD loss and/or osteoporosis. Moreover, some may also be predictive for response to therapies targeting related molecules or pathways, such as a human monoclonal antibody against receptor activator of nuclear factor κB ligand (RANKL) (denosumab), which was recently approved by the FDA for postmenopausal women at risk for fracture [16].

Among HCT recipients, rapid BMD loss may be due to an accelerated bone aging process after exposure to high doses of corticosteroids, chemotherapy and/or total body irradiation. Indeed, we have previously demonstrated that bone loss occurs within three months of HCT in both allogeneic and autologous HCT patients [6]. Therefore, predisposing genetic variants for low BMD and osteoporosis in the general population may also predispose carriers to risk of severe post-HCT BMD loss. Recently, McClune and colleagues proposed comprehensive guidelines for the screening, prevention and treatment of osteoporosis after HCT. They recommend dual-energy X-ray absorptiometry (DXA) scans for all adult patients 1 year post-HCT or earlier for patients at high risk of bone loss [17]. Bisphosphonates are effective in reducing or reversing HCT-related bone loss in several small randomized studies; however, they rarely resolve bone loss to pre-HCT levels and have a significant side-effect, osteonecrosis of the jaw. We hypothesized that genetic variants are associated with BMD loss in HCT patients, and sought to identify a panel of genetic biomarkers that can be incorporated into the above guidelines to personalize prevention and treatment strategy.

Methods

Ethics statement: Stem cell transplant patients at the Blood and Marrow Transplantation Program included in this study are part of an institution-level Data Bank and Biorepository (DBBR) at Roswell Park Cancer Institute (RPCI). All participants have provided written consent for their data and biospecimens to be used for research purposes. This study has been reviewed and approved by RPCI Institutional Review Board.

Patients, BMD measurement, and DNA specimens

A detailed description of the patient population has been published previously [6]. Briefly, between 1/2006 and 1/2009, 206 consecutive adult (≥18 years) patients underwent their first HCT in the Blood and Marrow Transplantation Program at Roswell Park Cancer Institute (RPCI). As part of routine clinical care, the average BMD at lumbar spine (L2–L4) and dual femurs were measured by DXA scans at baseline (pre-HCT) and day +100 post-HCT. The median time for 197 patients (96%) who had a baseline DXA scan was 20 days before HCT, and 98 days for 146 patients (74%) who had a second DXA scan after HCT. Reasons for not obtaining a follow-up DXA scan were unstable medical status (n = 14), or disease relapse/early death (n = 37). Before HCT, patients were invited to participate in the DataBank and BioRepository (DBBR), a comprehensive data and biospecimen core facility at RPCI [18]. Upon their consent to the DBBR, blood samples were drawn and genomic DNA was extracted and stored for multidisplinary research. For this study, 121 patients including 67 autologous and 54 allogeneic HCT patients, consented to the DBBR and had adequate DNA available for genotyping.

Candidate gene and SNP selection and genotyping

Candidate genes from bone metabolism pathways were selected based on the following criteria: (1) genes that have been well studied and established in association with osteoporosis or other bone phenotypes in the general population; (2) key genes in bone metabolism pathways, including osteoblast or osteoclast differentiation, proliferation and activation; calcitronic hormone metabolism and activation; and bone matrix formation and regulation. As listed in Table S1, a total of 45 candidate genes were clustered into 4 groups based on underlying biological function, including (1) RANKL-RANK-OPG central signaling axis and regulating cytokines, (2) bone matrix proteins and regulating factors, (3) vitamin D receptor and metabolizing enzymes, and (4) steroid hormones and receptors.

SNPs for each candidate gene were selected based on the following criteria: (1) minor allele frequency (MAF) ≥0.10 in the population of European ancestry; (2) SNPs that have been well studied and established in association with osteoporosis or other bone traits in the general population, including those identified in recent GWA studies and the large prospective study Genetic Factors for Osteoporosis (GEFOS) Consortium [10]; (3) coding SNPs and SNPs in the 3′ or 5′ untranslated region (UTR); and (4) tagSNPs selected by the Tagger program [19] from the HapMap Project data [20], if no functional SNPs or well studied SNPs were available. In all, 158 SNPs were initially selected from the 45 candidate genes. To remove redundant SNPs due to high linkage disequilibrium (LD), pair-wise r^2 was computed for SNPs in each gene and in genes clustered on the same chromosome by PLINK [21]; SNP_tools [22] was used for necessary data formatting. For SNP pairs in high LD ($r^2 ≥ 0.90$), one SNP was randomly selected from each pair for further consideration. As a result, a total of 122 SNPs were included in the final analysis (see Table S1).

Genotyping of DNA extracted from peripheral blood was performed in the Genomics Shared Resource at RPCI utilizing the MassARRAY® technology and iPLEX Gold assay (Sequenom). Nine percent duplicate samples and in-house Coriell trio samples were included within plates and across plates for genotyping quality assurance. The average qualified call rate was 98.1% for each SNP and 98.3% for each DNA sample. There was no discordance among duplicate pairs, and no SNPs violated Mendelian inheritance or Hardy-Weinberg equilibrium.

Statistical analysis

All analyses were performed stratified by autologous and allogeneic HCTs since these two treatments, and the characteristics of the patients given these two treatments, are significantly different. Change in BMD was standardized to 100 days (BMD change divided by the number of days between the two DXA scans then times 100) and used as a continuous variable; thus, a negative value indicates BMD loss and a positive value indicates BMD gain. We used linear regression models to analyze the association of clinical factors and genetic variants with four separate outcomes: BMD changes at the spine and at the femur in autologous and allogeneic HCT patients. Assuming an additive genetic model, 54 patients in the small allogeneic HCT group and two-sided p-value of 0.05, we had 80% power to detect a minimum BMD change of 0.023–0.040 g/cm^2 for a SNP with a minor allele frequency between 0.10–0.50. In the autologous HCT group which had a larger sample size of 67, we had 80% power to detect effect sizes <0.023 g/cm^2.

Single SNP analysis. SNPs associated with HCT-induced BMD change were identified as follows. First, each SNP was tested individually in a simple linear regression model without controlling for covariates; SNPs with p<0.10 were then added to regression models previously built with clinical factors for each of the four outcomes, including the cumulative dose of corticosteroids (in prednisone equivalents) between the two DXA scans for BMD loss in allogeneic HCT patients [6]. We measured the proportion of variance explained by all the covariates retained in a model, R^2, and determined, ΔR^2, an estimate of the proportion of variance that can be explained by the SNP(s) added to the base model, with adjustment for the number of covariates in the model. A SNP with a ΔR^2 of 5% or higher was deemed significant. Effect size (i.e., absolute BMD change) per copy of the variant allele and 95% confidence intervals (CI) were calculated for each significant SNP, with and without adjustment for clinical risk factors. The rate of annualized BMD change between pre- and post-HCT DXA scans was compared and plotted by the genotypes of each significant

SNP. To explore potential functionality of the significant SNPs, the SNP and CNV Annotation Database (SCAN) [23] was surveyed to explore whether it is a potential expression quantitative trait loci (eQTL) that has been associated with altered gene expression.

Multiple-SNP analysis. We examined the combined effects of multiple variants using backward elimination. SNPs with a p≤0.05 were retained in the final models. Adjusted R^2 was calculated for the complete models with both clinical and genetic factors and compared to the base models with only clinical factors,

to determine the overall contribution of genetic factors. For SNPs retained in the model, the number of risk alleles was summed for each patient, and the annualized rate of BMD change was compared across patients by number of risk alleles. Although we measured change in BMD between a set interval of approximately 100 days, we presented annualized BMD loss rates for comparisons to the general population. Prior reports of BMD loss post-HCT demonstrated that reversal of BMD loss takes several years after HCT [3]. Multiple-SNP analysis was not performed for spinal BMD loss after allogeneic HCT because only

Table 1. Characteristics of HCT patients with BMD measurement and genomic DNA samples.

Characteristics	Autologous HCT (n = 67)	Allogeneic HCT (n = 54)
Age at HCT in years	57 (25–74)	47 (18–71)
Spine BMD at baseline, median (range), g/cm²	1.23 (0.71–1.65)	1.20 (0.86–1.83)
Femur BMD at baseline, median (range), g/cm²	1.04 (0.60–1.41)	1.09 (0.71–1.45)
Gender		
Male	42 (63%)	30 (56%)
Female	25 (37%)	24 (44%)
Race		
White	59 (88%)	52 (96%)
Other	8 (12%)	2 (4%)
Diagnosis		
Acute leukemia	3 (4%)	34 (63%)
Lymphoma	37 (55%)	9 (17%)
Myeloma	27 (40%)	0
Other	0	11 (20%)
Disease status at HCT		
CR1/untreated MDS	29 (43%)	38 (70%)
CR2+/PIF/Relapse	38 (57%)	16 (30%)
Graft source		
Bone marrow ± PBSC	6 (9%)	8 (15%)
PBSC	61 (91%)	46 (85%)
Conditioning regimen		
Myeloblative	67 (100%)	19 (35%)
Reduced Intensity	0	32 (59%)
Non-myeloblative	0	3 (6%)
GvHD prophylaxis regimen		
CsMt/FKMt	-	19 (35%)
FK/FKMMF	-	15 (28%)
FKMtMMF		20 (37%)
Donor relation		
Unrelated	-	36 (67%)
Related	-	18 (33%)
HLA match		
Matched	-	45 (83%)
Mismatched	-	9 (17%)
Acute GvHD		
Grade 0–I	-	26 (48%)
Grade II–IV	-	28 (52%)

Abbreviations: BMD, bone mineral density; CR, complete remission; Cs, cyclosporine; FK, tacrolimus; GvHD, graft-versus-host disease; HCT, hematopoietic cell transplantation; HLA, human leukocyte antigen; MDS, myelodysplastic syndrome; MMF, mycophenolate mofetil; Mt, methotrexate; PIF, primary induction failure; PBSC, peripheral blood stem cell.

one SNP was retained in the final comprehensive model. All analyses were two-tailed and were performed with SAS 9.2 (SAS Institute, Cary, NC).

Results

Individual SNP analysis

Table 1 summarizes the demographic and clinical characteristics of the study population separately by auto- and allo-HCT groups, which were statistically similar to the overall patient population described in our prior report [6]. Unadjusted p-values for associations between individual SNPs and BMD change between pre- and post-HCT are shown in Figure S1. After controlling for clinical risk factors, at least one SNP remained significant for each of the four outcomes, with a total of 16 significant SNPs for all four outcomes. SNP rs2075555 in the COL1A1 gene remained significant after Bonferroni correction for multiple comparisons (p = 0.037).

Table 2 summarizes the unadjusted and adjusted BMD change associated with each of the 16 SNPs significant in individual SNP tests. Annualized rate of BMD change by genotype are shown in Figure 1. There was a significant dose-response trend between rate of BMD loss and number of risk alleles at the spine and the femur in autologous HCT and at the femur in allogeneic HCT. The

functions of these genes, SNPs and published literature are summarized in Table S2. Among these, three SNPs, including rs2075555 in COL1A1 gene [11,24], rs9594738 in RANKL gene [13] and rs4870044 in ESR1 gene [13], were significantly associated with bone phenotypes in GWA studies of the general population. Moreover, rs2075555 and rs9594738 were associated with altered gene expression in the SCAN (p<0.0001). Another 9 significant SNPs in our analysis were previously linked to bone phenotypes in candidate gene association studies, including rs4588 in GC, rs6256 in PTH, rs419598 in IL1RN, rs1801131 in MTHFR, rs1800896 in IL10, and rs1061624 in TNFRSF1B, rs1042358 in ALOX12, rs759330 in BGLAP, and rs2235579 in CLCN7. Four of these SNPs (rs759330, rs2235579, rs1800896 and rs1061624) were also associated with altered gene expression in the SCAN. The other 4 SNPs, including rs3787557 and rs2296241 in CYP24A1, rs25645 in CSF3, and rs1321080 in RUNX2, were selected as tagSNPs or SNPs in functional genomic regions, with no known associations with bone phenotypes. Two of these SNPs (rs2296241 and rs25645) were associated with altered gene expression in the SCAN.

Multiple-SNP analysis

The multiple-SNP models are shown in Table 3. For the spinal BMD change after autologous HCT, three SNPs (rs759330 in

Table 2. Change in bone mineral density per copy of the variant allele for individual SNPs which were significant in the multivariable models including clinical risk factors[1].

Gene	SNP	Unadjusted BMD change per copy of variant allele (95% CI), g/cm^2	Unadjusted P-value	Adjusted BMD change per copy of variant allele (95% CI), g/cm^2	Adjusted P-value
Spinal bone mineral density change after autologous hematopoietic cell transplantation					
BGLAP	rs759330	−0.024 (−0.045−0.002)	0.03	−0.026 (−0.047−0.006)	0.01
CLCN7	rs2235579	0.016 (−0.001−0.034)	0.07	0.019 (0.002−0.036)	0.03
GC	rs4588	−0.031 (−0.051−0.011)	0.003	−0.024 (−0.045−0.003)	0.02
CYP24A1	rs3787557	−0.055 (−0.095−0.016)	0.007	−0.049 (−0.087−0.010)	0.01
PTH	rs6256	0.036 (0.004−0.067)	0.03	0.032 (0.002−0.063)	0.04
Femoral bone mineral density change after autologous hematopoietic cell transplantation					
IL1RN	rs419598	−0.014 (−0.026−0.003)	0.01	−0.014 (−0.025−0.004)	0.009
CSF3	rs25645	0.011 (0.002−0.021)	0.02	0.011 (0.002−0.020)	0.02
MTHFR	rs1801131	0.022 (0.009−0.036)	0.001	0.020 (0.08−0.033)	0.008
ALOX12	rs1042357	−0.016 (−0.027−0.005)	0.004	−0.014 (−0.025−0.003)	0.01
CYP24A1	rs2296241	0.014 (0.004−0.024)	0.01	0.014 (0.004−0.024)	0.01
ESR1	rs4870044	−0.011 (−0.023−0.000)	0.06	−0.015 (−0.025−0.004)	0.008
Spinal bone mineral density change after allogeneic hematopoietic cell transplantation					
RANKL	rs9594738	−0.029 (−0.052−0.007)	0.01	−0.020 (−0.039−0.001)	0.04
Femoral bone mineral density change after allogeneic hematopoietic cell transplantation					
RANKL	rs9594738	−0.022 (−0.042−0.003)	0.02	−0.018 (−0.036−0.001)	0.05
IL10	rs1800896	−0.016 (−0.035−0.002)	0.08	−0.022 (−0.039−0.005)	0.01
TNFRSF1B	rs1061624	−0.023 (−0.041−0.004)	0.02	−0.021 (−0.039−0.003)	0.02
COL1A1	rs2075555	−0.052 (−0.080−0.024)	0.0003	−0.050 (−0.077−0.023)	0.0006
RUNX2	rs1321080	−0.028 (−0.051−0.006)	0.02	−0.024 (−0.047−0.002)	0.03

Footnote:
[1]The clinical risk factors included in the multivariable models are: (1) Spinal BMD change after autologous HCT: spinal BMD at baseline and diagnosis (lymphoma vs others); (2) Femoral BMD change after autologous HCT: age at HCT and diagnosis (lymphoma vs others); (3) Spinal BMD change after allogeneic HCT: spinal BMD at baseline, weight at baseline, and steroid dose; (4) Femoral BMD change after allogeneic HCT: femoral BMD at baseline, weight at baseline, and steroid dose. Please refer to Table S2 for description of functions of these genes and SNPs. Abbreviation: BMD, bone mineral density; CI, confidence interval; HCT, hematopoietic cell transplantation; SNP, single nucleotide polymorphism.

A. Annualized spinal BMD loss rate in autologous HCT patients

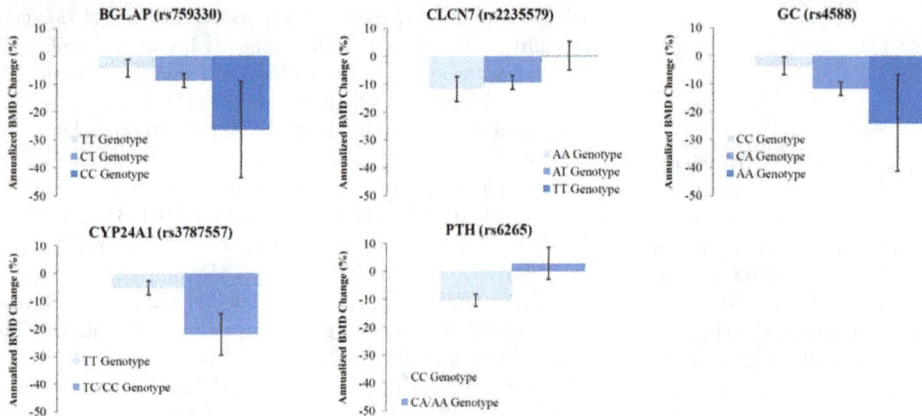

BGLAP (rs759330)

TT Genotype
CT Genotype
CC Genotype

CLCN7 (rs2235579)

AA Genotype
AT Genotype
TT Genotype

GC (rs4588)

CC Genotype
CA Genotype
AA Genotype

CYP24A1 (rs3787557)

TT Genotype
TC/CC Genotype

PTH (rs6265)

CC Genotype
CA/AA Genotype

B. Annualized femoral BMD loss rate in autologous HCT patients

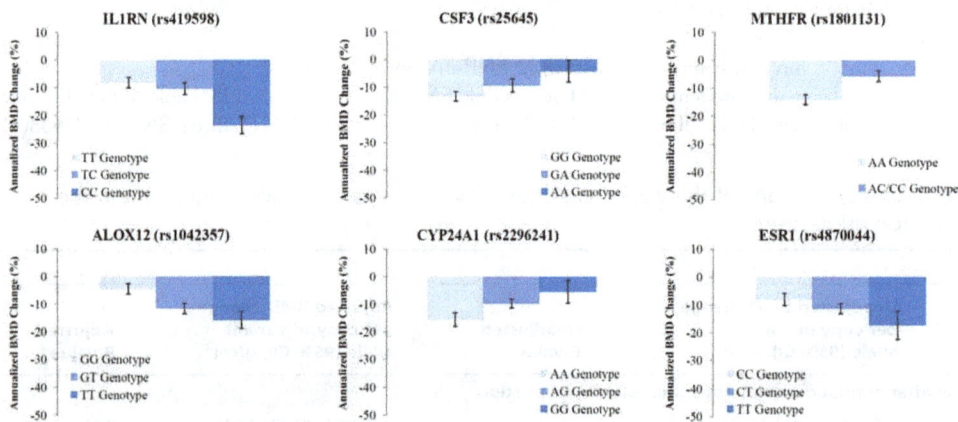

IL1RN (rs419598)

TT Genotype
TC Genotype
CC Genotype

CSF3 (rs25645)

GG Genotype
GA Genotype
AA Genotype

MTHFR (rs1801131)

AA Genotype
AC/CC Genotype

ALOX12 (rs1042357)

GG Genotype
GT Genotype
TT Genotype

CYP24A1 (rs2296241)

AA Genotype
AG Genotype
GG Genotype

ESR1 (rs4870044)

CC Genotype
CT Genotype
TT Genotype

C. Annualized spinal BMD loss rate in allogeneic HCT patients

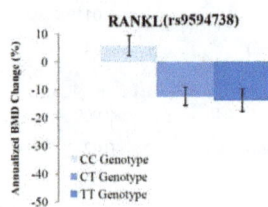

RANKL(rs9594738)

CC Genotype
CT Genotype
TT Genotype

D. Annualized femoral BMD loss rate in allogeneic HCT patients

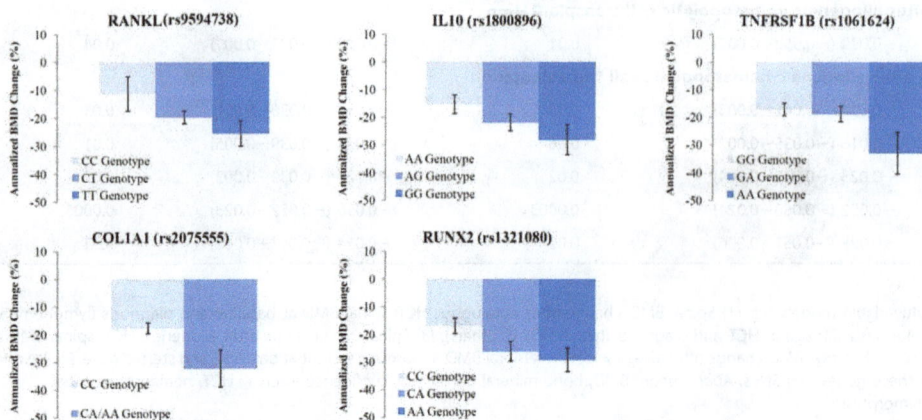

RANKL(rs9594738)

CC Genotype
CT Genotype
TT Genotype

IL10 (rs1800896)

AA Genotype
AG Genotype
GG Genotype

TNFRSF1B (rs1061624)

GG Genotype
GA Genotype
AA Genotype

COL1A1 (rs2075555)

CC Genotype
CA/AA Genotype

RUNX2 (rs1321080)

CC Genotype
CA Genotype
AA Genotype

Figure 1. Annualized rate of bone mineral density change after hematopoietic cell transplantation by genotype for SNPs significant in the multivariable models including clinical risk factors. Mean and standard error of the annualized rate of BMD change is plotted by genotype for significant SNPs in the multivariable models including clinical risk factors. If the frequency of the homozygous variant genotype was ≤5%, it was combined with the heterozygous genotype (includes rs3787557 [CYP24A1], rs6265 [PTH], rs1801131 [MTHFR] and rs2075555 [COL1A1]). Please refer to Table S2 for a description of functions of these genes and SNPs. *Abbreviation:* BMD, bone mineral density; HCT, hematopoietic cell transplantation; SNP, single nucleotide polymorphism.

BGLAP, rs4588 in *GC*, and rs3787557 in *CYP24A1*) remained in the final model and explained 16% of the variance in BMD loss, in addition to the 10% determined by the clinical risk factors. Similarly, SNPs retained in the final models explained an additional 35%, 5% and 29% of the variance in femoral BMD loss after autologous HCT, spinal BMD loss after allogeneic HCT, and femoral BMD loss after allogeneic HCT, respectively.

When the annualized rate of BMD loss was compared by the number of risk alleles, there was a significant association between higher number of risk alleles and higher BMD loss (Figure 2). In addition, the multiple-SNP models identified patients at the highest risk of BMD loss. Patients carrying the highest number of risk alleles had the most severe BMD loss.

Discussion

Our analysis identified a number of SNPs in bone metabolism pathways predictive for acute BMD loss following HCT. Because our candidate genes and SNPs have been previously implicated in age-related bone loss, osteoporosis and/or bone phenotypes in the general population, our findings support the hypothesis that HCT-related BMD loss is an acceleration of the normal bone aging process. Moreover, SNPs showed greater effects in HCT patients in our study than those identified in the general population for bone phenotypes. Four SNPs accounted for 35% of variance in femoral BMD change after autologous HCT, whereas the 12 most significant loci in a GWA study accounted for only about 3% of variance in hip and spine BMD in a healthy Icelandic population [13]. The stronger effect may be driven by potent exposures during HCT.

Among the 16 SNPs significant in our analysis, only rs9594738 in *RANKL* gene was related to BMD loss at both the spine and the femur in allogeneic patients. This marginal overlap could be attributed to differences in exposures related to allogeneic versus autologous transplant procedures, as well as to differences in susceptibility to HCT-induced BMD loss at these two anatomic

sites. The trabecular interconnection of the lumbar spine is much higher than that of the femur [25]. Thus, the difference in bone microarchitecture may explain the lack of overlap of SNPs associated with BMD and risk of fracture at the two sites in previous studies in the general populations [10] and the observations that femoral bone was more susceptible to HCT-induced bone loss than spinal bone [6,26].

A limitation of our study comes from the relatively small sample size and the large number of tests performed: 122 SNPs in relation to 4 quantitative outcomes in 121 patients stratified by autologous and allogeneic HCT. The statistical power was thus limited. Instead of using a Bonferroni correction, which would be over conservative, we propose a hierarchy of evidence in our findings based on curated knowledge of the SNPs in the literature.

The first level of evidence includes three SNPs implicated in two GWA studies of bone phenotypes. We found that rs2075555 in the intronic region of *COL1A1* is associated with femoral BMD loss after allogeneic HCT. The gene encodes for type I collagen, a major matrix protein for bone formation and this SNP has been previously associated with femoral neck width in women and shaft width in men [11]. Two other SNPs, rs9594738 near *RANKL* and rs4870044 near *ESR1* from a GWA study of BMD in an Icelandic population [13], and a meta-analysis of GWA studies of BMD[14], were also significant in our study. *RANKL* plays a central role in coupling the activities of osteoblasts and osteoclasts; and *ESR1* encodes for estrogen receptor alpha, which is key in estrogen-regulated activities.

The second level of evidence includes 9 SNPs, which have been previously studied in relation to various bone phenotypes using a candidate gene approach: rs4588 in *GC*, rs6256 in *PTH*, rs419598 in *IL1RN*, rs1801131 in *MTHFR*, rs1800896 in *IL10*, and rs1061624 in *TNFRSF1B*, and rs1042358 in *ALOX12*, rs759330 in *BGLAP*, and rs2235579 in *CLCN7* (Table S2). The first 5 SNPs are among the most widely studied candidates for osteoporosis and/or other bone phenotypes.

Table 3. Multiple SNP models of bone mineral density change after hematopoietic cell transplantation.

Outcome	Base model of clinical factors	Adjusted R^2	SNP (Gene)	Adjusted R^2	ΔR^2
Spinal BMD change after autologous HCT	Spinal BMD at baseline; lymphoma vs others	0.10	rs759330 (BGALP); rs4588 (GC); rs3787557 (CYP24A1)	0.26	0.16
Femoral BMD change after autologous HCT	Age at HCT; lymphoma vs others	0.12	rs419598 (IL1RN); rs1801131(MTHFR); rs1042357 (ALOX12); rs4870044 (ESR1)	0.46	0.35
Spinal BMD change after allogeneic HCT	Weight at HCT; spinal BMD at baseline; cortico-steroid dose	0.35	rs9594738 (RANKL)	0.40	0.05
Femoral BMD change after allogeneic HCT	Weight at HCT; femoral BMD at baseline; cortico-steroid dose	0.14	rs9594738 (RANKL); rs1061624 (TNFRSF1B); rs2075555(COL1A1); rs1321080 (RUNX2)	0.45	0.29

Footnote: R^2, coefficient of determination, provides an estimate of the proportion of BMD change that can be accounted for by all covariates in the model. ΔR^2 denotes the increase in model accountability by adding SNP(s) to the base clinical risk factor model. All R^2 are adjusted by the number of covariates in the model. A higher ΔR^2 suggests an important role of genetics in addition to clinical risk factors for HCT-inducted BMD loss. Please refer to Table S2 for a description of the functions of these genes and SNPs. *Abbreviation:* BMD, bone mineral density; HCT, hematopoietic cell transplantation; SNP, single nucleotide polymorphism. single nucleotide polymorphism.

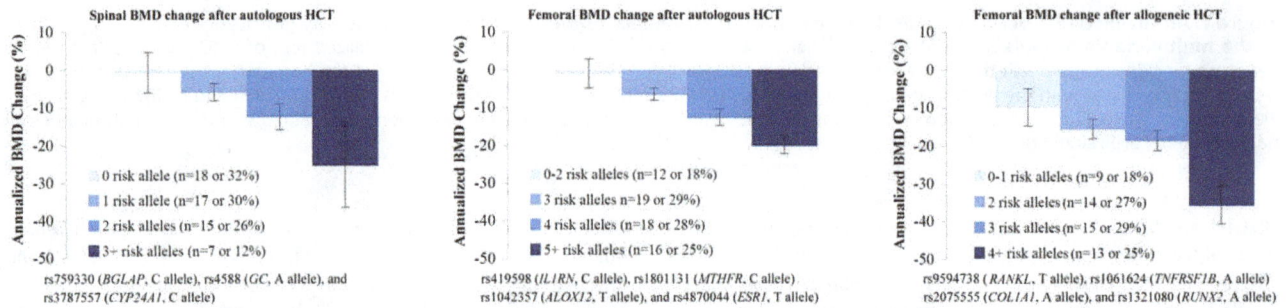

Figure 2. Annualized rate of bone mineral density change after hematopoietic cell transplantation by the number of risk alleles of the SNPs significant in the multiple SNP models. Mean and standard error of annualized rate of BMD change is plotted by the number of risk alleles in significant SNPs from the multiple SNP models as shown in Table 3. The p-values for a trend between the number of risk alleles and BMD change were ≤0.003 for all three outcomes. The proportion of HCT patients carrying the specified number of risk alleles is shown. The multiple SNP analysis was not performed for spinal BMD change after allogeneic HCT since only one SNP was significant in the multiple SNP model. Please refer to Table S2 for a description of these genes and SNPs. *Abbreviation:* BMD, bone mineral density; HCT, hematopoietic cell transplantation; SNP.

The third level of evidence includes 4 SNPs which have not been previously studied in relation to bone phenotypes: rs3787557 and rs2296241 in *CYP24A1*, rs25645 in *CSF3*, and rs1321080 in *RUNX2*. These SNPs are either tagSNPs or located in potentially functional regions, and these genes were selected for their importance in bone metabolism (Table S2).

As discussed above, we relied on *a priori* knowledge to rank our confidence in our results: those previously implicated in GWA studies were deemed most reliable, followed by those implicated in candidate gene studies, and lastly those without support from the literature. Although this knowledge-based hierarchy of evidence is not statistically stringent, and we cannot exclude the possibility of false positive (or negative) findings in our results, it aligns with our exploratory purpose and provides support that genetic variants contribute to post-HCT bone loss. Moreover, our findings may provide clues for future studies. Thus, in addition to rs2075555 in *COL1A1*, which remained significant in our analysis under the most stringent threshold of significance, we also reported other SNPs that may be interesting. Our study was designed to evaluate only one post-HCT BMD measurement (about +100 days); thus we do not know how the genetic variants described in our study affect long-term BMD post-HCT. We chose day +100 for post-HCT BMD measurement for three reasons. First, BMD loss occurs at the highest rate within the first 3–6 months after HCT [3], thus a true gene-exposure influence would be strongest in the time period closest to the exposure. Second, patients who were osteoporotic at their day +100 DXA scan were treated with a bisphosphonate soon afterwards which may distort the association between genotypes and BMD loss. Third, as an exploratory study, BMD loss at day +100 was an outcome immediately available, while we continue to follow-up patients with the plan to assess genotypes and long-term BMD loss.

It is of interest to investigate the association of donor genotype with BMD loss in allogeneic HCT recipients, considering their hematopoietic cells, and thus osteoclast precursors, are replaced by donors' hematopoietic cells once complete donor chimerism has been achieved. Unfortunately, donor DNA is not available from the allogeneic HCT patients in this study. However, given that the acute BMD loss we observed occurred quickly following transplantation, prior to complete donor chimerism, and that the acute BMD loss in our study was similar between autologous and allogeneic HCT recipients (ie., in the absence and presence of donor genomes), any effect of donor genotype may only be evidenced in chronic BMD loss with longer follow-up. This question warrants further investigation.

In summary, given the continuous bone loss due to normal aging, accelerated post-HCT bone loss may never recover without aggressive therapy, and HCT patients may be at much higher risk of fracture compared to their age-matched peers. Considering the well established relationship between low BMD and fracture risk in the general population, we support the routine post HCT surveillance guidelines developed by McClune et al [17]. Further studies are needed to determine the impact and timing of different prevention and/or intervention strategies.

Supporting Information

Figure S1 Log-transformed p-values for associations between bone mineral density change and individual SNPs without adjustment for clinical risk factors. Individual SNP (gene) remained significant in the multivariable models including clinical risk factors are labeled in circles. A number of other SNPs significant in univariate analysis but dropped out of multivariate analysis were not labeled. Please refer to Table S2 for description of functions of these genes and SNPs. *Abbreviation:* HCT, hematopoietic cell transplantation; SNP, single nucleotide polymorphism.

Table S1 Selected 122 single nucleotide polymorphisms from 46 candidate genes in bone metabolism pathways. [1]SNPs that have been previously studied in the large prospective study Genetic Markers for Osteoporosis (GENOMOS) Consortium were labeled as "GENOMOS SNPs". SNPs that have been identified in genome wide association (GWA) studies were labeled as "GWAS SNP". TagSNPs selected to represent genetic variations in genes that have not been previous studied and have no common SNPs in functional regions were labeled as "tagSNP". Functional regions include 3′ and 5′ untranslated region (UTR) and codon. For coding SNPs, amino acid changes are shown.

Table S2 Functions and summary of the published literature for genes and SNPs significant in the individual SNP models including clinical risk factors

Acknowledgments

The authors are grateful to the RPCI patients who agreed to participate in this study, the BMT nursing and laboratory staff, the nurse practitioners, physician assistants and the entire clinical team who cares for these patients, and the BMT data managers for assistance with data collection.

Author Contributions

Conceived and designed the experiments: SY LES SLS CBA PLM TH. Performed the experiments: SY WD JMC NJN. Analyzed the data: SY LES SLS CBA PLM TH. Contributed reagents/materials/analysis tools: WD JMC NJN CBA. Wrote the paper: SY LES SLS WD JMC NJN CBA PLM TH.

References

1. Benjamin RM (2010) Bone health: preventing osteoporosis. J Am Diet Assoc 110: 498.
2. Kelly PJ, Atkinson K, Ward RL, Sambrook PN, Biggs JC, et al. (1990) Reduced bone mineral density in men and women with allogeneic bone marrow transplantation. Transplantation 50: 881–883.
3. Schulte CM, Beelen DW (2004) Bone loss following hematopoietic stem cell transplantation: a long-term follow-up. Blood 103: 3635–3643.
4. Tauchmanova L, Serio B, Del Puente A, Risitano AM, Esposito A, et al. (2002) Long-lasting bone damage detected by dual-energy x-ray absorptiometry, phalangeal osteosonogrammetry, and in vitro growth of marrow stromal cells after allogeneic stem cell transplantation. J Clin Endocrinol Metab 87: 5058–5065.
5. Lee WY, Cho SW, Oh ES, Oh KW, Lee JM, et al. (2002) The effect of bone marrow transplantation on the osteoblastic differentiation of human bone marrow stromal cells. J Clin Endocrinol Metab 87: 329–335.
6. Yao S, Smiley SL, West K, Lamonica D, Battiwalla M, et al. (2010) Accelerated bone mineral density loss occurs with similar incidence and severity, but with different risk factors, after autologous versus allogeneic hematopoietic cell transplantation. Biol Blood Marrow Transplant 16: 1130–1137.
7. Peacock M, Turner CH, Econs MJ, Foroud T (2002) Genetics of osteoporosis. Endocr Rev 23: 303–326.
8. Eisman JA (1999) Genetics of osteoporosis. Endocr Rev 20: 788–804.
9. Liu YZ, Liu YJ, Recker RR, Deng HW (2003) Molecular studies of identification of genes for osteoporosis: the 2002 update. J Endocrinol 177: 147–196.
10. Richards JB, Kavvoura FK, Rivadeneira F, Styrkarsdottir U, Estrada K, et al. (2009) Collaborative meta-analysis: associations of 150 candidate genes with osteoporosis and osteoporotic fracture. Ann Intern Med 151: 528–537.
11. Kiel DP, Demissie S, Dupuis J, Lunetta KL, Murabito JM, et al. (2007) Genome-wide association with bone mass and geometry in the Framingham Heart Study. BMC Med Genet 8 Suppl 1: S14.
12. Richards JB, Rivadeneira F, Inouye M, Pastinen TM, Soranzo N, et al. (2008) Bone mineral density, osteoporosis, and osteoporotic fractures: a genome-wide association study. Lancet 371: 1505–1512.
13. Styrkarsdottir U, Halldorsson BV, Gretarsdottir S, Gudbjartsson DF, Walters GB, et al. (2008) Multiple genetic loci for bone mineral density and fractures. N Engl J Med 358: 2355–2365.
14. Rivadeneira F, Styrkarsdottir U, Estrada K, Halldorsson BV, Hsu YH, et al. (2009) Twenty bone-mineral-density loci identified by large-scale meta-analysis of genome-wide association studies. Nat Genet 41: 1199–1206.
15. Styrkarsdottir U, Halldorsson BV, Gretarsdottir S, Gudbjartsson DF, Walters GB, et al. (2009) New sequence variants associated with bone mineral density. Nat Genet 41: 15–17.
16. Perrone M (June 01, 2010) FDA clears Amgen's bone-strengthening drug Prolia. Available: http://www.biosciencetechnology.com/News/FeedsAP/2010/06/fda-clears-amgens-bone-strengthening-drug-prolia/ Accessed 2011 September 14.
17. McClune BL, Polgreen LE, Burmeister LA, Blaes AH, Mulrooney DA, et al. (2011) Screening, prevention and management of osteoporosis and bone loss in adult and pediatric hematopoietic cell transplant recipients. Bone Marrow Transplant 46: 1–9.
18. Ambrosone CB, Nesline MK, Davis W (2006) Establishing a cancer center data bank and biorepository for multidisciplinary research. Cancer Epidemiol Biomarkers Prev 15: 1575–1577.
19. de Bakker PI, Yelensky R, Pe'er I, Gabriel SB, Daly MJ, et al. (2005) Efficiency and power in genetic association studies. Nat Genet 37: 1217–1223.
20. The International HapMap Consortium (2003) The International HapMap Project. Nature 426: 789–796.
21. Purcell S, Neale B, Todd-Brown K, Thomas L, Ferreira MA, et al. (2007) PLINK: a tool set for whole-genome association and population-based linkage analyses. Am J Hum Genet 81: 559–575.
22. Chen B, Wilkening S, Drechsel M, Hemminki K (2009) SNP_tools: A compact tool package for analysis and conversion of genotype data for MS-Excel. BMC Res Notes 2: 214.
23. Gamazon ER, Zhang W, Konkashbaev A, Duan S, Kistner EO, et al. (2010) SCAN: SNP and copy number annotation. Bioinformatics 26: 259–262.
24. Murabito JM, Rosenberg CL, Finger D, Kreger BE, Levy D, et al. (2007) A genome-wide association study of breast and prostate cancer in the NHLBI's Framingham Heart Study. BMC Med Genet 8 Suppl 1: S6.
25. Amling M, Herden S, Posl M, Hahn M, Ritzel H, et al. (1996) Heterogeneity of the skeleton: comparison of the trabecular microarchitecture of the spine, the iliac crest, the femur, and the calcaneus. J Bone Miner Res 11: 36–45.
26. Yao S, McCarthy PL, Dunford LM, Roy DM, Brown K, et al. (2008) High prevalence of early-onset osteopenia/osteoporosis after allogeneic stem cell transplantation and improvement after bisphosphonate therapy. Bone Marrow Transplant 41: 393–398.

15

Calcitonin Inhibits SDCP-Induced Osteoclast Apoptosis and Increases Its Efficacy in a Rat Model of Osteoporosis

Yi-Jie Kuo[1,2], Fon-Yih Tsuang[3], Jui-Sheng Sun[4,5], Chi-Hung Lin[6], Chia-Hsien Chen[6], Jia-Ying Li[7], Yi-Chian Huang[8], Wei-Yu Chen[7], Chin-Bin Yeh[9], Jia-Fwu Shyu[7,9]*

1 Department of Orthopaedic, Taipei Medical University Hospital, Taipei, Taiwan, Republic of China, 2 Institute of Clinical Medicine, National Yang Ming University, Taipei, Taiwan, Republic of China, 3 Division of Neurosurgery, Department of Surgery, National Taiwan University Hospital, Taipei, Taiwan, Republic of China, 4 Department of Orthopaedic Surgery, National Taiwan University Hospital-Hsin Chu, Hsin-Chu, Taiwan, Republic of China, 5 Graduate Institute of Clinical Medicine, College of Medicine, Taipei Medical University, Taipei, Taiwan, Republic of China, 6 Institute of Microbiology and Immunology, National Yang Ming University, Taipei, Taiwan, Republic of China, 7 Department of Biology and Anatomy, National Defense Medical Center, Taipei, Taiwan, Republic of China, 8 Institute of Anatomy and Cell Biology National Yang Ming University, Taipei, Taiwan, Republic of China, 9 Department of Psychiatry, Tri-Service General Hospital, Taipei, Taiwan, Republic of China

Abstract

Introduction: Treatment for osteoporosis commonly includes the use of bisphosphonates. Serious side effects of these drugs are caused by the inhibition of bone resorption as a result of osteoclast apoptosis. Treatment using calcitonin along with bisphosphonates overcomes these side-effects in some patients. Calcitonin is known to inhibit bone resorption without reducing the number of osteoclasts and is thought to prolong osteoclast survival through the inhibition of apoptosis. Further understanding of how calcitonin inhibits apoptosis could prove useful to the development of alternative treatment regimens for osteoporosis. This study aimed to analyze the mechanism by which calcitonin influences osteoclast apoptosis induced by a bisphosphate analog, sintered dicalcium pyrophosphate (SDCP), and to determine the effects of co-treatment with calcitonin and SDCP on apoptotic signaling in osteoclasts.

Methods: Isolated osteoclasts were treated with CT, SDCP or both for 48 h. Osteoclast apoptosis assays, pit formation assays, and tartrate-resistant acid phosphatase (TRAP) staining were performed. Using an osteoporosis rat model, ovariectomized (OVX) rats received calcitonin, SDCP, or calcitonin + SDCP. The microarchitecture of the fifth lumbar trabecular bone was investigated, and histomorphometric and biochemical analyses were performed.

Results: Calcitonin inhibited SDCP-induced apoptosis in primary osteoclast cultures, increased Bcl-2 and Erk activity, and decreased Mcl-1 activity. Calcitonin prevented decreased osteoclast survival but not resorption induced by SDCP. Histomorphometric analysis of the tibia revealed increased bone formation, and microcomputed tomography of the fifth lumbar vertebrate showed an additive effect of calcitonin and SDCP on bone volume. Finally, analysis of the serum bone markers CTX-I and P1NP suggests that the increased bone volume induced by co-treatment with calcitonin and SDCP may be due to decreased bone resorption and increased bone formation.

Conclusions: Calcitonin reduces SDCP-induced osteoclast apoptosis and increases its efficacy in an in vivo model of osteoporosis.

Editor: Agustin Guerrero-Hernandez, Cinvestav-IPN, Mexico

Funding: This work was funded by National Defense Medical Center of Medical Research Grants (DOD-100-C-11-02) and Tri-Service General Hospital of Medical Research Grants (TSGH-C99-011-12-S03). The funders had no role in study design, data collection and analysis, decision to publish, or preparation of the manuscript.

Competing Interests: The authors have declared that no competing interests exist.

* E-mail: jiafwu.shyu@msa.hinet.net

Introduction

Bisphosphonates are the most commonly prescribed first line medication for osteoporosis despite causing side effects, including low bone turnover, hypocalcemia, and osteonecrosis of the jaw due to decreased bone formation as well as increased bone fracture due to reduced bone resorption [1,2]. Although the molecular mechanisms by which they inhibit bone resorption vary among the bisphosphonates, they collectively induce osteoclast apoptosis. Specifically, simple bisphosphonates are incorporated into non-hydrolysable adenosine triphosphate analogues, inducing osteo-clast apoptosis [3]. The more potent nitrogen-containing bisphos-phonates inhibit farnesyl pyrophosphate synthase, a key enzyme of the mevalonate pathway, which is essential for protein prenylation in osteoclasts [3,4]. Thus, bisphosphonates inhibit bone resorption by disrupting osteoclast function and survival.

Calcitonin has also been used as a therapy for osteoporosis, hypercalcemia, and Paget's disease. This 32-amino-acid peptide hormone induces hypocalcemia by inhibiting osteoclast-induced bone resorption. Although it has been used for nearly 30 years, it is less widely used than bisphosphonates and estrogen [5–7]. In addition, the physiological role of calcitonin in calcium homeostasis and bone remodeling as well as its effects on bone cells remains unclear. For example, studies using calcitonin-null mice indicate that it may be involved in protecting the skeleton during periods of "calcium stress", such as growth, pregnancy, and lactation [8]. However, in the basal state, only modest effects on regulating bone remodeling and calcium homeostasis were observed [9]. Furthermore, calcitonin primarily inhibits bone resorption [10,11] without reducing the number of osteoclasts [12]. Although the apoptotic signaling pathways regulated by calcitonin in osteoclasts remain to be fully elucidated, the phosphokinase A (PKA) pathway is likely involved [13]. In addition, calcitonin protects osteoclasts from the effects of a nitric oxide-releasing compound, a highly effective apoptotic stimulus [14]. Downregulation of Cox activity by calcitonin inhibits the function, but not survival of osteoclasts [15]. However, it may also interfere with bone remodeling by inhibiting bone formation [16,17] although not markedly in humans [1]. Combined use of calcitonin and anti-resorptive agents with different modes of action may overcome the side-effects experienced by some patients taking bisphosphonates.

Sintered dicalcium pyrophosphate (SDCP) is a pyrophosphate analog developed by Lin et al. [18]. It was proven biocompatible with bone in an in vivo animal model [18] and in vitro cell culture model [19]. Furthermore, in ovariectomized rats, SDCP increased bone mass [20] by inducing osteoclast apoptosis [21]. Moreover, the effects of SDCP were comparable to those observed for alendronate, a bisphosphonate commonly used clinically [20]. However, further studies are necessary to fully elucidate its mechanism of action.

Because calcitonin may prolong osteoclast survival through inhibition of apoptosis, this study aimed to analyze its influence on osteoclast apoptosis induced by a bisphosphate analog, SDCP. Specifically, the effects of calcitonin and SDCP co-treatment on osteoclast apoptosis and survival were assessed. In addition, the mechanism by which calcitonin influences SDCP-induced apoptosis of osteoclasts was determined. Finally, this study aimed to investigate the potential synergistic effects of calcitonin and SDCP co-treatment in ovariectomized rats by assessing bone volume, trabecular number, thickness, and separation as well as bone formation. Because the present osteoporosis treatments, including bisphosphonates, have side effects, the investigation of such potential alternative treatments is warranted. The examination of the effects of co-treatment with calcitonin and SDCP on osteoclast apoptotic signaling may help elucidate the mechanism by which calcitonin exerts its antiapoptotic effect in osteoclasts.

Results

Effects of Calcitonin and SDCP on Osteoclast Apoptosis

As shown in Fig. 1, osteoclast apoptosis was assessed using the TUNEL assay. Confocal analysis of osteoclasts cultured in control medium for 48 h revealed approximately 5% of TUNEL stain-positive cells (Fig. 1A and B). SDCP induced a time-dependent increase in TUNEL stain-positive cells, which became apparent after 12 hours and reached a maximum level at 48 hours of treatment. Both DNase and SDCP treatment increased TUNEL stain-positive cells to 100.0±0% and 72.8±11.6%, respectively (Fig. 1B). As compared to control and SCDP-treated cells, addition of calcitonin significantly decreased the number of TUNEL-positive osteoclasts (2.0±0.9 vs. 5.2±2.3% and 27.0±11.1 vs. 72.8±11.6%, respectively; Fig. 1B).

Apoptosis was also assessed using annexin-V staining (Fig. 2). In osteoclasts cultured for 18 h, treatment with TGF-β1, the positive control, and SDCP increased annexin-V-positive cells by

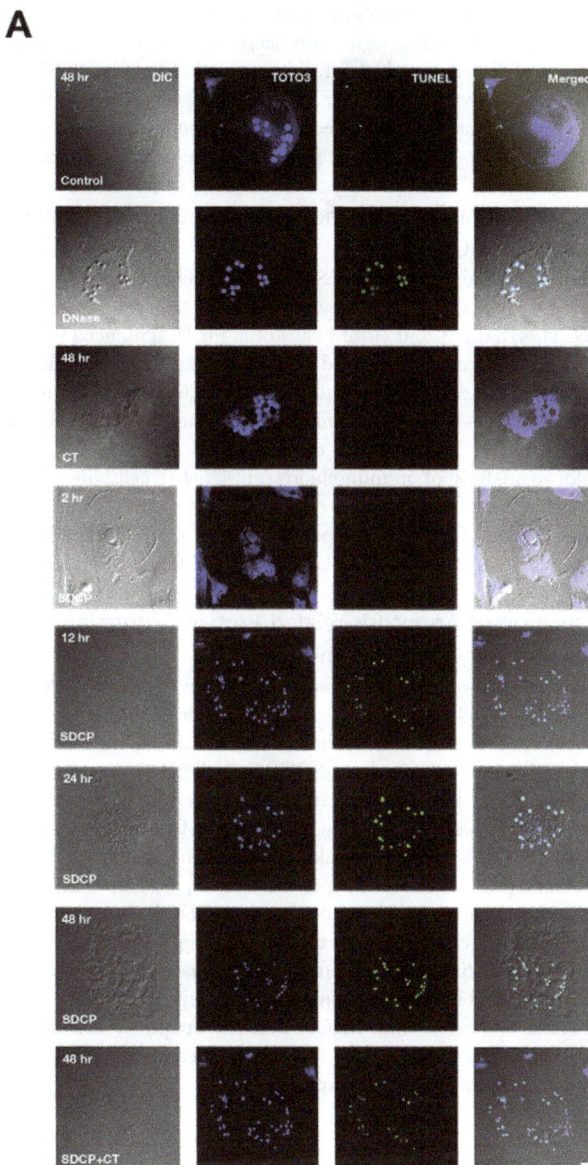

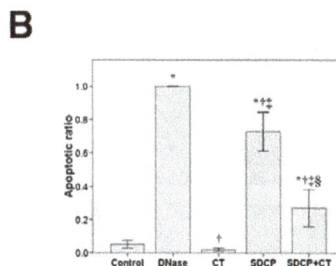

Figure 1. Detection of osteoclast apoptosis using TUNEL analysis. (A) Osteoclasts were treated with CT (10 nM), SDCP (10 µM), or both for the times indicated. Osteoclasts treated with DNase I (3 U/mL) were included as positive controls. Green nuclear labeling indicates apoptotic cells. Nuclei were counterstained using TOTO-3 (blue). Difference interference contrast (DIC) images show morphology of the cells. Bar = 20 µm. (B) Quantitative results of the experiment shown in panel A. $P<0.05$ compared to *control group, †DNase group, ‡CT group, and §SDCP group after Bonferroni adjustment, mean ± SD, n = 6 in each group.

24.9±4.6% and 14.6±4.0%, respectively. Upon cotreatment with calcitonin and SDCP, a significant decrease in annexin-V-positive cells was observed as compared with those cells treated with SDCP alone (6.7±0.6 vs. 14.6±0.4%; Fig. 2A and B). Because these data demonstrate that SDCP induced osteoclast apoptosis, the TGF-β1 treatment group was eliminated from subsequent experiments.

Calcitonin Inhibits SDCP-induced Expression of Cleaved Caspase 3 in Osteoclasts

To determine the effects of SDCP and calcitonin on caspase-3 cleavage, Western blot analysis was employed (Fig. 3). Exposure of osteoclasts to 0.1, 1 and 10 nM calcitonin for 18 h induced a dose-dependent decrease of cleaved caspase-3 (Fig. 3A). In addition, exposure of osteoclasts to 10 μM SDCP induced an increase in cleaved caspase-3, which was inhibited with the addition of 10 nM calcitonin (Fig. 3A). Cleaved caspase-3 was also assessed using confocal analysis of immunofluorescent-labeled cells; decreased cleaved caspase-3 labeling was observed in osteoclasts treated with calcitonin and SDCP as compared to those treated with SDCP alone (13.4±1.5 vs. 32.9±3.2%; Fig. 3B and C).

Regulation of Apoptosis-related Protein Expression and Activation by Calcitonin and SDCP

The effects of calcitonin and SDCP on Bcl-2 and Mcl-1 expression as well as caspase cleavage were assessed using Western blot analysis (Fig. 4). Calcitonin alone and with SDCP increased Bcl-2 expression in osteoclasts; SDCP only slightly increased Bcl-2 expression (Fig. 4A). However, SDCP decreased Mcl-1 expression, which was partially reversed by the addition of calcitonin with the SDCP (Fig. 4A); calcitonin alone only slightly reduced Mcl-1 expression (Fig. 4A). FasL, the positive control, increased caspase-8 cleavage whereas both calcitonin and SDCP induced little activation of caspase-8 in osteoclasts (Fig. 4B). Calcitonin decreased and SDCP increased caspase-9 cleavage in osteoclasts, which was inhibited by calcitonin co-treatment (Fig. 4B). Because this data indicates that SDCP induces apoptosis through a pathway distinct from FasL, the FasL treatment group was eliminated from subsequent experiments.

Calcitonin Inhibits Osteoclast Apoptosis through Bcl-2 and Erk Signaling Pathway

As shown in Fig. 5, the effects of calcitonin and SDCP treatment on apoptosis-related signaling pathways were determined by Western blot analysis. Pretreatment of osteoclasts with HA14-1, a Bcl-2 inhibitor, blocked the reduction in cleaved caspase-3 and -9 induced by calcitonin treatment (Fig. 5A). In addition, pretreatment of osteoclasts with PD98059, an Erk1/2 inhibitor, blocked the calcitonin-induced increase of Bcl-2 and SDCP-induced decrease of Mcl-1 (Fig. 5B). The SDCP-induced increase of cleaved caspase-9 was also blocked by PD98059 pre-treatment, but the calcitonin-induced decrease was not. Finally, the decreased cleaved caspase-9 by cotreatment with calcitonin and SDCP as well as the calcitonin-induced decrease of cleaved caspase-3 were sensitive to PD98059 pretreatment (Fig. 5B).

Calcitonin Reduces the Inhibitory Effect of SDCP on Osteoclast Survival but not Activity

The effects of calcitonin and SDCP cotreatment on osteoclast number, size and bone resorption were determined (Fig. 6). In osteoclasts treated with calcitonin, TRAP staining revealed a significant decrease in cell number and size as compared to those cells in control medium, which was further decreased with SDCP treatment alone. However, combined treatment of calcitonin and SDCP alleviated the SDCP-induced decrease in osteoclast number and size (Fig. 6A). A similar inhibitory effect on pit number and area was observed on dentine discs in the calcitonin and SDCP alone groups. Combined treatment of calcitonin and SDCP induced a further decrease in pit number (Fig. 6B).

Calcitonin Increases the Therapeutic Efficacy of SDCP in an in vivo Osteoporosis Model

The influence of calcitonin-SDCP cotreatment on bone deposition was determined in an in vivo model of osteoporosis (Fig. 7). Ovariectomy or sham operation was performed in 3-month-old female Sprague Dawley rats. After four weeks, ovariectomized rats received normal saline, calcitonin, SDCP, or calcitonin plus SDCP treatment for four additional weeks after which micro-computed tomography analysis of the fifth lumbar vertebrae and histomorphometric analysis of the tibia were

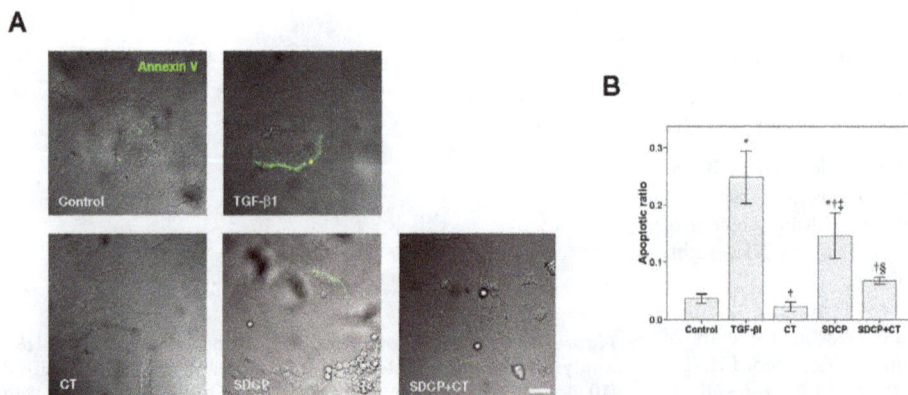

Figure 2. Detection of apoptosis by annexin V labeling in osteoclasts. (A) Osteoclasts were treated with CT (10 nM), SDCP (10 μM), or both for 18 h. Osteoclasts treated with TGF-βI (10 ng/mL) were included as positive controls. Green cellular membrane labeling indicates apoptotic cells. Only cells without propidium iodide (red) labeling were considered to be apoptotic. DIC images and nucleus stain were performed as described in Fig. 1. Bar = 10 μm. (B) Quantitative results of the experiment shown in panel A. The measurement of apoptosis was calculated as the percentage of positive annexin V labeling cells in a total of at least 500 osteoclasts. P<0.05 compared to *control group, †TGF-β1 group, ‡CT group; and §SDCP group after Bonferroni adjustment, mean ± SD, n = 6 in each group.

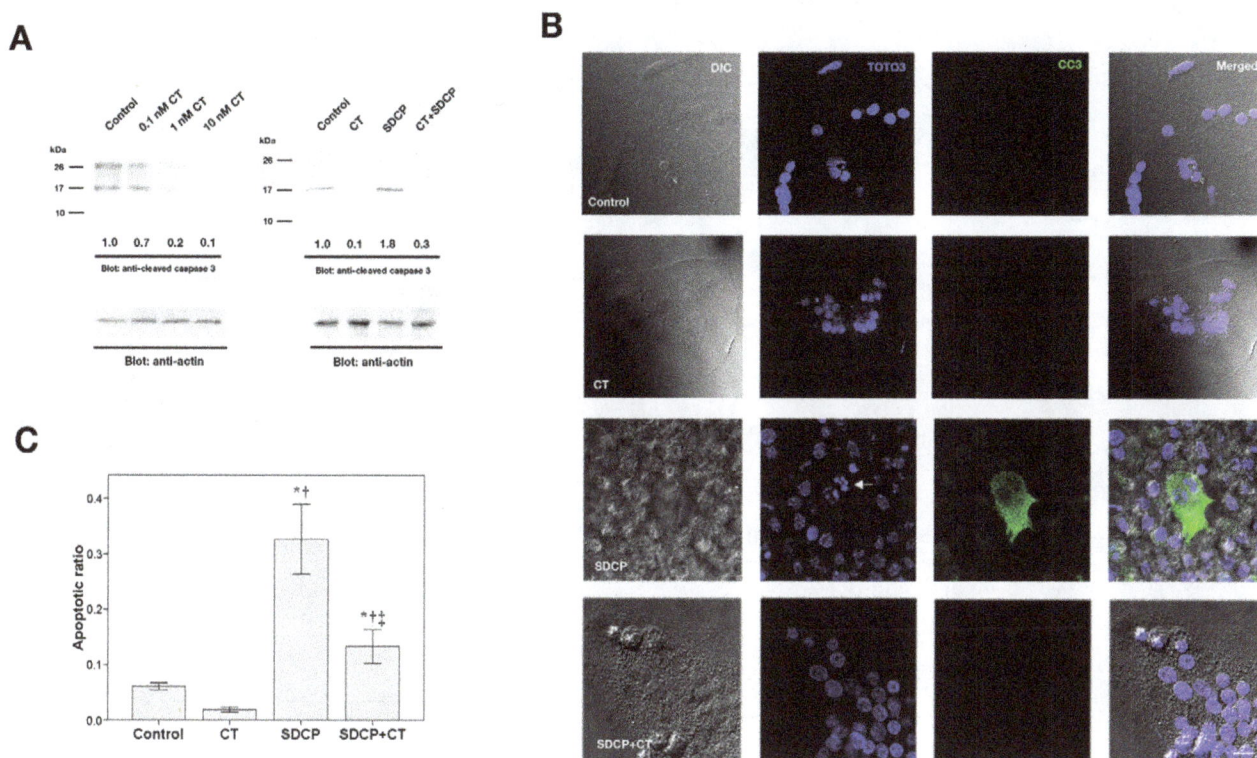

Figure 3. Calcitonin inhibits SDCP-induced expression of cleaved caspase 3 in osteoclasts. (A) Western blot analysis of cleaved caspase 3 expression in osteoclasts treated with CT (10 nM), SDCP (10 µM), or both. Protein levels were quantified by densitometry, corrected for the sample load based on actin expression, and expressed as fold-increase or decrease relative to the control lane. Each blot is representative of at least three replicate experiments. (B) Confocal analysis of immunofluorescent labeling of cleaved caspase 3 in calcitonin- or SDCP-treated osteoclast. Green intracellular cleaved caspase 3 labeling and blue TOTO3-labeled nuclear chromatin condensation (white arrow) indicate cells that underwent apoptosis. Bar = 10 µm. (C) Quantitative results of the experiment shown in panel B. The measurement of apoptosis was calculated as a percentage of positive cleaved caspase-3–labelled cells in a total of at least 500 osteoclasts. $P < 0.05$ compared to *control group, † CT group, and ‡SDCP group after Bonferroni adjustment, mean $\pm$ SD, $n = 6$ in each group.

undertaken on the five-month-old rats. Although the 2D images also included cortical bone, regions of interest containing trabecular bone were selected for subsequent quantification. Significant increases in bone loss were observed in ovariectomized rats as compared to those of the sham controls (Fig. 7A and B). As compared to untreated ovariectomized rats, calcitonin treatment significantly increased percent bone volume and trabecular number. Compared to calcitonin treatment, SDCP induced further but not significant changes in these bone parameters; however, cotreatment with calcitonin and SDCP significantly increased percent bone volume and trabecular number in ovariectomized rats (Fig. 7A and 7B). No additional benefits in trabecular separation and thickness were observed upon cotreatment with calcitonin and SDCP. As shown in Figure 7C, a significant increase in bone formation was observed in ovariectomized rats, which was further increased upon calcitonin treatment. SDCP treatment in ovariectomized rats decreased bone formation, which was reversed by cotreatment with calcitonin (Fig. 7C).

Analysis of bone resorption and formation markers was next carried out after various treatments with calcitonin and SDCP (Fig. 7D). Analysis of a serum bone resorption marker, CTX-I, revealed increased bone resorption in ovariectomized rats as compared to those receiving the sham operation (Fig. 7D). Significant decreases in CTX-I were found in the calcitonin treatment group as compared to the untreated group. In both SDCP treatment and cotreatment groups, a further reduction in CTX-I was observed. Increases in the serum bone formation

marker, P1NP, were observed in ovariectomized rats as compared to those receiving the sham operation (Fig. 7D). Further increases in P1NP levels were observed in ovariectomized rats receiving calcitonin. Although decreased P1NP levels were observed in the SDCP treatment group as compared to the calcitonin and vehicle groups, a significant increase was found in ovariectomized rats receiving the combination treatment of calcitonin and SDCP.

Discussion

[LOSSEST]Because calcitonin may prolong osteoclast survival through inhibition of apoptosis, this study aimed to analyze its influence on osteoclast apoptosis induced by a bisphosphate analog, SDCP. Cotreatment of calcitonin and SDCP was chosen because the in vivo therapeutic effects of SDCP were comparable to those observed for alendronate, a conventional bisphosphonate [20]. In addition, the efficacy of cotreatment with these agents was explored in ovariectomized rats. In primary osteoclast cultures, calcitonin inhibited SDCP-induced apoptosis, resulting in increased osteoclast number and size. However, the SDCP-induced reduction in bone resorption was not affected by calcitonin. Furthermore, an additive effect of calcitonin and SDCP on increased bone formation, increasing bone volume, was observed in ovariectomized rats.

In contrast to most other antiresorptive agents, calcitonin treatment inhibits the function but not the survival of osteoclasts

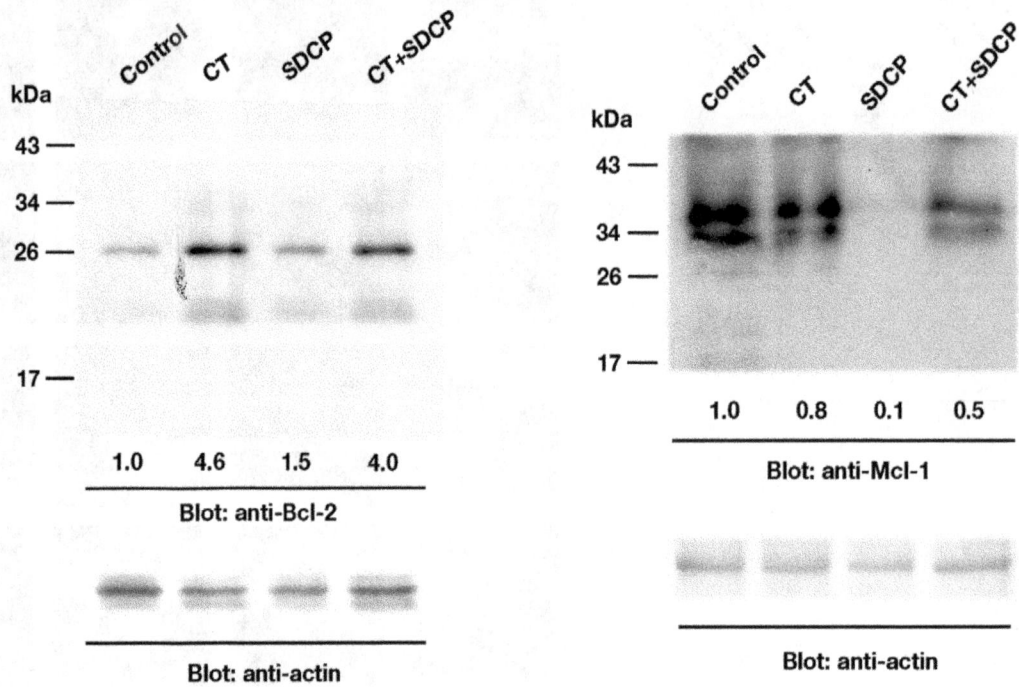

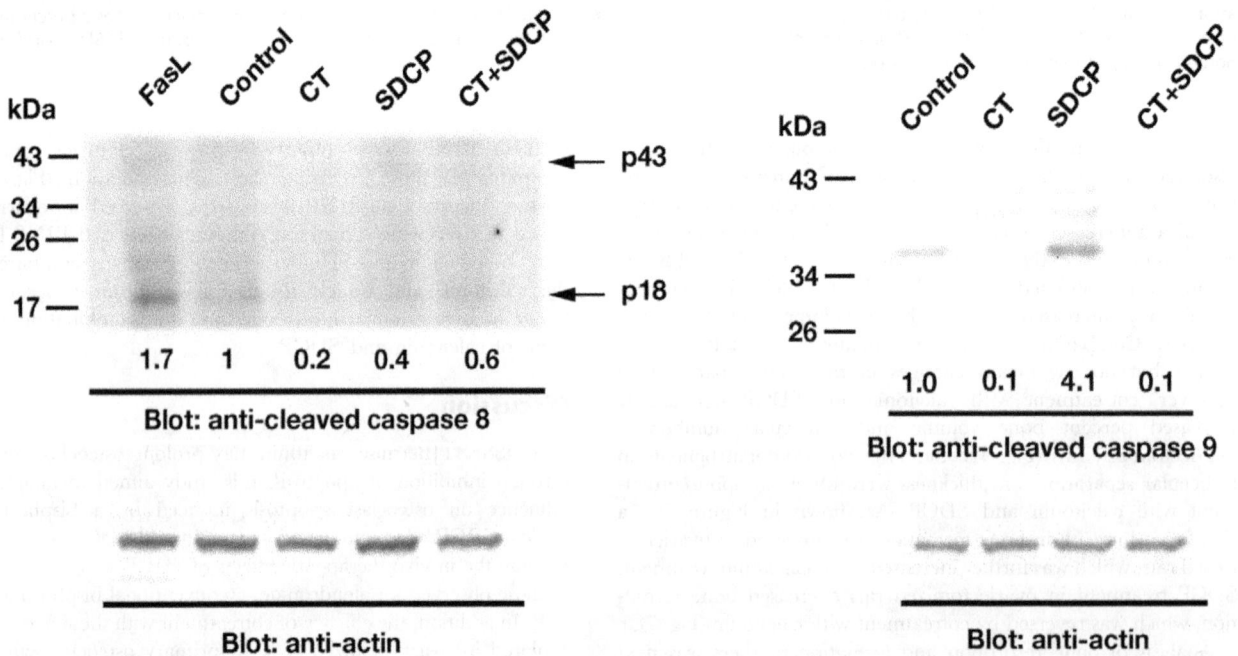

Figure 4. Regulation of apoptotic signaling by calcitonin and SDCP. (A) Western blot analysis of Bcl-2 and Mcl-1 expression in osteoclasts treated with CT (10 nM), SDCP (10 μM), or both. (B) Caspase 8 and 9 activation in response to CT (10 nM) or SDCP (10 μM) stimulation. Western blot analysis revealed the presence of two fragments (p43 and p18), corresponding to the cleaved caspase 8 under the treatment of FasL (10 ng/mL). Western blot analysis of cleaved caspase 9 was shown in the right panel. Protein levels were quantified by densitometry, corrected for the sample load based on actin expression, and expressed as fold-increase or decrease relative to the control lane. Each blot is representative of at least three replicate experiments.

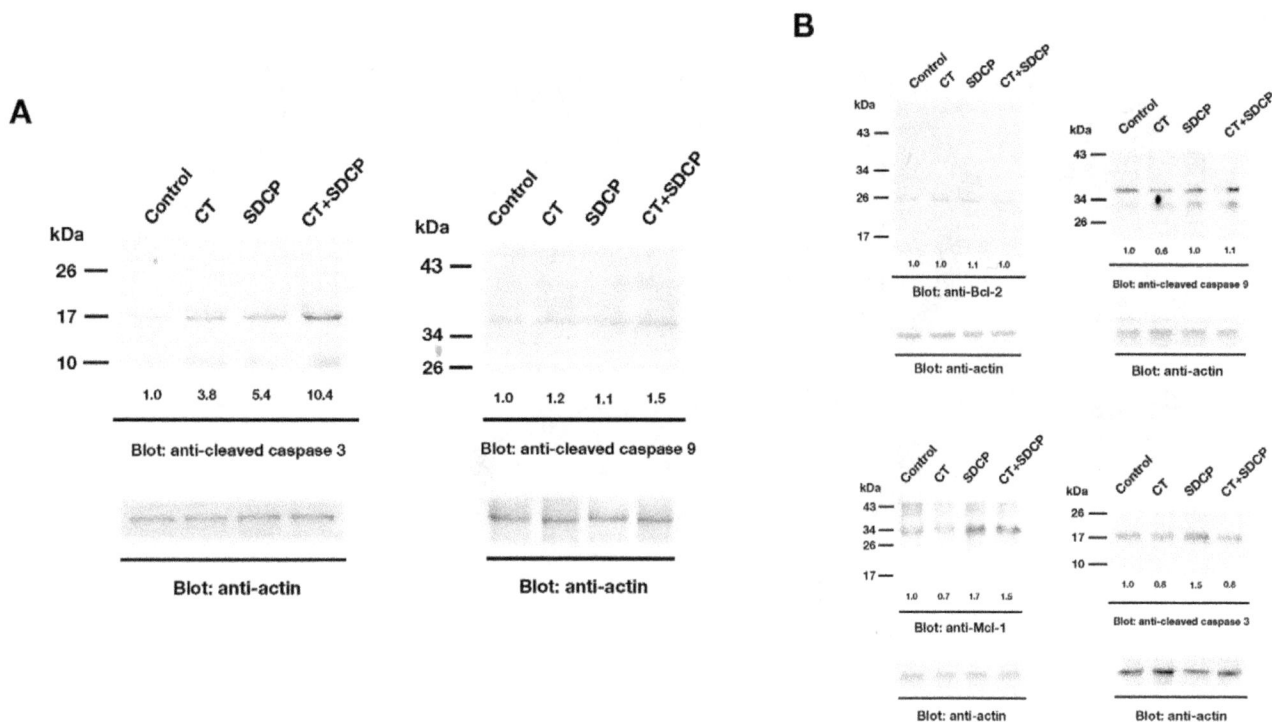

Figure 5. Calcitonin inhibits osteoclast apoptosis through Bcl-2 and Erk signaling. (A) Western blot analysis of expression of caspase 3 and 9. Osteoclasts were first treated with HA14-1 (50 μM) for 2 h and then CT (10 nM), SDCP (10 μM), or both were added to the culture medium. (B) Examination of apoptotic signaling regulated by calcitonin and SDCP in the presence of an Erk inhibitor. Osteoclasts were first treated with PD98059 (5 μM) for 2 h and then CT (10 nM), SDCP (10 μM), or both were added to the culture medium. Protein levels were quantified by densitometry, corrected for the sample load based on actin expression, and expressed as fold-increase or decrease relative to the control lane. Each blot is representative of at least three replicate experiments.

[22]. Indeed, calcitonin may play an important role in osteoclast survival by preventing apoptosis [10,13–15]. To decrease bone resorption by osteoclasts, calcitonin induces cytoskeletal changes [23], causing cell detachment [11], decreasing mobility [24], and interaction with integrin-related signaling [10]. As in osteoclasts cultured on glass or bone [13], the present study showed that calcitonin promoted osteoclast survival in cells treated with SDCP by reducing apoptosis as observed by reduced chromatin condensation and DNA degradation, annexin-V staining, and caspase-3 cleavage. However, little activation of caspase 8 was observed in osteoclasts treat with calcitonin or SDCP, indicating that calcitonin and SDCP may not function through the extrinsic apoptotic pathway. This notion is corroborated by the effect of these agents on Bcl-2 family proteins. Specifically, calcitonin alone and combined with SDCP increased Bcl-2 expression in osteoclasts. In addition, SDCP reduced Mcl-1 expression, which was partially reversed with calcitonin cotreatment. These results indicate that calcitonin inhibits osteoclast apoptosis at least in part by increasing Bcl-2 expression, whereas SDCP treatment induces apoptosis by decreasing Mcl-1 expression. Consistent with these results, Sutherland et al. [25] reported that alendronate induced osteoclast apoptosis by decreasing Mcl-1 levels, which is prevented by co-treatment with RANKL. Further studies will be undertaken to elucidate the mechanism by which SDCP reduces Mcl-1 expression.

The antiapoptotic proteins Mcl-1, Bcl-2, and Bcl-xL differentially inhibit activator BH3-only proteins Bim, Bid, and Puma, which can directly activate Bak and Bax [26]. In the present study, the BH3-mimetic molecule, HA14-1, blocked the calcitonin-mediated reduction in caspase-3 and -9 activation. Thus,

upregulation of Bcl-2 by calcitonin is likely the mechanism by which calcitonin prevents SDCP-induced osteoclast apoptosis.

Calcitonin receptor couples to multiple G proteins and activates multiple signaling pathways [27]. In osteoclasts, calcitonin activates Erk1/2 [15], mediating osteoclast survival [28]. Erk promotes cell survival by direct phosphorylation and inhibition of caspase-9 during development and tissue homeostasis [29]. In the present study, calcitonin-induced Bcl-2 expression, and inhibition of caspase-3 and -9 activation were sensitive to the Erk1/2 inhibitor, PD98059, confirming that Erk1/2 is involved in the antiapoptotic signaling induced by calcitonin in osteoclasts.

To achieve more powerful therapeutic effects, a combination of multiple anti-resorption agents might be needed for osteoporosis patients. Ogawa et al. [30] showed an additive effect on trabecular architecture and bone strength in ovariectomized rats after cotreatment with calcitonin and alendronate. In addition, a combined therapy of calcitonin and alendronate in patients with rheumatoid arthritis for 12 months had additive effects, significantly increasing lumbar and hip bone mineral density [31]. However, Iwamoto et al. [32] reported no significant changes in lumbar bone mineral density in postmenopausal osteoporotic women treated with alendronate and calcitonin compared to those receiving alendronate alone. This may be due to the short treatment period (6 months) [32]. In the present study, both calcitonin and SDCP increased the percent bone volume and trabecular number and thickness, and decreased trabecular separation in ovariectomized rats although not all these parameters reached significance. Calcitonin-SDCP cotreatment further increased percent bone volume, illustrating an additive effect by the combined treatment for osteoporosis. Further studies are

A

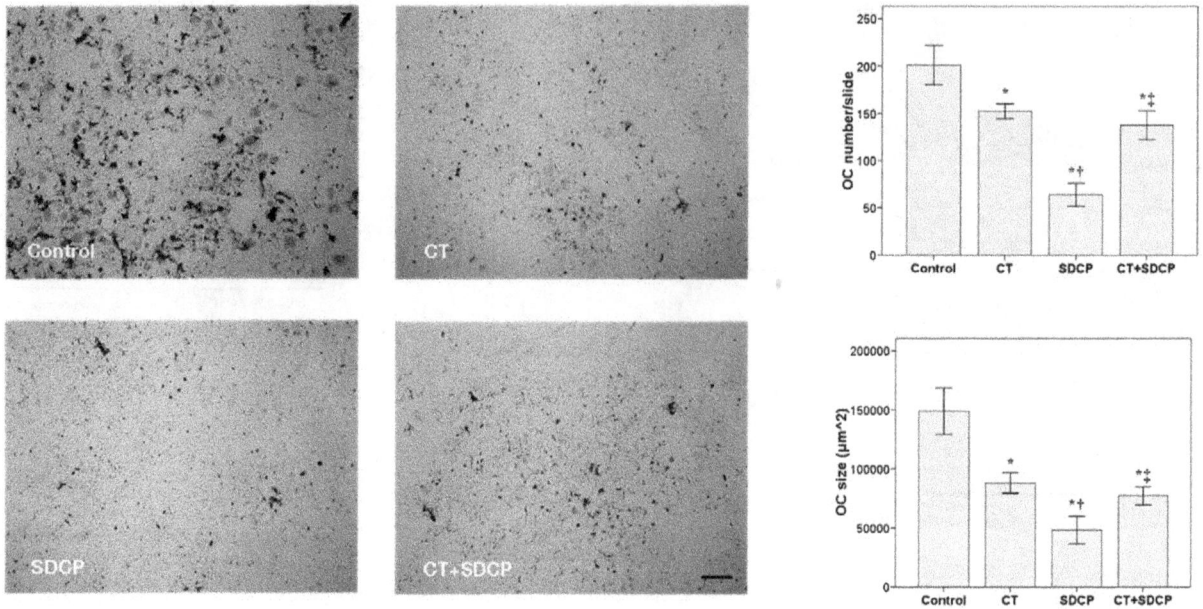

B

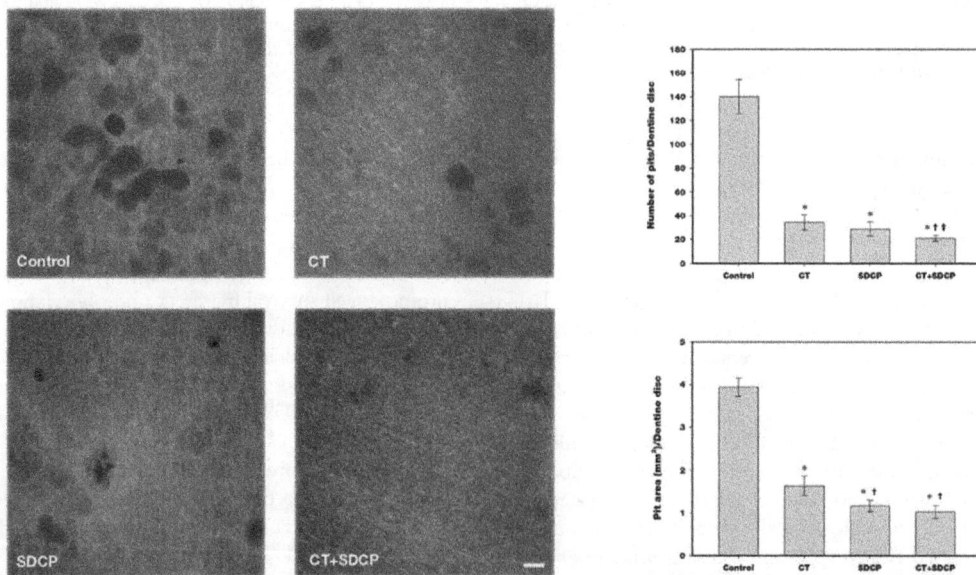

Figure 6. Calcitonin reduces inhibitory effect of SDCP on osteoclast survival but not activity. (A) TRAP stain of osteoclasts treated with CT (10 nM), SDCP (10 µM), or both. Red intracellular stain with multiple nuclei indicates positive labeling. Quantitative results of cell number and size were shown in right panel. Bar = 500 µm. (B) Pit formation assay. Osteoclasts were cultured on dentine discs and treated with CT (10 nM), SDCP (10 µM), or both. Quantitative results of the number and area of resorption pits were shown in right panel. Bar = 50 mm. $P<0.05$ compared to *control group, † CT group, and ‡SDCP group after Bonferroni adjustment, mean ± SD, n = 6 in each group.

necessary to determine whether combined therapy of pyrophosphate analog and calcitonin may represent a new strategy for osteoporosis treatment.

A balance between osteoblast and osteoclast activity is required for normal bone formation and maintenance. A coupling mechanism has been described in which resorption products and osteoclast-derived factors stimulate bone formation by osteoblast lineage cells [33]. Similarly, osteoblast lineage cells regulate osteoclast formation and activity [33]. Therefore, because of the coupled nature of remodeling, most of the anti-resorptive agents available also reduce bone formation directly or indirectly, limiting their effect on bone mass. Drugs that uncouple bone resorption from bone formation (e.g. inhibitors of chloride channels, cathepsin K, vacuolar H+ATPase and Src) may have a greater

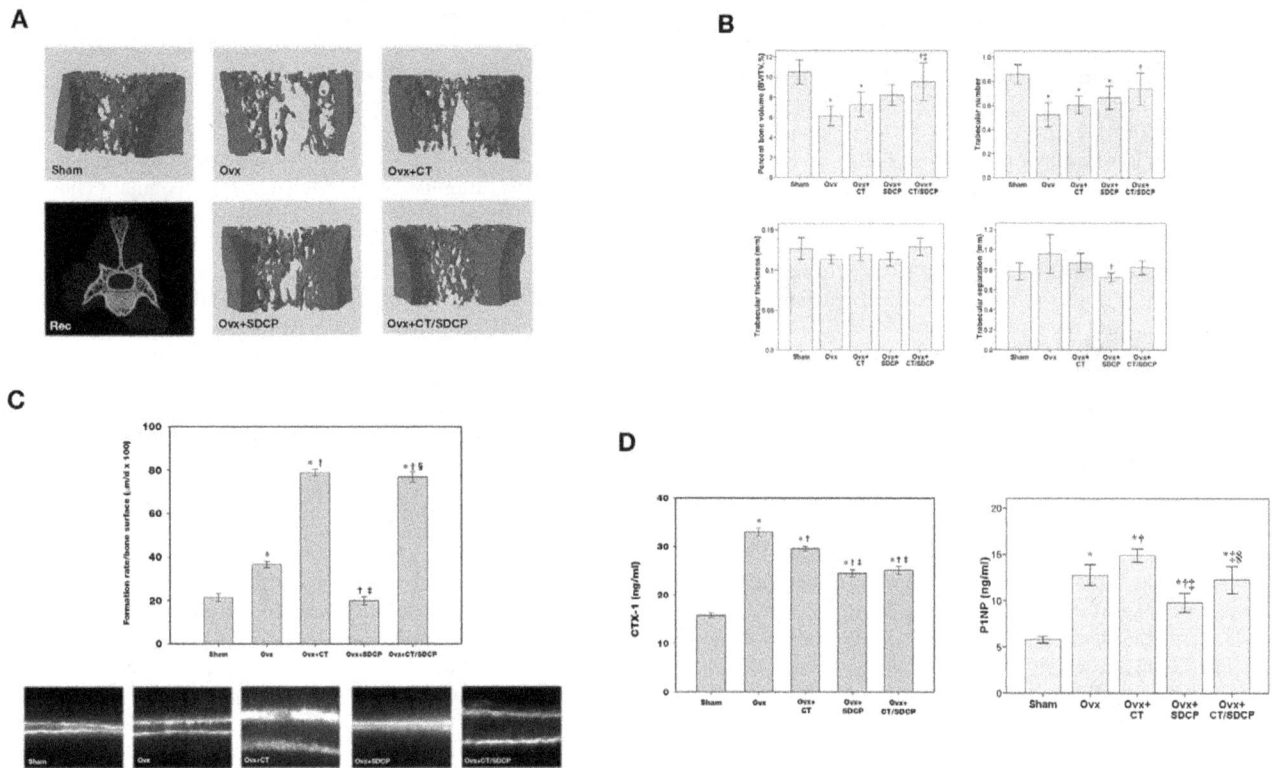

Figure 7. Calcitonin increases therapeutic efficacy of SDCP to treat osteoporotic rats. (A) Micro-computed tomography analysis of 5th lumbar vertebrate in ovariectomized (OVX) rats treated with CT (5 IU/kg/day), SDCP (1 mg/kg/day), or both. Figures are representative 3D reconstruction images from each treatment groups except lower left panel which is 2D reconstruction image shows the contouring method used to delineate the trabecular bone region. (B) Quantitative results of the experiment shown in panel A. (C) Calcein double-labeling in OVX rats. Representative fluorescent micrographs show that the distance between the two labeled mineralization fronts. The quantification of the bone formation rate per bone surface is shown in the right panel. (D) Serum bone resorption marker (CTX-1) and bone formation marker (P1NP) were determined by ELISA. P<0.05 compared to *sham group, †Ovx group, ‡Ovx+CT group, and §Ovx+SDCP group after Bonferroni adjustment, mean ± SD, n = 6 in each group.

effect in terms of increasing bone mass. In the present study, combined therapy of calcitonin and SDCP had less of an effect on inhibiting bone resorption and induced more bone formation as compared to SDCP treatment alone as observed by pit formation assay, CTX-1 and P1NP expression, and calcein double labeling. Consistent with these results, calcitonin increased bone formation in ovariectomized rats [34,35] and anabolic effect was observed in glucocorticoid-induced osteopenia [36]. Though results from calcitonin and calcitonin receptor-null mice suggest that it is a physiologic inhibitor of bone formation, the mechanism of how calcitonin regulates bone formation remains unknown [37]. The results from the present study suggest that calcitonin-induced inhibition of osteoclast apoptosis may be an important factor in this process.

There are some study limitations that warrant further discussion. For example, this study analyzes the effect of combination therapy using the bisphosphonate analog, SDCP, without comparing them with a conventional bisphosphonate, such as alendronate. In addition, the effects of SDCP alone or with calcitonin on osteoblasts were not assessed in the present study. However, Sun et al. [38] reported that SDCP inhibited osteoblast proliferation, which was mediated by the promotion of osteoblast differentiation and the increased synthesis of prostaglandin E2. Also, the effect of calcitonin and SDCP on apoptosis was only addressed in vitro without further studies seeding the osteoclasts on bone. Because this study will permit a correlation of anti-resorptive

effects versus apoptosis, it will be carried out in future studies. Furthermore, 3-month old rats were used for the in vivo study. Because their skeletons are immature, the effect of bone growth cannot be separated from the effect of calcitonin or SDCP treatment to the rat skeleton. However, by the end of the study, the rats were five months of age. In conclusion, this study confirmed that calcitonin inhibits osteoclast apoptosis; it inhibited SDCP-induced apoptosis in primary osteoclast cultures. In addition, calcitonin-SDCP combination therapy inhibited bone resorption to a lesser extent and induced more bone formation as compared to SDCP alone. The benefits of combination therapy for osteoporosis warrant further investigation as a possible treatment for postmenopausal osteoporosis.

Materials and Methods

Reagents

Salmon calcitonin was purchased from Sigma-Aldrich (St. Louis, MO, USA). SDCP was purchased from Purzer Pharmaceutical Co., Taipei, Taiwan. TGF-βI was obtained from Peprotech (Rockey Hill, NJ, USA). HA14-1, a Bcl-2 inhibitor, was purchased from Enzo Life Science (Plymouth Meeting, PA, USA). PD98059, a MEK1 inhibitor, was purchased from Cell Signaling Technology (Danvers, MA, USA). Fas ligand (FasL) was purchased from R&D System (Minneapolis, MN, USA).

Isolation and Treatment of Rabbit Osteoclasts

New Zealand white rabbits approximately 7-day-old (90–120 g) were used as the source of bone cells for purification of osteoclasts as previously described [11]. For subsequent imaging analyses, unpurified cultures were employed; however, purified cultures (>90% purity) were used for the molecular analysis. Purification of the cultures was performed using 0.02% EDTA and 0.001% pronase E for 5 min at 37°C. The experiment was performed with the approval of the Laboratory Animal Center of the National Defense Medical Center in Taipei, Taiwan. Purified osteoclasts were cultured in alpha-minimum essential medium (α-MEM, Sigma-Aldrich), pH 6.9, supplemented with 26 mM sodium bicarbonate, 10 mM HEPES, 1% penicillin/streptomycin, and 5% fetal bovine serum (FBS, HyClone, Logan, Utah, USA). Unless otherwise indicated, osteoclasts were treated with CT (10 nM), SDCP (10 μM), or both for 18 h for short-term changes including analysis of signaling molecules to 48 h for TUNEL and TRAP analysis.

Confocal Microscopic Analysis of Osteoclast Apoptosis

1.5×10^4 osteoclasts were cultured on 22×22 mm glass cover-slips for 18 h after which they were treated with CT (10 nM), SDCP (10 μM) or both for 48 h. After the cells were washed with phosphate buffered saline (PBS), they were fixed in 4% parafor-maldehyde for 10 min and permeabilized with 0.1% Triton X-100 in PBS for 5 min. The cells were subsequently incubated in 1% bovine serum albumin (BSA) in PBS for 1 h. Apoptosis was determined using an In Situ Cell Death Kit (Roche Applied Science, Mannheim, Germany) based on the TdT-mediated fluorescein dUTP nick-end labeling (TUNEL) method, according to the recommendations of the manufacturer. Negative controls included omission of TdT, and positive controls included DNase I treatments. Nuclei were counterstained using TOTO-3 diluted 1:5000 (Molecular Probes, Inc., Eugene, OR, USA). For each treatment, at least 500 osteoclasts in three glass coverslips were counted. Measurement of apoptosis was calculated as a percentage of apoptotic nuclei versus total nuclei [39].

Apoptosis of cells was also determined by analysis of Annexin V as well as cleaved caspase staining. 1.5×10^4 osteoclasts were cultured on 22×22 mm glass coverslips for 18 h after which they were treated with CT (10 nM), SDCP (10 μM) or both for 18 h. For Annexin V staining, an Annexin V-FITC Apoptosis Detection kit (BioVision, Mountain View, CA, USA) was used, according to the recommendation of the manufacturer. Propidium iodide (50 μg/ml) was added to the binding buffer to detect necrosis. For analysis of cleaved caspase-3, cells were incubated with anticleaved caspase-3 polyclonal antibody (Cell Signaling Technology) in 1% BSA PBS at 4°C for 16 h, and then with Cy-3-conjugated anti-rabbit IgG antibody (Jackson Immunoresearch Laboratories, West Grove, PA, USA) in PBS for 1 h. Microscopy was performed using a confocal microscope equipped with difference interference contrast light path (LSM 510, Zeiss, Göttingen, Germany). Annexin V- and active caspase-3–positive osteoclasts were counted manually as stated above, and the apoptosis rate was statistically analyzed. Multi-nucleated cells were considered osteoclasts if they had more than three nuclei.

Tartrate-resistant Acid Phosphatase (TRAP) Staining

1.5×10^4 osteoclasts were cultured on 22×22 mm glass coverslips for 18 h after which they were treated with CT (10 nM), SDCP (10 μM) or both for 72 h. They were then stained for TRAP using a kit that uses 50 mM tartrate and following the manufacturer's instructions (Sigma-Aldrich). For each treatment, at least 500 osteoclasts in three glass coverslips were counted.

Osteoclasts were defined as cells with more than three nuclei. The number of TRAP$^+$ cells per coverslip was determined by light microscope (Axio Imager A2, Zeiss).

Pit Formation Assay

In the Pit formation assay, 1×10^3 osteoclasts were cultured on dentine discs (Immunodiagnostic Systems Inc, Fountain Hills, AR) in a 96-well plate for 18 h after which they were treated with CT (10 nM), SDCP (10 μM), or both for 72 h. For most groups, there were 4 dentine discs per group. To measure the areas containing resorption lacunae, cells were removed, and the dentine discs were incubated in 0.25 M ammonium hydroxide, washed with distilled water, and then stained with 0.5% (wt/vol) toluidine blue. The images of the resorbed areas were measured using a reflective optical microscope (LSM 510, Zeiss), and the results were expressed as the number of resorption pits and total area resorbed per dentine disc.

Western Blot Analysis

Purified osteoclasts ($1.5 \pm 0.5 \times 10^5$/10 cm dish) were cultured in α-MEM for 18 h after which they were treated with CT (10 nM), SDCP (10 μM), or both for 18 h. They were then washed twice with PBS, and lysed with cold lysis buffer (150 mM NaCl, 50 mM Tris, pH 7.5, 0.25% sodium deoxycholate, 0.1% Nonidet P-40, 1 mM sodium orthovanadate, 1 mM sodium fluoride, 1 mM phenylmethylsulfonyl fluoride, 10 μg/mL aprotinin, and 10 μg/mL leupeptin). The cell lysate was obtained by centrifugation at $16,000 \times g$ at 4°C for 30 min. The protein concentration was measured with a Bicinconinic acid kit (Pierce, Rockford, IL, USA), and 30 μg of total protein was separated on a 12% SDS-polyacrylamide gel. After the proteins were transferred to nitrocellulose membranes (Whatman, Dassel, Germany), the membranes were blocked with 5% skim milk in TBS-T (20 mM Tris, pH 7.6, 137 mM NaCl, and 0.1% Tween-20) and incubated with antibodies specific for cleaved caspase-3, 8, and 9 (Cell Signaling Technology) or anti-Bcl-2 and anti-Mcl-1(Santa Cruz, CA, USA). Proteins were visualized using the appropriate secondary antibody conjugated to horseradish peroxidase (HRP; Santa Cruz), followed by the application of ECL reagents (Amersham, Buckinghamshire, UK). The bands were quantified by densitometry (ProXPRESS Proteomic Imaging System, Perkin Elmer, Melbourne, VIC, Australia), and normalized to the loading control, actin. The influence of various treatments was expressed as fold-increase or decrease relative to the control lane. Each analysis was carried out in at least three independent experiments.

In vivo Osteoporosis Model

Fifty 3-month-old female Sprague–Dawley rats were purchased from the Laboratory Animal Center, National Defense Medical Center (Taipei, Taiwan) and acclimated under standard laboratory conditions at 22 ± 2°C and 50 ± 10% humidity. Food and water were available ad libitum during the acclimatization period. A sham-operation (n = 10) or ovariectomy (OVX, n = 40) was performed. Four weeks after the surgery, OVX rats were divided into four groups: vehicle, calcitonin (50 IU/ml, subcutaneous injection of 5 IU/kg/day), SDCP (2.5 mg/ml, oral administration of 1 mg/kg/day), and calcitonin+SDCP (n = 10 for each group). Rats were treated five times per week for four weeks. The sham and OVX vehicle groups received the vehicle, an isotonic sodium chloride solution, orally. SDCP was administered orally by catheter at 1.0 mg/kg/day five times per week as previously described [20]. Salmon calcitonin (Miacalcic by Novartis-Pharma) was administered by subcutaneously injection at 5 IU/kg/day five times per week. The vehicle and drug were given on the same days, and the treatment period lasted 4 weeks. The animal study was carried out in accordance with ethical guidelines for animal care, and the experimental protocols were approved by the animal care committee of National Defense Medical Center.

Whole blood samples were obtained with plastic syringes via intracardiac puncture immediately following sacrifice at five months of age (8 weeks after surgery). The blood samples were allowed to clot at room temperature after which the serum was separated by centrifugation, divided into 500-μL aliquots, and stored at −80°C until further analysis. The lumbar vertebrae were also removed and stored at −80°C for subsequent assessment of trabecular microstructure.

Micro-computed Tomography

Microarchitecture of the fifth lumbar trabecular bone was investigated using a microcomputed tomography (Skyscan 1174; Skyscan, Aartselaar, Belgium) as previously described [40]. The X-ray source was set at 50 kV, with a pixel size at 11 μm. Four hundred projections were acquired over an angular range of 180° (angular step of 0.45°). The image slices were reconstructed using the cone-beam reconstruction software version 2.6 based on the Feldkamp algorithm (Skyscan). The registered data sets were segmented into binary images. Simple global thresholding methods were used due to the low noise and relatively good resolution of the data sets. The trabecular bone was extracted by drawing ellipsoid contours with the CT analyzer software (Skyscan). Trabecular bone volume (BV/TV; percentage), trabecular number, and trabecular separation were calculated by the mean intercept length method. Trabecular thickness was calculated according to the method of Hildebrand and Ruegsegger [41].

Histomorphometric Analysis

Eight weeks after ovariectomy, the rats received an intraperitoneal injection of calcein (30 mg/kg) and another injection 8 days later. Two days later they were sacrificed [42]. The proximal tibia were dehydrated in graded ethanol, defatted in acetone, and embedded undecalcified in London resin (London Resin Co., London, United Kingdom) after staining with Villanueva bone stain (Polyscience Ltd, Warrington, PA, USA). Frontal sections of the tibiae (7 μm thick) were prepared. Measurements were performed on the entire marrow region within the cortical shell of the proximal tibia metaphysis from 1–4 mm distal to the growth plate-metaphyseal junction using an Image Analysis System (Osteomeasure, Inc., Atlanta, GA, USA). Bone area, perimeter, single- and double-labeling surface were measured, and trabecular number, thickness, and separation as well as the bone formation rate/bone surface (BFR/BS) were calculated.

Biochemical Analyses

Serum type 1 carboxyterminal collagen fragments (CTX-1) were measured using the RatLaps enzyme immunoassay (EIA; Immunodiagnostic Systems, UK), and the amino-terminal propeptide of type 1 procollagen (P1NP) was measured using the Rat PINP EIA (Immunodiagnostic Systems), according to the manufacturer's instructions.

Statistical Analysis

Means and standard deviations (SDs) were calculated for each group. Comparisons were performed using ANOVA with post-hoc comparison adjusted by the Bonferroni method. Data were analyzed with SAS 9.0 (SAS Institute Inc., Cary, NC), and a P value <0.05 was considered statistically significant.

Acknowledgments

We would like to thank Tzu-Hui Chu for her expert technical assistance.

Author Contributions

Conceived and designed the experiments: J-FS Y-JK J-SS C-HL. Performed the experiments: J-FS Y-JK F-YT C-HC J-YL Y-CH W-YC C-BY. Analyzed the data: J-FS Y-JK C-HL C-HC J-YL Y-CH W-YC C-BY. Contributed reagents/materials/analysis tools: J-FS Y-JK F-YT J-SS C-HL. Wrote the paper: J-FS Y-JK.

References

1. Rogers MJ, Frith JC, Luckman SP, Coxon FP, Benford HL, et al. (1999) Molecular mechanisms of action of bisphosphonates. Bone 24: 73S–79S.
2. Drake MT, Clarke BL, Khosla S (2008) Bisphosphonates: mechanism of action and role in clinical practice. Mayo Clin Proc 83: 1032–1045.
3. Rogers MJ, Crockett JC, Coxon FP, Mönkkönen J (2011) Biochemical and molecular mechanisms of action of bisphosphonates. Bone 49: 34–41.
4. Luckman SP, Hughes DE, Coxon FP, Graham R, Russell G, et al. (1998) Nitrogen-containing bisphosphonates inhibit the mevalonate pathway and prevent post-translational prenylation of GTP-binding proteins, including Ras. J Bone Miner Res 13: 581–589.
5. Karsdal MA, Henriksen K, Arnold M, Christiansen C (2008) Calcitonin: a drug of the past or for the future? Physiologic inhibition of bone resorption while sustaining osteoclast numbers improves bone quality. BioDrugs 22: 137–144.
6. de Paula FJ, Rosen CJ (2010) Back to the future: revisiting parathyroid hormone and calcitonin control of bone remodeling. Horm Metab Res 42: 299–306.
7. Gallagher JC, Sai AJ (2010) Molecular biology of bone remodeling: implications for new therapeutic targets for osteoporosis. Maturitas 65: 301–307.
8. Woodrow JP, Sharpe CJ, Fudge NJ, Hoff AO, Gagel RF, et al. (2006) Calcitonin plays a critical role in regulating skeletal mineral metabolism during lactation. Endocrinology 147: 4010–4021.
9. Davey RA, Turner AG, McManus JF, Chiu WS, Tjahyono F, et al. (2008) Calcitonin receptor plays a physiological role to protect against hypercalcemia in mice. J Bone Miner Res 23: 1182–1193.
10. Marzia M, Chiusaroli R, Neff L, Kim NY, Chishti AH, et al. (2006) Calpain is required for normal osteoclast function and is down-regulated by calcitonin. J Biol Chem 281: 9745–9754.
11. Shyu JF, Shih C, Tseng CY, Lin CH, Sun DT, et al. (2007) Calcitonin induces podosome disassembly and detachment of osteoclasts by modulating Pyk2 and Src activities. Bone 40: 1329–1342.
12. Stern PH (2007) Antiresorptive agents and osteoclast apoptosis. J Cell Biochem 101: 1087–1096.
13. Selander KS, Härkönen PL, Valve E, Mönkkönen J, Hannuniemi R, et al. (1996) Calcitonin promotes osteoclast survival in vitro. Mol Cell Endocrinol 122: 119–129.
14. Kanaoka K, Kobayashi Y, Hashimoto F, Nakashima T, Shibata M, et al. (2000) A common downstream signaling activity of osteoclast survival factors that prevent nitric oxide-promoted osteoclast apoptosis. Endocrinology 141: 2995–3005.
15. Miyazaki T, Neff L, Tanaka S, Horne WC, Baron R (2003) Regulation of cytochrome c oxidase activity by c-Src in osteoclasts. J Cell Biol 160: 709–718.
16. Hoff AO, Catala-Lehnen P, Thomas PM, Priemel M, Rueger JM, et al. (2002) Increased bone mass is an unexpected phenotype associated with deletion of the calcitonin gene. J Clin Invest 110: 1849–1857.
17. Huebner AK, Schinke T, Priemel M, Schilling S, Schilling AF, et al. (2006) Calcitonin deficiency in mice progressively results in high bone turnover. J Bone Miner Res 2006; 21: 1924–1934.
18. Lin FH, Lin CC, Lu CM, Liu HC, Sun JS, et al. (1995) Mechanical properties and histological evaluation of sintered beta-Ca2P2O7 with Na4P2O7.10H2O addition. Biomaterials 16: 793–802.
19. Sun JS, Tsuang YH, Liao CJ, Liu HC, Hang YS, et al. (1997) The effects of calcium phosphate particles on the growth of osteoblasts. J Biomed Mater Res 37: 324–334.
20. Sun JS, Huang YC, Tsuang YH, Chen LT, Lin FH (2002) Sintered dicalcium pyrophosphate increases bone mass in ovariectomized rats. J Biomed Mater Res59: 246–253.
21. Sun JS, Huang YC, Lin FH, Chen LT (2003) The effect of sintered dicalcium pyrophosphate on osteoclast metabolism: an ultrastructural study. J Biomed Mater Res A 64: 616–621.
22. Karsdal MA, Henriksen K, Arnold M, Christiansen C (2008) Calcitonin- A drug of the Past or for the Future? BioDrugs 22: 137–144.
23. Chambers TJ, Athanasou NA, Fuller K (1984) Effect of parathyroid hormone and calcitonin on the cytoplasmic spreading of isolated osteoclasts. J Endocrinol 102: 281–286.

24. Zaidi M, Chambers TJ, Moonga BS, Oldoni T, Passarella E, et al. (1990) A new approach for calcitonin determination based on target cell responsiveness. J Endocrinol Invest 13: 119–126.

25. Sutherland KA, Rogers HL, Tosh D, Rogers MJ (2009) RANKL increases the level of Mcl-1 in osteoclasts and reduces bisphosphonate-induced osteoclast apoptosis in vitro. Arthritis Res Ther 11: R58.

26. Tanaka S, Wakeyama H, Akiyama T, Takahashi K, Amano H, et al. (2010) Regulation of osteoclast apoptosis by bcl-2 family protein bim and caspase-3. Adv Exp Med Biol 658: 111–116.

27. Horne WC, Sanjay A, Baron R (2008) Regulating Bone Resorption: Targeting Integrins, Calcitonin Receptor, and Cathepsin K, in: J.P. Bilezikian, T.J. Martin (Eds.) Principles of Bone Biology 3rd ed., Academic Press, New York, NY, USA, 221–236.

28. Miyazaki T, Katagiri H, Kanegae Y, Takayanagi H, Sawada Y, et al. (2000) Reciprocal role of ERK and NF-kappaB pathways in survival and activation of osteoclasts. J Cell Biol 148: 333–342.

29. Allan LA, Morrice N, Brady S, Magee G, Pathak S, et al. (2003) Inhibition of caspase-9 through phosphorylation at Thr 125 by ERK MAPK. Nat Cell Biol 5: 647–654.

30. Ogawa K, Hori M, Takao R, Sakurada T (2005) Effects of combined elcatonin and alendronate treatment on the architecture and strength of bone in ovariectomized rats. J Bone Miner Metab 23: 351–358.

31. Ozoran K, Yildirim M, ÖNDER M, Sivas F, Inanir A (2007) The bone mineral density effects of calcitonin and alendronate combined therapy in patients with rheumatoid arthritis. APLAR J Rheumatol 10: 17–22.

32. Iwamoto J, Uzawa M, Sato Y, Takeda T, Matsumoto H. (2009) Effects of short-term combined treatment with alendronate and elcatonin on bone mineral density and bone turnover in postmenopausal women with osteoporosis. Ther Clin Risk Manag 5: 499–505.

33. Martin T, Gooi JH, Sims NA. (2009) Molecular mechanisms in coupling of bone formation to resorption. Crit Rev Eukaryot Gene Expr 19: 73–88.

34. Mochizuki K, Inoue T. (2000) Effect of salmon calcitonin on experimental osteoporosis induced by ovariectomy and low-calcium diet in the rat. J Bone Miner Metab 18: 194–207.

35. Davey RA, Morris HA. (2005) The effects of salmon calcitonin-induced hypocalcemia on bone metabolism in ovariectomized rats. J Bone Miner Metab 23: 359–365.

36. Furuichi H, Fukuyama R, Izumo N, Fujita T, Kohno T, et al. (2000) Bone-anabolic effect of salmon calcitonin on glucocorticoid-induced osteopenia in rats. Biol Pharm Bull 23: 946–951.

37. Huebner AK, Keller J, Catala-Lehnen P, Perkovic S, Streichert T, et al. (2008) The role of calcitonin and alpha-calcitonin gene-related peptide in bone formation. Arch Biochem Biophys 473: 210–217.

38. Sun JS, Tsuang YH, Liao CJ, Liu HC, Hang YS, et al. (1999) The effect of sintered beta-dicalcium pyrophosphate particle size on newborn Wistar rat osteoblasts. Artif Organs 23: 331–338.

39. Penolazzi L, Lampronti I, Borgatti M, Khan MT, Zennaro M, et al. (2008) Induction of apoptosis of human primary osteoclasts treated with extracts from the medicinal plant Emblica officinalis. BMC Complement Altern Med 8: 59.

40. Bouxsein ML, Boyd SK, Christiansen BA, Guldberg RE, Jepsen KJ, et al. (2010) Guidelines for assessment of bone microstructure in rodents using micro-computed tomography. J Bone Miner Res 25: 1468–1486.

41. Hildebrand T, Ruegsegger P. (1997) Quantification of Bone Microarchitecture with the Structure Model Index. Comput Methods Biomech Biomed Engin 1: 15–23.

42. Lin C, Moniz C, Chambers TJ, Chow JWM (1996) Colitis causes bone loss in rats through suppression of bone formation. Gastroenterol; 11: 1263–1271.

16

Parathyroid Hormone versus Bisphosphonate Treatment on Bone Mineral Density in Osteoporosis Therapy

Longxiang Shen, Xuetao Xie, Yan Su, Congfeng Luo, Changqing Zhang, Bingfang Zeng*

Department of Orthopedic Surgery, Shanghai Sixth People's Hospital, Shanghai Jiaotong University, Shanghai, People's Republic of China

Abstract

Background: Bisphosphonates and parathyroid hormone (PTH) represent the antiresorptive and anabolic classes of drugs for osteoporosis treatment. Bone mineral density (BMD) is an essential parameter for the evaluation of anti-osteoporotic drugs. The aim of this study was to evaluate the effects of PTH versus bisphosphonates on BMD for the treatment of osteoporosis.

Methods/Principal Findings: We performed a literature search to identify studies that investigated the effects of PTH versus bisphosphonates treatment on BMD. A total of 7 articles were included in this study, representing data on 944 subjects. The pooled data showed that the percent change of increased BMD in the spine is higher with PTH compared to bisphosphonates (WMD = 5.90, 95% CI: 3.69–8.10, $p < 0.01$,). In the hip, high dose (40 µg) PTH (1–34) showed significantly higher increments of BMD compared to alendronate (femoral neck: WMD = 5.67, 95% CI: 3.47–7.87, $p < 0.01$; total hip: WMD = 2.40, 95%CI: 0.49–4.31, $p < 0.05$). PTH treatment has yielded significantly higher increments than bisphosphonates with a duration of over 12 months (femoral neck: WMD = 5.67, 95% CI: 3.47–7.86, $p < 0.01$; total hip: WMD = 2.40, 95% CI: 0.49–4.31, $P < 0.05$) and significantly lower increments at 12 months (femoral neck: WMD = −1.05, 95% CI: −2.26–0.16, $p < 0.01$; total hip: WMD: −1.69, 95% CI: −3.05–0.34, $p < 0.05$). In the distal radius, a reduction in BMD was significant between PTH and alendronate treatment. (WMD = −3.68, 95% CI: −5.57–1.79, $p < 0.01$).

Discussion: Our results demonstrated that PTH significantly increased lumbar spine BMD as compared to treatment with bisphosphonates and PTH treatment induced duration- and dose-dependent increases in hip BMD as compared to bisphosphonates treatment. This study has also disclosed that for the distal radius, BMD was significantly lower from PTH treatment than alendronate treatment.

Editor: Maria Moran, Hospital Universitario 12 de Octubre, Spain

Funding: Funding provided by China Postdoctoral Science Foundation (20100470700) http://www.chinapostdoctor.org.cn/. The funders had no role in study design, data collection and analysis, decision to publish, or preparation of the manuscript.

Competing Interests: The authors have declared that no competing interests exist.

* E-mail: xiang9669@yahoo.com

Introduction

Osteoporosis is a common skeletal disease characterized by low bone mass and deterioration in bone micro-architecture, which induces bone fragility and increased risk of fracture [1]. Increasing bone mass and improving bone architecture and strength reduces skeletal fragility and the risk of fracture and are the optimal treatments for osteoporosis.

Antiresorptive agents, such as bisphosphonates, are the most widely used group of drugs for osteoporosis treatment [2,3,4]. Bisphosphonates directly reduce the number of active osteoclasts by inhibiting their recruitment and also by inhibiting the osteoclast-stimulating activity of osteoblasts [5,6]. bisphosphonate therapy normalizes bone turnover, reduces the number of bone remodeling units, restores the balance of bone remodeling, prevents bone loss and deterioration of bone structure and reduces fracture risk in patients with osteoporosis [6,7,8].

Parathyroid hormone (PTH) is used clinically as an anabolic agent [9,10,11,12,13]. Two forms of recombinant human PTH

have been evaluated: teriparatide, the 34 residue amino-terminal fragment of human PTH (1–34) and the intact 84-amino acid form of PTH (1–84), which is marketed as Preotact® [14]. PTH directly increases osteoblast production rate and inhibits apoptosis of osteoblasts, thereby leading to a rapid increase in skeletal mass as well as improvement of bone micro-architecture and strength [15].

A decrease in bone mineral density (BMD) is a significant risk factor for fracture and is of similar importance in both women and men [16,17]. The measurement of BMD is a major determinant of fracture and an essential parameter for the evaluation of anti-osteoporotic drugs used in clinical therapy. As more studies comparing the effects of PTH and bisphosphonates on BMD in patients with osteoporosis are now becoming available, we decided to perform a meta-analysis on the effects of PTH and bisphosphonates on BMD for the treatment of osteoporosis. Our main goal was to study the effects of PTH and bisphosphonates on BMD separately at various skeletal sites (lumbar spine, total hip, femoral neck and distal radius).

Methods

Search Strategy

This meta-analysis followed the PRISMA statement guidelines [18]. A literature search was performed on August 17, 2010 and an updated search was performed on 14 April 2011 using the phrase, "parathyroid hormone AND bisphosphonate AND osteoporosis" with the limits "humans" and "randomized controlled trial". A second search was performed using the phrase, "parathyroid hormone AND bisphosphonate AND bone mineral" with the limits "humans" and "randomized controlled trial" using PubMed (1990–2010), Ovid's MEDLINE (1990–2010), MEDLINE In Process &. Other Non-Indexed Citations (1990-2010), Web of Knowledge and EMBASE (1991–2010). Further searches using the same keywords and limitations did not provide additional references. We also performed a search of the Cochrane Central Register of Controlled Trials and a conference abstract search of the Journal of Bone and Mineral Research. Review articles were also scanned to find additional eligible studies. In addition, reference lists of all original articles and previous systematic reviews were hand searched for other relevant papers. The searches were not restricted to English language literature. Duplicates were removed. Information was carefully extracted from all eligible publications independently by two of the authors of the present study (LS and XX). Differences in the extraction of data were inspected by a third investigator (CL). All the searched studies were retrieved and their references were checked for other relevant publications. The search results were then screened on the basis of the following inclusion criteria: (a) randomized controlled studies with a duration of at least 6 months, (b) The active treatment arm of the study had to include PTH and bisphosphonate, and (c) Studies on patients with postmenopausal or gonadal osteoporosis. Exclusion criteria included non-randomized trials or duration of less than 6 months and studies on any secondary osteoporosis (for example, glucocorticoid-induced). Reports were excluded if the subjects had prior treatment with PTH or a PTH analogue or treatment with bisphosphonates within the previous 12 months. Both area BMD data measured by dual X-ray absorptiometry (DXA) and volumetric BMD data measured by quantitative controlled trials were eligible. The Jadad scale was used to assess the quality of included randomly controlled trials (RCTs), where a score of <3 indicated low quality [19].

Statistical analysis

Changes in BMD values were expressed in percent change vs. baseline for both PTH and bisphosphonate treatment groups. We calculated the weighted mean differences (WMD) for percent changes in BMD. We conducted a random-effects model meta-analysis for heterogeneous outcomes and a fixed-effects model meta-analysis for homogeneous outcomes. The pooled analyses were performed using the Stata/SE 10.0 program for Windows (Stata Corporation, College Station, TX, USA). Statistical heterogeneity was investigated using the χ^2 test and I^2 statistic (I^2 represents the percentage of variability due to between-study variability). Funnel plots and the Egger's tests were used to estimate possible publication bias. A sensitivity analysis was conducted using the trim and fill method, to detect possible publication bias. A p-value less than 0.05 was considered to be statistically significant.

Results

Selected studies and characteristics

A total of 782 potentially relevant citations were identified and screened, of which only 7 published RCTs met the inclusion criteria and were selected for this meta-analysis [10,20,21,22, 23,24,25] (Figure 1). The main characteristics of the 7 studies are shown in Table 1. The level of evidence for each article was graded from scores 3 to 5 according to the Jadad quality score. A total of 944 patients, 896 women and 48 men were included in this analysis. Six trials involved postmenopausal women with osteoporosis [10,20,21,22,24,25] and one trial involved osteoporotic men [23]. Of the 7 included trials, 5 had demonstrated the effects of alendronate [10,20,22,23,24], one showed results from risedronate [21] and the last showed the effects of zoledronic acid [25]. Allocation concealment was adequately reported in 4 trials [19,20,22,24] and unclear in the remaining trials. Four trials were double-blind or partially double-blind [10,22,24,25].

Effects of PTH versus bisphosphonates on spinal BMD

All of the 7 RCTs studied lumbar spine areal BMD. Finkelstein et al. [23] reported BMD data in both posteroanterior spine and lateral spine. The pooled data showed that the percent change of increased BMD in the spine is higher with PTH in comparison to treatment with bisphosphonates after 12–30 months (WMD = 5.90, 95% CI: 3.69–8.10, $p<0.01$, n = 953). These estimates were heterogeneous. To explore this heterogeneity, we assessed the data within subgroups based on the gender of the participants and the type of agent used. For women, the pooled data from 6 studies showed that increases in BMD was higher in PTH treatment than that of bisphosphonates (WMD = 4.27, 95% CI: 2.46–6.08, $p<0.01$; n = 865). Whereas for men, Finkelstein et al. [23] reported that PTH treatment resulted in statistically significant increases in both posteroanterior spine and lateral spine BMD values as compared to that of alendronate. Comparing PTH treatment to alendronate, the increase in spine BMD was significantly higher in the PTH group (WMD = 7.42, 95% CI: 4.21–10.62, $p<0.01$; five studies, n = 649). Comparing PTH values to other types of bisphosphonates, the results were consistent (WMD = 2.74, 95% CI: 1.68–3.74, $p<0.01$; two studies, n = 304). The effects of 20–40 µg of PTH (1–34) compared to those of the bisphosphonate groups showed a significantly higher increase in BMD values (WMD = 4.41, 95% CI: 3.60–5.21, $p<0.01$; six studies, n = 774). Heterogeneity remained in the above analysis. To further explore this heterogeneity, subgroup analysis showed that the effects of both 20 µg and 40 µg of PTH (1–34) treatment increased lumbar spine BMD values significantly higher than bisphosphonates (WMD = 3.31, 95% CI: 2.42–4.21, $p<0.01$; three studies, n = 491; WMD = 8.92, 95% CI: 7.10–10.75, $p<0.01$; three studies, n = 283, respectively). Heterogeneity was not found in both subgroups (Figure 2A). In addition, we also grouped the studies on the basis of the duration of treatment. PTH treatment has yielded consistently and significantly higher increments as compared to the bisphosphonate groups (12 months: WMD = 3.00, 95% CI: 1.69–4.32, $p<0.01$; four studies, n = 670; over 12 months: WMD = 9.85, 95% CI: 6.70–13.01, $p<0.01$; three studies, n = 283) (Figure 2B). Heterogeneity was not found in either duration subgroup. The shape of the funnel plot showed slight asymmetry and the Egger's test indicated publication bias ($P<0.05$) (Figure 3A). We conducted a trim and fill method to further investigate the publication bias. The imputed studies produced a symmetrical funnel plot (Figure 3B) and the pooled analysis incorporating the hypothetical studies continued to show statistically significant higher increments in BMD values with PTH treatment over those using bisphosphonates (WMD = 3.48, 95% CI: 1.09–5.88, $p<0.01$).

Four of the 6 RCTs reported volumetric BMD data of the lumbar spine. The overall pooled results by random-effects analysis showed that the increase was higher with PTH treatment

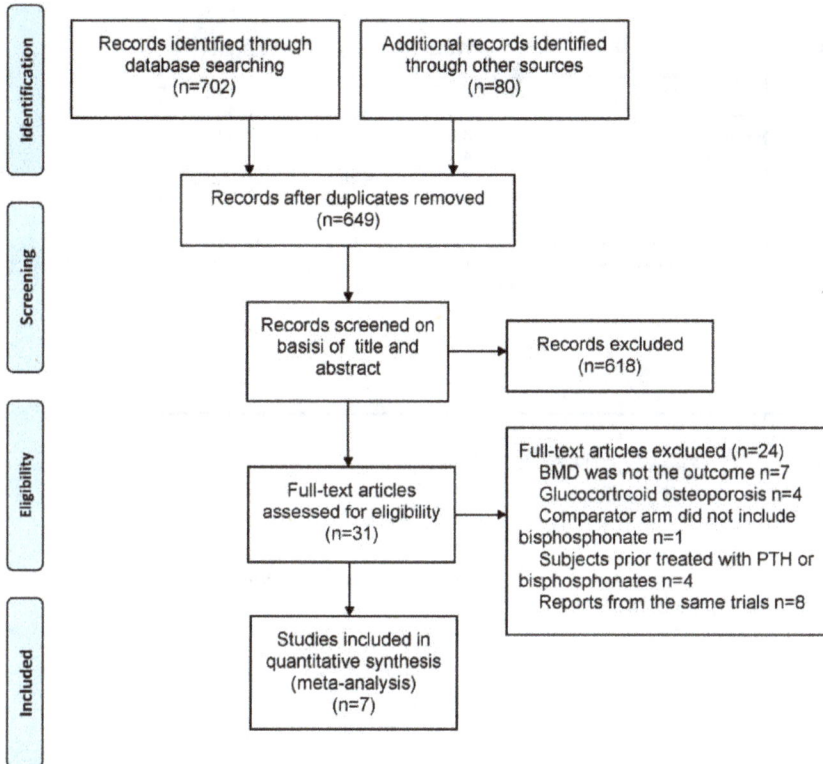

Figure 1. Flowchart of the meta-analysis.

Table 1. Basal characteristics of clinical trials enrolled in the analysis.

Author (Ref.)	Year	Gender (F/M)	Number of patients (PTH/ bisphosphonate)	Intervention (calcium and/or vitamin D)	Duration (months)	Outcomes measured: Areal BMD, volumetric BMD	Jadad score [19]
Cosman et al. [25]	2011	F	138 vs.137	20 µg PTH (1–34)/day + placebo infusion of zoledronic acid vs. a single intravenous infusion of zoledronic acid 5 mg. No placebo PTH. All: 1000–1200 mg calcium/day +400–800 IU vitamin D/day	12	Areal BMD: lumbar spine, total hip, femoral neck	3
Finkelstein et al. [20]	2010	F	20 vs. 29	40 µg PTH (1–34)/day vs. alendronate 10 mg/day. No placebo PTH. All: 1000–1200 mg calcium/day (diet or suppl.) +400 IU vitamin D/day	30	Areal BMD: lumbar spine, total hip, femoral neck, distal radius. Volumetric BMD: lumbar spine.	3
Anastasilakis et al. [21]	2008	F	22 vs. 22	35 mg Risedronate/week vs. 20 µg PTH (1–34)/day. No placebo PTH. All: 500 mg elemental calcium/day+400 IU vitamin D/day	12	Areal BMD: lumbar spine.	3
McClung et al. [22]	2005	F	102 vs. 101	20 µg PTH (1–34)/day+oral placebo vs. 10 mg alendronate 10/day+placebo injection. All: 1000 mg calcium/day (diet or suppl.) +400 to 800 IU vitamin D/day	12	Areal BMD: lumbar spine and femoral neck. Volumetric BMD: lumbar spine	3
Finkelstein et al. [23]	2003	M	20 vs. 28	40 µg PTH (1–34)/day vs. alendronate 10 mg/day. No placebo PTH. All: 1000 to 1200 mg calcium/day (diet or suppl.) +400 IU vitamin D/day	30	Areal BMD: lumbar spine (posteroanterior and lateral), total hip, femoral neck, distal radius. Volumetric BMD: lumbar spine.	3
Black et al. [10]	2003	F	119 vs. 60	100 µg PTH (1–84)/day vs. alendronate 10 mg/day. Placebo PTH All: 500 mg calcium/day+400 IU vitamin D/day	12	Areal BMD: lumbar spine, total hip, femoral neck, distal radius . Volumetric BMD: lumbar spine	4
Body et al. [24]	2002	F	73 vs. 73	40 µg rPTH (1–34) +oral placebo vs. alendronate+placebo inj. All: calcium 1000 mg/day+vitamin D 400 to 1200 IU/day	14	Areal BMD: lumbar spine, total hip, femoral neck, distal radius	4

A

Study ID		WMD (95% CI)	Weight (%)
20μg PTH			
Cosman (2010)		2.70 (1.57, 3.83)	18.27
Anastasilakis (2008)		3.00 (−0.09, 6.09)	14.78
McClung (2005)		4.80 (3.10, 6.50)	17.47
Subtotal (I−squared = 51.6%, p = 0.127)		3.49 (2.01, 4.98)	50.52
40μg PTH			
Finkelstein (2010)		11.00 (5.98, 16.02)	10.86
Finkelstein (2003)		10.20 (6.88, 13.52)	14.28
Finkelstein♦ (2003)		14.70 (8.32, 21.08)	8.58
Body (2002)		6.60 (3.98, 9.22)	15.76
Subtotal (I−squared = 59.5%, p = 0.060)		9.85 (6.70, 13.01)	49.48
Overall (I−squared = 85.3%, p = 0.000)		6.73 (4.20, 9.26)	100.00

-5   0   5   10   15

Favours bisphosphonates   Favours PTH

B

Study ID		WMD (95% CI)	Weight (%)
12 months			
Cosman (2010)		2.70 (1.57, 3.83)	15.86
Anastasilakis (2008)		3.00 (−0.09, 6.09)	12.50
McClung (2005)		4.80 (3.10, 6.50)	15.07
Black (2003)		1.70 (0.14, 3.26)	15.29
Subtotal (I−squared = 58.5%, p = 0.065)		3.00 (1.69, 4.32)	58.72
>12months			
Finkelstein♦ (2003)		14.70 (8.32, 21.08)	6.93
Body (2002)		6.60 (3.98, 9.22)	13.42
Finkelstein (2010)		11.00 (5.98, 16.02)	8.91
Finkelstein (2003)		10.20 (6.88, 13.52)	12.02
Subtotal (I−squared = 59.5%, p = 0.060)		9.85 (6.70, 13.01)	41.28
Overall (I−squared = 86.0%, p = 0.000)		5.90 (3.69, 8.10)	100.00

-5   0   5   10   15

Favours bisphosphonates   Favours PTH

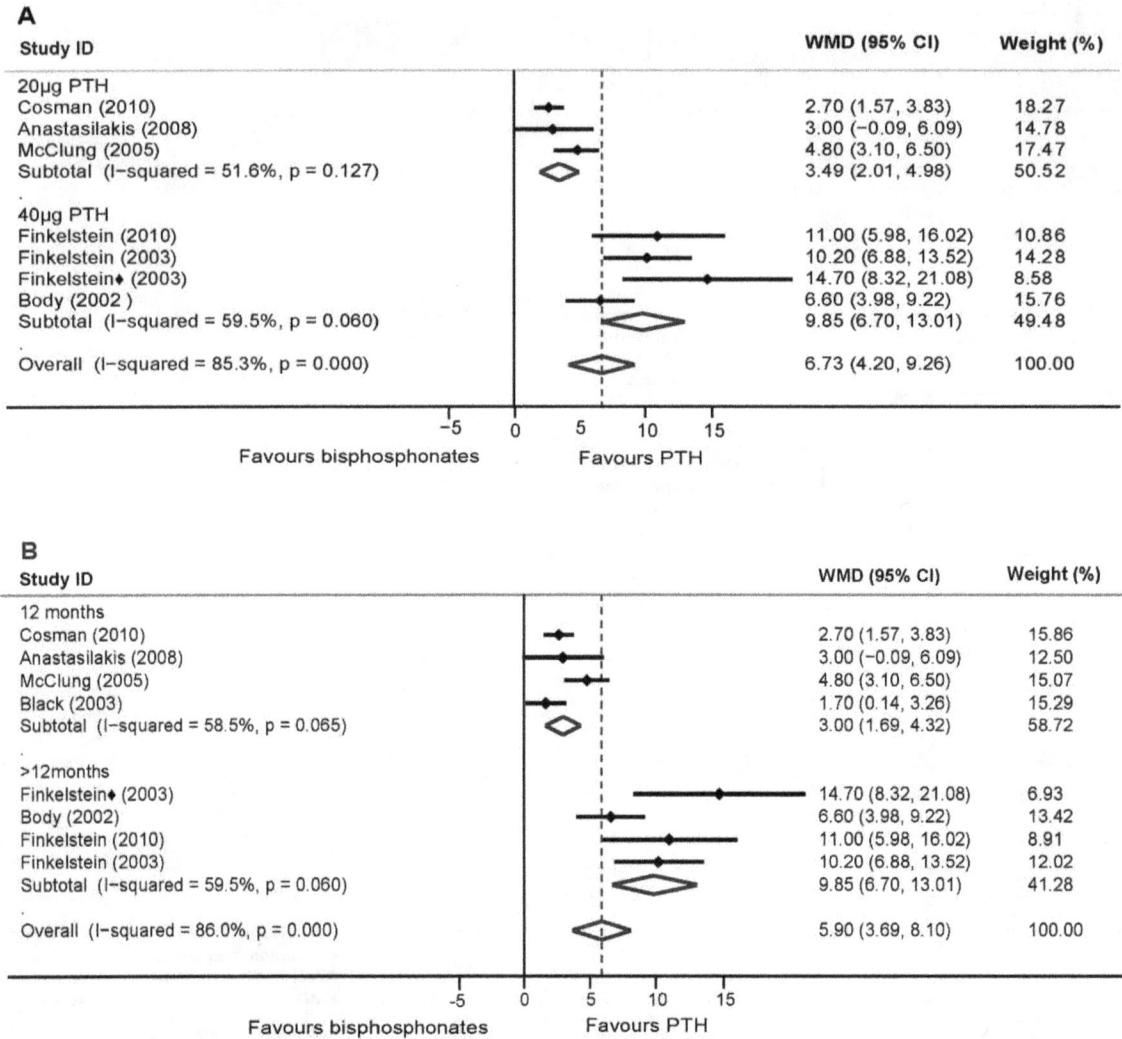

Figure 2. Assessment of the effects of PTH versus bisphosphonates on BMD of the lumbar spine. A: Subgrouped analysis of dosage of PTH (1–34) versus bisphosphonates treatment on spinal BMD. B: Subgrouped analysis of the duration of PTH (1–34) versus bisphosphonates treatment on spinal BMD. ♦: The study reported BMD data in lateral spine.

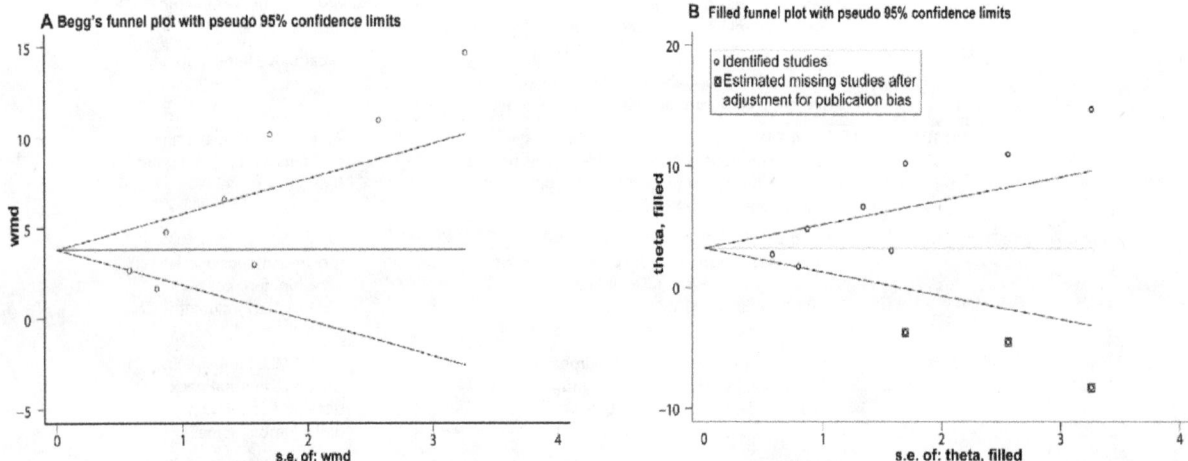

Figure 3. Funnel plot of all studies on the effects of PTH and bisphosphonates on spine BMD. A: Begg's funnel plot with pseudo 95% confidence limits. B: Filled funnel plot with pseudo 95% confidence limits. WMD, weighted mean difference; S.E., standard error.

compared to bisphosphonates during 12–30 months of follow-up (95% CI: 13.81–52.12, $p<0.01$; four studies, n = 325). This comparison showed significant heterogeneity (Table 2). Funnel plot and Egger's test results did not reveal signs of publication bias (plot not shown).

Effects of PTH versus alendronate on BMD of the hip

In this pooled analysis, the increases in the femoral neck BMD values were not significant between PTH and bisphosphonate treatments (WMD = 2.24, 95% CI: −0.48–4.97, $p=0.11$, n = 824). In women, no significant difference was observed between the PTH and bisphosphonate groups (WMD = 1.54, 95% CI: −1.25–4.33, $p=0.28$; five studies, n = 777). Nonetheless, statistical heterogeneity was large both in overall pooled analysis and in the analysis of women ($I^2 > 80\%$, $p<0.01$). For men, there was only one trial (n = 47) that investigated the effects of 40 µg PTH (1–34) versus 10 mg alendronate daily on the femoral neck BMD during osteoporosis treatment [23]; therefore, we were unable to estimate a pooled effect. A sensitivity analysis excluding the trial using full-length PTH (1–84) [10] indicated that PTH (1–34) increased femoral neck BMD with no significant difference to the bisphosphonate group (WMD = 3.09, 95%CI: −0.30–6.48, $p=0.07$, five studies, n = 645). Statistical heterogeneity was found in the analysis ($I^2 = 93\%$, $p<0.01$). We then grouped the studies on the basis of the dose of PTH (1–34) used for treatment. 20 µg of PTH (1–34) yielded lower increments compared to bisphosphonates without statistical significance (WMD = −0.78, 95% CI: −2.93–1.37, $p=0.48$; two studies, n = 403), while 40 µg PTH (1–34) showed significantly higher increments of BMD than alendronate (WMD = 5.67, 95% CI: 3.47–7.87, $p<0.01$; three studies, n = 242). Heterogeneity was found in the 20 µg treatment subgroup ($I^2 = 77.3\%$, $p<0.05$), but not in the 40 µg subgroup ($I^2 = 51.0\%$, $p=0.13$) (Figure 4A). In the grouped studies comparing the duration of treatment, PTH treatment has yielded significantly higher increments than bisphosphonates with a duration of over 12 months (WMD = 5.67, 95% CI: 3.47–7.86, $p<0.01$; three studies, n = 242), and significantly lower increments at 12 months (WMD = −1.05, 95% CI: −2.26–0.16, $p<0.01$; three studies, n = 682). Heterogeneity was not found in either of the duration subgroups ($I^2 = 51\%$, $p=0.13$; $I^2 = 56\%$, $p=0.09$, respectively) (Figure 4B). The shape of the funnel plot showed slight asymmetry and the Egger's test indicated publication bias ($p<0.05$). The trimmed and filled funnel plot was symmetrical (plot not shown). The pooled analysis, incorporating the two hypothetical studies, continued to show statistically non-significant

increments of BMD between the PTH and bisphosphonate groups (WMD = 0.01, 95% CI: −2.84–2.84, $p=0.10$).

The pooled data showed there was no significant difference between PTH and bisphosphonates in increasing total hip BMD (WMD = 0.59, 95% CI: −1.42–2.60, $p=0.57$, five studies, n = 683). For PTH (1–34) treatment, the pooled data showed that BMD increase in the total hip was not significant as compared to bisphosphonates (WMD = 1.48, 95%CI: −0.91–3.87, $p<0.05$, four studies, n = 504). Heterogeneity was found among the studies. A sensitivity analysis conducted by removing the 20 µg PTH study [26] indicated that treatment with 40 µg of PTH (1–34) increased total hip BMD significantly higher than alendronate treatment (WMD = 2.40, 95%CI: 0.49–4.31, $p<0.05$, three studies, n = 242). Heterogeneity was not found among these studies ($I^2 = 52.8\%$, $p=0.12$) (Figure 5A). In addition, subgroup analysis indicated that PTH treatment for the duration of 12 months increased the total hip BMD significantly less than bisphosphonates while higher than bisphosphonates with a duration of over 12 months (WMD: −1.69, 95% CI: −3.05–0.34, $p<0.05$, two studies, n = 441; WMD = 2.40, 95% CI: 0.49–4.31, $P<0.05$, three studies, n = 242; respectively). Heterogeneity was not found in either subgroup ($I^2 = 52.8\%$, $p=0.12$; $I^2 = 66.3\%$, $p=0.08$, respectively) (Figure 5B). The shapes of the funnel plots showed symmetry and the Egger's test indicated the absence of publication bias ($p=0.14$) (plot not shown).

Effects of PTH versus alendronate on BMD of the distal radius

A significant reduction in distal radius BMD was observed with PTH as compared to alendronate in the pooled analysis (WMD = −3.68, 95% CI: −5.57–1.79, $p<0.01$, four studies, n = 422). For the three studies involving women, the pooled effects presented the same result (WMD = −4.38, 95% CI: −6.83–1.93, $p<0.01$, n = 374). Heterogeneity was found in the above estimates. For PTH and alendronate treatment in men, data from the study by Finkelstein et al. [23] showed PTH decreased and alendronate increased BMD in the distal radius (n = 48, $p<0.01$) (Figure 6A). For PTH (1–34) treatment, the pooled data showed that PTH (1–34) significantly reduced BMD in the distal radius as compared to alendronate (WMD = −4.12, 95% CI: −6.69–1.26, p=0.46, three studies, n = 243). The study by Black et al. [10] showed that distal radius BMD decreased with PTH (1–84) treatment, while BMD values increased with alendronate treatment (n = 179, $p<0.01$) (Figure 6B). The funnel plot did not reveal any signs of symmetry and the Egger's test indicated the absence of publication bias ($p=0.07$) (plot not shown).

Table 2. Effects of PTH versus bisphosphonates on volumetric BMD of the spine.

Author (Ref.)	Volumetric BMD of the spine				Weight (%)	Weighted mean difference (WMD) of BMD (95%CI)
	PTH		bisphosphonates			
	n	percent change(%)	n	percent change(%)		
Finkelstein 2003 [23]	20	48.0±27.9	28	3.0±7.8	24.19	45.00 [32.44, 57.56]
Black 2003 [10]	119	25.3±15.1	60	10.3±8.1	26.78	15.00 [11.60, 18.40]
McClung 2005 [22]	26	19.0±17.3	23	3.8±16.3	25.35	15.20 [5.79, 24.61]
Finkelstein 2010 [20]	20	61.0±31.0	29	1.0±7.0	23.68	60.00 [46.18, 73.82]
Pooled	185		140		100	32.96 [13.81, 52.12]
Heterogeneity	Tau^2 =353.63; Chi^2 =56.19, df = 3; I^2 =95% p<0.01					

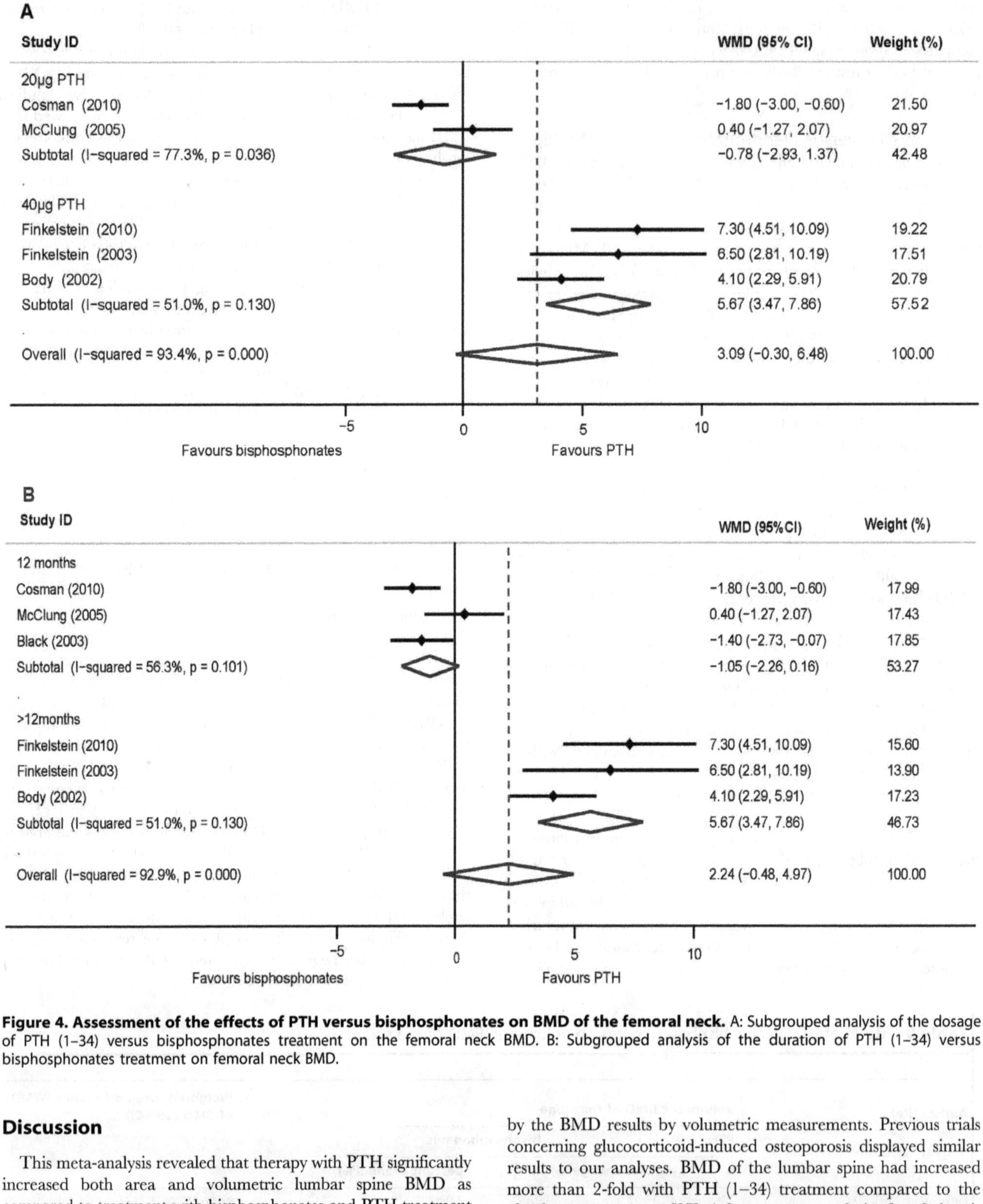

A

B

Figure 4. Assessment of the effects of PTH versus bisphosphonates on BMD of the femoral neck. A: Subgrouped analysis of the dosage of PTH (1–34) versus bisphosphonates treatment on the femoral neck BMD. B: Subgrouped analysis of the duration of PTH (1–34) versus bisphosphonates treatment on femoral neck BMD.

Discussion

This meta-analysis revealed that therapy with PTH significantly increased both area and volumetric lumbar spine BMD as compared to treatment with bisphosphonates and PTH treatment induced duration- and dose-dependent increases of hip BMD as compared to bisphosphonates treatment. This analysis has also disclosed that for the distal radius, BMD was significantly lower from PTH treatment than alendronate treatment.

The overall results indicated that PTH therapy displayed higher gain in areal BMD than therapy with bisphosphonates in respect to dose and duration of PTH and gender of patients as supported

by the BMD results by volumetric measurements. Previous trials concerning glucocorticoid-induced osteoporosis displayed similar results to our analyses. BMD of the lumbar spine had increased more than 2-fold with PTH (1–34) treatment compared to the alendronate treatment [27]. A former meta-analysis of pooled anti-resorptive comparative trials including alendronate showed significant reductions in PTH treated patients (1–34) for back pain, which was possibly caused by vertebral fracture [28]. Our analyses indicated that compared to low does of PTH treatment, greater BMD gains were obtained with high doses of PTH compared to treatment with bisphosphonates for the spine (WMD = 8.92 versus WMD = 3.31). This finding is in agreement

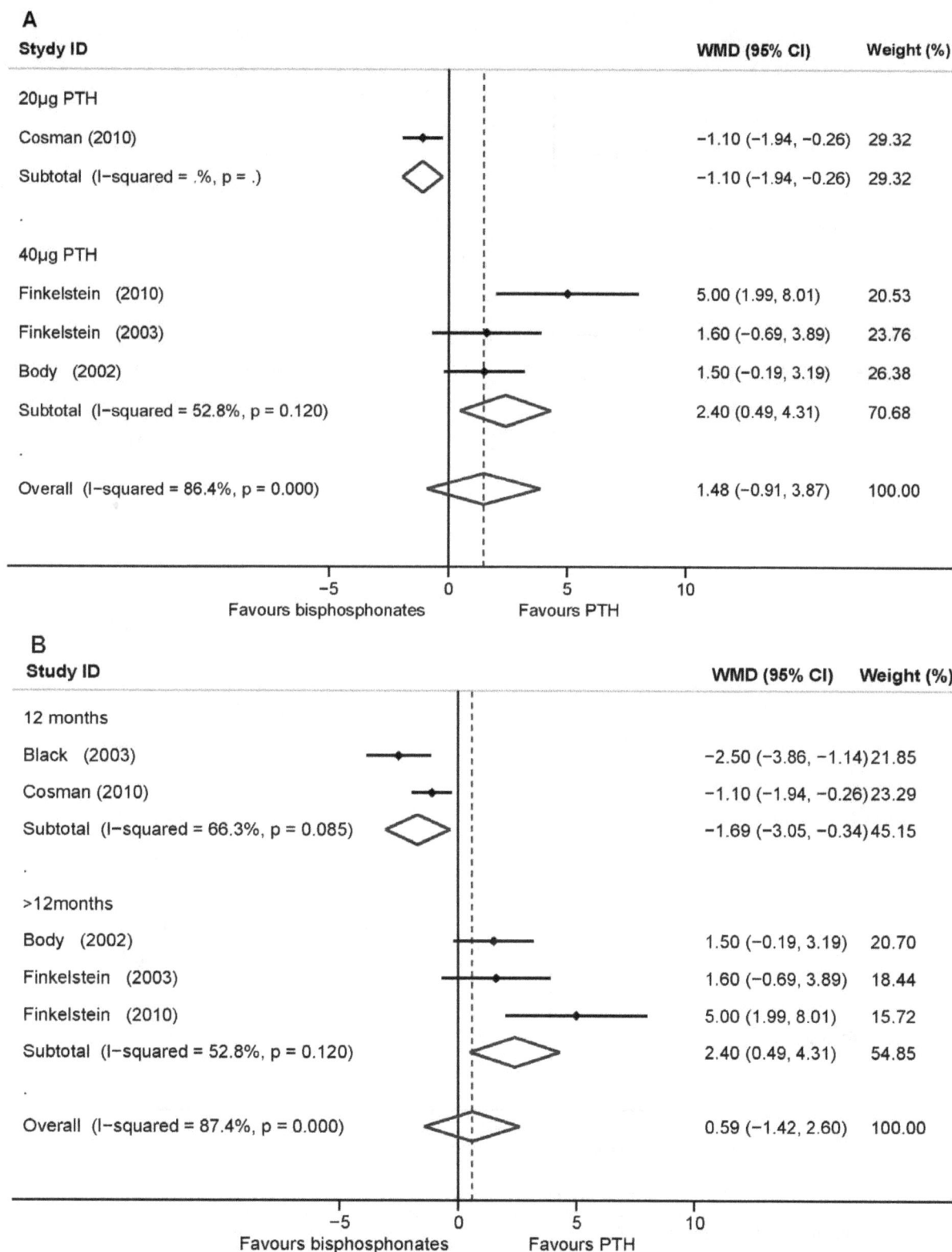

Figure 5. Assessment of the effects of PTH versus bisphosphonates on BMD of the total hip. A: Subgrouped analysis of the dosage of PTH (1–34) versus bisphosphonates treatment on total hip BMD. B: Subgrouped analysis of the duration of PTH (1–34) versus bisphosphonates treatment on total hip BMD.

with previous clinical trials involving PTH (1–34) [9,29] and PTH (1–84) [12]. A former meta-analysis also disclosed a dose response relationship for BMD in the spine with both PTH (1–34) and PTH

(1–84) treatments [30]. Previous placebo-controlled trials showed that spine BMD was significantly increased after 3 months of PTH therapy [12,29]. Body et al. [24] revealed that the difference in

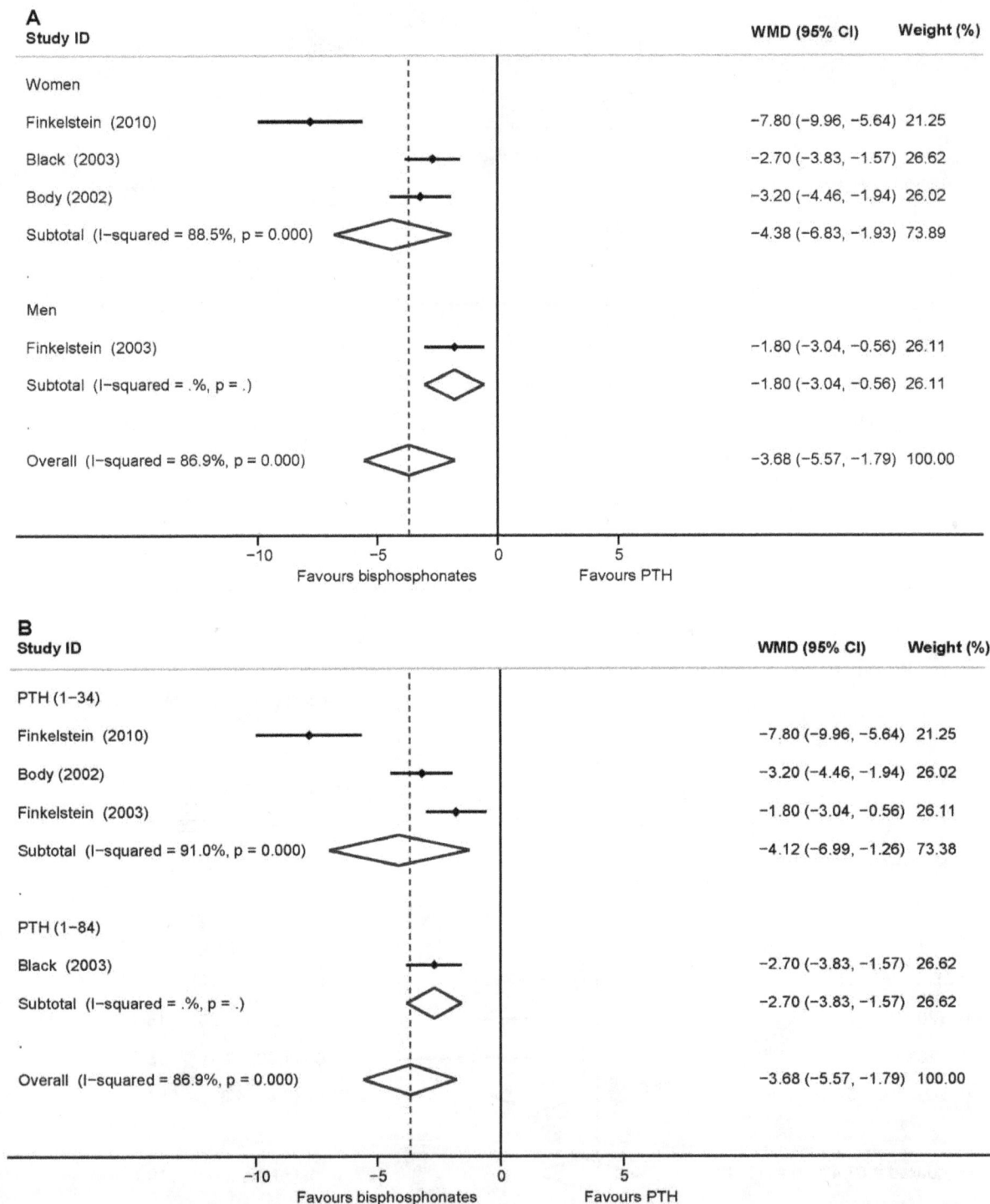

Figure 6. Assessment of the effects of PTH versus bisphosphonates on BMD of the distal radius. A: Subgrouped analysis of PTH versus bisphosphonates treatment on BMD of the distal radius in women and men. B: Subgrouped analysis of PTH (1–34) and PTH (1–84) versus bisphosphonates treatment on BMD of the distal radius.

lumbar spine BMD values between PTH (1–34) and alendronate treatment was statistically significant at 3 months. The alendronate-treated women required 12 months of treatment to increase lumbar spine BMD to a level equilvilant to women treated with PTH (1–34) for only 3 months.

In contrast to the spine, PTH treatment-induced changes in BMD of the hip were relatively inconsistent as compared to treatment with bisphosphonates. The former meta-analysis failed to draw a conclusion on the effect of PTH compared to bisphosphonates on hip BMD because of the low number of studies available [30]. In our meta-analysis, the overall analysis did not show significant differences between PTH and bisphosphonates. Former studies showed a trend towards higher hip BMD with higher PTH doses in both women and men [9,12,29].

Similarly, our subgroup analysis based on dosage of PTH (1–34) showed that compared to bisphosphonates, BMD increases of the femoral neck and total hip were significantly higher with treatment of high doses (40 μg/day) of PTH (1–34). On the other hand, analysis on the basis of duration indicated that the effect of PTH on hip BMD was inferior to bisphosphonates after treatment for 12 months, and was superior for over 12 months. This duration-related BMD change of PTH versus bisphosphonates could be explained by the different effects of PTH on trabecular and cortical bone. In trabecular bone, PTH adds new bone by increasing active bone remodeling units, which promotes new bone formation on quiescent bone surfaces. In cortical bone, PTH stimulates new bone formation mainly on the endocortical surface and to a lesser extent on the periosteal surface. One of the potential limitations is that it also increases intracortical (Haversian) remodeling and cortical porosity, thereby decreasing cortical BMD. Because the hip contains roughly equal amounts of cortical and trabecular bone, and BMD measured by DXA is a composite of these two bone types, the effect of PTH treatment on the hip BMD is the overall result of increased trabecular BMD and decreased cortical BMD. A transiently increased cortical remodeling space may lead to early reduction of cortical BMD. However, other competing effects within the periosteal, endocortical, and Haversian systems gradually allow the anabolic effects of PTH to predominate over the observed effects of an enlarged intracortical remodeling space. In this scenario, increased hip BMD during the second year of therapy showed a net gain in BMD.

In our meta-analysis, the distal radius was the only site at which the pooled data displayed BMD had decreased and was significantly lower in the PTH group as compared to the alendronate group. Previous observations disclosed that PTH therapy reduces BMD of the distal radius [9,29]. On the other hand, in postmenopausal women, a significant correlation was observed between changes in percentage from baseline in bone strength of the ultradistal radius site in the alendronate treated group [31]. Using animal models, the decrease in areal density measured by DXA is likely due to increased Haversian remodeling. As compared to the hip, the distal radius consists mainly of cortical bone. Increased remodeling transiently increases cortical porosity, which does not affect biomechanical strength [32,33]. In Neer's large placebo-controlled study, PTH therapy showed no increase in wrist fractures, which was consistent with the observations of preserved biomechanical strength in animal models [9].

For the present meta-analysis, most of the data originated from PTH (1–34) therapy, whereas the amount of data concerning PTH (1–84) is limited. Former studies showed a convincing reduction of vertebral fractures in both PTH (1–84) and PTH (1–34) treatment, but a reduction of non-vertebral fractures was shown in cases of treatment with PTH (1–34) only [34,35]. No clear conclusions can be made about the potential differences in effectiveness on BMD of PTH (1–34) and PTH (1–84) because of the lack of directly comparative studies. The 100 μg PTH (1–84) trial should

correspond to 43 μg of PTH (1–34) calculated on molecular basis [34]. We conducted grouped analysis with trials using 40 μg of PTH (1–34) and 100 μg PTH (1–84) both on the spine and hip BMD, but the results displayed large heterogeneity among trials. Thus, more data are needed on PTH (1–84) to establish if any clinically significant differences exist between these two types of PTH agents currently available. In our meta-analysis, dose and duration of PTH (1–34) was a main source of the heterogeneity. It was reported that adverse effects were more frequent in the 40 μg group compared to the 20 μg group [29]. Currently, the dose of PTH (1–34) approved by the US Food and Drug Administration is 20 μg. Even though BMD increased more with 40 μg for PTH treatment, fracture rates were similar [9]. Thus, only the lower dosage is approved for clinical administration. On the other hand, PTH (1–34) has been associated with the development of osteosarcoma in experimental animal models [36]; therefore, the safety of long-term clinical administration of PTH has yet to be determined. The use of PTH leads to new bone formation, but the skeletal response wanes over time, thereby limiting its anabolic effect. Sequential treatment with PTH and bisphosphonate showed benefits in maintaining gains in BMD [13,37,38].

Certain limitations in the present meta-analysis need to be addressed. First, the analysis is only based on published data and no unpublished data were included. Further, heterogeneity of the patients' ages and ethnic origin should be expected because it is impossible to match the cohorts completely for the analyses. On the other hand, our meta-analysis did not reveal gender-specific effects between PTH and bisphosphonates on BMD due to the limited number of trials on men. These factors limit the ability to elucidate the age-, ethnic- and gender- specific effects of PTH and bisphosphonates on BMD in osteoporosis treatment. Finally, the presented analysis was not designed to assess incident fractures.

We conclude that the bone-formation agent PTH substantially increased BMD of the lumbar spine compared to bisphosphonates as indicated in the current clinical reports on osteoporosis treatment. High doses of PTH (1–34) over 12 months of treatment duration increased BMD in the hip more effectively than bisphosphonates. PTH treatment reduced BMD of the distal radius significantly more than alendronate treatment. Further research could compare the effects of approved doses of PTH to bisphosphonates on BMD at vital sites in multicentric trials containing both women and men to attain robust clinical evidence.

Acknowledgments

The authors are grateful to Dr. Shuanhu Zhou at Orthopedic Surgery, Brigham and Women's Hospital, Harvard Medical School, Boston, MA, USA for helpful conversations and advice.

Author Contributions

Conceived and designed the experiments: LS XX CL CZ BZ. Analyzed the data: LS XX YS CZ. Contributed reagents/materials/analysis tools: LS XX YS CL. Wrote the paper: LS XX YS CL BZ.

References

1. (1993) Consensus development conference: diagnosis, prophylaxis, and treatment of osteoporosis. Am J Med 94: 646–650.
2. Cremers SC, Pillai G, Papapoulos SE (2005) Pharmacokinetics/pharmacodynamics of bisphosphonates: use for optimisation of intermittent therapy for osteoporosis. Clin Pharmacokinet 44: 551–570.
3. Mulder JE, Kolatkar NS, LeBoff MS (2006) Drug insight: Existing and emerging therapies for osteoporosis. Nat Clin Pract Endocrinol Metab 2: 670–680.
4. Macedo JM, Macedo CR, Elkis H, De Oliveira IR (1998) Meta-analysis about efficacy of anti-resorptive drugs in post-menopausal osteoporosis. J Clin Pharm Ther 23: 345–352.
5. Miller PD (2005) Optimizing the management of postmenopausal osteoporosis with bisphosphonates: the emerging role of intermittent therapy. Clin Ther 27: 361–376.
6. Reszka AA, Rodan GA (2003) Mechanism of action of bisphosphonates. Curr Osteoporos Rep 1: 45–52.
7. Heaney RP, Yates AJ, Santora AC (1997) Bisphosphonate effects and the bone remodeling transient. J Bone Miner Res 12: 1143–1151.
8. Boonen S, Vanderschueren D, Venken K, Milisen K, Delforge M, et al. (2008) Recent developments in the management of postmenopausal osteoporosis with bisphosphonates: enhanced efficacy by enhanced compliance. J Intern Med 264: 315–332.

9. Neer RM, Arnaud CD, Zanchetta JR, Prince R, Gaich GA, et al. (2001) Effect of parathyroid hormone (1-34) on fractures and bone mineral density in postmenopausal women with osteoporosis. N Engl J Med 344: 1434–1441.

10. Black DM, Greenspan SL, Ensrud KE, Palermo L, McGowan JA, et al. (2003) The effects of parathyroid hormone and alendronate alone or in combination in postmenopausal osteoporosis. N Engl J Med 349: 1207–1215.

11. Jodar-Gimeno E (2007) Full length parathyroid hormone (1-84) in the treatment of osteoporosis in postmenopausal women. Clin Interv Aging 2: 163–174.

12. Hodsman AB, Hanley DA, Ettinger MP, Bolognese MA, Fox J, et al. (2003) Efficacy and safety of human parathyroid hormone-(1-84) in increasing bone mineral density in postmenopausal osteoporosis. J Clin Endocrinol Metab 88: 5212–5220.

13. Adami S, Brandi ML, Canonico PL, Minisola G, Minisola S, et al. (2010) Appropriate use of anabolic treatment for severe osteoporosis. Clin Cases Miner Bone Metab 7: 114–122.

14. Moricke R, Rettig K, Bethke TD (2011) Use of recombinant human parathyroid hormone(1-84) in patients with postmenopausal osteoporosis: a prospective, open-label, single-arm, multicentre, observational cohort study of the effects of treatment on quality of life and pain–the PROPOSE study. Clin Drug Investig 31: 87–99.

15. Lyritis GP, Georgoulas T, Zafeiris CP (2010) Bone anabolic versus bone anticatabolic treatment of postmenopausal osteoporosis. Ann N Y Acad Sci 1205: 277–283.

16. Johnell O, Kanis JA, Oden A, Johansson H, De Laet C, et al. (2005) Predictive value of BMD for hip and other fractures. J Bone Miner Res 20: 1185–1194.

17. Papaioannou A, Morin S, Cheung AM, Atkinson S, Brown JP, et al. (2010) 2010 clinical practice guidelines for the diagnosis and management of osteoporosis in Canada: summary. CMAJ 182: 1864–1873.

18. Liberati A, Altman DG, Tetzlaff J, Mulrow C, Gotzsche PC, et al. (2009) The PRISMA statement for reporting systematic reviews and meta-analyses of studies that evaluate health care interventions: explanation and elaboration. PLoS Med 6: e1000100.

19. Jadad AR, Moore RA, Carroll D, Jenkinson C, Reynolds DJ, et al. (1996) Assessing the quality of reports of randomized clinical trials: is blinding necessary? Control Clin Trials 17: 1–12.

20. Finkelstein JS, Wyland JJ, Lee H, Neer RM (2010) Effects of teriparatide, alendronate, or both in women with postmenopausal osteoporosis. J Clin Endocrinol Metab 95: 1838–1845.

21. Anastasilakis AD, Goulis DG, Polyzos SA, Gerou S, Koukoulis GN, et al. (2008) Head-to-head comparison of risedronate vs. teriparatide on bone turnover markers in women with postmenopausal osteoporosis: a randomised trial. Int J Clin Pract 62: 919–924.

22. McClung MR, San Martin J, Miller PD, Civitelli R, Bandeira F, et al. (2005) Opposite bone remodeling effects of teriparatide and alendronate in increasing bone mass. Arch Intern Med 165: 1762–1768.

23. Finkelstein JS, Hayes A, Hunzelman JL, Wyland JJ, Lee H, et al. (2003) The effects of parathyroid hormone, alendronate, or both in men with osteoporosis. N Engl J Med 349: 1216–1226.

24. Body JJ, Gaich GA, Scheele WH, Kulkarni PM, Miller PD, et al. (2002) A randomized double-blind trial to compare the efficacy of teriparatide [recombinant human parathyroid hormone (1-34)] with alendronate in postmenopausal women with osteoporosis. J Clin Endocrinol Metab 87: 4528–4535.

25. Cosman F, Eriksen EF, Recknor C, Miller PD, Guanabens N, et al. (2011) Effects of intravenous zoledronic acid plus subcutaneous teriparatide [rhPTH(1-34)] in postmenopausal osteoporosis. J Bone Miner Res 26: 503–511.

26. Cosman F, Nieves J, Zion M, Woelfert L, Luckey M, et al. (2005) Daily and cyclic parathyroid hormone in women receiving alendronate. N Engl J Med 353: 566–575.

27. Saag KG, Shane E, Boonen S, Marin F, Donley DW, et al. (2007) Teriparatide or alendronate in glucocorticoid-induced osteoporosis. N Engl J Med 357: 2028–2039.

28. Nevitt MC, Chen P, Dore RK, Reginster JY, Kiel DP, et al. (2006) Reduced risk of back pain following teriparatide treatment: a meta-analysis. Osteoporos Int 17: 273–280.

29. Orwoll ES, Scheele WH, Paul S, Adami S, Syversen U, et al. (2003) The effect of teriparatide [human parathyroid hormone (1-34)] therapy on bone density in men with osteoporosis. J Bone Miner Res 18: 9–17.

30. Vestergaard P, Jorgensen NR, Mosekilde L, Schwarz P (2007) Effects of parathyroid hormone alone or in combination with antiresorptive therapy on bone mineral density and fracture risk–a meta-analysis. Osteoporos Int 18: 45–57.

31. Schneider PF, Fischer M, Allolio B, Felsenberg D, Schroder U, et al. (1999) Alendronate increases bone density and bone strength at the distal radius in postmenopausal women. J Bone Miner Res 14: 1387–1393.

32. Hirano T, Burr DB, Turner CH, Sato M, Cain RL, et al. (1999) Anabolic effects of human biosynthetic parathyroid hormone fragment (1-34), LY333334, on remodeling and mechanical properties of cortical bone in rabbits. J Bone Miner Res 14: 536–545.

33. Mashiba T, Burr DB, Turner CH, Sato M, Cain RL, et al. (2001) Effects of human parathyroid hormone (1-34), LY333334, on bone mass, remodeling, and mechanical properties of cortical bone during the first remodeling cycle in rabbits. Bone 28: 538–547.

34. Borba VZ, Manas NC (2010) The use of PTH in the treatment of osteoporosis. Arq Bras Endocrinol Metabol 54: 213–219.

35. Verhaar HJ, Lems WF (2009) PTH-analogs: comparable or different? Arch Gerontol Geriatr 49: e130–132.

36. Vahle JL, Sato M, Long GG, Young JK, Francis PC, et al. (2002) Skeletal changes in rats given daily subcutaneous injections of recombinant human parathyroid hormone (1-34) for 2 years and relevance to human safety. Toxicol Pathol 30: 312–321.

37. Black DM, Bilezikian JP, Ensrud KE, Greenspan SL, Palermo L, et al. (2005) One year of alendronate after one year of parathyroid hormone (1-84) for osteoporosis. N Engl J Med 353: 555–565.

38. Rittmaster RS, Bolognese M, Ettinger MP, Hanley DA, Hodsman AB, et al. (2000) Enhancement of bone mass in osteoporotic women with parathyroid hormone followed by alendronate. J Clin Endocrinol Metab 85: 2129–2134.

Protection by Salidroside against Bone Loss via Inhibition of Oxidative Stress and Bone-Resorbing Mediators

Jin-Kang Zhang[1,⑨], Liu Yang[1,⑨], Guo-Lin Meng[1,⑨], Zhi Yuan[1], Jing Fan[1], Dan Li[1], Jian-Zong Chen[2], Tian-Yao Shi[3], Hui-Min Hu[1], Bo-Yuan Wei[1], Zhuo-Jing Luo[1]*, Jian Liu[1]*

1 Institute of Orthopedic Surgery, Xijing Hospital, Fourth Military Medical University, Xi'an, People's Republic of China, 2 Research Center of Traditional Chinese Medicine, Xijing Hospital, Fourth Military Medical University, Xi'an, People's Republic of China, 3 Department of Pharmacology, School of Pharmacy, Fourth Military Medical University, Xi'an, People's Republic of China

Abstract

Oxidative stress is a pivotal pathogenic factor for bone loss in mouse model. Salidroside, a phenylpropanoid glycoside extracted from Rhodiola rosea L, exhibits potent antioxidative effects. In the present study, we used an in vitro oxidative stress model induced by hydrogen peroxide (H_2O_2) in MC3T3-E1 cells and a murine ovariectomized (OVX) osteoporosis model to investigate the protective effects of salidroside on bone loss and the related mechanisms. We demonstrated that salidroside caused a significant ($P<0.05$) elevation of cell survival, alkaline phosphatase (ALP) staining and activity, calcium deposition, and the transcriptional expression of *Alp*, *Col1a1* and *Osteocalcin* (*Ocn*) in the presence of H_2O_2. Moreover, salidroside decreased the production of intracellular reactive oxygen species (ROS), and osteoclast differentiation inducing factors such as receptor activator of nuclear factor-kB ligand (RANKL) and IL-6 induced by H_2O_2. In vivo studies further demonstrated that salidroside supplementation for 3 months caused a decrease in malondialdehyde (MDA) and an increase in reduced glutathione (GSH) concentration in blood of ovariectomized mouse ($P<0.05$), it also improved trabecular bone microarchitecture and bone mineral density in the fourth lumbar vertebra and distal femur. Our study indicated that the protection provided by salidroside in alleviating bone loss was mediated, at least in part, via inhibition of the release of bone-resorbing mediators and oxidative damage to bone-forming cells, suggesting that salidroside can be used as an effective remedy in the treatment or prevention of osteoporosis.

Editor: Zhongjun Zhou, The University of Hong Kong, Hong Kong

Funding: This work was supported by Ministry of Science and Technology of China (2011CB964703), National High Technology Research and Development Program 863 (2012AA020502), China Postdoctoral Science Foundation (20100480093) and National Natural Science Foundation of China (30901504). The funders had no role in study design, data collection and analysis, decision to publish, or preparation of the manuscript.

Competing Interests: The authors have declared that no competing interests exist.

* E-mail: zjk1271984@21cn.com (JL); zjluo@fmmu.edu.cn (ZJL)

⑨ These authors contributed equally to this work.

Introduction

Osteoporosis is a degenerative bone disease characterized by low bone mass and structural deterioration of bone tissue, leading to bone fragility [1]. Oxidative stress, resulting from excessive generation of reactive oxygen species, can damage all components of the cell. At present, numerous studies have shown the positive correlation between oxidative stress and osteoporotic status. For instance, in osteoporotic postmenopausal women, decreased bone mineral density was shown to be associated with higher plasma lipid oxidation [2], and catalase and glutathione peroxidase activity were found to be lowered [3,4]. Ovariectomy induces oxidative stress in rat femurs together with a decreased activity of antioxidant systems [5]. Evidence mainly obtained from the studies in mouse model provides a paradigm shift from the 'estrogen-centric' account of the pathogenesis of involutional osteoporosis to one in which age-related mechanisms intrinsic to bone and oxidative stress are protagonists, and moreover, age-related changes in other organs and tissues, such as ovaries, accentuate them [6].

Bone mass is maintained through a dynamic balance between osteoblastic bone formation and osteoclastic bone resorption [7]. Evolving evidence suggests that reactive oxygen species can enhance bone resorption by directly or indirectly promoting osteoclasts formation and activity [8]. However, it can induce apoptosis of osteoblasts and decrease their activity leading to reduced osteoblastic bone formation [9]. As a result, the imbalance between these two types of cell leads to bone metabolic diseases, such as osteoporosis. Postmenopausal osteoporosis is associated with significant changes in bone turnover: bone formation decreases and bone resorption increases or remains unchanged, leading to a net bone loss [10]. Therefore, therapeutic strategies aimed at preventing or delaying reactive oxygen species might be a reasonable choice for the treatment of osteoporosis. Recently, attention has been focused on searching for natural substances with antioxidative potential that can scavenge free radicals and protect cells from oxidative damage.

Salidroside (structure shown in Fig. 1) is an active constituent extracted from the root of Rhodiola rosea L, which has been used as a medicinal herb for a long time. Reports have existed in the literature that salidroside possesses anti-aging, anti-cancer, anti-inflammatory, anti-hypoxia and antioxidative properties [11,12,13,14]. Moreover, recent studies have shown that salidroside protects human erythrocytes against hydrogen peroxide (H_2O_2) -induced apoptosis and protects against H_2O_2-induced injury in cardiac H9c2 cells via PI3K-Akt dependent pathway [15,16]. Our previous studies revealed that salidroside protects against 1-methyl-4-phenylpyridinium (MPP+)-induced apoptosis in PC12 cells by inhibiting the NO pathway, it can also provide neuroprotective effects against focal cerebral ischemia in vivo and H_2O_2-induced neurotoxicity in vitro [17,18].

However, whether salidroside can provide protection against bone loss associated with oxidative stress remains unknown. Therefore, in this study, we used an in vitro oxidative stress model induced by H_2O_2 in MC3T3-E1 cells, which are preosteoblastic cells from mouse calvariae commonly used in studying osteogenic development [19], and an in vivo ovariectomized (OVX) osteoporosis model in mouse to investigate the protective effects of salidroside on bone loss as well as the underlying mechanisms.

Materials and Methods

Materials

Salidroside extracted from Rhodiola rosea L (purity>99%) was obtained from National Institute for the Control of Pharmaceutical and Biological Products (Beijing, China). Fetal bovine serum (FBS) and α-Modified minimal essential medium (α-MEM) were purchased from Gibco Life Technologies (Grand Island, USA). ALP activity assay kit was purchased from GENMED scientific Inc. (USA). RANKL and IL-6 ELISA kit were purchased from R&D system Inc. (Minneapolis, MN, USA). PrimeScript RT reagent kit and SYBR Premix Ex Taq were obtained from TaKaRa Biotechnology (Dalian, China). Oligonucleotide primers were synthesized by Sangon Biological Engineering Technology Co. (Shanghai, China). BCIP/NBT Alkaline Phosphatase Color Development Kit,RIPA Lysis Buffer, Reactive Oxygen Species Assay Kit, GSH and MDA Assay kit were purchased from the Beyotime Institute of Biotechnology (Shanghai, China). All other chemicals and reagents were of analytical grade.

Cell culture

Murine osteoblastic MC3T3-E1 cells were obtained from the Center Laboratory for Tissue Engineering, College of Stomatology, Fourth Military Medical University, Xi'an, China [20,21]. MC3T3-E1 cells were maintained in a-MEM with 10% heat-inactivated FBS and 100 U/ml penicillin and 100μg/ml streptomycin under conditions of 5% CO_2 and 37°C. H_2O_2 was used as the exogenous ROS source, and N-acetyl-L-cysteine (NAC) was used as an ROS scavenger. When reaching confluence, MC3T3-E1 cells were treated with culture medium containing 10 mM β-glycerophosphate and 50μg/ml ascorbic acid to initiate differentiation. After 6 or 14 days, the cells were pre-incubated with serum-free regular culture medium containing salidroside for 24 h before treatment with 300μM H_2O_2 for another 24 h. In all the experiments, salidroside treatment continued after the pretreatment. Each experiment was performed in duplicate wells and repeated three times.

Assays of cell viability

In the experiments, cells were treated with different concentrations of H_2O_2 (0, 100, 200, 300, 400μM) for 2, 6, 12, 24h or salidroside (0, 0.1, 1, 10μM) for 24, 72h to investigate the toxicity of H_2O_2 and salidroside. Then, cells were cultured with serum-free regular culture medium containing salidroside (0, 0.1, 1, 10μM) for 24 h followed by treatment with 300μM H_2O_2 for 24 h. Cell viability was measured by MTT assay. In brief, 0.02 ml MTT solution was added to each well and the plates were incubated at 37 °C for 4 h. Then DMSO was added and the plates were shaken for 5 min to dissolve formazan products. The absorbance of each well was recorded on a microplate reader at a wavelength of 492 nm. Cell viability of the control group not exposed to either H_2O_2 or salidroside was defined as 100%.

Alkaline phosphatase (ALP) staining and activity assay

After 6 days, the cells were cultured with serum-free medium containing salidroside and/or H_2O_2 for 2 days. At harvesting, cells were washed twice with phosphate-buffered saline (PBS), fixed with 10% formalin in PBS for 30 s, rinsed with deionized water, and stained with BCIP/NBT Alkaline Phosphatase Color Development Kit under protection from direct light. To measure ALP activity, the cell monolayer was lysed with RIPA. The lysate was centrifuged at 10,000×g for 5 min. The clear supernatant was used to measure the ALP activity, which was determined using an ALP activity assay kit. Total protein concentrations were determined by Bradford protein assay method. ALP activity was normalized to total protein measured with the Bradford protein assay method.

Calcium deposition assay

After 14 days, the cells were cultured with serum-free medium containing salidroside and/or H_2O_2 for 2 days. At harvesting, the cells were fixed in ice-cold 10% formalin for 20 min and stained with 40 mM Alizarin Red S (pH 4.4, Sigma) for 45 min at room temperature. For matrix calcification estimate, the stain was solubilized with 10% cetylpyridinum chloride by shaking for 15 min. The absorbance of the released Alizarin red S was measured at the wave length of 562 nm [22].

Quantitative real-time PCR

After 6 days, the cells were cultured with serum-free medium containing salidroside and/or H_2O_2 for 2 days. Total cellular RNA was extracted using the Trizol reagent according to the manufacturer's instructions (OMEGA). Single strand cDNA synthesis was performed by using PrimeScript RT reagent kit (TaKaRa). Real-time quantitative RT-PCR was performed using the CFX96 (BIO-RAD) instrument and individual PCRs were carried out in 96-well optical reaction plates with SYBR Green-I (TaKaRa) in accordance with the manufacturer's instructions. Briefly, PCR was carried out in a 25-μl final volume containing the following reagents: 12.5 μl of 2× SYBR Green-I master mix, 1 μl of 10 μM each primer, 2.5 μl of 1 μg/μl cDNA template, and 8 μl

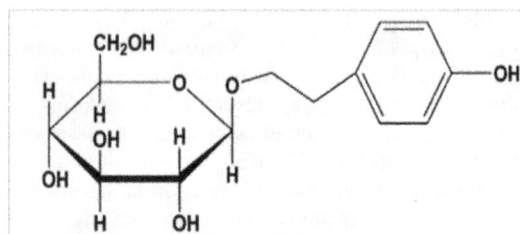

Figure 1. Chemical structure of salidroside.

of double deionized water. PCR conditions were as follows: initial denaturation at 95°C for 30 s, followed by 40 cycles of denaturation at 95°C for 5 s, and annealing at 58°C for 15 s. Fluorescent product was measured by a single acquisition mode at 58°C after each cycle. Target genes (*Alp*, *Col1a1*, *Osteocalcin* (*Ocn*)) expression was normalized to the reference gene β-actin. The $2^{-\Delta\Delta Ct}$ method was applied to calculate relative gene expression. The PCR products were subjected to melting curve analysis and standard curve to confirm the correct amplification. All the RT-PCRs were performed in triplicates and the primers used for PCR are listed in Table 1.

Measurement of RANKL and IL-6

After 6 days, the cells were cultured with serum-free medium containing salidroside and/or H_2O_2 for 2 days. RANKL and IL-6 contents in culture medium were measured using sandwich ELISA assay kit, according to the manufacturer's recommendation. Total protein concentrations were determined by Bradford protein assay method.

Measurement of intracellular ROS

The level of intracellular ROS was quantified using Reactive Oxygen Species Assay Kit. DCFH-DA is oxidized by ROS in viable cells to 2′,7′-dichlorofluorescein (DCF) which is highly fluorescent at 530 nm. The cells were washed three times with PBS. DCFH-DA, diluted to a final concentration of 10 μM, was added and incubated for 30 min at 37°C in the dark. After being washed three times with PBS, the relative levels of fluorescence were quantified using a multi-detection microplate reader (485 nm excitation and 535 nm emission).

Animals and salidroside treatments

Thirty-two 9-week-old and weighing 20.3 ± 1.34 g BALB/c female mice were purchased from the Experimental Animal Center of The Fourth Military Medical University (Xi'an, China) and were acclimated to laboratory conditions for 1 week before the experiment. The initial body weight of the mice was no significant difference among the four groups in this study. They were maintained in a well-ventilated controlled room at 20°C on a 12-h light/dark cycle with free access to water and food. Mice underwent sham-operation (n = 8) or were surgically ovariectomized (OVX; n = 24) under anesthesia by pentobarbital sodium (50 mg/kg body weight, i.p.). OVX was performed by removing the bilateral ovaries through a dorsal approach and sham surgery was performed by identifying the bilateral ovaries. The mice were randomly divided into four groups: (1) untreated (Sham: sham-operated controls); (2) untreated (OVX controls); (3) OVX administered intraperitoneally with salidroside (5 mg/kg body weight) daily; (4) OVX administered intraperitoneally with salidroside (20 mg/kg body weight) daily. Salidroside were

Table 1. Real-time PCR primers for amplification of specific MC3T3-E1 mRNA.

Gene	Forward (5′-3′)	Reverse (5′-3′)
Alp	aacccagacacaagcattcc	ccagcaagaagaagcctttg
Col1a1	gcatggccaagaagacatcc	cctcgggtttccacgtctc
Ocn	ctgacaaagccttcatgtccaa	gcgccggagtctgttcacta
β-actin	ctggcaccacacacacttctaca	ggtacgaccagaggcataca

dissolved in distilled water and distilled water alone was administered to untreated mice. The treatments started 1week after the surgery and lasted for 15 weeks. Blood samples were taken from the heart in anesthetized mice and serum was then prepared by centrifugation. The left femur and the 4 th lumbar vertebra (L4) from each mouse were removed and cleaned of adherent tissue. All experimental procedures in animals were approved by the Ethics in Animal Research Committee of the Fourth Military Medical University (permission code 2010C00843).

Measurements of serum reduced glutathione (GSH) and malondialdehyde (MDA)

The GSH in whole blood samples were determined using a GSH Assay kit following the manufacturer's instructions. Determination of GSH is based on the reaction of GSH with 5.50-dithiobis-2-nitrobenzoic acid (DTNB) to form a product that can be detected by a spectrophotometer at 412 nm. The MDA in whole blood samples were determined using a Lipid peroxidation MDA Assay Kit following the manufacturer's instructions. The binding of thiobarbituric acid to MDA which was formed during lipid peroxidation results in a chromogenic complex.

Bone microarchitecture assessment by micro-computed tomography

Bone microarchitecture in the 4 th lumbar vertebra (L4) and distal femur was scanned using explore Locus SP Pre-Clinical Specimen micro-computed tomography (GE Healthcare, USA) with 8-μm resolution, tube voltage of 50 kV and tube current of 0.1 mA. The reconstruction and 3D quantitative analyses were performed by using software provided by a desktop micro-CT system (GE Healthcare, USA). The same settings for scan and analysis were used for all samples. In the femora, scanning regions were confined to the distal metaphysis, extending proximally 2.0 mm from the proximal tip of the primary spongiosa. Trabecular bone region from the vertebral body was outlined for each micro-CT slice, excluding both the cranial and caudal endplate regions. Within these regions, trabecular bone was separated from cortical bone with boundaries defined by the endocortical bone surfaces. The following 3D indices in the defined region of interest (ROI) were analyzed: relative bone volume over total volume (BV/TV, %), trabecular number (Tb.N), trabecular separation (Tb.Sp), trabecular thickness (Tb.Th), connectivity density (Conn.D), structure model index (SMI) and bone mineral density (BMD).The operator conducting the scan analysis was blinded to the treatments associated with the specimens.

Undecalcified histological examination

The left femur of each mouse was collected and fixed in 4% paraformaldehyde for 48 hours. All samples were dehydrated in graded alcohols and embedded in polymethyl-methacrylate (PMMA). The distal femurs were cut into sections of 5 and 240μm in thickness in the coronal plane on a rotation microtome. The 5μm sections were stained with Von kossa staining to visualize calcium deposition and 240μm sections were hand grounded to a thickness of 20μm for Van Gieson staining, which is used to stain collagen fiber.

Statistical analysis

Data were expressed as means ± S.D. of multiple repeats of the same experiment (n = 5). The data for these measurements were analyzed with one-way analysis of variance (ANOVA) with subsequent post hoc multiple comparison by Dunnett's test. Statistically significant values defined as $P<0.05$.

Results

Protective effect of salidroside on H_2O_2 induced cytotoxicity in MC3T3-E1 cells

Cell viability was analyzed to determine the protective effect of salidroside on the response of MC3T3-E1 cells to oxidative stress induced by H_2O_2. As shown in Fig.2A, 100 to 400μM of H_2O_2 induced significant decrease in cell survival in a dose- and time-dependent manner. In the group treated with 300 μM H_2O_2 for 24 h, cell viability was significantly decreased by approximately 50% as compared with the control group($P<0.01$). Therefore, the treatment of 300 μM H_2O_2 for 24 h was used to induce MC3T3-E1 cell injury in subsequent experiments. As shown in Fig. 2B, salidroside alone was non-toxic to cells at the concentrations used in this study ($P>0.05$). When the cells were pretreated with salidroside for 24 h before the addition of H_2O_2 (300μM) for 24 h, salidroside (0.1~10μM) significantly increased the survival of MC3T3-E1 cells as compared to H_2O_2 alone treated cells ($P<0.05$), suggesting that salidroside suppressed H_2O_2 induced cytotoxicity (Fig. 2C). NAC, which significantly inhibited H_2O_2–induced cytotoxicity at 1mM as a potent antioxidant, was used here serving as a positive control.

Protective effect of salidroside on osteoblast dysfunction induced by H_2O_2

In order to assess the effect of salidroside on osteoblast dysfunction induced by H_2O_2, ALP staining and activity, calcium deposition and osteogenic differentiation genes (*Alp, Col1a1, Ocn*) were determined. Compared with the control cells, the presence of H_2O_2 significantly decreased cellular ALP activity, mineralization and expression of osteogenic differentiation genes (Fig.3). When osteoblasts were pretreated with salidroside in the presence of H_2O_2, salidroside (0.1-10μM) significantly increased cellular ALP activity, which is one of the major osteoblast differentiation markers (Fig. 3B). We further investigated the effect of salidroside on mineralization in the presence of H_2O_2 by measuring calcium deposition by Alizarin Red staining. As shown in Fig. 3C, salidroside (0.1–1μM) showed significant recovery effect on mineralization inhibited by H_2O_2. Moreover, salidroside supplementation significantly enhanced the expression of osteogenic differentiation genes (*Alp, Col1a1, Ocn*) compared with the group treated with H_2O_2 alone (Fig. 3D). Our results demonstrated that salidroside attenuates osteoblast dysfunction induced by H_2O_2.

Inhibition of salidroside on RANKL and IL-6 production of MC3T3-E1 cells in the presence of H_2O_2

In order to determine the possible regulation of osteoclast differentiation by osteoblasts, we examined the production of RANKL and IL-6, which are primarily released from osteoblast cells. Osteoblast-derived RANKL binds to RANK on osteoclasts, resulting in osteoclast activation, and IL-6 have also been demonstrated to increase osteoclastic activity. When 0.3 mM H_2O_2 was added to the cells, the production of RANKL and IL-6 increased significantly. However, H_2O_2-induced RANKL and IL-6 production was significantly inhibited by pretreatment of salidroside at concentrations of 0.1–10μM and 0.1–1μM, respectively (Fig.4).

Salidroside reduces the production of ROS induced by H_2O_2

To investigate whether cell-protective action of salidroside is related to its antioxidant activity, the production of ROS detected by fluorescent probe DCFH-DA was assessed. As shown in Fig. 5, the production of ROS was increased significantly by treatment of 0.3 mM H_2O_2. These results suggest that H_2O_2 enhanced oxidant generation and may cause damage to osteoblastic MC3T3-E1 cells. However, the production of ROS was significantly inhibited when pretreated with salidroside at concentrations of 0.1–10μM (Fig.5). These data support the hypothesis that the cytoprotective effect offered by salidroside may be associated with its antioxidant capacity.

Inhibition of salidroside on oxidative status in serum

Serum MDA and GSH levels are potential biomarkers for measurement of oxidative stress. As shown in Fig. 6, serum MDA level was increased and GSH level was decreased in OVX mice when compared with sham groups ($P<0.05$). Salidroside supplementation (20 mg/kg) significantly decreased serum MDA concentrations and increased GSH level ($P<0.05$). No differences in MDA and GSH levels were observed in OVX mice treated with different concentrations of salidroside ($P>0.05$).

Protective effect of salidroside against bone loss in OVX mice

We administered salidroside as early as 7 days after ovariectomy to evaluate its effects on trabecular bone microarchitecture. We sacrificed all the animals 16 weeks after the operation. No significant difference in body weight of the mice in four groups was noted. The analysis of the properties of trabecular bone in distal femoral metaphyses and lumber vertebrate (L4) indicated that ovariectomy induced deterioration of the trabecular bone microarchitecture in mice, as demonstrated by the reduction in BV/TV, Conn.D, Tb.N, Tb.Th and BMD when compared with the sham group mice ($P<0.01$) (Table 2). In contrast, as shown in Table 2, SMI and Tb.Sp were significantly increased in response to OVX ($P<0.05$ for both). However, treating OVX mice with a high dose of salidroside at 20 mg/kg could significantly ($P<0.05$) reverse the changes in these parameters induced by ovariectomy and could maintain the microarchitecture of trabecular bone in distal femoral metaphyses and lumber vertebrate (L4).These increments in trabecular bone parameters were readily observable in micro-CT images of the distal femur (Fig. 7). Salidroside at 5 mg/kg improved the trabecular bone mass loss and microarchitecture deterioration, but no significant difference was noticed ($P>0.05$) when compared with the OVX group. Van Gieson and Von Kossa staining also showed similar results (Fig. 8). Compared with the sham group, the trabecular number was reduced and spaces between trabecules were broader in the OVX groups. Salidroside supplementation inhibited these deleterious effects, as demonstrated by an increase in the trabecular number and a decrease in the trabecular space in the OVX+salidroside groups (Fig. 8).

Discussion

Oxidative stress is characterized by an increased level of reactive oxygen species (ROS) that disrupts the intracellular reduction–oxidation (redox) balance. Numerous studies have suggested that increased oxidative stress is involved in the pathogenesis of osteoporosis, caused by aging and estrogen deficiency [23,24]. H_2O_2 is generated from nearly all sources of oxidative stress and has been demonstrated to play a crucial role in estrogen deficiency osteoporosis [25]. Therefore, we used H_2O_2-induced oxidative

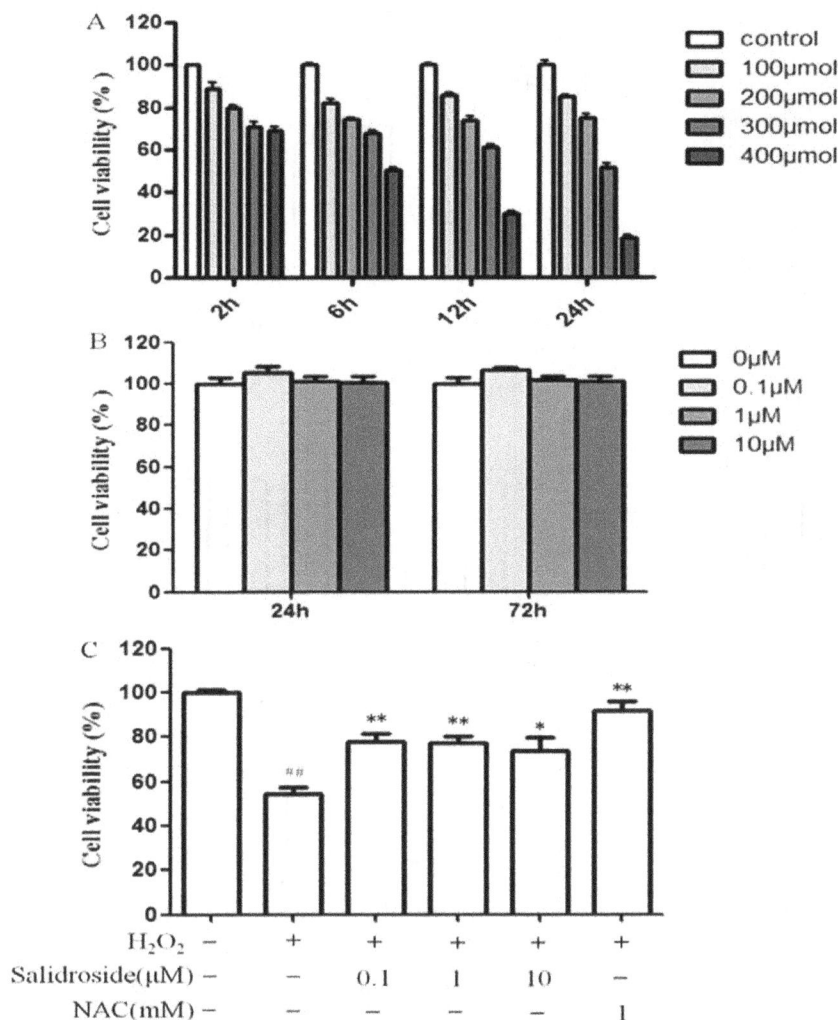

Figure 2. Protective effect of salidroside on H_2O_2 induced cytotoxicity in MC3T3-E1 cells. A: Concentration- and time-dependent effects of H_2O_2 on cell viability. B: Cells were incubated in different concentrations of salidroside alone. C: Cells were pretreated with salidroside for 24 h before treatment with 0.3 mM H_2O_2 for 24 h. NAC was used as positive control. The control value for cell viability was 0.431±0.05 OD. ##$P<0.01$ versus untreated control cells; *$P<0.05$ and **$P<0.01$ compared with the group treated with H_2O_2 alone.

stress model in the present study. Fatokun reported that exposure of MC3T3-E1 cells to a concentration of at least 0.2 mM H_2O_2 for 1 h was required to produce significant lethality involving both apoptosis and necrosis [26].Our results showed that H_2O_2 substantially reduced cell viability in a dose-dependent manner, but the toxic effect was reversed to some degree when pretreated with different concentrations of salidroside for 24 h. Our previous studies revealed that salidroside protects against (MPP+)-induced apoptosis in PC12 cells, it can provide neuroprotective effects against focal cerebral ischemia in vivo and H_2O_2-induced neurotoxicity in vitro [17,18]. The present study indicated that salidroside reduced the cytotoxicity induced by H_2O_2 in osteoblastic MC3T3-E1 cells.

Apart from affecting cell viability, oxidative stress also influences osteoblast differentiation. Liu et al. showed that H_2O_2 induced oxidative stress and suppressed the osteoblastic differentiation in primary mouse BMSCs [27]. This inhibition of cell differentiation was characterized by a reduction in ALP activity, which is an early differentiation marker and is important to regulate mineralization of bone matrix [28]. Subsequently, Bai et al. reported that H_2O_2-treated osteoblasts exhibited a reduction in levels of differentiation

markers including *Alp*, *Co1a1*, colony-forming unit-osteoprogenitor (CFU-O) formation, and nuclear phosphorylation of the transcription factor *Runx2* [29]. More recently, it was indicated that H_2O_2 diminished mineralization and decreased the expression of osteogenic genes *Runx2*, *Alp* and bone sialoprotein in MC3T3-E1cells [30]. The present study has demonstrated that H_2O_2 significantly decreased cellular ALP activity, mineralization and expression of osteogenic differentiation genes *Alp*, *Col1a1* and *Ocn*, which confirms the previous observations that H_2O_2 toxicity leads to dysfunction of osteoblasts. Meanwhile, we found that the inhibition induced by H_2O_2 of osteogenic differentiation can be reversed by salidroside. According to our unpublished date, salidroside alone could not improve the proliferation and osteogenic differentiation of MC3T3-E1 cells significantly within the observed concentration. Therefore, we deduced that the protection of salidroside may mainly contribute to its antioxidant ability, suggesting that salidroside may be a beneficial agent in preventing osteoporosis associated with oxidative stress by enhancing osteoblast function.

Osteoblasts are coupled with osteoclasts in terms of the release of various bone-resorbing cytokines, such as receptor activator of

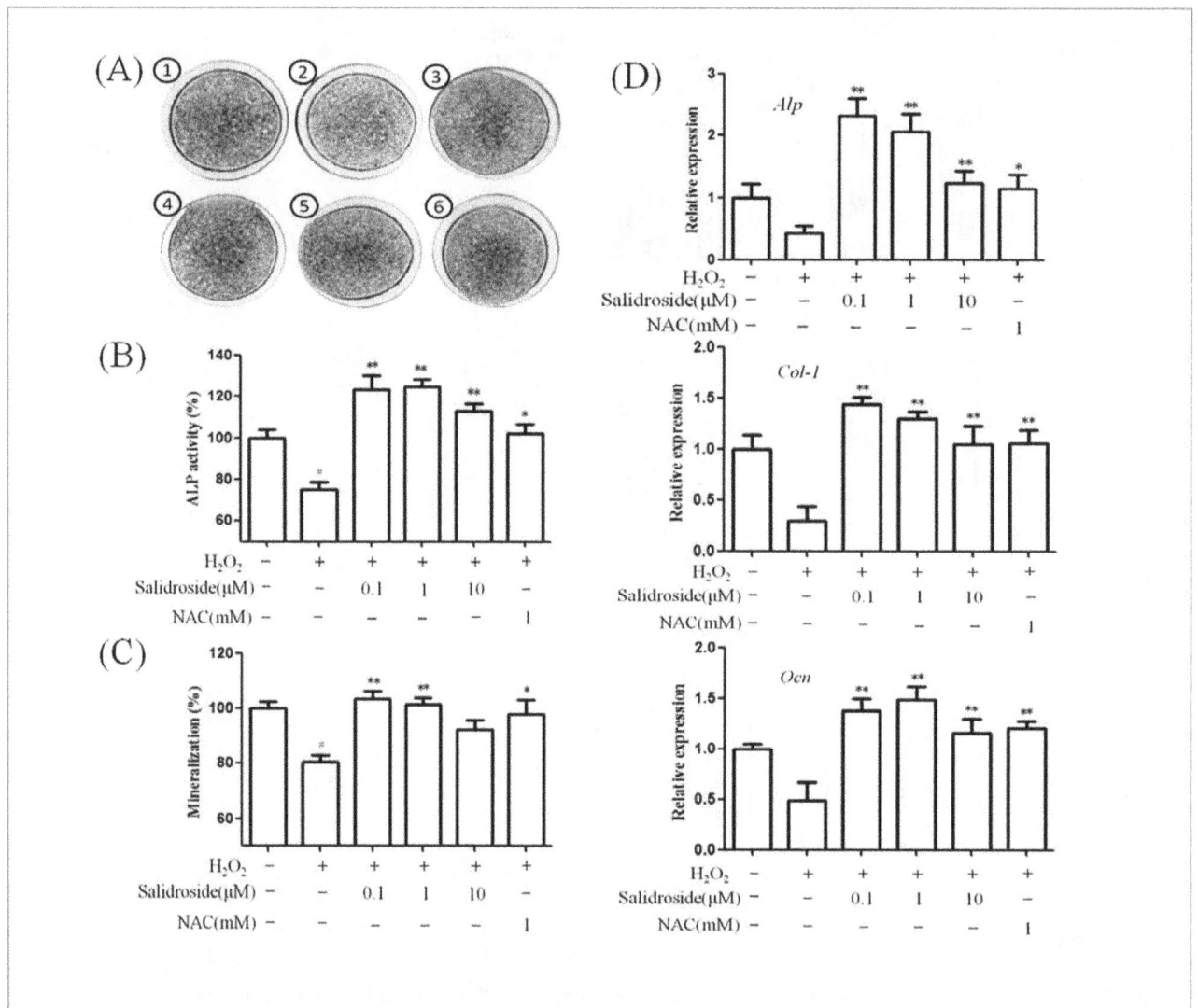

Figure 3. Protective effect of salidroside on H₂O₂ induced osteoblast dysfunction. After differentiation induction of 6 or 14 days, MC3T3-E1 cells were pretreated with salidroside for 24 h before treatment with 0.3 mM H₂O₂ for 24 h. NAC was used as positive control. A: Effect of salidroside on the ALP staining of MC3T3-E1 cells in the presence of H₂O₂. ① the control group; ② H₂O₂; ③ H₂O₂+ salidroside (0.1μM); ④ H₂O₂+ salidroside (1μM); ⑤ H₂O₂+ salidroside (10μM); ⑥ H₂O₂+NAC(1 mM). B: Effect of salidroside on the ALP activity of MC3T3-E1 cells in the presence of H₂O₂. The control value for ALP activity was 0.682 ± 0.021 unit /μg protein. C: Effect of salidroside on the mineralization of MC3T3-E1 cells in the presence of H₂O₂. The control value for mineralization was 1.392±0.31 OD. D: Effect of salidroside on the mRNA expression of Alp, Col-1 and Ocn in the presence of H₂O₂. #P<0.05 versus untreated control cells;*P<0.05 and **P<0.01 compared with the group treated with H₂O₂ alone.

nuclear factor (NFκB) ligand (RANKL) and IL-6. RANKL, highly expressed on osteoblasts, marrow stromal cells and T cells, is an essential cytokine involved in osteoclastogenesis. RANKL acts by binding to the RANK receptor on osteoclast progenitor cells, leading to expression of osteoclast differentiation genes, prolonged survival of osteoclasts and increased bone resorption [31]. RANKL is prevented by osteoprotegerin (OPG), a soluble decoy receptor that competes with RANK for binding to RANKL and is also expressed by osteoblasts [32]. Bai et al. reported that ROS stimulates RANKL expression in mouse osteoblasts and human MG63 cells [33]. IL-6 was also reported to be produced by osteoblasts [34] and can induce RANKL mRNA expression, promote the differentiation of osteoclasts from its precursor and play an important role in the pathogenesis of osteoporosis due to estrogen deficiency [35,36]. ROS might indirectly stimulate osteoclasts by augmenting expression of resorptive cytokines such

as RANKL, TNF-α and IL-6 that have been strongly implicated in estrogen deficiency bone loss [37]. In this study, salidroside inhibited the production of RANKL and IL-6 induced by H₂O₂ in osteoblastic cells. The inhibitory effect on RANKL and IL-6 production may contribute to bone anti-resorbing effect of salidroside, and may play a role in the reduction of bone loss.

Reactive oxygen species (ROS) such as superoxides anions, hydroxyl radicals, and H₂O₂ can cause severe damage to DNA, protein, and lipids [38]. High levels of oxidant produced during normal cellular metabolism or from environmental stimuli perturb the normal redox balance and shift cells into a state of oxidative stress. Accumulating evidence suggests that ROS may play its role in bone loss-related diseases in two ways: suppression of bone formation and stimulation of bone resorption. Salidroside is extracted from Rhodiola rosea L, which is one of Chinese traditional medicine, has been reported to possess antioxidative

A
B

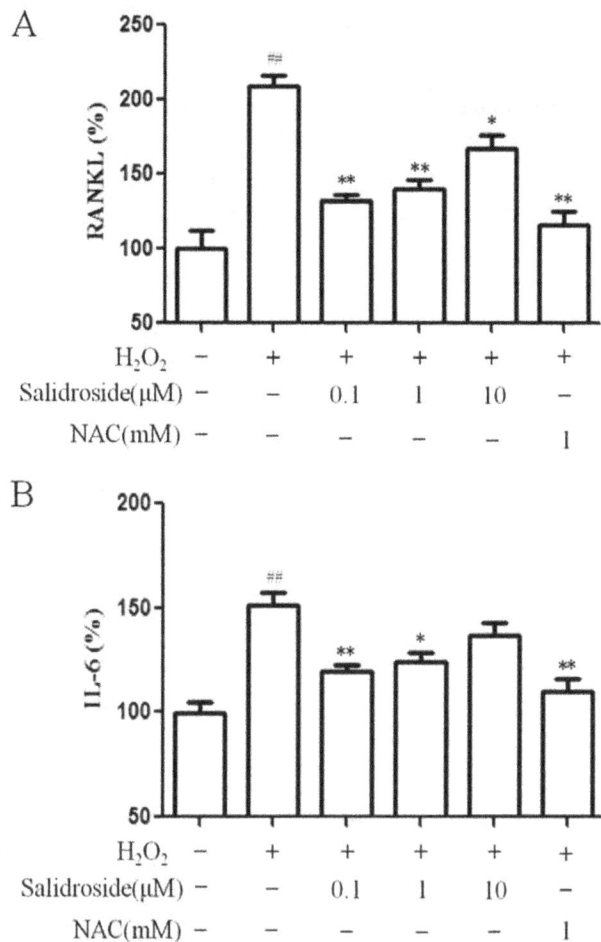

Figure 4. Inhibition of salidroside on RANKL and IL-6 production of MC3T3-E1 cells in the presence of H₂O₂. After differentiation induction of 6 days, MC3T3-E1 cells were pretreated with salidroside for 24 h before treatment with 0.3 mM H₂O₂ for 24 h. NAC was used as positive control. A: The production of RANKL in the presence of salidroside and/or H₂O₂. The control value for RANKL was 3.792 ± 0.271ng/mg. B: The production of IL-6 in the presence of salidroside and/or H₂O₂. The control value for IL-6 was 0.429 ± 0.391 ng/mg. $^{\#\#}P<0.01$ versus untreated control cells;$^{*}P<0.05$ and $^{**}P<0.01$ compared with the group treated with H₂O₂ alone.

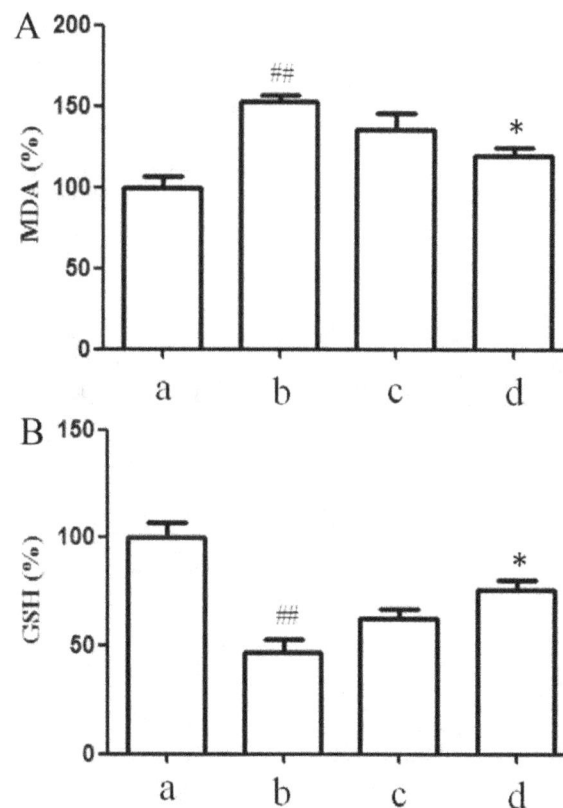

Figure 5. Inhibition of salidroside on reactive oxygen species generation induced by H₂O₂ in MC3T3-E1 cells. After differentiation induction of 6 days, MC3T3-E1 cells were pretreated with salidroside for 24 h before treatment with 0.3 mM H₂O₂ for 24 h. NAC was used as positive control. The data shows changes in levels of ROS, which was measured by DCF fluorescence method. $^{\#\#}P<0.01$ versus untreated control cells;$^{*}P<0.05$ and $^{**}P<0.01$ compared with the group treated with H₂O₂ alone.

Figure 6. Inhibition of salidroside on oxidative status in serum of ovariectomized mice. A: Serum MDA concentrations in ovariectomized mice supplemented with different concentration of salidroside. B: Serum GSH concentrations in ovariectomized mice supplemented with different concentration of salidroside. a: sham; b: OVX; c: OVX+salidroside (5 mg/kg); d: OVX+salidroside (20 mg/kg). The control value for MDA and GSH was 7.692 ± 0.928 nM/mg and 13.24 ± 1.391 nM/mg.$^{\#\#}P<0.01$ versus sham group;$^{*}P<0.05$ compared with OVX group.

properties [14]. In the present study, pretreatment with salidroside for 24 h could reverse the production of ROS induced by H₂O₂ to some degree. Therefore, the results of the present study demonstrated that salidroside can act as a biological antioxidant and protect cells from oxidative stress-induced toxicity. Accordingly, the protective effect provided by salidroside to osteoblastic MC3T3-E1 cells might be mediated, at least in part, via its antioxidant ability.

Protection against oxidative stress is a possible mechanism explaining salidroside's beneficial effects. However, there is a paucity of knowledge regarding its molecular mode of action. We speculated that it may degrade H₂O₂ directly, elevate the endogenous antioxidant defenses or through ROS-irrelevant mechanisms. Wiegant et al. reported that Rhodiola rosea L. could increase expression of hemeoxygenase-1 (HO-1), a protein that can be activated by the antioxidant-response element (ARE) in response to oxidative challenge [39]. ARE is a *cis*-acting enhancer element in the 5′flanking region of the cytoprotective enzymes.

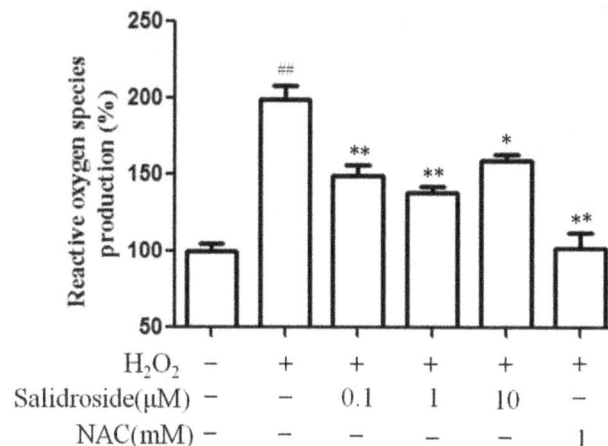

Table 2. Effect of salidroside on bone microarchitecture indices in mice measured by Micro-CT.

Indices	Sham	OVX	OVX+salidroside(5)	OVX+salidroside(20)
Distal femur				
BV/TV (%)	0.107±0.029	0.031±0.004##	0.041±0.002*	0.073±0.011**
Tb.Th. (mm)	0.032±0.003	0.021±0.002##	0.025±0.002	0.028±0.004*
Tb.N. (1/mm)	3.59±0.331	1.441±0.111##	1.762±0.136	2.96±0.433**
Tb.Sp. (mm)	0.250±0.024	0.676±0.053##	0.579±0.048*	0.317±0.047**
Conn.D (1/mm^3)	107.004±15.928	32.739±9.391##	45.551±7.697	66.516±10.429**
SMI	2.346±0.079	3.299±0.249##	2.925±0.187**	2.658±0.143**
BMD (mg/cm^3)	213.043±22.29	120.028±14.94##	139.135±20.283	161.576±27.259**
Lumbar vertebra				
BV/TV (%)	0.189±0.562	0.093±0.031##	0.128±0.007**	0.145±0.081**
Tb.Th. (mm)	0.049±0.015	0.028±0.007##	0.036±0.011	0.043±0.009*
Tb.N. (1/mm)	4.753±1.427	2.897±0.678#	3.745±1.087	4.054±0.873
Tb.Sp. (mm)	0.184±0.065	0.365±0.083##	0.277±0.088	0.218±0.053*
Conn.D (1/mm^3)	154.732±17.973	68.537±12.338##	85.447±13.46	119.781±15.749**
SMI	1.649±0.183	2.524±0.12##	2.171±0.21**	1.867±0.159**
BMD (mg/cm^3)	183.984±20.14	92.661±15.592##	121.059±26.827	143.759±22.349*

Data were expressed as means ± S.D., n=8 in each group.
#$P<0.05$ and ##$P<0.01$vs. the sham group.
*$P<0.05$ and **$P<0.01$vs. the OVX group.

This element regulates many antioxidant enzymes including the glutathione S-transferases, HO-1 and NQO1, and its activation by transcription factor nuclear erythroid-2 related factor-2 (Nrf-2) confers a resistance to oxidative damage. Salidroside is an active constituent extracted from Rhodiola rosea L. Therefore, we speculate that salidroside provided protection effects against H_2O_2-induced cytotoxicity and osteoblast dysfunction in MC3T3-E1 cells may through the HO-1 and Nrf-2 signaling pathways. We will confirm this molecular mechanism in the further study.

The mechanisms through which estrogen deficiency stimulates bone loss remain controversial. Recently, oxidative stress has been suggested to be responsible for the development of postmenopausal osteoporosis. Serum MDA levels is one of the potential

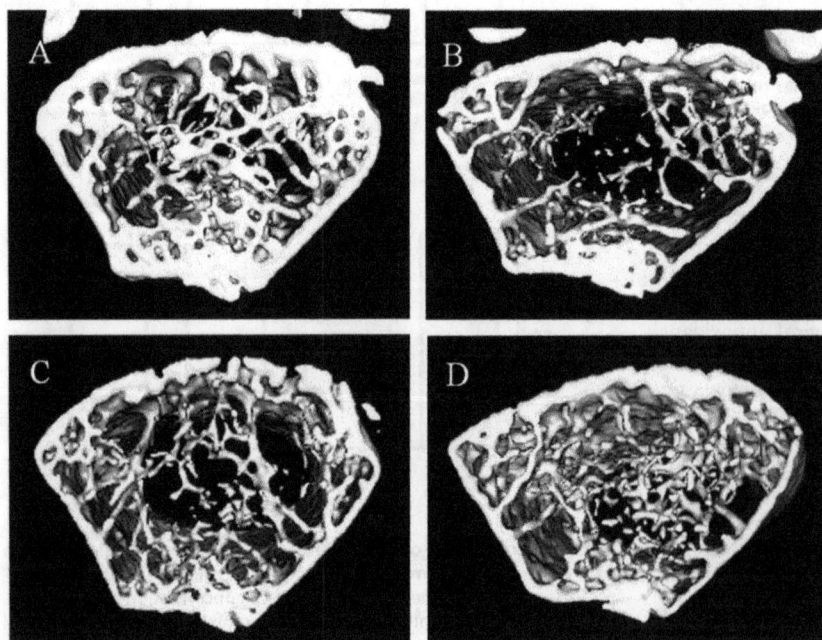

Figure 7. Analysis of micro-computed tomography within the distal metaphyseal femur region. A: sham, B: OVX, C: OVX+salidroside(5 mg/kg), D: OVX+salidroside(20 mg/kg).

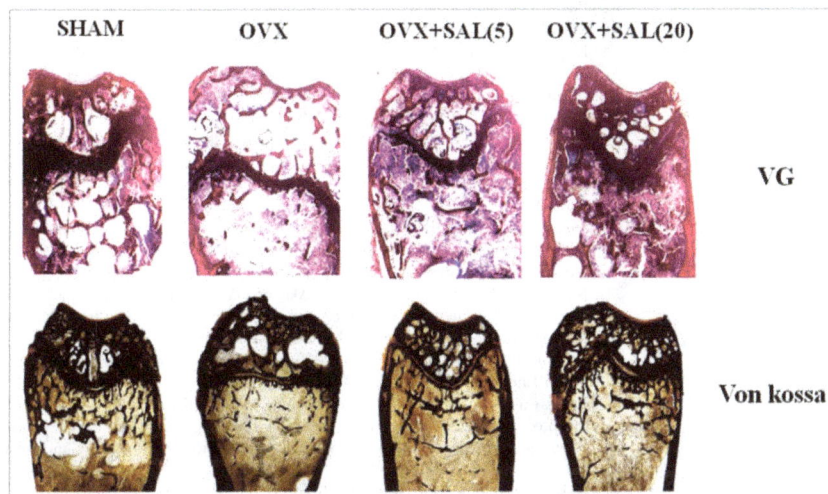

Figure 8. Van Gieson (VG) and Von Kossa (Silver nitrate) staining of the distal femur. The figure was 40× of the original section.

biomarkers for oxidative stress [40]. Lipid peroxides (MDA) is the end product of lipid peroxidation caused by ROS. It can cause increased cell membrane permeability [41]. Reduced glutathione is one of the most important reducer agents which maintain the intracellular redox balance [42]. Decrease of GSH level is also a marker for oxidative stress [43]. In our study, salidroside treatment for 3 months prevented the increased serum MDA level and decreased GSH level resulting from OVX. Our results indicated that salidroside could improve the oxidative status in estrogen deficient osteoporosis model. Bone quality is determined by microarchitecture, geometry and material properties of the bone. Measuring such microarchitectural parameters as BV/TV, Tb.N, Tb.Sp, Tb.Th, Conn.D, SMI and BMD may improve our ability to estimate bone strength [44,45]. The effects of ovariectomy on bone are smaller in cortical compartments than in trabecular compartments [46].Therefore, we observed the effect of salidro-side on trabecular microarchitecture by scanning with Micro-CT. All parameters, such as BMD, BV/TV, Tb.N, and Tb.Sp, showed that salidroside treatment with 20 mg/kg for 3 months improved bone structural indices, bone mineral density and trabecular thickness compromised by OVX. Meanwhile, histological exam-ination also showed that ovariectomy had negative effects on the microarchitecture of the trabecular bone. However, this effect could be reversed by supplementation of salidroside to some degree. These data implied that salidroside may significantly increase trabecular bone mass in ovariectomized mouse model and salidroside has a therapeutic effect in prevention of estrogen-deficient osteoporosis.

In conclusion, our studies demonstrated that salidroside protects MC3T3-E1 cells from H_2O_2-induced cell damage and dysfunction of osteoblasts via inhibition of oxidative stress and bone-resorbing mediators. Moreover, salidroside reduces the oxidative status in serum and prevents bone loss and deterioration of trabecular microarchitecture in OVX-induced osteoporosis mouse model. Our results suggest that salidroside could be used as a good candidate for preventing and treating osteoporosis. Further investigation is required in order to clarify the detailed molecular mechanisms of action of salidroside in bone.

Acknowledgments

We would like to thank Jun Wang from the institute of orthopedic surgery in Xijing hospital for Micro-CT scanning and analysis.

Author Contributions

Conceived and designed the experiments: JZ ZJL JL. Performed the experiments: JKZ LY GLM ZY JF. Analyzed the data: JZC HMH BYW. Contributed reagents/materials/analysis tools: TYS DL. Wrote the paper: JKZ LY.

References

1. (2001) Osteoporosis prevention, diagnosis, and therapy. JAMA 285: 785–795.
2. Sendur OF, Turan Y, Tastaban E, Serter M (2009) Antioxidant status in patients with osteoporosis: a controlled study. Joint Bone Spine 76: 514–518.
3. Ozgocmen S, Kaya H, Fadillioglu E, Aydogan R, Yilmaz Z (2007) Role of antioxidant systems, lipid peroxidation, and nitric oxide in postmenopausal osteoporosis. Mol Cell Biochem 295: 45–52.
4. Ozgocmen S, Kaya H, Fadillioglu E, Yilmaz Z (2007) Effects of calcitonin, risedronate, and raloxifene on erythrocyte antioxidant enzyme activity, lipid peroxidation, and nitric oxide in postmenopausal osteoporosis. Arch Med Res 38: 196–205.
5. Muthusami S, Ramachandran I, Muthusamy B, Vasudevan G, Prabhu V, et al. (2005) Ovariectomy induces oxidative stress and impairs bone antioxidant system in adult rats. Clin Chim Acta 360: 81–86.
6. Manolagas SC (2010) From estrogen-centric to aging and oxidative stress: a revised perspective of the pathogenesis of osteoporosis. Endocr Rev 31: 266–300.
7. Seeman E, Delmas PD (2006) Bone quality--the material and structural basis of bone strength and fragility. N Engl J Med 354: 2250–2261.

8. Lee NK, Choi YG, Baik JY, Han SY, Jeong DW, et al. (2005) A crucial role for reactive oxygen species in RANKL-induced osteoclast differentiation. Blood 106: 852–859.
9. Arai M, Shibata Y, Pugdee K, Abiko Y, Ogata Y (2007) Effects of reactive oxygen species (ROS) on antioxidant system and osteoblastic differentiation in MC3T3-E1 cells. IUBMB Life 59: 27–33.
10. Isomura H, Fujie K, Shibata K, Inoue N, Iizuka T, et al. (2004) Bone metabolism and oxidative stress in postmenopausal rats with iron overload. Toxicology 197: 93–100.
11. Mao GX, Deng HB, Yuan LG, Li DD, Li YY, et al. (2010) Protective role of salidroside against aging in a mouse model induced by D-galactose. Biomed Environ Sci 23: 161–166.
12. Skopinska-Rozewska E, Malinowski M, Wasiutynski A, Sommer E, Furmanowa M, et al. (2008) The influence of Rhodiola quadrifida 50% hydro-alcoholic extract and salidroside on tumor-induced angiogenesis in mice. Pol J Vet Sci 11: 97–104.
13. Yu S, Liu M, Gu X, Ding F (2008) Neuroprotective effects of salidroside in the PC12 cell model exposed to hypoglycemia and serum limitation. Cell Mol Neurobiol 28: 1067–1078.

14. Yu P, Hu C, Meehan EJ, Chen L (2007) X-ray crystal structure and antioxidant activity of salidroside, a phenylethanoid glycoside. Chem Biodivers 4: 508–513.

15. Qian EW, Ge DT, Kong SK (2012) Salidroside Protects Human Erythrocytes against Hydrogen Peroxide-Induced Apoptosis. J Nat Prod 75: 531–537.

16. Zhu Y, Shi YP, Wu D, Ji YJ, Wang X, et al. (2011) Salidroside protects against hydrogen peroxide-induced injury in cardiac H9c2 cells via PI3K-Akt dependent pathway. DNA Cell Biol 30: 809–819.

17. Li X, Ye X, Li X, Sun X, Liang Q, et al. (2011) Salidroside protects against MPP(+)-induced apoptosis in PC12 cells by inhibiting the NO pathway. Brain Res 1382: 9-18.

18. Shi TY, Feng SF, Xing JH, Wu YM, Li XQ, et al. (2012) Neuroprotective effects of Salidroside and its analogue tyrosol galactoside against focal cerebral ischemia in vivo and H2O2-induced neurotoxicity in vitro. Neurotox Res 21: 358–367.

19. Fatokun AA, Stone TW, Smith RA (2008) Responses of differentiated MC3T3-E1 osteoblast-like cells to reactive oxygen species. Eur J Pharmacol 587: 35–41.

20. Li Y, Tang L, Duan Y, Ding Y (2010) Upregulation of MMP-13 and TIMP-1 expression in response to mechanical strain in MC3T3-E1 osteoblastic cells. BMC Res Notes 3: 309.

21. Li Y, Ma W, Feng Z, Wang Z, Zha N, et al. (2012) Effects of irradiation on osteoblast-like cells on different titanium surfaces in vitro. J Biomed Mater Res B Appl Biomater.

22. Stanford CM, Jacobson PA, Eanes ED, Lembke LA, Midura RJ (1995) Rapidly forming apatitic mineral in an osteoblastic cell line (UMR 106-01 BSP). J Biol Chem 270: 9420–9428.

23. Baek KH, Oh KW, Lee WY, Lee SS, Kim MK, et al. (2010) Association of oxidative stress with postmenopausal osteoporosis and the effects of hydrogen peroxide on osteoclast formation in human bone marrow cell cultures. Calcif Tissue Int 87: 226–235.

24. Maggio D, Barabani M, Pierandrei M, Polidori MC, Catani M, et al. (2003) Marked decrease in plasma antioxidants in aged osteoporotic women: results of a cross-sectional study. J Clin Endocrinol Metab 88: 1523–1527.

25. Lean JM, Jagger CJ, Kirstein B, Fuller K, Chambers TJ (2005) Hydrogen peroxide is essential for estrogen-deficiency bone loss and osteoclast formation. Endocrinology 146: 728–735.

26. Fatokun AA, Stone TW, Smith RA (2006) Hydrogen peroxide-induced oxidative stress in MC3T3-E1 cells: The effects of glutamate and protection by purines. Bone 39: 542–551.

27. Liu AL, Zhang ZM, Zhu BF, Liao ZH, Liu Z (2004) Metallothionein protects bone marrow stromal cells against hydrogen peroxide-induced inhibition of osteoblastic differentiation. Cell Biol Int 28: 905–911.

28. Hessle L, Johnson KA, Anderson HC, Narisawa S, Sali A, et al. (2002) Tissue-nonspecific alkaline phosphatase and plasma cell membrane glycoprotein-1 are central antagonistic regulators of bone mineralization. Proc Natl Acad Sci U S A 99: 9445–9449.

29. Bai XC, Lu D, Bai J, Zheng H, Ke ZY, et al. (2004) Oxidative stress inhibits osteoblastic differentiation of bone cells by ERK and NF-kappaB. Biochem Biophys Res Commun 314: 197–207.

30. Arai M, Shibata Y, Pugdee K, Abiko Y, Ogata Y (2007) Effects of reactive oxygen species (ROS) on antioxidant system and osteoblastic differentiation in MC3T3-E1 cells. IUBMB Life 59: 27–33.

31. Boyle WJ, Simonet WS, Lacey DL (2003) Osteoclast differentiation and activation. Nature 423: 337–342.

32. Li J, Sarosi I, Yan XQ, Morony S, Capparelli C, et al. (2000) RANK is the intrinsic hematopoietic cell surface receptor that controls osteoclastogenesis and regulation of bone mass and calcium metabolism. Proc Natl Acad Sci U S A 97: 1566–1571.

33. Bai XC, Lu D, Liu AL, Zhang ZM, Li XM, et al. (2005) Reactive oxygen species stimulates receptor activator of NF-kappaB ligand expression in osteoblast. J Biol Chem 280: 17497–17506.

34. Girasole G, Jilka RL, Passeri G, Boswell S, Boder G, et al. (1992) 17 beta-estradiol inhibits interleukin-6 production by bone marrow-derived stromal cells and osteoblasts in vitro: a potential mechanism for the antiosteoporotic effect of estrogens. J Clin Invest 89: 883–891.

35. Kurihara N, Bertolini D, Suda T, Akiyama Y, Roodman GD (1990) IL-6 stimulates osteoclast-like multinucleated cell formation in long term human marrow cultures by inducing IL-1 release. J Immunol 144: 4226–4230.

36. Papanicolaou DA, Vgontzas AN (2000) Interleukin-6: the endocrine cytokine. J Clin Endocrinol Metab 85: 1331–1333.

37. Kitazawa R, Kimble RB, Vannice JL, Kung VT, Pacifici R (1994) Interleukin-1 receptor antagonist and tumor necrosis factor binding protein decrease osteoclast formation and bone resorption in ovariectomized mice. J Clin Invest 94: 2397–2406.

38. Naka K, Muraguchi T, Hoshii T, Hirao A (2008) Regulation of reactive oxygen species and genomic stability in hematopoietic stem cells. Antioxid Redox Signal 10: 1883–1894.

39. Wiegant FA, Surinova S, Ytsma E, Langelaar-Makkinje M, Wikman G, et al. (2009) Plant adaptogens increase lifespan and stress resistance in C. elegans. Biogerontology 10: 27–42.

40. Nielsen F, Mikkelsen BB, Nielsen JB, Andersen HR, Grandjean P (1997) Plasma malondialdehyde as biomarker for oxidative stress: reference interval and effects of life-style factors. Clin Chem 43: 1209–1214.

41. Yang P, He XQ, Peng L, Li AP, Wang XR, et al. (2007) The role of oxidative stress in hormesis induced by sodium arsenite in human embryo lung fibroblast (HELF) cellular proliferation model. J Toxicol Environ Health A 70: 976–983.

42. Ning J, Grant MH (2000) The role of reduced glutathione and glutathione reductase in the cytotoxicity of chromium (VI) in osteoblasts. Toxicol In Vitro 14: 329–335.

43. Kinov P, Leithner A, Radl R, Bodo K, Khoschsorur GA, et al. (2006) Role of free radicals in aseptic loosening of hip arthroplasty. J Orthop Res 24: 55–62.

44. Kazakia GJ, Majumdar S (2006) New imaging technologies in the diagnosis of osteoporosis. Rev Endocr Metab Disord 7: 67–74.

45. Teo JC, Si-Hoe KM, Keh JE, Teoh SH (2006) Relationship between CT intensity, micro-architecture and mechanical properties of porcine vertebral cancellous bone. Clin Biomech (Bristol, Avon) 21: 235–244.

46. Peng ZQ, Vaananen HK, Zhang HX, Tuukkanen J (1997) Long-term effects of ovariectomy on the mechanical properties and chemical composition of rat bone. Bone 20: 207–212.

18

Periodontal Regeneration Using Strontium-Loaded Mesoporous Bioactive Glass Scaffolds in Osteoporotic Rats

Yufeng Zhang[1], Lingfei Wei[1], Chengtie Wu[2]*, Richard J. Miron[1,3]*

1 The State Key Laboratory Breeding Base of Basic Science of Stomatology (Hubei-MOST) & Key Laboratory of Oral Biomedicine Ministry of Education, Wuhan University, Wuhan, People's Republic of China, 2 State Key Laboratory of High Performance Ceramics and Superfine Microstructure, Shanghai Institute of Ceramics, Shanghai, People's Republic of China, 3 Faculté de medecine dentaire, Université Laval, Québec, Canada

Abstract

Recent studies demonstrate that the rate of periodontal breakdown significantly increased in patients compromised from both periodontal disease and osteoporosis. One pharmacological agent used for their treatment is strontium renalate due to its simultaneous ability to increase bone formation and halt bone resorption. The aim of the present study was to achieve periodontal regeneration of strontium-incorporated mesoporous bioactive glass (Sr-MBG) scaffolds in an osteoporotic animal model carried out by bilateral ovariectomy (OVX). 15 female Wistar rats were randomly assigned to three groups: control unfilled periodontal defects, 2) MBG alone and 3) Sr-MBG scaffolds. 10 weeks after OVX, bilateral fenestration defects were created at the buccal aspect of the first mandibular molar and assessed by micro-CT and histomorphometric analysis after 28 days. Periodontal fenestration defects treated with Sr-MBG scaffolds showed greater new bone formation (46.67%) when compared to MBG scaffolds (39.33%) and control unfilled samples (17.50%). The number of TRAP-positive osteoclasts was also significantly reduced in defects receiving Sr-MBG scaffolds. The results from the present study suggest that Sr-MBG scaffolds may provide greater periondontal regeneration. Clinical studies are required to fully characterize the possible beneficial effect of Sr-releasing scaffolds for patients suffering from a combination of both periodontal disease and osteoporosis.

Editor: Michael Glogauer, University of Toronto, Canada

Funding: This project was supported by Program for New Century Excellent Talents in University (NCET-11-0414), Excellent Youth Foundation of Hubei and the funds of the National Natural Science Foundation of China (81271108). Shanghai Pujiang Talent Program (12PJ1409500) and Natural Science Foundation of China (Grant 31370963). The funders had no role in study design, data collection and analysis, decision to publish, or preparation of the manuscript.

Competing Interests: The authors have declared that no competing interests exist.

* Email: richard.miron@zmk.unibe.ch (RM); chengtiewu@mail.sic.ac.cn (CW)

Introduction

Osteoporosis is a worldwide chronic disease which now affects over 200 million people worldwide characterized by low bone mass, poor bone strength and microarchitectural deterioration of bone [1]. The primary cause is governed by the imbalance between bone forming osteoblasts and bone resorbing osteoclasts commonly resulting from postmenopausal oestrogen deficiency [2,3]. At present, the two major therapies include the use of anabolic agents such as parathyroid hormone that stimulate bone formation, and anti-resorptive agents including bisphosphonates, calcitonin, raloxifene, RANKL inhibitors and estrogen which act by inhibiting osteoclast differentiation and activity [4,5]. In relation to periodontal tissues, osteoporosis is believed to contribute to periodontal breakdown given that it may increase bone resorption and prevent proper healing ultimately increasing the severity of the pre-existing periodontal disease [6–8]. Diminished bone density as seen in osteoporotic bone leads to an increase in susceptibility towards alveolar bone loss and further complicates regenerative periodontal procedures.

One agent that is clinically used to prevent bone loss in osteoporotic patients is strontium renalate [9–14]. Studies have demonstrated that it simultaneous acts by both increasing bone formation and decreasing bone resorption [15–20] thus demonstrating increases in bone mineral density in the lumbar spine, the femoral neck and in total hip reconstruction following its use in clinical trials [21–25]. Its dual mechanism of action makes it advantageous over other leading therapies. While the great majority of research in the field of osteoporosis is currently focused on the preventative measures of disease progression, less study on the therapeutic effect of local transplantation of bioactive scaffolds has been investigated following osteoporotic-related fractures. The advancements in tissue engineering over the last several decades warrant the discovery and application of new therapeutic options carrying bioactive and pharmacological agents within scaffolds capable of guiding cell tissue response upon implantation.

One bone grafting material that has gained awareness in recent years is mesoporous bioactive glass (MBG); a synthetic bone graft capable of bone regeneration [26,27]. Recently it has been demonstrated that the chemical composition in MBG (CaO-P2O5-SiO2) improves the in vitro cell activity of cells seeded on MBG scaffolds and improves bone osseointegration in vivo [28,29]. Furthermore, MBG scaffolds have optimal degradation properties making them slowly resorbed over time and replaced by native bone and provide the additional benefit of easily carrying pharmacological agents capable of being released over time to the surrounding tissues [28-31]. Recently we have demonstrated that the advantages of MBG scaffolds incorporated with trace element Strontium (Sr-MBG) were a suitable scaffold for the delivery of strontium to bone defects in a rat osteoporosis model [30,31]. The aim of the present study was to determine if the advantages of Sr-containing mesoporous bioactive glass scaffolds could also be advantageous for the repair of alveolar bone defects created in periodontal tissues. Acute type fenestration defects were created on the buccal aspect of first mandibular molars in 15 ovariectomised rats to generate an osteoporotic phenotype. Healing was assessed 4 weeks post implantation by micro-CT, hematoxylin and eosin staining, and Mason staining.

Materials and Methods

Animals and surgical procedures

15 mature female Wistar rats (10 weeks old, mean body weight 230 g) were purchased and used for this study with all handling and surgical procedure approved by the Ethics Committee for Animal Research, Wuhan University, China. Animals had food and water ad libitum with constant temperature at 22 degrees Celsius.

After one week for acclimatizing to the new laboratory surroundings, an osteoporosis animal model was carried out by bilateral ovariectomy (OVX) under sterile conditions with a minimally invasive surgical technique as previously described [32,33]. Briefly, when general anesthesia by intraperitoneal injection of chloral hydrate (10%, 4 ml/kg body weight) was achieved, rats were operated with 10 mm linear bilateral lumbar lateral skin incisions. Then the enterocoelia was exposed by blunt dissection of muscle and peritoneum. The bilateral ovaries were removed gently following ligation of the ovarian artery and vein. Then the overlying muscles and epithelial tissues were sutured in multi-layers. Postoperatively, penicillin (40,000 IU/ml, 1 ml/kg) was injected for 3 days and there was no sign of inflammation or other notable anomaly.

Periodontal fenestration defects (standardized with 2.8 mm in length, 1.4 mm in height and ≈0.5 mm in deep) were created 2 months later when an osteoporosis model was established as previously described [34]. Briefly, under general anesthesia, rats were subjected to bilateral extra-oral incision at the base of the mandible. The buccal mandibular bone overlying the first molar roots was removed to create a defect (2.8 mm in length, 1.4 mm in height and ≈0.5 mm in depth) using a size-4 round bur. The procedure was performed under an operating microscope to avoid perforation of intraoral mucosa. The roots of the first molar were carefully denuded of their periodontal ligament, overlying cementum, and superficial dentin. The height was standardized to the width of the round bur (diameter 1.4 mm) and extended longitudinally to either side. Then, bilateral defects were created in 15 animals for a total of 30 defects and divided into three groups of 10 defects as follows: 1) non-treated control, 2) MBG alone and 3) Sr-MBG group. Porous strontium-incorporated mesopore-bioglass (Sr-MBG) scaffolds were prepared according to the method as previously described [35]. Following implantation of scaffolds, the

muscle and the skin were repositioned and sutured separately. Postoperatively, penicillin (40,000 IU/ml, 1 ml/kg) was injected intramuscularly for 3 days. Four weeks after surgery, the animals were sacrificed by an overdose of chloral hydrate and samples were removed and prepared for analysis.

μCT analysis

The samples were fixed in 4% formaldehyde for 12 h at 4°C. A μCT imaging system (μCT50, Scanco Medical, Bassersdorf, Switzerland) was used to reveal new bone formation within the defect region. Scanning parameters was performed at 70 kV and 114 μA with a thickness of 0.048 mm per slice in medium-resolution mode. For 3D reconstruction, the mineralized bone tissue was differentially segmented with a fixed low threshold (value = 212). Representative sections were cut out from buccal and mesial-distal view. After 3D reconstruction, the bone volume faction (BV/TV) was determined in defect regions to evaluate new bone formation, using a protocol provided by the manufacturer.

Histological analysis

The mandibles were decalcified in 10% EDTA for 4 weeks. Gradient dehydration was performed for embedding in paraffin followed by perpendicular sectioning to the long axis of the molar roots as previously described [36]. Serial sections of 5 μm were cut and mounted on polylysine-coated slides and then performed for H&E staining, Masson trichrome staining (Sigma #HT15; Sigma-Aldrich, St. Louis, USA.) and tartrate-resistant acid phosphatase (TRAP) staining (Sigma #387A; Sigma-Aldrich, St. Louis, USA.) in accordance with the manufacturer's protocol. For histomorphometry, six individual sections were selected from three different locations, which were situated in the middle, coronal and apical levels of the defect (with 400 μm apart from the central). The histometric measurements were determined by processing the images, which were captured with an Olympus DP72 microscope, in Adobe Photoshop CS5 (Adobe Systems, Inc.). New mineralized tissue was identified by Masson trichrome staining and the defect fill was defined as the ratio of area of new mineralized tissue within bony envelope and the total defect area. The number of TRAP-positive cells was performed in a 500 μm square of the defect area.

Statistical analysis

All data analysis was performed using SPSS software and statistically significant values were adopted as p <0.05. Based on the sample size, a Kolmogorov-Smirnow Test was used to confirm the asymptotic normality of our data. For the bone density, bone thickness and percentage of angiogenesis, mean and standard deviation (SD) were calculated and statistical inference was made by one-way ANOVA and Student t-test (Newman Keuls Test).

Results

Establishment of rat osteoporotic model

Both 2D representation and 3D μ-CT images of the ovariectomized rat animal model was confirmed by demonstrating a decrease in trabecular bone volume, thickness and density (Fig. 1). Furthermore, OVX animals also demonstrated a significant increase in trabecular separation, a reduced thickness of cortical bone and enlarged marrow cavities when compared to control animals (Fig. 1). After analysis of 3D reconstruction, BV/TV in the distal femur region was significantly decreased in OVX rats confirming the established osteoporotic model (data not shown).

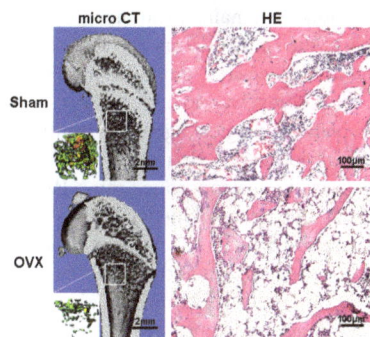

Figure 1. Establishment of rat osteoporotic model created by OVX. 3D μ-CT images of normal bone and osteoporotic bone as well as their representative H&E staining.

H&E staining also supported the establishment of an osteoporotic model by demonstrating evident deterioration of trabecular patterns with fat-rich bone marrow-like tissue in ovariectomized rats (Fig. 1).

3D reconstruction observations and analysis

Following establishment of an osteoporotic model, representative images of osteogenesis in the periodontal fenestration defect performed by 3D reconstruction for each group were shown in ways of buccal holistic view (Fig. 2 A, D and G) and cutaway view from both horizontal (Fig. 2 B, E and H) and vertical (Fig. 2 C, F and I) directions. Only minimal regenerated bone was visible in the control group, where both defects treated with scaffolds demonstrated newly formed bone following implantation with either MBG or Sr-MBG. The groups receiving Sr-MBG scaffolds exhibited statistically higher newly mineralized tissue when compared to the other modalities (Fig. 3A; $17.50\pm3.94\%$, $39.33\pm4.13\%$ and $46.67\pm3.67\%$, $P<0.01$, for control, MBG and Sr-MBG, respectively).

Histological observation and analysis

The histological observation demonstrated that little bone was observed in control defects (Fig. 4A). Within the defects receiving MBG or Sr-MBG scaffolds, a fibrous tissue of woven bone occurred around at the edges as well as around the scaffolds themselves (Fig. 4C and E). Consistently, no new cementum was observed on the root surface among all three groups at a time point of 28 days. It was noted that osteoblasts clustered on the surface of MBG and Sr-MBG and participated aided in the osteogenesis and mineralization (Fig. 4D and F). Noteworthy, more mature alveolar bone was generated around the Sr-MBG when compared to MBG scaffolds. Histomorphometric analysis additionally revealed that the area of new bone was statistically higher in Sr-MBG group (0.52 ± 0.08 mm^2) when compared to other modalities (Fig. 3B). Interestingly, little difference was observed between MBG and Sr-MBG for defect fill indicating that the speed of new bone formation was slightly faster in the defects receiving Sr-MBG scaffolds (Fig. 3C).

TRAP-staining was used to determine the number of multi-nucleated cells laying at the edges of the alveolar bone defect in all three groups (Fig. 5). Large multi-nucleated cells stained for TRAP were observed around both MBG and Sr-MBG scaffolds. The

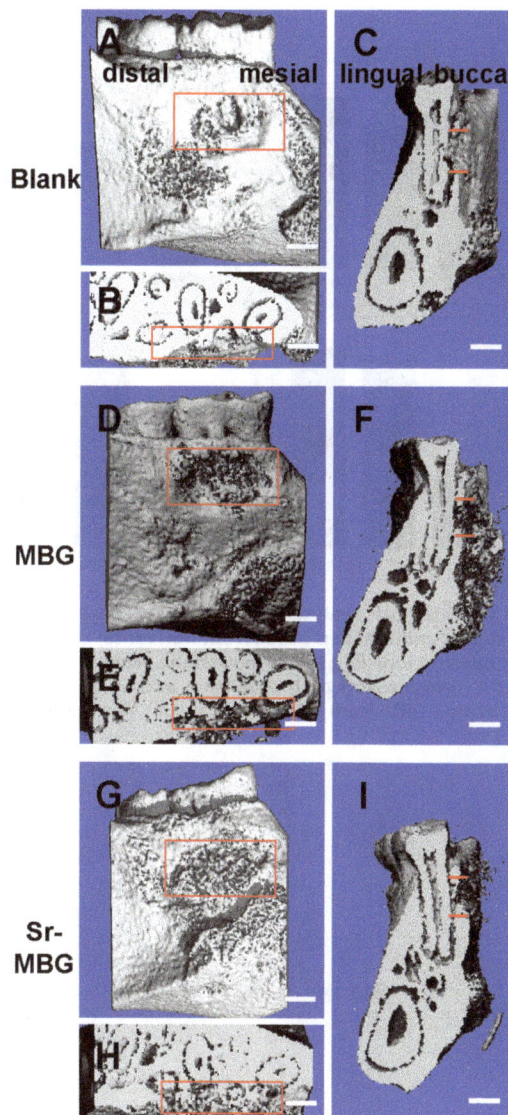

Figure 2. The overall state of bone regeneration was exhibited by 3D reconstruction. The red box represented the original extent of surgical defect in general. A, D and G: buccal view; B, E and H: screenshot in horizontal; C, F and I: screenshot in vertical. Bar: 1 mm.

addition of Sr to MBG significantly decreased the number of TRAP-positive stained cells when compared to MBG scaffolds alone. Both scaffold groups showed higher values when compared to control unfilled defects (Fig. 3D, $P<0.01$).

Discussion

The aim of the present study was to investigate the effect of Sr-containing scaffolds on the biological response of periodontal defects created in OVX rats. As the prevalence of osteoporosis continues to rise along with a high number of patients with periodontal disease in the elderly population, the need for treatment modalities directed at patients suffering from precise

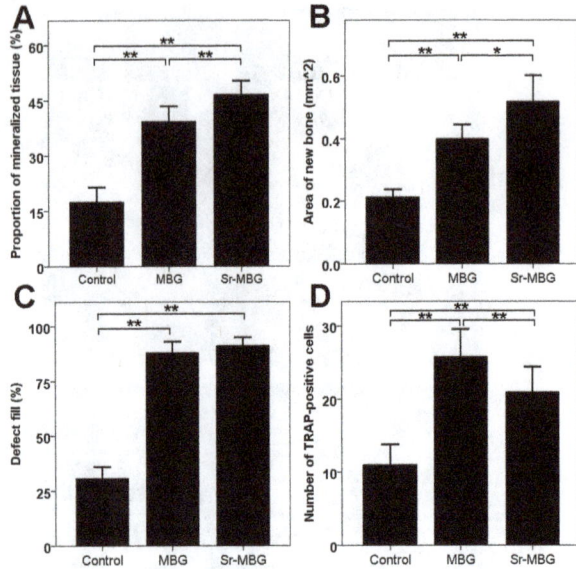

Figure 3. Statistical analysis of periodontal regeneration: A) proportion of mineralized tissue from horizontal cutaway view of 3D construction, B) area of new bone from H&E stain, C) defect fill from Masson trichrome stain and D) the number of TRAP-positive cells from TRAP stain. Results were given by mean ±SD. *: p<0.05, **: p<0.01.

combination of diseases remains prominent. The ability to direct therapy to meet the patient's individual needs remains the clinician's optimal and desired outcome. For these reasons, the goal of the present study was to utilize the therapeutic benefits from the active pharmacological agent in strontium renalate, and fabricate a scaffold containing Sr to assist in the regeneration of periodontal defects in osteoporotic rats. Recently we have demonstrated that the release kinetics and in vitro behavior of these scaffolds demonstrates ideal release of Sr ions over time and supports osteoblast proliferation and differentiation as well as bone regeneration in a rat femur defect model [31]. The goal therefore of the present study was to further investigate the ability for these scaffolds to fully regenerate the more complicated periodontal defect in OVX animals.

The benefit and future incorporation of Sr into pharmacological agents and biomaterials stems from previous studies indicating that Sr ions is a safe and effective way to stimulate proliferation and differentiation of bone mesenchymal stem cells, osteoblasts and periodontal ligament cells harvested [19,37]. It has previously been demonstrated that Sr significantly influences osteoblastic differentiation by increasing alkaline phosphatase activity, real-time PCR for ALP and osteocalcin mRNA expression, and alizarin red staining for mineralization. Furthermore, recent investigations have also demonstrated a positive correlation of Sr incorporation into biomaterials [38,39].

In order to verify our hypothesis that Sr would be advantage in combination with a carrier scaffold, we created Sr-MBG scaffolds

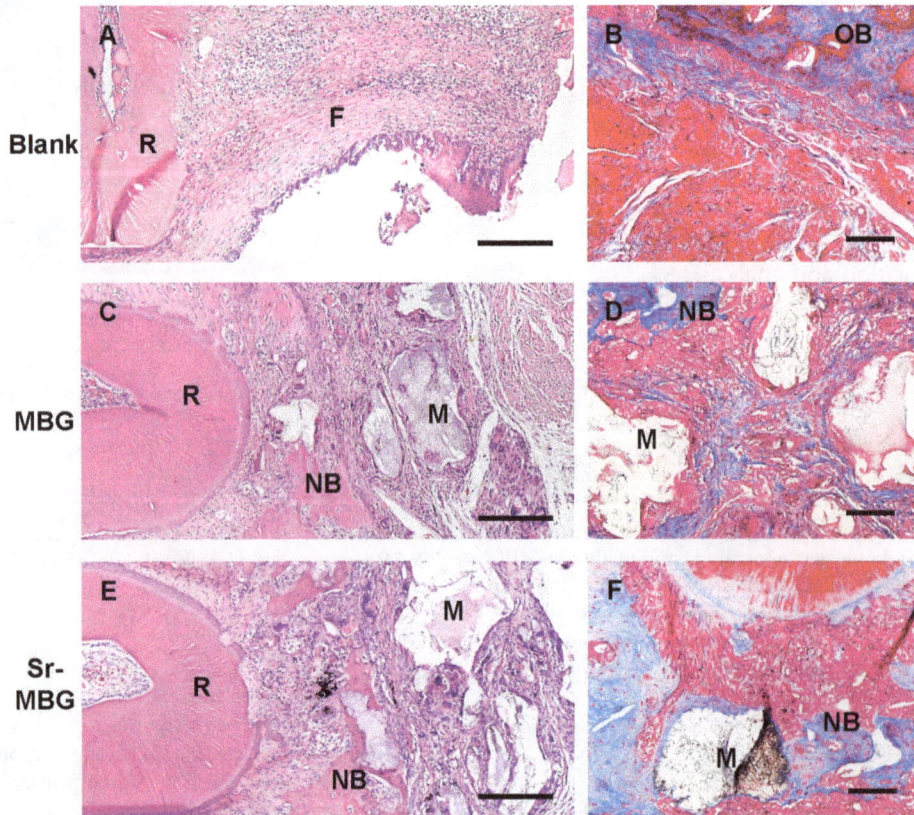

Figure 4. Representative sections of H&E stain (A, C and E) revealed the osteogenesis among the defects. New bone was visible in the area adjacent to the old bone and implanted scaffolds. Representative sections of Masson trichrome stain (B, D and F) revealed the compound of collagen in the osteogenic active zone. Bar: 200 μm. R: Root, F = Fibroblasts, NB = New bone, OB = Old bone, M = Material.

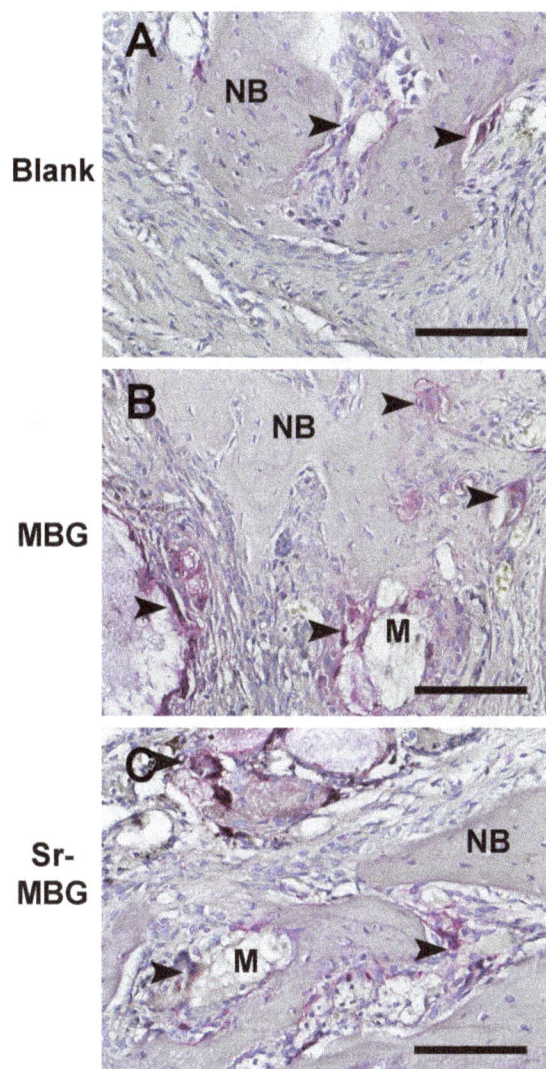

Figure 5. TRAP-staining for A) control, B) MBG alone and C) Sr-MBG scaffolds. Positive cells were visible in the surface of bone (control, MBG and Sr-MBG) and scaffolds (MBG and Sr-MBG). Bar: 100 μm. Arrows depict areas of TRAP-staining, NB = New bone, M = Material.

and implanted them in acute type periodontal defects in ovariectomised rats to mimic the osteoporotic phenotype. The micro-CT analysis demonstrated that Sr-MBG scaffolds induced more mineralization than MBG scaffolds alone or control samples.

The morphological and histormorphometry analysis based on the HE and Mason staining suggested that the Sr-MBG stimulated a more effectively osteoconductive and anti-osteoporotic phenotype which increased the speed and quality of bone regeneration. Furthermore it was shown from TRAP staining that the number of multi-nucleated giant cells was significantly reduced when Sr was administered in MBG scaffolds (Fig. 4). This finding is in accordance with studies from the literature that demonstrate that Sr is able to suppress osteoclastogenesis [40–44]. It has been shown that Sr is able to reduce osteoclast resorption in vitro [40] by decreasing receptor activator of nuclear factor-KappaB ligand (RANKL)-induced osteoclast differentiation [41,44].

The incorporation of strontium into biomaterials has become a hot topic in recent years. Investigators have now demonstrated positive results for the incorporation of Sr into calcium phosphate [45,46], osseointegration of titanium implants [47,48], hydro-xyappatite implants [49–51] and bioactive glass [52]. These investigations utilize the bone formation capabilities of Sr not only for osteoporotic related defects and patients but also for the general public. Thus, it is plausible that the use of Sr may become mainstream within the next decade for a large variety of dental application. The desirable outcome of simultaneously improving bone formation while decreasing bone resorption by incorporating Sr into biomaterials presents many future options for a large variety of applications.

In conclusion, the results from the present study demonstrates that Sr-releasing MBG scaffolds are capable of significantly increasing alveolar bone regeneration in periodontal tissues in OVX rats 28 days post-surgery when compared to control and MBG groups. To the best of our knowledge, we demonstrate for the first time the ability for Sr-containing scaffolds to support bone formation in periodontal tissues in vivo. The scaffolds utilized in this study demonstrate that the release of Sr2+ ions is capable of improving osteoblast function by increasing new bone formation. Simultaneously, the release of Sr also significantly decreased the number of multi-nucleated osteoclasts as demonstrated by TRAP staining. Taken together, these results suggest that the use of Sr-containing scaffolds may provide greater defect healing in osteoporotic related periodontal defects. Additional clinical studies are required to fully characterize the possible beneficial effect of Sr-MBG scaffolds for patients suffering from both periodontal disease and osteoporosis.

Author Contributions

Conceived and designed the experiments: YZ LW CW RM. Performed the experiments: YZ LW CW RM. Analyzed the data: YZ LW CW RM. Contributed reagents/materials/analysis tools: YZ CW. Wrote the paper: YZ LW CW RM.

References

1. Genant HK, Cooper C, Poor G, Reid I, Ehrlich G, et al. (1999) Interim report and recommendations of the World Health Organization Task-Force for Osteoporosis. Osteoporos Int 10: 259–264.
2. Tontonoz P, Pei LM (2004) Fat's loss is bone's gain. Journal of Clinical Investigation 113: 805–806.
3. Rodan GA, Martin TJ (2000) Therapeutic approaches to bone diseases. Science 289: 1508–1514.
4. Silva BC, Bilezikian JP (2011) New approaches to the treatment of osteoporosis. Annu Rev Med 62: 307–322.
5. Boonen S, Ferrari S, Miller PD, Eriksen EF, Sambrook PN, et al. (2012) Postmenopausal osteoporosis treatment with antiresorptives: effects of discontinuation or long-term continuation on bone turnover and fracture risk–a perspective. J Bone Miner Res 27: 963–974.
6. Passos Jde S, Gomes-Filho IS, Vianna MI, da Cruz SS, Barreto ML, et al. (2010) Outcome measurements in studies on the association between osteoporosis and periodontal disease. J Periodontol 81: 1773–1780.
7. Sultan N, Rao J (2011) Association between periodontal disease and bone mineral density in postmenopausal women: a cross sectional study. Med Oral Patol Oral Cir Bucal 16: e440–447.
8. von Wowern N, Klausen B, Kollerup G (1994) Osteoporosis: a risk factor in periodontal disease. J Periodontol 65: 1134–1138.
9. Chung CJ, Long HY (2011) Systematic strontium substitution in hydroxyapatite coatings on titanium via micro-arc treatment and their osteoblast/osteoclast responses. Acta Biomater 7: 4081–4087.
10. Hao J, Acharya A, Chen K, Chou J, Kasugai S, et al. (2013) Novel bioresorbable strontium hydroxyapatite membrane for guided bone regeneration. Clin Oral Implants Res.

11. Gallacher SJ, Dixon T (2010) Impact of treatments for postmenopausal osteoporosis (bisphosphonates, parathyroid hormone, strontium ranelate, and denosumab) on bone quality: a systematic review. Calcif Tissue Int 87: 469–484.

12. Marie PJ (2010) Strontium ranelate in osteoporosis and beyond: identifying molecular targets in bone cell biology. Mol Interv 10: 305–312.

13. Mentaverri R, Brazier M, Kamel S, Fardellone P (2012) Potential anti-catabolic and anabolic properties of strontium ranelate. Curr Mol Pharmacol 5: 189–194.

14. Rizzoli R, Reginster JY (2011) Adverse drug reactions to osteoporosis treatments. Expert Rev Clin Pharmacol 4: 593–604.

15. Marie PJ, Ammann P, Boivin G, Rey C (2001) Mechanisms of action and therapeutic potential of strontium in bone. Calcif Tissue Int 69: 121–129.

16. Verberckmoes SC, De Broe ME, D'Haese PC (2003) Dose-dependent effects of strontium on osteoblast function and mineralization. Kidney Int 64: 534–543.

17. Qiu K, Zhao XJ, Wan CX, Zhao CS, Chen YW (2006) Effect of strontium ions on the growth of ROS17/2.8 cells on porous calcium polyphosphate scaffolds. Biomaterials 27: 1277–1286.

18. Peng S, Liu XS, Zhou G, Li Z, Luk KD, et al. (2011) Osteoprotegerin deficiency attenuates strontium-mediated inhibition of osteoclastogenesis and bone resorption. J Bone Miner Res 26: 1272–1282.

19. Choudhary S, Halbout P, Alander C, Raisz L, Pilbeam C (2007) Strontium ranelate promotes osteoblastic differentiation and mineralization of murine bone marrow stromal cells: involvement of prostaglandins. J Bone Miner Res 22: 1002–1010.

20. Blake GM, Compston JE, Fogelman I (2009) Could strontium ranelate have a synergistic role in the treatment of osteoporosis? J Bone Miner Res 24: 1354–1357.

21. Meunier PJ, Slosman DO, Delmas PD, Sebert JL, Brandi ML, et al. (2002) Strontium ranelate: dose-dependent effects in established postmenopausal vertebral osteoporosis–a 2-year randomized placebo controlled trial. J Clin Endocrinol Metab 87: 2060–2066.

22. Meunier PJ, Roux C, Seeman E, Ortolani S, Badurski JE, et al. (2004) The effects of strontium ranelate on the risk of vertebral fracture in women with postmenopausal osteoporosis. N Engl J Med 350: 459–468.

23. Reginster JY, Seeman E, De Vernejoul MC, Adami S, Compston J, et al. (2005) Strontium ranelate reduces the risk of nonvertebral fractures in postmenopausal women with osteoporosis: Treatment of Peripheral Osteoporosis (TROPOS) study. J Clin Endocrinol Metab 90: 2816–2822.

24. Seeman E, Devogelaer JP, Lorenc R, Spector T, Brixen K, et al. (2008) Strontium ranelate reduces the risk of vertebral fractures in patients with osteopenia. J Bone Miner Res 23: 433–438.

25. Ammann P, Badoud I, Barraud S, Dayer R, Rizzoli R (2007) Strontium ranelate treatment improves trabecular and cortical intrinsic bone tissue quality, a determinant of bone strength. J Bone Miner Res 22: 1419–1425.

26. Yan X, Huang X, Yu C, Deng H, Wang Y, et al. (2006) The in-vitro bioactivity of mesoporous bioactive glasses. Biomaterials 27: 3396–3403.

27. Li X, Shi J, Dong X, Zhang L, Zeng H (2008) A mesoporous bioactive glass/polycaprolactone composite scaffold and its bioactivity behavior. J Biomed Mater Res A 84: 84–91.

28. Wu C, Ramaswamy Y, Zhu Y, Zheng R, Appleyard R, et al. (2009) The effect of mesoporous bioactive glass on the physiochemical, biological and drug-release properties of poly(DL-lactide-co-glycolide) films. Biomaterials 30: 2199–2208.

29. Wu C, Zhang Y, Zhou Y, Fan W, Xiao Y (2011) A comparative study of mesoporous glass/silk and non-mesoporous glass/silk scaffolds: physiochemistry and in vivo osteogenesis. Acta Biomater 7: 2229–2236.

30. Wei L, Ke J, Prasadam I, Miron RJ, Lin S, et al. (2014) A comparative study of Sr-incorporated mesoporous bioactive glass scaffolds for regeneration of osteopenic bone defects. Osteoporos Int.

31. Zhang Y, Wei L, Chang J, Miron RJ, Shi B, et al. (2013) Strontium-incorporated mesoporous bioactive glass scaffolds stimulating in vitro proliferation and differentiation of bone marrow stromal cells and in vivo regeneration of osteoporotic bone defects. Journal of Materials Chemistry B 1: 5711–5722.

32. Cheng N, Dai J, Cheng X, Li S, Miron RJ, et al. (2013) Porous CaP/silk composite scaffolds to repair femur defects in an osteoporotic model. J Mater Sci Mater Med 24: 1963–1975.

33. Zhang Y, Cheng N, Miron R, Shi B, Cheng X (2012) Delivery of PDGF-B and BMP-7 by mesoporous bioglass/silk fibrin scaffolds for the repair of osteoporotic defects. Biomaterials 33: 6698–6708.

34. Miron RJ, Wei L, Yang S, Caluseru OM, Sculean A, et al. (2014) Effect of an Enamel Matrix Derivative on Periodontal Wound Healing/Regeneration in an Osteoporotic Model. J Periodontol: 1–12.

35. Wu C, Zhou Y, Lin C, Chang J, Xiao Y (2012) Strontium-containing mesoporous bioactive glass scaffolds with improved osteogenic/cementogenic differentiation of periodontal ligament cells for periodontal tissue engineering. Acta Biomater 8: 3805–3815.

36. Zhao M, Jin Q, Berry JE, Nociti FH, Jr., Giannobile WV, et al. (2004) Cementoblast delivery for periodontal tissue engineering. J Periodontol 75: 154–161.

37. Chattopadhyay N, Quinn SJ, Kifor O, Ye C, Brown EM (2007) The calcium-sensing receptor (CaR) is involved in strontium ranelate-induced osteoblast proliferation. Biochem Pharmacol 74: 438–447.

38. Han L, Okiji T (2011) Evaluation of the ions release / incorporation of the prototype S-PRG filler-containing endodontic sealer. Dent Mater J.

39. Sakai A, Valanezahad A, Ozaki M, Ishikawa K, Matsuya S (2012) Preparation of Sr-containing carbonate apatite as a bone substitute and its properties. Dent Mater J 31: 197–205.

40. Bonnelye E, Chabadel A, Saltel F, Jurdic P (2008) Dual effect of strontium ranelate: stimulation of osteoblast differentiation and inhibition of osteoclast formation and resorption in vitro. Bone 42: 129–138.

41. Caudrillier A, Hurtel-Lemaire AS, Wattel A, Cournarie F, Godin C, et al. (2010) Strontium ranelate decreases receptor activator of nuclear factor-KappaB ligand-induced osteoclastic differentiation in vitro: involvement of the calcium-sensing receptor. Mol Pharmacol 78: 569–576.

42. Peng S, Liu XS, Huang S, Li Z, Pan H, et al. (2011) The cross-talk between osteoclasts and osteoblasts in response to strontium treatment: involvement of osteoprotegerin. Bone 49: 1290–1298.

43. Roy M, Bose S (2012) Osteoclastogenesis and osteoclastic resorption of tricalcium phosphate: effect of strontium and magnesium doping. J Biomed Mater Res A 100: 2450–2461.

44. Yamaguchi M, Weitzmann MN (2012) The intact strontium ranelate complex stimulates osteoblastogenesis and suppresses osteoclastogenesis by antagonizing NF-kappaB activation. Mol Cell Biochem 359: 399–407.

45. Baier M, Staudt P, Klein R, Sommer U, Wenz R, et al. (2013) Strontium enhances osseointegration of calcium phosphate cement: a histomorphometric pilot study in ovariectomized rats. J Orthop Surg Res 8: 16.

46. Mohan BG, Shenoy SJ, Babu SS, Varma HK, John A (2013) Strontium calcium phosphate for the repair of leporine (Oryctolagus cuniculus) ulna segmental defect. J Biomed Mater Res A 101: 261–271.

47. Andersen OZ, Offermanns V, Sillassen M, Almtoft KP, Andersen IH, et al. (2013) Accelerated bone ingrowth by local delivery of strontium from surface functionalized titanium implants. Biomaterials 34: 5883–5890.

48. Lopa S, Mercuri D, Colombini A, De Conti G, Segatti F, et al. (2013) Orthopedic bioactive implants: Hydrogel enrichment of macroporous titanium for the delivery of mesenchymal stem cells and strontium. J Biomed Mater Res A.

49. Yang GL, Song LN, Jiang QH, Wang XX, Zhao SF, et al. (2012) Effect of strontium-substituted nanohydroxyapatite coating of porous implant surfaces on implant osseointegration in a rabbit model. Int J Oral Maxillofac Implants 27: 1332–1339.

50. Berglund IS, Brar HS, Dolgova N, Acharya AP, Keselowsky BG, et al. (2012) Synthesis and characterization of Mg-Ca-Sr alloys for biodegradable orthopedic implant applications. J Biomed Mater Res B Appl Biomater 100: 1524–1534.

51. Fu DL, Jiang QH, He FM, Yang GL, Liu L (2012) Fluorescence microscopic analysis of bone osseointegration of strontium-substituted hydroxyapatite implants. J Zhejiang Univ Sci B 13: 364–371.

52. Brauer DS, Karpukhina N, Kedia G, Bhat A, Law RV, et al. (2012) Bactericidal strontium-releasing injectable bone cements based on bioactive glasses. J R Soc Interface.

19

Hovenia dulcis Thunb Extract and Its Ingredient Methyl Vanillate Activate Wnt/β-Catenin Pathway and Increase Bone Mass in Growing or Ovariectomized Mice

Pu-Hyeon Cha[1,2], Wookjin Shin[1,2], Muhammad Zahoor[1,2], Hyun-Yi Kim[1,2], Do Sik Min[1,3], Kang-Yell Choi[1,2]*

1 Translational Research Center for Protein Function Control, College of Life Science and Biotechnology, Yonsei University, Seoul, Korea, 2 Department of Biotechnology, College of Life Science and Biotechnology, Yonsei University, Seoul, Korea, 3 Department of Molecular Biology, College of Natural Science, Pusan National University, Pusan, Korea

Abstract

The Wnt/β-catenin pathway is a potential target for development of anabolic agents to treat osteoporosis because of its role in osteoblast differentiation and bone formation. However, there is no clinically available anti-osteoporosis drug that targets this Wnt/β-catenin pathway. In this study, we screened a library of aqueous extracts of 350 plants and identified *Hovenia dulcis* Thunb (HDT) extract as a Wnt/β-catenin pathway activator. HDT extract induced osteogenic differentiation of calvarial osteoblasts without cytotoxicity. In addition, HDT extract increased femoral bone mass without inducing significant weight changes in normal mice. In addition, thickness and area of femoral cortical bone were also significantly increased by the HDT extract. Methyl vanillate (MV), one of the ingredients in HDT, also activated the Wnt/β-catenin pathway and induced osteoblast differentiation *in vitro*. MV rescued trabecular or cortical femoral bone loss in the ovariectomized mice without inducing any significant weight changes or abnormality in liver tissue when administrated orally. Thus, natural HDT extract and its ingredient MV are potential anabolic agents for treating osteoporosis.

Editor: Brenda Smith, Oklahoma State University, United States of America

Funding: This work was supported by grants from the National Research Foundation (NRF), funded by the Ministry of Future Creation and Science (MFCS) of Korea; Mid-career Researcher Program (2012R1A2A1A01010285), Translational Research Center for Protein Function Control; (2009-0083522), and Stem Research Project (2010-0020235). This work was also partly supported by a grant from the Ministry of Knowledge Economy through the Korea Research Institute of Chemical Technology (SI-095). The funders had no role in study design, data collection and analysis, decision to publish, or preparation of the manuscript.

Competing Interests: The authors have declared that no competing interests exist.

* E-mail: kychoi@yonsei.ac.kr

Introduction

Bone homeostasis is maintained by a balance between osteoblast-mediated bone formation and osteoclast-mediated bone resorption [1]. An imbalance in bone homeostasis causes various diseases including osteoporosis, which is characterized by low bone mass and increased risk of bone fractures [2]. Osteoporosis frequently occurs in the elderly and in menopausal woman, and the most wildly used anti-osteoporosis drugs are anti-resorptive bisphosphonates that inhibit the activity of osteoclasts. Bisphosphonates, including alendronate (ALN), efficiently prevent bone loss; however, they have various adverse effects including upset stomach, inflammation of the esophagus, and osteonecrosis of the jaw [3–5]. In addition, bisphosphonates also elevate the risk of bone fractures caused by accumulation of microfractures [6]. Another class of anti-resorptive drugs includes estrogens and selective estrogen receptor modulators (SERMs). However, sustained treatment with these therapies results in higher risk of breast cancer, uterine bleeding, and cardiovascular events [7]. These adverse effects of anti-resorptive drugs warrant development of anabolic agents to treat osteoporosis.

Unlike anti-resorptive agents, anabolic agents stimulate proliferation or differentiation of osteoblasts, and consequently, improve both quality and quantity of bone [8]. Parathyroid hormone (PTH) drugs such as PTH (1–34) and PTH (1–84) are only approved anabolic agents by the US Food and Drug Administration (FDA) and/or European Union (EU) [9]. PTH drugs increase BMD and decrease vertebral fracture risk in humans compared to the anti-resorptive drugs, ALN and a SERM raloxifene, respectively [10,11]. However, these protein drugs can be applied by only subcutaneous injection on the daily basis, and relatively expensive. In addition, treatment with PTH drugs is approved for a maximum of 2 years for continuous usage in humans, because of increased osteosarcoma incidence and hyperparathyroidism [8,12]. Therefore, novel and safe anabolic agents for treating osteoporosis are increasingly needed.

The Wnt/β-catenin signaling pathway is of interest as a novel therapeutic target for development of osteoporosis treatment. Growing evidence suggests that activation of this pathway increases osteoblast differentiation and subsequent bone formation, while suppressing osteoclastogenesis [13,14]. The drugs activating Wnt/β-catenin pathway are often suspected to induce human cancers, because aberrant activation of this pathway is known to relate various cancer developments. However, involvement of the Wnt/β-catenin pathway activation in osteosarcoma occurrence was not reported unlike bone morphogenetic protein (BMP) or transforming growth factor signaling [15–17]. Wnt/

β-catenin pathway is inactive in osteosarcoma, and inhibition of this pathway contributes to the tumorigenesis of osteosarcoma [18]. Therefore, activation of the Wnt/β-catenin pathway is relatively safe for bone anabolic agent development compared with PTH or BMP pathway activators. Inhibitors for GSK3β or antibodies against dickkopf-1 (DKK1), sclerostin and secreted frizzled-related protein-1 (sFRP1), antagonists of Wnt/β-catenin pathway, increase bone formation and bone mass in mice, rats or humans [19]. A sclerostin neutralizing antibody entered phase I clinical trials in 2007 as the first osteoporosis treatment candidate in the Wnt/β-catenin pathway. However, clinically available osteoporosis drugs, especially small molecular drugs that target Wnt/β-catenin pathway are not available.

Natural products such as plant extracts and their individual ingredients have been used traditionally to treat various diseases including obesity and inflammation in eastern Asia and western Africa [20,21]. These natural products are regarded as relatively safe for drug development and are increasingly being used in medicines. The global market of medicinal plants was estimated at approximately 83 billion US dollars in 2008, and the World Health Organization reports that over 80% of the world's population use natural products for medicinal treatment of primary health care needs [22,23]. This resource, however, has not been fully exploited and many more natural products remain to be identified.

In this study, we searched plant extracts that activate Wnt/β-catenin signaling pathway and induce osteoblast differentiation. Through the screening of plant extracts library, we identified an extract from *Hovenia Dulcis* Thunb (HDT) as an activator of the Wnt/β-catenin pathway, and characterized its ability to modulate osteoblast differentiation and bone mass *in vitro* and *in vivo*, respectively. We determined that methyl vanillate (MV), an ingredient of HDT, activates the Wnt/β-catenin pathway and is involved in osteoblast differentiation. The non-toxic concentration of MV rescued femoral bone loss in ovariectomized mice after oral administration, and the effect was equivalent to that of intraperitoneal PTH (1–34) injection. HDT extract and the small molecule MV have potential for development as anabolic agents to treat osteoporosis.

Materials and Methods

Cell culture, transfection and reagents

Human embryonic kidney 293 (HEK293) cells and HEK293 reporter cells (containing the chromosomally incorporated TCF reporter (TOPflash) gene) [24] were grown in Dulbecco's Modified Eagle Medium (DMEM; Gibco BRL, Carlsbad, CA, USA) supplemented with 10% fetal bovine serum (FBS; Gibco BRL), and 100 U/ml penicillin G and 100 µg/ml streptomycin (Gibco BRL). Calvarial osteoblasts were extracted from calvaria of ICR mice at postnatal day 4. The calvaria were digested with 0.32 mg/ml collagenase type II (Worthington, Lakewood, NJ, USA) for 20 min at 37°C, and the extracted cells were collected by centrifugation at 1500 RPM for 2 min. These steps were repeated five times. This calvarial cells and mouse osteoblastic cell line, MC3T3E1, were cultured in basic medium (α-Minimum Essential Medium (α–MEM; Gibco BRL) supplemented with 10% FBS and antibiotics. For differentiation of osteoblast cells, 100 µg/ml ascorbic acid (Sigma Aldrich, St. Louis, MO, USA) and 10 mM β-glycerophosphate (Sigma Aldrich) were added to the basic media. Transfection of plasmid or siRNA (β-catenin and control GFP; Bioneer, Daejeon, Korea) was performed with Lipofectamine Plus (Invitrogen, Carlsbad, CA, USA) according to the manufacturer's instructions. Plant extracts, including the HDT extract and its 8

ingredients (vanillic acid (VA), methyl vanillate (MV), ferulic acid (FA), myricetin, taxifolin, 2,3,4-trihydrobenzoic acid (2,3,4-TA), dihydrokaempferol (DH) and gallocatechin (GC)) were purchased from the Korea Plant Extract Bank and Sigma Aldrich, respectively, and those were dissolved in dimethyl sulfoxide (DMSO; Sigma Aldrich) for *in vitro* studies.

Reporter assay

For plant extracts screening, HEK293 reporter cells were seeded onto 96-well black polystyrene plates (Greiner Bio-One, Stonehouse, UK) at 2×10^4 cells per well and grown for 24 h. Each plant extract or DMSO (control) was added at a final concentration of 1 µg/ml. After 24 h, firefly luciferase activity was measured and the relative reporter activity was determined by normalizing to the control [24]. For quantitative analysis of TOPflash activity induced by the HDT extract or its individual ingredients, HEK293 reporter cells were seeded into 24-well plates at a density of 5×10^4 cells/well. After 24 h, the HDT extract (5 or 50 µg/ml) or the 8 ingredients (each 20 µM) were individually added to the cells for 24 h. Reporter activity was measured as described previously [24]. TOPflash and FOPflash assays were performed in calvarial osteoblasts. The pTOPflash or pFOPflash [25] vector was transfected with pCMV–β-galactosidase (β-gal; Clontech, Mountain View, CA, USA) reporter plasmids using Lipofectamine Plus. After 24 h, HDT extract (5 µg/ml) or DMSO (control) was added to the calvarial osteoblasts for another 24 h. Luciferase activity was measured in whole cell lysates and normalized to the internal control β-gal.

Ex vivo culture and morphometric analysis of mouse calvaria

Calvaria were extracted from ICR mice at postnatal day 4, and cultured on a grid in a 12-well plate with α–MEM for 24 h. Plant extracts or MV in differentiation media were treated to calvaria for 7 days, and those were changed with identical fresh media every 2 days. The calvaria were fixed in 4% paraformaldehyde (PFA) for 2 days, and decalcified in 4% HCl and 4% formic acid for 2 days. After decalcification, the calvaria were dehydrated, embedded in paraffin, and sagittally sectioned to a thickness of 4 µm (Leica Microsystems, Wetzlar, Germany) from the midline [26]. The sectioned tissues were rehydrated and hematoxylin and eosin (H&E) staining was performed.

Animals and experimental treatments

ICR mice were purchased from KOATECH (Pyeongtaek, Gyeonggido, Korea), and animal care and experiments were carried out according to the guidelines of the Korean Food and Drug Administration. Protocols were reviewed and approved by the Institutional Review Board of Severance Hospital, Yonsei University College of Medicine (09-013). Animals were maintained under a 12 h light/12 h darkness cycle at 22–25°C in a conventional conditions and fed with standard rodent chow and water.

Normal 8-week-old male mice were given intraperitoneal (i.p.) injection of 200 mg/kg of HDT extract for 5 sequential days each week for 4 weeks. Each group included 5 mice, and the weight of mice was measured every 4 days. Calcein (10 mg/kg; Sigma Aldrich) was i.p. injected into at least 3 mice per a group at 15 days and 5 days prior to sacrifice, respectively. At 8 weeks of age, females were ovariectomized (OVX) under anesthesia with avertin (2,2,2-tribromoethanol; Worthington). Dorsal incisions, approximately 1-cm long, were made with dissection scissors into the dermal layer above both sides of the ovaries. The connection between the fallopian tube and the uterine horn was cut and the ovary was removed. The incision was then sutured with 3 single catgut stitches. Sham-operated (Sham) mice were used as controls. After 2 or 4 weeks, the OVX group was divided into several groups according to experimental designs (n = 5–7 per group). PTH (1–34) (80 μg/kg; BACHEM, Bubendorf, Switzerland) was i.p. injected into mice, while MV was dissolved in corn oil and orally applied. Treatment of both PTH (1–34) and MV was given for 5 sequential days each week for 4 weeks. Animals were sacrificed and organs were obtained for analysis.

Bone histomorphometric analysis and Immunohistochemistry (IHC)

The tissues were fixed in 4% PFA for 3 days at 4°C for histological evaluation. After fixation, femurs were decalcified in 10% ethylenediaminetetraacetic acid (EDTA; Sigma Aldrich), dehydrated, embedded in paraffin and sectioned to 4 μm thickness (Leica Microsystem). The tissues were rehydrated and used for further analyses including H&E and IHC staining. Florescence IHC analyses were described previously [27]. For fluorescent IHC, sections were incubated with primary antibody (anti-β-catenin; Santa Cruz Biotechnology, Santa Cruz, CA, USA) overnight at 4°C, followed by incubation with anti-mouse Alexa Flour 488 (Life Technologies, Carlsbad, CA, USA; 1:500) or anti-rabbit Alex Flour 555 (Life Technologies; 1:500) secondary antibodies for 1 h at room temperature. The sections were then counterstained with 4′, 6-diamidino-2-phenylindole (DAPI; Sigma Aldrich, St. Louis, MO, USA) and mounted in Gel/Mount media (Biomeda Corporation, Foster City, CA, USA). All incubations were conducted in dark, humid chambers. The fluorescence signals were visualized using confocal microscopy (LSM510; Carl Zeiss Inc., Thornwood, NY) at excitation wavelengths of 488 nm (Alexa Fluor 488), 543 nm (Alexa Fluor 555) and 405 nm (DAPI). At least 3 fields per section were analyzed.

Microcomputated tomography analysis and cortical bone measurement

After sacrifice, mouse femurs were harvested and stored in 70% ethanol (Duksan Pure Chemical Co., Ansan, Gyeonggido, Korea) until analysis. To analyze the femoral trabecular bone, standardized cone-beam microcomputed tomography (μCT) scanning of the right limb was performed using a μCT system for small animal imaging (Skyscan 1076; Skyscan, Kontich, Belgium). Scanning was performed with a 10 μm thick at the region of the distal femur from growth plate and extended proximally along the femur diaphysis. One hundred continuous slices were scanned and analyzed stating at 0.1 mm from the most proximal aspect of the growth plate until both condyles were no longer visible were selected for analysis. All trabecular bone from each selected slice was segmented for three dimensional reconstruction to calculate the bone parameters such as bone volume/tissue volume (BV/TV), trabecular number (Tb.N), trabecular separation (Tb.Sp), and trabecular thickness (Tb.Th) [28]. Cortical bone parameters such as outer diameter of x-axis (C.Od), outer diameter of y-axis, inner diameter or thickness (C.Th) were evaluated using NIS elements AR 3.1 software (Nikon) in μCT 3D images. The cortical bone area (C.Ar) was calculated by mathematical formula for ellipse by multiplication of x-axis diameter, y-axis diameter and pi (π) value.

RNA extraction, cDNA synthesis and reverse transcriptase polymerase chain reaction (RT-PCR)

Total RNA was isolated using Trizol (Invitrogen) and 2 μg of total RNA was reverse transcribed using 200 U of reverse transcriptase (Invitrogen) according to the manufacturer's instructions. The following primer sets were used: *runt-related transcription factor 2 (RUNX2)*, forward 5′-GAGGCCGCCGCACGA-CAACCG-3′ and reverse 5′- CTCCGGCCCACAAATCT-CAGA-3′; *bone morphogenetic protein 2 (BMP2)*, forward 5′-AGA-GATGAGTGGGAAAACGG-3′ and reverse 5′-GAAGTCCACATACAAAGGGT-3′; *alkaline phosphatase (ALP)*, forward 5′-GGGACTGGTACTCGGATAACGA-3′ and reverse 5′- CTGATATGCGATGTCCTTGCA-3′; *osteocalcin (OCN)*, forward 5′-GCAGCTTGGTGCACACCTAG-3′ and reverse 5′-ACCTTATTGCCCTCCTGCTT-3′; *receptor activator of nuclear factor kappa-B ligand (RANKL)*, forward 5′-CCAGTGAAGCAG-CAGCCAGC-3′ and reverse 5′-CCCTCTCAT-CAGCCCTGTCC-3′; *osteoprotegerin (OPG)*, forward 5′-ACGGA-CAGCTGGCACACCAG-3′ and reverse 5′-CTCACACACTCGGTTGTGGG-3′; *GAPDH*, forward 5′-CCATGGAGAAGGCTGGGG′ and reverse 5′–CAAAGTTGT-CATGGATGACC-3′.

Immunoblotting

Cells were washed with ice-cold phosphate-buffered saline (PBS; Gibco BRL, Carlsbad, CA, USA) and lysed in radio immunoprecipitation assay (RIPA) buffer (Millipore, Bedford, MA, USA). Proteins were separated on a 6–15% sodium dodecyl sulfate (SDS) polyacrylamide gel and transferred to a nitrocellulose membrane (Whatman, Florham Park, NJ, USA). Immunoblotting was performed with the following primary antibodies: anti-β-catenin (Santa Cruz Biotechnology, Santa Cruz, CA, USA) and anti-α-tubulin (Oncogene Research Products, Cambridge, MA, USA). Horseradish peroxidase-conjugated anti-mouse (Cell Signaling, Beverly, MA, USA) or anti-rabbit (Bio-Rad Laboratories, Hercules, CA, USA) antibodies were used as secondary antibodies.

Immunofluorescence staining

Calvarial osteoblasts were seeded onto a coverslip in 12-well plates at a density of 3×10^4 cells/well. After 24 h, HDT extract or MV was added for another 24 h and the cells were subsequently fixed with 4% PFA for 10 min. Cells were permeabilized with 0.2% Triton X-100 for 15 min and incubated for 30 min with 5% bovine serum albumin (BSA) blocking solution. The cells were incubated with the primary antibody (β-catenin) overnight at 4°C and then washed with PBS three times. Cells were then incubated with Alexa Fluor 502-conjugated IgG secondary antibody (Life Technologies, Carlsbad, CA, USA) was incubated for 1 h, followed by incubation with 4′, 6-diamidino-2-phenylindole (DAPI; Sigma Aldrich, St. Louis, MO, USA) for 5 min. The cells were mounted in Gel/Mount media (Biomeda Corporation, Foster City, CA, USA). The fluorescence signal was captured using confocal microscopy (LSM510; Carl Zeiss Inc., Thornwood, NY). To measure the fluorescence signal, we detected intensities of β-catenin in the fluorescence staining images using NIS elements AR 3.1 software (Nikon).

Cytotoxicity assay

Calvarial osteoblasts were plated at a density of 5×10^3 cells per 24-well plate. The cells were then treated with DMSO (control) or HDT extract for 72 h. Next, 3-(4,5-Dimethylthiazol-2-yl)-2, 5-diphenyltetrazolium bromide (MTT; AMRESCO, Solon, Ohio, U) was added to each well at a concentration of 0.25 mg/ml. After incubation for 2 h at 37°C, insoluble purple formazan was obtained by media removal. The formazan was dissolved in 1 ml DMSO for 1 h. The absorbance of the formazan product was measured at 590 nm.

Alkaline phosphatase (ALP) assay and staining

Calvarial osteoblasts were seeded in 24-well plates at a density of 5×10^4 cells/well. The HDT extract or MV in differentiation media was added to the cells for 5 days. The basic media was used as a negative control. The media with DMSO alone, HDT extract, or MV was changed after 3 days. To measure ALP activity, the cells were washed with cold PBS and lysed in 55 μl of buffer containing 0.2 M Tris-HCl (pH 8.0) and 0.1% Triton X-100. After centrifugation at 13,000 RPM for 15 min at 4°C, the supernatant (15 μl) was incubated with 30 μl of p-nitrophenylphosphate (pNPP, Sigma Aldrich), a substrate used to quantify ALP activity. To stop the reaction, 20 μl of 0.2 N NaOH was used and the absorbance was read at 405 nm. Whole cell lysates were analyzed for protein concentration using the Bradford assay (Bio-Rad Laboratories), and ALP activity was normalized to the protein concentration. ALP was stained using the TRACP & ALP double-stain kit (Takara Bio Inc., Shiga, Japan) according to the manufacturer's instructions.

Alizarin Red S staining

Calvarial osteoblasts were seeded into 24-well plates at a density of 5×10^4 cells/well. The HDT extract or MV in differentiation medium was treated into the cells for 21 days. Media changes occurred every 3 days. At the end of incubation period, the cells were washed with cold PBS and fixed with 4% PFA for 10 min. The cells were stained with 40 mM Alizarin staining solution (pH 4.2; Sigma Aldrich) for 30 min at room temperature and washed with water three times. Colorimetric staining was extracted and quantified at 550 nm [29].

Statistical analyses

Data are presented as mean ± standard deviation (S.D.) unless otherwise indicated. Significance was analyzed using a Student's t test.

Results

Identification of HDT extract as an activator of Wnt/β-catenin signaling

To identify plant extracts that activate the Wnt/β-catenin pathway, we screened aqueous extracts of 350 plants using the HEK293 reporter cells containing TOPflash. Fourteen plant

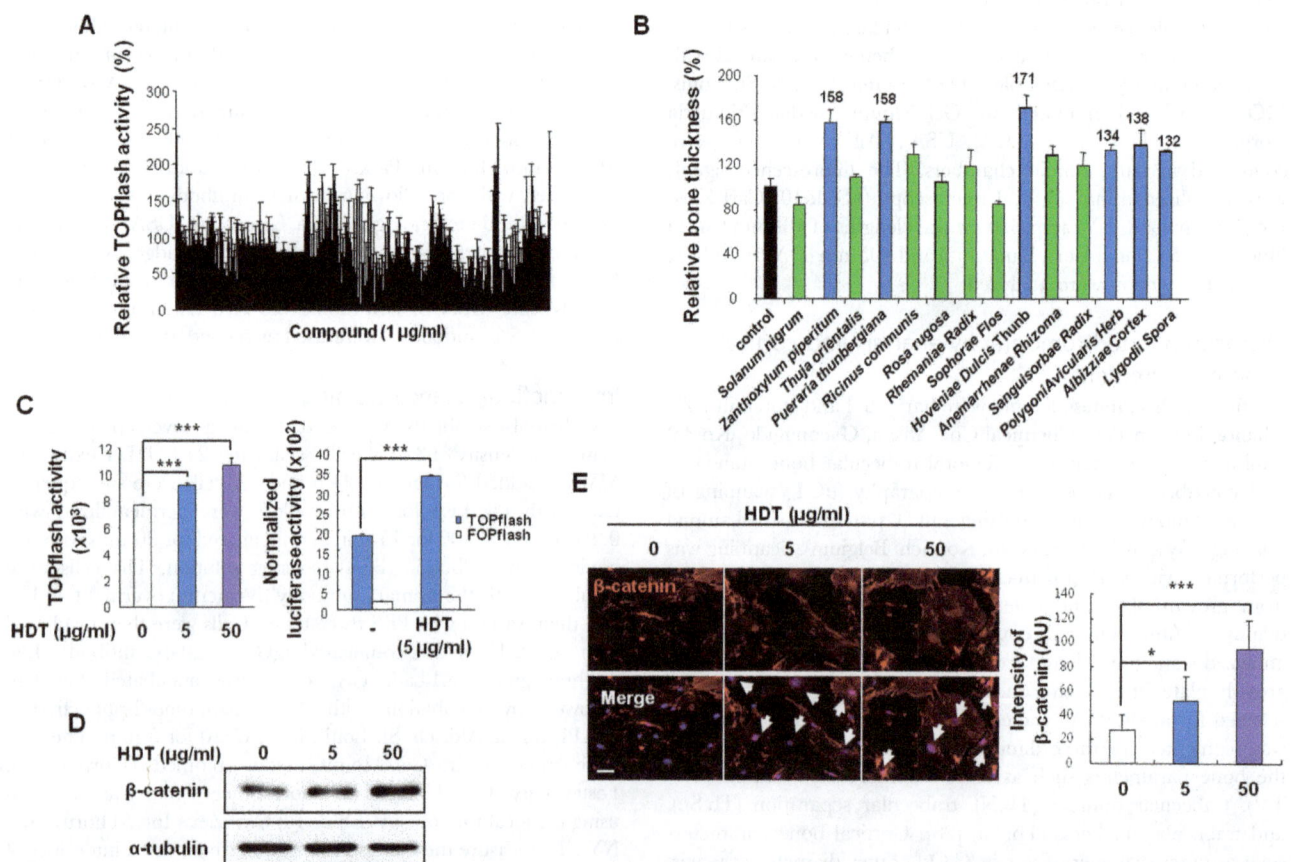

Figure 1. Identification of *Hovenia dulcis* Thunb (HDT) extract as an activator of Wnt/β-catenin signaling pathway. (A) Each of the 350 plant extracts (1 μg/ml each) was added to HEK293 reporter cells for 24 h, and TOPflash activity was measured. (n = 3). (B) Fourteen plant extracts, which showed increased TOPflash activity compared with control, were subjected to calvaria *ex vivo* assay. Of 14 plant extracts, six plant extracts, which increased the thickness of the *ex-vivo* cultured calvaria, were marked by blue bars (n = 2). (C–E) HDT extract was added to HEK293 reporter cells (C) or calvarial osteoblasts (D, and E) for 24 h. (C) Luciferase activity of HEK293 reporter cells (left) and calvarial osteoblasts transfected with TOPflash or FOPflash (right) was measured, respectively (n = 3). (D–E) β-catenin proteins were detected by immunoblotting (D) and immunofluorescence staining (E, left), respectively (white arrows indicate nuclear localized β-catenin). Scale bars, 50 μm. Intensities of β-catenin were measured from the immunofluorescence staining images (E, right) (n>3). (C, and E) *p<0.05, ***p<0.001 *versus* control.

extracts showed the >150% TOPflash activity compared with the control (Figure 1A). Using *ex vivo* calvaria assays, we found that six plant extracts stimulated bone formation (>130% compared with the control). The HDT extract revealed the highest increase in bone thickness of calvaria among the 6 plant extracts (Figure 1B). We further confirmed that the HDT extract dose-dependently increased TOPflash activity in HEK293 reporter cells and increased the activity of TOPflash but not the FOPflash harboring mutant TCF binding site in calvarial osteoblasts (Figure 1C). Expression of β-catenin and translocation of β-catenin into nuclei were also dose-dependently increased with exposure to the HDT extract in calvarial osteoblasts (Figure 1D, and E). HDT extract as high as 50 μg/ml was not cytotoxic in calvarial osteoblasts for 72 h (Figure S1). HDT extract activates the Wnt/β-catenin pathway without significant toxicity in calvarial osteoblasts.

HDT extract induces osteoblast differentiation of primary calvarial osteoblasts

Because activation of the Wnt/β-catenin pathway stimulates osteoblast differentiation, we investigated whether HDT extract can induce osteoblast differentiation of primary calvarial osteoblasts. HDT extract dose-dependently increased mRNA levels of the osteoblast differentiation markers such as *RUNX2*, *BMP2*, *ALP* and *OCN* (Figure 2A). Gene expression of two genes related to osteoclast activity, *RANKL*, a secreted osteoclastogenesis activator, and *OPG*, a secreted osteoclastogenesis inhibitor, was reduced and increased dose-dependently, respectively (Figure 2A). HDT extract also elevated ALP activity compared with the control in a dose-dependent manner (Figure 2B). Alizarin Red S staining revealed that the HDT extract induced terminal osteogenic differentiation (Figure 2C). We confirmed the effect of HDT extract on bone formation *ex vivo* using calvaria from neonatal mice. H&E staining showed that HDT extract increased calvaria thickness in a dose-dependent manner (Figure 2D).

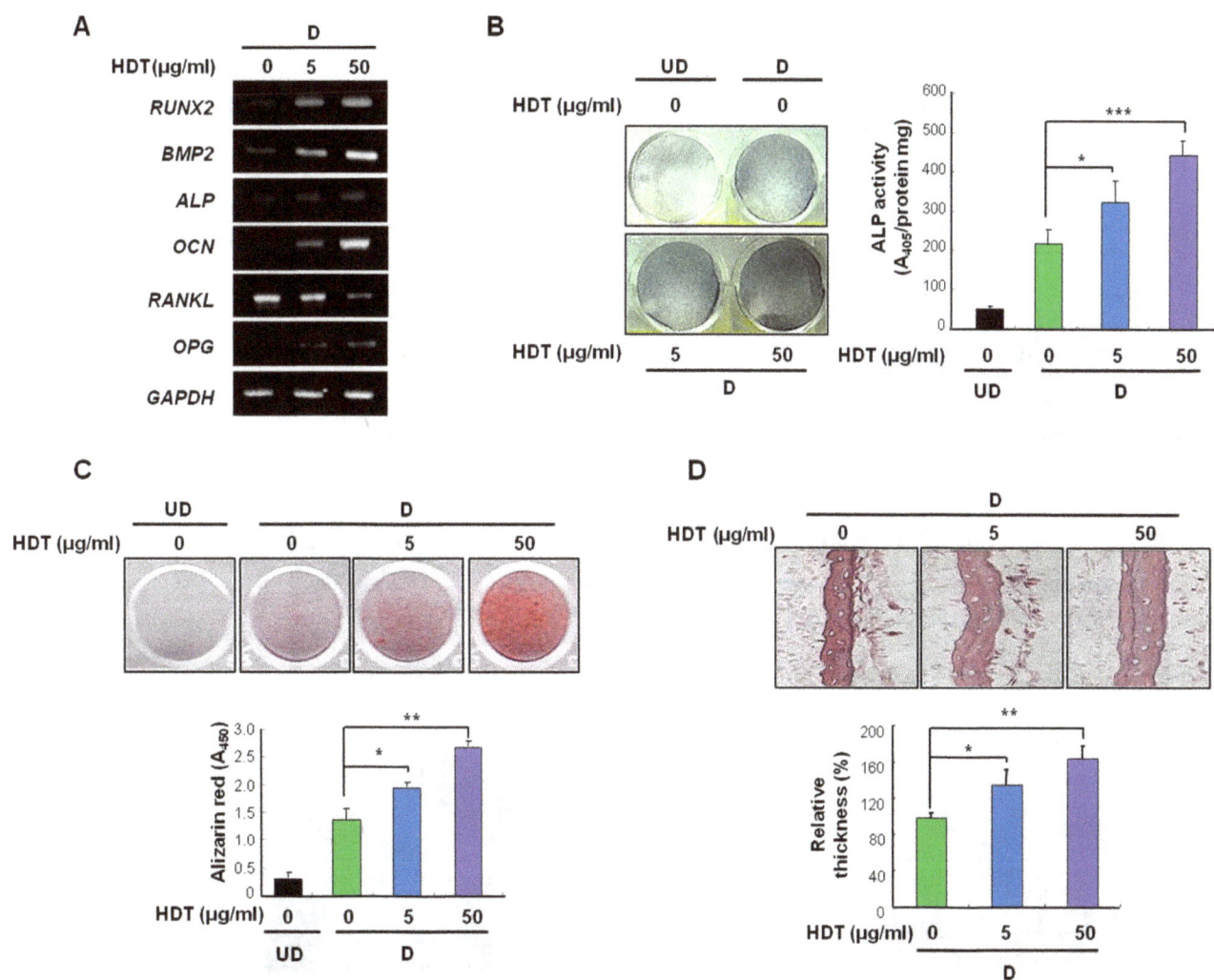

Figure 2. HDT extract has osteogenic effects on calvarial osteoblasts and mouse calvaria. (A–C) Calvarial osteoblast cells were treated with HDT extract or DMSO (control) in osteogenic differentiation (D) or the basic undifferentiation (UD) medium. (A) Calvarial osteoblasts were treated with HDT extract for 3 days followed by harvesting for RT-PCR analyses. (B) Calvarial osteoblasts were treated with HDT extract for 5 days and then subjected to ALP staining (left) or ALP activity measurements (right). (C) Calvarial osteoblasts were treated with HDT extract for 21 days. The cells were then stained with Alizarin Red S solution (up) and quantification was performed by measuring absorbance at 450 nm (n = 3; down). (D) Calvaria were treated with HDT extract in osteogenic differentiation (D) media for 7 days. Thickness of the calvaria was assessed by H&E staining (up) and quantified (down; n = 3). (B–D) *p<0.05, **p<0.01, ***p<0.001 *versus* control of differentiation medium.

Intraperitoneal application of HDT extract stimulated bone mass of normal ICR mice

To investigate the effects of HDT extract on bone mass *in vivo*, 200 mg/kg of HDT extract was i.p. injected into 8-week-old male mice for 4 weeks. Femurs from mice injected with vehicle or HDT extract were analyzed using μCT generated 3D images (Figure 3A). HDT extract increased trabecular bone parameters such as BV/TV and Tb.N, but not Tb.Th (Figure 3B). Reversely, Tb.Sp was significantly reduced by HDT extract treatment (Figure 3B). Increase in trabecular bone by HDT extract treatment was also shown by H&E staining (Figure 3C).

Trabecular bone is related to metabolism and strength of bone. Cortical bone maintains the correct architecture and stiffness of bone [30]. Both trabecular and cortical bone volumes or thickness were increased in the mice harboring the Wnt/β-catenin pathway activation (GSK3β$^{+/-}$, Sfrp3$^{-/-}$, or Sost$^{-/-}$ mice) [31–33]. To evaluate effects of HDT extract on femoral cortical bone, we analyzed cortical bone parameters such as outer diameter and thickness from the μCT 3D images. HDT extracts stimulated

increment of thickness and area of femoral cortical bones as well as those of trabecular bones (Figure 3D). Calcein double labeling showed dynamic increase in bone formation of femoral trabecular (Figure 3E) or cortical bones (Figure 3F) of HDT extract-treated mice compared with those of the vehicle-treated mice. Compared with the vehicle-treated mice, we also confirmed that HDT extract-treated mice showed an increased expression of β-catenin in trabecular and cortical bones of femurs, respectively (Figure 3G, and H). Overall, HDT extract activated the Wnt/β-catenin pathway and increased femoral bone mass through elevation of bone formation in normal mouse model. Significant weight differences were not observed between the vehicle and HDT extract-treated groups (Figure S2).

MV induced osteoblast differentiation of primary calvarial osteoblasts

To identify which HDT ingredients activate the Wnt/β-catenin pathway and induce osteoblast differentiation, we obtained 8 available ingredients that make up HDT; VA, MV, FA, myricetin,

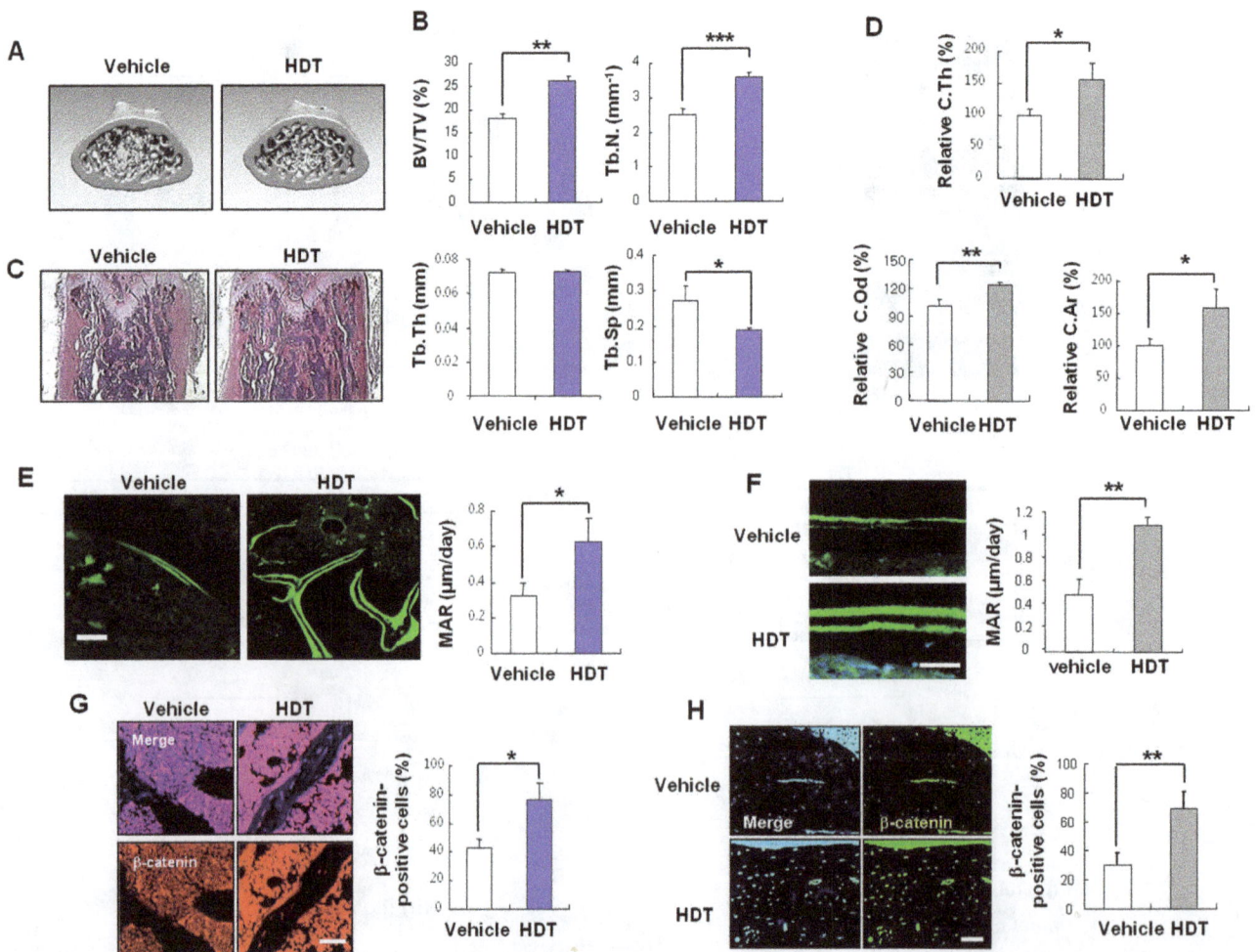

Figure 3. HDT extract enhances bone mass in normal mice. (A–H) HDT extract (200 mg/kg) was i.p. injected into 8-weeks-old male mice (n = 5) and the femurs were analyzed. (A) The representative μCT images are shown. (B) Trabecular bone parameters, such as BV/TV (%), Tb.N. (mm^{-1}), Tb. Th (mm) and Tb.Sp (mm) from the μCT analysis are presented. (C) Photomicrographs of H&E stained-femur from vehicle- and HDT extract-treated mice are shown (original magnification: ×40). (D) Cortical bone parameters such as C.Th, C.Od, and C.Ar were measured from μCT 3D images and were normalized by the values of vehicle, respectively. (E–F) Calcein double staining (left) and mineral appositional rate (MAR; right) of trabecular bone (E) and endocortical surface (F) at femurs (n = 3). Scale bars, 20 μm. (G–H) Florescence staining of β-catenin (left) in the femoral trabecular (G) and cortical bones (H) and quantification data are shown (n = 3; right). Scale bars, 50 μm. (B, and D–H) *p<0.05, **p<0.01, ***p<0.001 *versus* vehicle.

Hovenia dulcis Thunb Extract and Its Ingredient Methyl Vanillate Activate Wnt/β-Catenin Pathway...

165

tasifolin, 2,3,4-TA, DH and GC [34–36]. Of these ingredients, MV, 2,3,4-TA and GC increased TOPflash activity in HEK293 reporter cells (Figure S3A) and MV most significantly increased the ALP activity (Figure S3B). MV did not cause any significant cytotoxicity when treated to calvarial osteoblasts as high as 20 μM for 72 h (Figure S4). Therefore, we chose MV for further characterization of its osteogenic capacity (Figure 4A). We observed that MV increased the expression and nuclear translocation of β-catenin in calvarial osteoblasts (Figure 4B). Like the HDT extract, MV increased the expression of differentiation markers *RUNX2*, *BMP2*, *ALP*, and *OCN* in a dose-dependent manner (Figure 4C). MV decreased and increased the expression of *RANKL* and *OPG*, respectively (Figure 4C). We confirmed that MV dose-dependently elevated ALP activity in calvarial osteoblasts (Figure 4D). Furthermore, calvarial thickness was dose-dependently increased with MV treatment (Figure 4E). Collectively, MV increased the β-catenin expression and induced osteoblasts differentiation, leading to the enhanced bone formation *ex vivo*. In addition, siRNA-mediated β-catenin knockdown abolished the increment of β-catenin (Figure S5A) and ALP activity (Figure S5B) by MV. These results indicated that the Wnt/β-catenin pathway signaling is involved in MV-induced ALP activation.

Orally administrated MV rescues osteopenia-induced by ovariectomy

To investigate whether MV reverses bone loss *in vivo*, we performed ovariectomies on mice and induced bone loss for 2 weeks. Lower bone mass in vehicle-treated OVX mice was confirmed through bone histomorphometric analyses by μCT (Figure 5A). Trabecular bone parameters such as BV/TV, Tb.N and Tb.Th were significantly reduced in OVX-vehicle mice compared with Sham-vehicle mice. Oral administration of MV rescued the reduced parameters in a dose-dependent manner (Figure 5B). In contrast, Tb.Sp was increased in OVX-vehicle mice. Following MV treatment, this parameter decreased in dose-dependent fashion (Figure 5B). We observed increase of trabecular bone volume at femurs with MV treatment by H&E staining (Figure 5C). MV also showed anabolic effects on femoral cortical bones (Figure 5D). MV dose-dependently elevated the expression of β-catenin in femoral trabecular and cortical bones, respectively (Figure 5E, Figure S6A, and B), however, no significant difference was observed in the expression of β-catenin between the vehicle-treated Sham and vehicle-treated OVX mice (Figure 5E).

The body weights of the MV-treated mice did not significantly differ compared to those of non-treated mice (Figure S7A). No discernible abnormalities were observed in H&E-stained liver tissue of MV-treated mice (Figure S7B). Because estrogen is limited in clinical applications due to its tumor-promoting characteristics, we checked whether MV has estrogenicity by

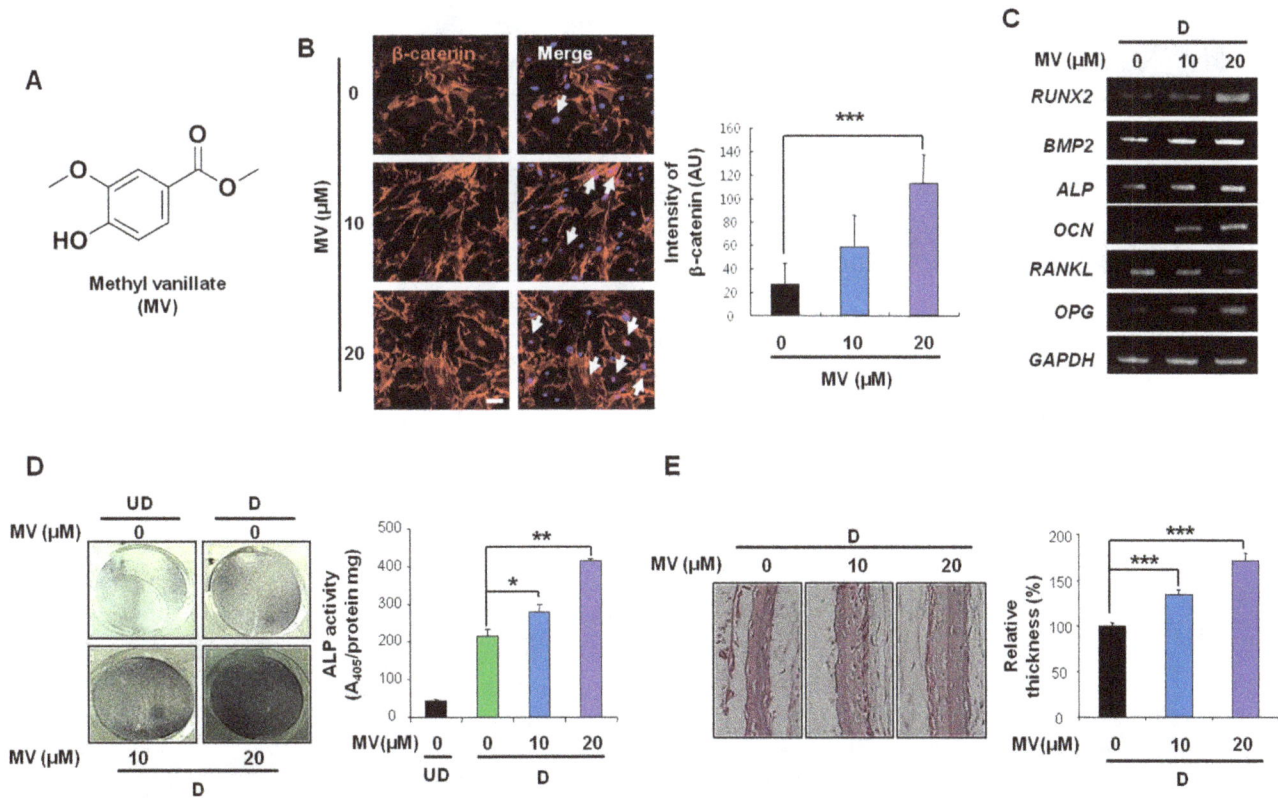

Figure 4. MV activates the Wnt/β-catenin signaling pathway and induces calvarial osteoblast differentiation. (A) A structure of MV. (B) Immunofluorescence staining of β-catenin in calvarial osteoblasts is shown (left, white arrows indicate nuclear β-catenin). Scale bars, 50 μm. Intensities of β-catenin were measured (right, n>3). (C–E) Osteogenic differentiation (D) or the basic (UD) medium was used. (C) Calvarial osteoblasts were treated with MV for 72 h and mRNA levels of the indicated genes were analyzed. (D) Calvarial osteoblasts treated with MV were stained for ALP (left) and ALP activity was measured (n = 3; right). (E) Calvaria isolated from postnatal day 4 mice were incubated with MV for 7 days. H&E staining revealed the thickness of the calvaria (left), and the thickness was quantified (n = 3; right). (B, D–E) *p<0.05, **p<0.01, ***p<0.001 *versus* control of differentiation medium.

assessing the wet weights and histomorphometry of the uterus [37]. The weight of wet uterine in OVX-mice was reduced by 84% compared with that of the Sham-mice, however, oral administration of MV did not exhibit increase in uterine weights compared to OVX-vehicle-treated mice (Figure S7C). We also confirmed that MV does not have any estrogenic effects by histomorphometric analyses showing maintenance of atrophic histological characteristics in the uterine of MV-treated OVX mice (Figure S7D). Overall, MV rescued bone loss induced by OVX without resulting in any significant changes of the weights or status of liver and uterine tissue.

MV rescued bone loss in OVX-mice as efficiently as PTH drug

We compared the efficacies of MV with PTH (1–34) in bone formation because PTH (1–34) is the only anabolic agent approved by the FDA for osteoporosis treatment [38]. We performed ovariectomies on mice and allowed them to develop severe osteopenia over a period of 4 weeks to induce (Figure 6A). In these mice, MV increased the BV/TV, Tb.N and Tb.Th, while decreasing Tb.Sp similar to PTH (1–34) treatment in OVX-mice

compared to vehicle-treated OVX-mice (Figure 6A, and B). Interestingly, orally administered MV at 100 mg/kg revealed equivalent effects on bone mass to those observed with i.p. injection of PTH (1–34; 80 μg/kg) in femurs (Figure 6A, and B). No significant changes of weight were observed for mice used in the experiments (Figure 6C).

Discussion

Because activation of the Wnt/β-catenin pathway induces osteoblast differentiation and bone mass, the pathway is of recent interest as a major target for development of anabolic agents to treat osteoporosis. Here, we screened 350 plant extracts to find novel activators of the Wnt/β-catenin pathway and identified HDT extract as a candidate for anabolic bone formation. HDT, also known as the Japanese raisin tree, has been used as a traditional medicine for treatment of liver diseases and for detoxification of alcoholic poisoning in eastern Asian countries such as Japan, China and Korea [39,40]. The HDT extract also has anti-diabetic and anti-cancer effects, neuroprotective effects, and regenerative effects in damaged liver [36,39]. However, the

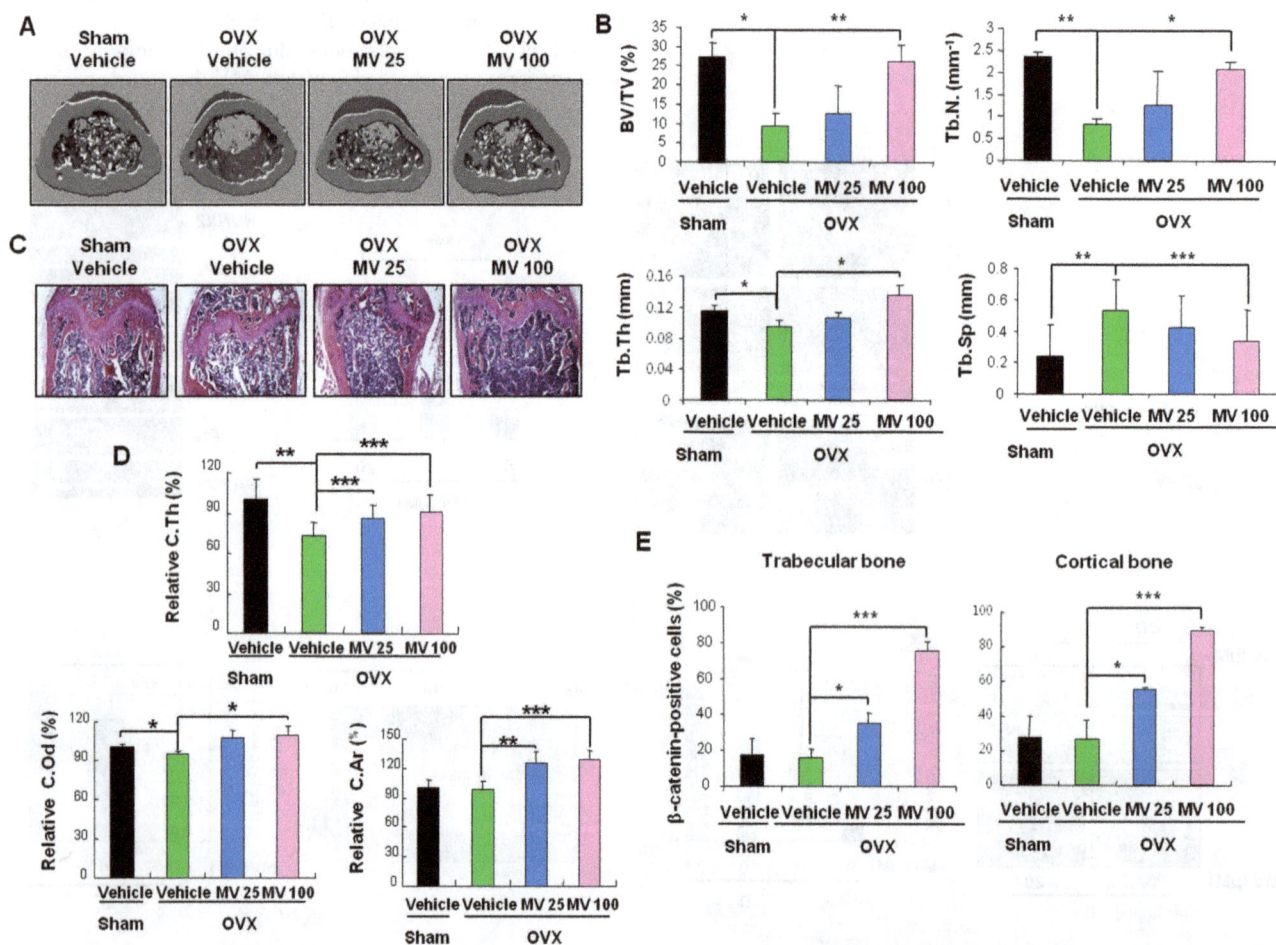

Figure 5. MV rescues bone loss induced by ovariectomy. (A–E) MV was orally administered to Sham- or OVX-mice for 4 weeks and femurs were used for further analysis (n=5). (A) The representative μCT analysis images are presented. (B) The μCT analyses for femoral trabecular bone parameters are presented. (C) Femurs from the SHAM-vehicle, OVX-vehicle, or OVX-MV mice were stained with H&E (original magnification: ×40). (D) Cortical bone parameters were measured from μCT 3D images and were normalized by those of Sham-vehicle mice. (E) Florescence staining of β-catenin in the femoral trabecular and cortical bones (Figure S6) were quantified (n=3). (B, D–E) *p<0.05, **p<0.01, ***p<0.001 between indicated samples.

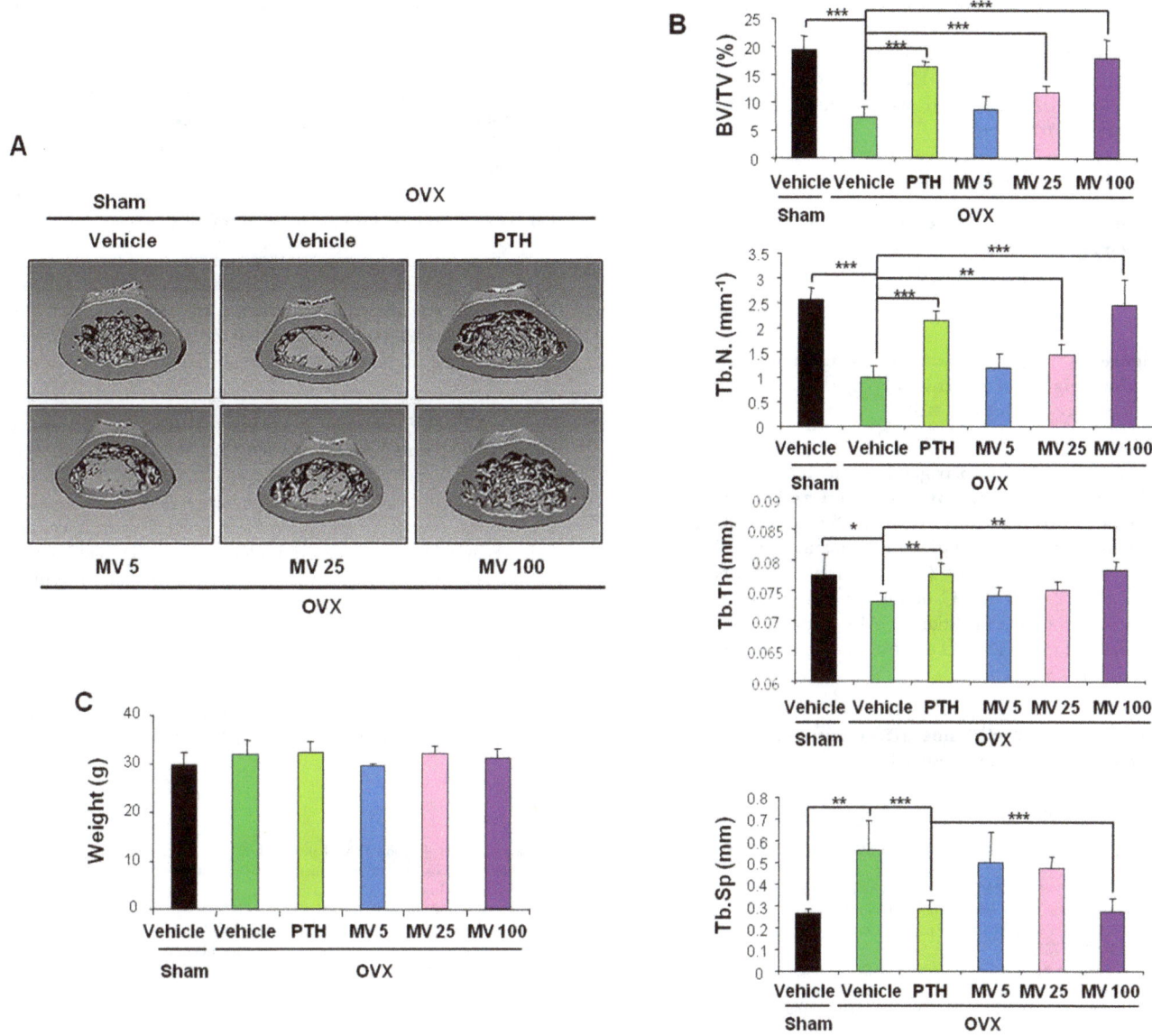

Figure 6. Effects of MV or PTH on the bone loss induced by ovariectomy. (A–D) MV or PTH (80 µg/kg) was administered to the Sham- or OVX-mice. The femurs were used for further analyses (n = 5–7). (A) The representative µCT analysis images are presented. (B) Femoral trabecular bone parameters were obtained for µCT analyses *p<0.05, **p<0.01, ***p<0.001 between indicated samples. (C) The relative weights of mice after final treatment with PTH or MV are shown.

effect of HDT extract on skeletal physiology has not been reported. We investigated whether the HDT extract increases bone mass, following our identification of its function in the activation of Wnt/β-catenin pathway. We found that HDT extract induces osteogenic differentiation *in vitro* and increases femoral bone mass *in vivo*.

To identify the ingredients responsible for activating the Wnt/β-catenin pathway and inducing osteoblast differentiation, we tested the 8 known ingredients in HDT to determine whether they modulate Wnt/β-catenin signaling and osteoblast differentiation. Of those, we determined that MV is as the most effective active ingredient that increases osteoblast differentiation with activation of the Wnt/β-catenin pathway. MV is present in many plants, including the stem bark of *Zanthoxylum scandens* and HDT, and has been reported to have anti-platelet and anti-oxidant activity

[36,41–43]. Here, we showed that MV induces osteoblast differentiation *in vitro* and the oral administration of MV rescues femoral trabecular and cortical bone loss caused by OVX. Moreover, when orally administered at 100 mg/kg, MV possesses an efficacy similar to PTH (1–34; 80 µg/kg) [44] for recovering bone loss in OVX-mice. PTH drugs are a standard anabolic treatment for osteoporosis approved by the FDA. However, PTH drugs can only be administrated by injection and for only 2 years due to the risk of cancer [45]. Unlike PTH drugs, MV could be administrated orally and is considered safe because it is a natural plant-derived ingredient. We show that treatment with HDT extract or MV is not critically cytotoxic to calvarial osteoblasts and does not significantly affect the weights of mice used *in vivo* experiments. Medicinal plants and their active ingredients have been used in traditional medicines for centuries [20,21,46]. HDT extract from stem barks, leaves, and fruits is not cytotoxic to mammalian cells [36,47]. HDT extract and its active ingredients are used as additives to food in Asian countries without inducing cytotoxicity [48,49]. Thus, HDT extract and its active ingredient MV could be developed as potential anabolic agents for osteoporosis treatment.

Supporting Information

Figure S1 HDT extract did not affect cytotoxicity in calvarial osteoblasts. Calvarial osteoblasts were treated with HDT extract for 72 h and the cytotoxicity was assessed by MTT assay (n = 3).

Figure S2 HDT extract did not induce critical changes to the weights of the mice. Weight difference of mice used in Figure 3 are presented (n = 5).

Figure S3 MV is an ingredient in HDT responsible for Wnt/β-catenin pathway activation and increased osteoblasts differentiation. (A) HEK293 reporter cells were treated with its 8 ingredients (20 μM) for 24 h, and subjected to TOPflash activity measurement (n = 3). (B) Calvarial osteoblasts were treated with MV, 2,3,4-TA, GC or FA for 3 days, and the cells were harvested for determination of ALP activity. ALP activity was normalized to the DMSO (control), and FA was used as a positive control (n = 3).

Figure S4 MV did not affect cytotoxicity in calvarial osteoblasts. Calvarial osteoblasts were incubated with MV for

72 h and the cytotoxicity of MV was determined by MTT assay (n = 3).

Figure S5 MV increases ALP activity via activation of Wnt/β-catenin pathway in MC3T3E1 cell lines. (A–B) The siRNA for β-catenin or a control (siRNA for GFP) was transfected into MC3T3E1 cells. After 12 h, MV was treated with differentiation media for 72 h and the cells were subjected to immunoblotting (A) and measurement of ALP activity (B; n = 3).

Figure S6 MV increases β-catenin expression at femur. (A–B) Data are shown from mice used in Fig. 5. (n = 5). Representative images of IHC staining for β-catenin in trabecular (A) and cortical (B) bone at femur. Scale bars, 50 μm.

Figure S7 MV causes no critical abnormalities in weight, live, and uterine. (A–D) Data are shown from mice used in Fig. 5. (n = 5). (A) The weights of mice were measured every 4 days. (B) Liver tissue from the mice was stained with H&E (CV; central veins). (C) The uteri were isolated from mice, and their wet weights were measured after sacrifice. (D) The uteri in (C) were subjected to H&E staining. (B, D) Scale bars, 100 μm.

Author Contributions

Conceived and designed the experiments: PHC WJS MZ HYK DSM KYC. Performed the experiments: PHC WJS MZ. Contributed reagents/materials/analysis tools: PHC WJS MZ HYK. Wrote the paper: PHC KYC.

References

1. Rodan GA (1998) Bone homeostasis. Proc Natl Acad Sci U S A 95: 13361–13362.
2. Khosla S, Riggs BL (2005) Pathophysiology of age-related bone loss and osteoporosis. Endocrinol Metab Clin North Am 34: 1015–1030, xi.
3. McGrath H Jr (1996) Alendronate in postmenopausal osteoporosis. N Engl J Med 334: 734–735.
4. Cummings SR, Black DM, Thompson DE, Applegate WB, Barrett-Connor E, et al. (1998) Effect of alendronate on risk of fracture in women with low bone density but without vertebral fractures: results from the Fracture Intervention Trial. JAMA 280: 2077–2082.
5. Woo SB, Hellstein JW, Kalmar JR (2006) Narrative [corrected] review: bisphosphonates and osteonecrosis of the jaws. Ann Intern Med 144: 753–761.
6. Kennel KA, Drake MT (2009) Adverse effects of bisphosphonates: implications for osteoporosis management. Mayo Clin Proc 84: 632–637; quiz 638.
7. Tang DZ, Hou W, Zhou Q, Zhang M, Holz J, et al. (2010) Osthole stimulates osteoblast differentiation and bone formation by activation of beta-catenin-BMP signaling. J Bone Miner Res 25: 1234–1245.
8. Khan AW, Khan A (2006) Anabolic agents: a new chapter in the management of osteoporosis. J Obstet Gynaecol Can 28: 136–141.
9. Rachner TD, Khosla S, Hofbauer LC (2011) Osteoporosis: now and the future. Lancet 377: 1276–1287.
10. Saag KG, Zanchetta JR, Devogelaer JP, Adler RA, Eastell R, et al. (2009) Effects of teriparatide versus alendronate for treating glucocorticoid-induced osteoporosis: thirty-six-month results of a randomized, double-blind, controlled trial. Arthritis Rheum 60: 3346–3355.
11. Bouxsein ML, Chen P, Glass EV, Kallmes DF, Delmas PD, et al. (2009) Teriparatide and raloxifene reduce the risk of new adjacent vertebral fractures in postmenopausal women with osteoporosis. Results from two randomized controlled trials. J Bone Joint Surg Am 91: 1329–1338.
12. Tashjian AH Jr, Gagel RF (2006) Teriparatide [human PTH(1–34)]: 2.5 years of experience on the use and safety of the drug for the treatment of osteoporosis. J Bone Miner Res 21: 354–365.
13. Holmen SL, Zylstra CR, Mukherjee A, Sigler RE, Faugere MC, et al. (2005) Essential role of beta-catenin in postnatal bone acquisition. J Biol Chem 280: 21162–21168.
14. Glass DA 2nd, Bialek P, Ahn JD, Starbuck M, Patel MS, et al. (2005) Canonical Wnt signaling in differentiated osteoblasts controls osteoclast differentiation. Dev Cell 8: 751–764.
15. Luo X, Chen J, Song WX, Tang N, Luo J, et al. (2008) Osteogenic BMPs promote tumor growth of human osteosarcomas that harbor differentiation defects. Lab Invest 88: 1264–1277.
16. Massague J, Blain SW, Lo RS (2000) TGFbeta signaling in growth control, cancer, and heritable disorders. Cell 103: 295–309.
17. Kloen P, Gebhardt MC, Perez-Atayde A, Rosenberg AE, Springfield DS, et al. (1997) Expression of transforming growth factor-beta (TGF-beta) isoforms in osteosarcomas: TGF-beta3 is related to disease progression. Cancer 80: 2230–2239.
18. Cai Y, Mohseny AB, Karperien M, Hogendoorn PC, Zhou G, et al. (2010) Inactive Wnt/beta-catenin pathway in conventional high-grade osteosarcoma. J Pathol 220: 24–33.
19. Hoeppner LH, Secreto FJ, Westendorf JJ (2009) Wnt signaling as a therapeutic target for bone diseases. Expert Opin Ther Targets 13: 485–496.
20. Vasudeva N, Yadav N, Sharma SK (2012) Natural products: a safest approach for obesity. Chin J Integr Med 18: 473–480.
21. Sawadogo WR, Schumacher M, Teiten MH, Dicato M, Diederich M (2012) Traditional West African pharmacopeia, plants and derived compounds for cancer therapy. Biochem Pharmacol 84: 1225–1240.
22. Zhang J, Wider B, Shang H, Li X, Ernst E (2012) Quality of herbal medicines: challenges and solutions. Complement Ther Med 20: 100–106.
23. Sheng-Ji P (2001) Ethnobotanical approaches of traditional medicine studies: some experiences from Asia. Pharm Biol 39 Suppl 1: 74–79.
24. Yun MS, Kim SE, Jeon SH, Lee JS, Choi KY (2005) Both ERK and Wnt/beta-catenin pathways are involved in Wnt3a-induced proliferation. J Cell Sci 118: 313–322.
25. Korinek V, Barker N, Morin PJ, van Wichen D, de Weger R, et al. (1997) Constitutive transcriptional activation by a beta-catenin-Tcf complex in APC-/- colon carcinoma. Science 275: 1784–1787.
26. Gong Y, Slee RB, Fukai N, Rawadi G, Roman-Roman S, et al. (2001) LDL receptor-related protein 5 (LRP5) affects bone accrual and eye development. Cell 107: 513–523.
27. Jeong WJ, Yoon J, Park JC, Lee SH, Lee SH, et al. (2012) Ras stabilization through aberrant activation of Wnt/beta-catenin signaling promotes intestinal tumorigenesis. Sci Signal 5: ra30.
28. Iwaniec UT, Wronski TJ, Liu J, Rivera MF, Arzaga RR, et al. (2007) PTH stimulates bone formation in mice deficient in Lrp5. J Bone Miner Res 22: 394–402.

29. Trivedi R, Kumar S, Kumar A, Siddiqui JA, Swarnkar G, et al. (2008) Kaempferol has osteogenic effect in ovariectomized adult Sprague-Dawley rats. Mol Cell Endocrinol 289: 85–93.

30. Seeman E (2009) Bone modeling and remodeling. Crit Rev Eukaryot Gene Expr 19: 219–233.

31. Arioka M, Takahashi-Yanaga F, Sasaki M, Yoshihara T, Morimoto S, et al. (2013) Acceleration of bone development and regeneration through the Wnt/beta-catenin signaling pathway in mice heterozygously deficient for GSK-3beta. Biochem Biophys Res Commun.

32. Li X, Ominsky MS, Niu QT, Sun N, Daugherty B, et al. (2008) Targeted deletion of the sclerostin gene in mice results in increased bone formation and bone strength. J Bone Miner Res 23: 860–869.

33. Lories RJ, Peeters J, Bakker A, Tylzanowski P, Derese I, et al. (2007) Articular cartilage and biomechanical properties of the long bones in Frzb-knockout mice. Arthritis Rheum 56: 4095–4103.

34. Ding LS, Liang QL, Teng YF (1997) [Study on flavonoids in seeds of Hovenia dulcis]. Yao Xue Xue Bao 32: 600–602.

35. Yoshikawa M, Murakami T, Ueda T, Yoshizumi S, Ninomiya K, et al. (1997) [Bioactive constituents of Chinese natural medicines. III. Absolute stereostructures of new dihydroflavonols, hovenitins I, II, and III, isolated from hoveniae semen seu fructus, the seed and fruit of Hovenia dulcis THUNB. (Rhamnaceae): inhibitory effect on alcohol-induced muscular relaxation and hepatoprotective activity]. Yakugaku Zasshi 117: 108–118.

36. Li G, Min BS, Zheng C, Lee J, Oh SR, et al. (2005) Neuroprotective and free radical scavenging activities of phenolic compounds from Hovenia dulcis. Arch Pharm Res 28: 804–809.

37. Finan B, Yang B, Ottaway N, Stemmer K, Muller TD, et al. (2012) Targeted estrogen delivery reverses the metabolic syndrome. Nat Med 18: 1847–1856.

38. Sibai T, Morgan EF, Einhorn TA (2011) Anabolic agents and bone quality. Clin Orthop Relat Res 469: 2215–2224.

39. Hyun TK, Eom SH, Yu CY, Roitsch T (2010) Hovenia dulcis–an Asian traditional herb. Planta Med 76: 943–949.

40. Chen SH, Zhong GS, Li AL, Li SH, Wu LK (2006) [Influence of Hovenia dulcis on alcohol concentration in blood and activity of alcohol dehydrogenase (ADH) of animals after drinking]. Zhongguo Zhong Yao Za Zhi 31: 1094–1096.

41. Yun-Choi HS, Kim JH, Lee JR (1987) Potential inhibitors of platelet aggregation from plant sources, III. J Nat Prod 50: 1059–1064.

42. Ming-Jen Cheng C-FL, Huun-Shuo Chang, Ih-Sheng Chen (2008) CHEMICAL CONSTITUENTS FROM THE STEM BARK OF ZNTHOWYLUM SCANDENS. J Chil Chem Soc 53: 1631–1634.

43. Tai A, Sawano T, Ito H (2012) Antioxidative properties of vanillic acid esters in multiple antioxidant assays. Biosci Biotechnol Biochem 76: 314–318.

44. Yadav VK, Balaji S, Suresh PS, Liu XS, Lu X, et al. (2010) Pharmacological inhibition of gut-derived serotonin synthesis is a potential bone anabolic treatment for osteoporosis. Nat Med 16: 308–312.

45. Bilezikian JP, Matsumoto T, Bellido T, Khosla S, Martin J, et al. (2009) Targeting bone remodeling for the treatment of osteoporosis: summary of the proceedings of an ASBMR workshop. J Bone Miner Res 24: 373–385.

46. Yang SP, Yue JM (2012) Discovery of structurally diverse and bioactive compounds from plant resources in China. Acta Pharmacol Sin 33: 1147–1158.

47. Gadelha AP, Vidal F, Castro TM, Lopes CS, Albarello N, et al. (2005) Susceptibility of Giardia lamblia to Hovenia dulcis extracts. Parasitol Res 97: 399–407.

48. Hussain RA, Lin YM, Poveda LJ, Bordas E, Chung BS, et al. (1990) Plant-derived sweetening agents: saccharide and polyol constituents of some sweet-tasting plants. J Ethnopharmacol 28: 103–115.

49. Yoshikawa K, Nagai M, Wakabayashi M, Arihara S (1993) Aroma glycosides from Hovenia dulsis. Phytochemistry 34: 1431–1433.

20

Palmitoyl Acyltransferase, *Zdhhc13,* Facilitates Bone Mass Acquisition by Regulating Postnatal Epiphyseal Development and Endochondral Ossification

I-Wen Song[1,2], Wei-Ru Li[1], Li-Ying Chen[1], Li-Fen Shen[1], Kai-Ming Liu[1,3], Jeffrey J. Y. Yen[1], Yi-Ju Chen[4], Yu-Ju Chen[4], Virginia Byers Kraus[5], Jer-Yuarn Wu[1], M. T. Michael Lee[1,6,7]*, Yuan-Tsong Chen[1,2,8]*

1 Institute of Biomedical Sciences, Academia Sinica, Taipei, Taiwan, 2 Graduate Institute of Life Sciences, National Defense Medical Center, Taipei, Taiwan, 3 Institute of Clinical Medicine, National Yang-Ming University, Taipei, Taiwan, 4 Institute of Chemistry, Academia Sinica, Taipei, Taiwan, 5 Department of Medicine, Division of Rheumatology, Duke University Medical Center, Durham, North Carolina, United States of America, 6 Laboratory for International Alliance on Genomic Research, RIKEN Center for Integrative Medical Sciences, Yokohama, Japan, 7 Graduate Institute of Chinese Medical Science, China Medical University, Taichung, Taiwan, 8 Department of Pediatrics, Duke University Medical Center, Durham, North Carolina, United States of America

Abstract

ZDHHC13 is a member of DHHC-containing palmitoyl acyltransferases (PATs) family of enzymes. It functions by post-translationally adding 16-carbon palmitate to proteins through a thioester linkage. We have previously shown that mice carrying a recessive *Zdhhc13* nonsense mutation causing a *Zdhcc13* deficiency develop alopecia, amyloidosis and osteoporosis. Our goal was to investigate the pathogenic mechanism of osteoporosis in the context of this mutation in mice. Body size, skeletal structure and trabecular bone were similar in *Zdhhc13* WT and mutant mice at birth. Growth retardation and delayed secondary ossification center formation were first observed at day 10 and at 4 weeks of age, disorganization in growth plate structure and osteoporosis became evident in mutant mice. Serial microCT from 4-20 week-olds revealed that *Zdhhc13* mutant mice had reduced bone mineral density. Through co-immunoprecipitation and acyl-biotin exchange, MT1-MMP was identified as a direct substrate of ZDHHC13. In cells, reduction of MT1-MMP palmitoylation affected its subcellular distribution and was associated with decreased VEGF and osteocalcin expression in chondrocytes and osteoblasts. In *Zdhhc13* mutant mice epiphysis where MT1-MMP was under palmitoylated, VEGF in hypertrophic chondrocytes and osteocalcin at the cartilage-bone interface were reduced based on immunohistochemical analyses. Our results suggest that *Zdhhc13* is a novel regulator of postnatal skeletal development and bone mass acquisition. To our knowledge, these are the first data to suggest that ZDHHC13-mediated MT1-MMP palmitoylation is a key modulator of bone homeostasis. These data may provide novel insights into the role of palmitoylation in the pathogenesis of human osteoporosis.

Editor: Damian Christopher Genetos, University of California Davis, United States of America

Funding: This study was supported by the Academia Sinica Genomic Medicine Multicenter Study (40-05-GMM), the National Research Program for Genomic Medicine, National Science Council, Taiwan (National Center for Genome Medicine, NSC101-2319-B-001-001). The funders had no role in study design, data collection and analysis, decision to publish, or preparation of the manuscript.

Competing Interests: The authors have declared that no competing interests exist.

* E-mail: mikelee@ibms.sinica.edu.tw (MTML); chen0010@ibms.sinica.edu.tw (YTC)

Introduction

Palmitoylation is a post-translational lipid modification involving the addition of a 16-carbon palmitate on specific cysteine residues of proteins through a thioester linkage [1]. Palmitoylation is unique for being the only lipid modification that has been shown to be reversible; this confers upon it the capability being a dynamic modulator of physiologic and pathologic conditions. To date, numerous proteins have been reported to be palmitoylated including scaffold proteins, ion channels, signaling molecules, cell adhesion molecules, and receptors. Palmitoylation has been shown to be an important regulator of protein trafficking, protein stability, protein-protein interactions and signal transduction [2–4].

A family of proteins with palmitoyl acyltransferase (PAT) activity was recently identified in yeast [5,6]; these proteins contain aspartate-histidine-histidine-cysteine (DHHC) motifs that mediate the PAT enzymatic activity. There are at least 23 DHHC PATs in the mammalian genome [7]. Current knowledge is limited of the involvement of the DHHC family in disease processes. Although *DHHC2* and *DHHC11* were reported to relate to cancers [8–10], most of the evidence concerning *DHHC* gene functions has been gleaned in the context of neurological development [11]. To date, 4 mouse models have been generated: *Zdhhc5* gene-trap mice show a reduction in contextual fear [12]; *Zdhhc8* knockout mice manifest a schizophrenia phenotype [13]; mice with a F233 deletion in *Zdhhc21* show abnormalities of skin homeostasis and hair defects [14]; and as described in our previous report, a nonsense mutation was generated in the Zdhhc13 gene by ENU mutagenesis. This mutation resulted in nonsense mediated mRNA decay of Zdhhc13 mRNA. The *Zdhhc13* deficient mice show the most severe phenotype with amyloidosis, alopecia, and osteoporosis [15]. The detailed pathogenic mechanisms of all these phenotypes still remain unclear.

Our goal in this study was to investigate the pathogenic mechanisms underlying osteoporosis in the *Zdhhc13* deficient mice. We aimed to understand how a palmitoylation enzyme, *Zdhhc13*, can affect bone homeostasis with the hope of providing new insights into the biological functions of palmitoylation and the pathogenic mechanisms of human osteoporosis.

Materials and Methods

Mice and genotyping

The *Zdhhc13* mutant mice were generated by ENU mutagenesis as described previously [15]. Genotype was analyzed by sequencing tail genomic DNA. Newborn mice were sacrificed by incubation in CO_2 for 15–20 minutes. All the animals and protocols (IACUC number: 11-05-187) used in this study were approved by the Institutional Animal Care and Utilization Committee of Academia Sinica.

Skeletal preparation

Newborn mice were skinned and eviscerated. The remaining skeletons were fixed overnight in 1% acetic acid and 95% ethanol, then stained with Alcian blue 8GX (0.05%) for 72 hours, followed by dehydration in 95% ethanol for 24 hours. The solution was changed to 1% KOH until the bone became visible. The skeletons were stained overnight with Alizarin red (0.005%). Specimens were cleared, dehydrated in 70% ethanol/glycerol (1:1), and finally stored in 100% glycerol.

Micro-Computed Tomography (MicroCT)

Tissues were fixed in 4% paraformaldehyde overnight and transferred to 70% alcohol. The microCT scan was performed as described previously [15].

Pathology and Immunohistochemistry (IHC)

Tissues were fixed in 4% paraformaldehyde and decalcified in 10% EDTA. Paraffin sections were stained with Masson's trichrome stain for morphological analysis. For IHC, antigens of de-paraffinized sections were retrieved by 0.05% trypsin or hyaluronidase (10 mg/ml) and treated with 3% H_2O_2. After blocking with 5% normal goat serum, tissues were incubated with primary antibodies in 4°C, overnight. The following rabbit polyclonal antibodies against mouse were used, anti-VEGF (Abcam, Cambridge, UK), anti-PECAM (Abcam), and anti-Osteocalcin (Millipore, Billerica, MA, USA). Sections were then incubated with anti-rabbit secondary antibody (Vectastain ABC system, Vector Laboratories, Servion, Switzerland) and developed with 0.1% 3, 39-diaminobenzidine. Images were captured using standard light microscopy (Zeiss, Oberkochen, Germany) and quantified using Image-Pro Plus software (Rockville, MD, USA). Data from three independent mice staining were used for statistical analysis.

In situ hybridization

RNA *in situ* hybridizations were performed on paraffin sections as previously described [16]. The PCR product (501 bp) generated with primers specific to mouse *Zdhhc13* (Forward: GGGCCATCCGACAAGGGCAT, and Reverse: TGTGCAGC-CATCGCCAAAGC) was inserted into pGEM-T Easy vector

(Promega, Madison, WI, USA). Digoxigenin (DIG)-labeled single-strand sense and anti-sense RNA probes were prepared with a DIG-RNA labeling kit (Roche, Indianapolis, IN, USA). The hybridized probe-RNA was then detected by anti-DIG-AP (alkaline phosphatase) (Roche) and visualized by NBT/BCIP (Roche) with a developing time of 3 hours.

RNA isolation and real-time PCR (Q-PCR)

Total RNA was extracted from tissue using the RNeasy kit (Qiagen, Hilden, Germany). cDNA was synthesized from 2 μg total RNA using the SuperScript III First-Strand cDNA Synthesis Kit (Invitrogen, Grand Island, NY, USA) and 15 ng of the cDNA was amplified in a final volume of 15 μl for Q-PCR. Q-PCR was performed using Power SYBER green PCR Master Mix with ABI PRISM 7700 Sequence Detection System (Applied Biosystems, Grand Island, NY, USA). The level of gene expression was normalized to *Gapdh* for the fold change calculation. Primers: *Zdhhc13* F- CAGCAGCATCCATCTGCGGT; R- GCCGA-TAGCATGAGCGGCGT; *Gapdh* F-TGCCAAGGCTGTGGG-CAAGG; R-TCTCCAGGCGGCACGTCAGA.

Cell culture

HEK293 and MC3T3E1 cells were purchased and cultured as described by the American Tissue Culture Collection (ATCC). ATDC5 chondrocytic cells were purchased from RIKEN and cultured using F12/DMEM medium (Sigma-Aldrich, Louis, MO, USA) with 10% FBS, 1% penicillin and streptomycin. The primary osteoblasts were isolated by modifying of a previous method [17]. Mainly, femur and tibia were collected from WT and mutant mice at age P14. Bone marrow was flushed out with PBS. The bone tissues were then dissected into 1–2 mm^2 fragments and digested in collagenase type II solution (Worthington, Lakewood, NJ, USA) for 4 hours. After washing with DMEM, the digested bone fragments were placed in culture dishes or chamber slides for following experiments. Primary epiphyseal chondrocytes were isolated as previously described [18] with several modifications. Briefly, P10 mice were scarified, the epiphysis region was dissected, and the connective tissues were removed. The connective tissue free epiphysis was then digested with type II collagenase (Worthington) overnight. Chondrocytes were separated by 70 μm mesh (BD Biosciences, San Jose, CA, USA) and cultured in DMEM containing 10% FCS. No subculture was performed to avoid transformation of the cell phenotype. Cell lysates were generated with RIPA (Millipore).

Western blotting (WB)

Tissue or cell lysates were separated by SDS-PAGE gel and transferred to PVDF membrane (Millipore). After blocking with 5% milk, the same antibodies used for VEGF and osteocalcin IHC were used for WB detection. Signals were developed by film after incubating with appropriate horseradish peroxidase (HRP) - conjugated secondary antibodies (Millipore). Densitometry quantification was performed using software in BioSpectrum Imaging System (UVP, Upland, CA, USA). Intensity for all selected bands was all normalized to their actin (loading control) intensity then calculated as fold change to vector group. Data from three independent repeat experiments were used for statistical analysis.

Co-immunoprecipitation (Co-IP)

Mouse Zdhhc13 cDNA was cloned into a pcDNA4/myc-His expression vector (Invitrogen); mouse MT1-MMP was cloned into a pcDNA3.1/V5-His TOPO TA Expression Vector (Invtrogen). These vectors were co-transfected into HEK293 cells using

Lipofectamine 2000 (Invitrogen). 24 to 48 hours after transfection, cells were harvested and lysed with lysis buffer (150 mM Nacl, 50 mM Tris-HCl pH 7.4, 5 mM EDTA, 1 mM PMSF, 1X protease inhibitor cocktail (Roche), 1% TritonX-100). Total Zdhhc13 and MT1-MMP proteins were immunoprecipitated using anti-V5 (Invitrogen) or anti-myc (Millipore) antibodies, respectively with protein G sepharose beads (GE Healthcare, Giles, Buckinghamshire, UK). The Co-IP results were analyzed by WB with the antibodies used for IP.

Palmitoylation assay (Acyl-biotin exchange assay)

WT and mutant mouse Zdhhc13 cDNA were subcloned into the p3XFLAG-CMV14 vector (Sigma-Aldrich). The MT1-MMP-V5-His plasmid was subsequently co-transfected with the WT Zdhhc13 or mutant Zdhhc13 construct into HEK293 cells using Lipofectamine 2000. Cells and tissues were harvested and lysed in lysis buffer containing 50 mM N-ethylmaleimide. Overexpressed MT1-MMP-V5 was purified from 500 μg total cell lysate by immunoprecipitation with anti-V5 antibody (Invitrogen) and protein G sepharose beads (GE Healthcare) in 4°C overnight. Endogenous MT1-MMP was purified from 1 mg epiphysis tissue lysate by immunoprecipitation with anti-MT1-MMP antibody (Abcam) and protein G sepharose beads (GE Healthcare) in 4°C overnight. The antibody-beads purified MT1-MMP was then used for the acyl-biotin exchange assay as described previously [15,18]. Palmitoylation level was quantified through biotin signal WB using streptavidin-HRP. Palmitoylation level quantification was performed using BioSpectrum Imaging System (UVP, Upland, CA, USA). For cell base analysis, the MT1-MMP palmitoylation intensity (streptavidin intensity) was first normalized to MT1-MMP loading (myc intensity) and then presented as fold change to vector group. For direct tissue *in vivo* analysis, the palmitoylation level was presented as percentage. It was calculated as streptavidin intensity divided by MT1-MMP intensity.

Immunofluorescence

Cells were fixed with 4% paraformaldehyde in PBS followed by 0.1% Triton X-100 (in PBS) permeabilized for 10 minutes at room temperature. After blocking with 5% normal goat serum for 1 hour, cells were incubated with primary antibodies overnight. Antibodies and their dilutions used: rabbit anti-MT1-MMP (1:250; Abcam). The secondary antibodies used here were anti-mouse Alexa Fluor 594 or anti-rabbit Alexa Fluor 488 correspondence to species of primary antibody (1:500; Molecular Probes, Grand Island, NY, USA). Nuclei were stained by DAPI using ProLong Gold Antifade Reagent (Invitrogen). Images were captured by UltraVIEW (PerkinElmer, Waltham, MA, USA). Granularity and nuclear intensity were calculated by MetaMorph software (Molecular Devices, Sunnyvale, CA, USA). Granularity represented the average speckle number per cell. Nuclear intensity was quantified as average intensity of green fluorescence which was overlapped with blue (DAPI) fluorescence. The quantitative and statistic data was calculated from a total 140 primary cultured osteoblasts or 122 primary chondrocytes from three littermate pairs.

Statistical analysis

Statistical significance was determined by two-tailed Student's t-test. A P-value <0.05 was considered statistically significant (*P-value <0.05, **P-value <0.01, ***P-value <0.001)

Results

A *Zdhhc13* mutation results in poor postnatal bone mass accumulation and early onset osteoporosis in mice

We previously reported that *Zdhhc13* deficient mutant mice had severe osteoporosis at 26 weeks of age [15]. To understand whether the osteoporosis was due to an embryonic or postnatal defect, we first analysed the mice at birth. The appearance of WT and mutant mice was indistinguishable at birth (Figure 1A left). Skeletal staining showed similar bone structure. All the bony components were intact in the mutant mice (Figure 1A middle). The size of long bones was not significantly different between WT and mutant (Figure 1A right). Notable growth differences first appeared on postnatal day 10 (P10) and persisted through the lifespan (P70) (Figure S1). Length of femur showed no significant difference in WT and mutant at P0. At age P14 and P28, the femur was significantly shorter in mutant. (Figure S2). Bone mineral density (BMD) and trabecular bone were similar between WT and mutant mice at birth (Figure 1B left, Table S1). At P14 of age, mutant mice showed significantly lower bone volume, thinner and fewer trabecular bone with larger inter space comparing to WT. The BMD was also significantly lower in mutant (Figure 1B middle, Table S1). By P28, a more severe low bone mass and loosened trabecular bone phenotype was observed in mutant mice. The bone volume and bone density were significantly lower, trabeculaes were thinner and trabecular number was extremely low (Figure 1B right, Table 1). Based on bone mineral density (BMD) by MicroCT, accumulation of bone mass was impaired in mutant mice from 4 to 20 weeks of age (Figure 1C). These results suggest that *Zdhhc13* deficiency impacts postnatal not prenatal bone mass and bone accumulation. Similar bone changes were also observed in *Zdhhc13* gene-trap mice (Figure S3).

Zdhhc13 mutant mice showed delayed epiphyseal maturation, disorganized growth plate structure, and reduced endochondral bone

Histology of the distal femur from birth (P0) to P28 showed a delay in formation of the secondary ossification center (SOC) in mutant mice (Figure 2A). From P0 to P5 the epiphyseal structure was similar between the WT and mutant. Compared to WT, at P10, fewer cartilage canals appeared at epiphyses of mutant mice. By P14, when the SOC cavity was clearly present at WT epiphyses, the SOC cavity remained immature at mutant mouse epiphyses, and was underdeveloped though P28 (Figure 2A bottom). The orientation of the epiphyseal growth plate depends on well-controlled chondrocyte differentiation and proper SOC formation. Even though the SOC was formed at P28 in mutant mice, the well-organized column structure of resting, proliferating and hypertrophic chondrocytes started to be disrupted at P28 (Figure 2B top). Severity of growth plate disorganization increased with age P42 and P84 (Figure 2B). In accord with the microCT data, a significantly reduced endochondral bone was also observed (Figure 2C) suggesting a defect in endochondral ossification. Thus, *Zdhhc13* appears to be crucial for the establishment of appropriate epiphyseal growth plate structure and facilitates endochondral bone formation.

Zdhhc13 is detected in a wide range of bone cells with a high level in proliferating and hypertrophic chondrocytes

In situ hybridization was performed to analyze the expression pattern of *Zdhhc13*. *Zdhhc13* expression signals in P14 WT distal femur (Figure 3A-D and I) and mutant proximal tibia (Figure 3E-H and J) were compared to the negative sense control (Figure 3K).

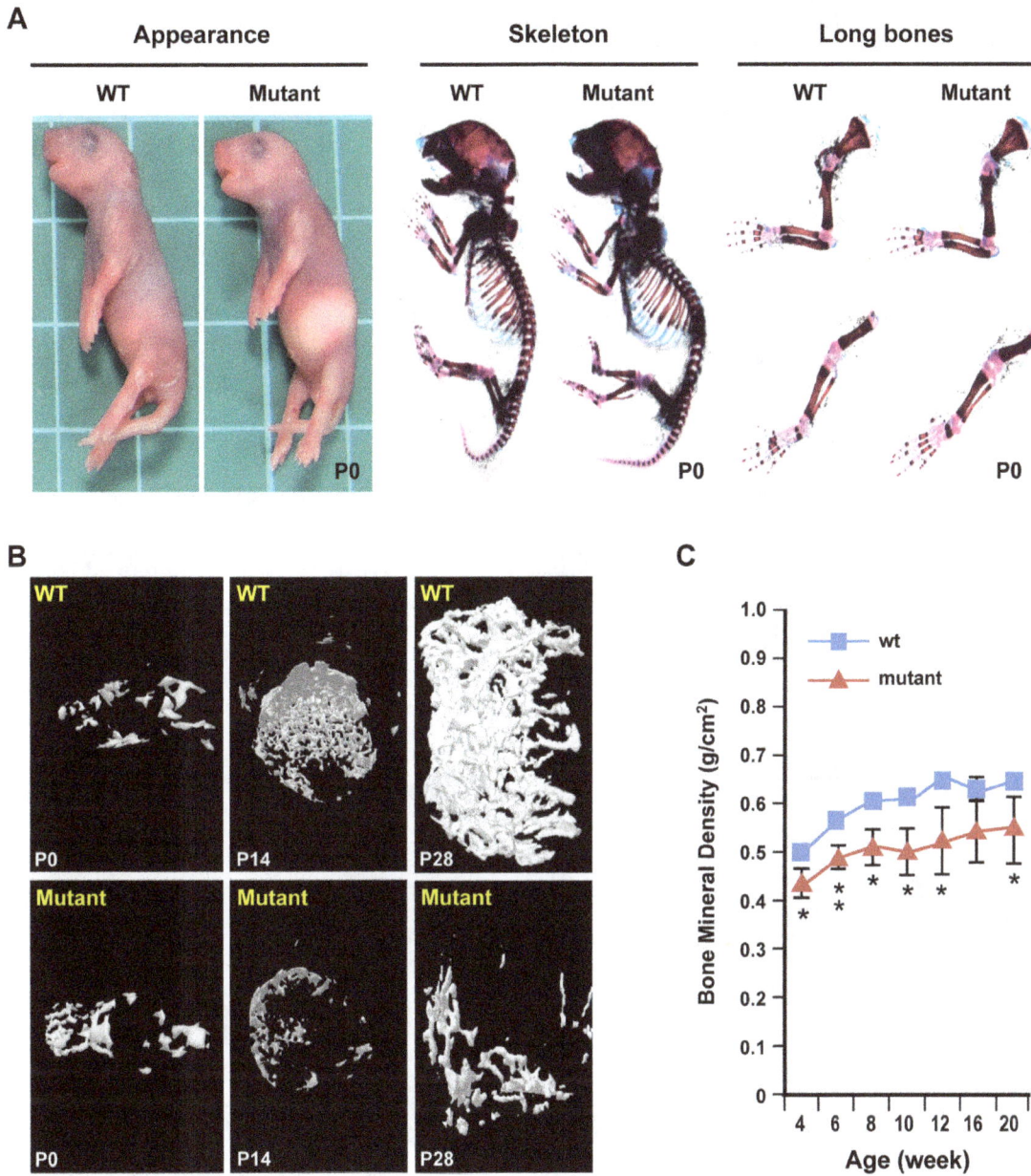

Figure 1. Reduced postnatal skeletal growth and less bone density accumulation in *Zdhhc13* deficient mutation mice. (**A**) WT and mutant mice appearance (left), whole skeleton (middle), and long bone (right) staining with alcian blue (cartilage) and alizarin red S (bone). (**B**) 3D images of trabecular bone constructed μCT scan of P0 (left), P14 (middle), and P28 (right) WT and mutant mice. (**C**) Bone mineral density (BMD) of WT and mutant mice from 4 to 20 weeks of age. Femur BMD was analyzed by μCT. CT scan was performed every 2 weeks starting from 4-week-old to 12-week-old and then every 4 weeks from 12-week-old to 20-week-old. The data were acquired from the same 3 WT and mutant littermate pairs at certain ages. μCT: Microcomputer Tomography. *$P<0.05$;**$P<0.01$.

Zdhhc13 was detected predominantly in proliferating and hypertrophic chondrocytes (Figure 3B). It was also detected in chondrocytes near the perichondrium (Figure 3C) and in osteoblasts surrounding trabecular bone (Figure 3D). Some bone lining cells also showed positive signals (Figure 3I). Since our mutant mice carried a non-sense mutation that led to Zdhhc13 mRNA premature degradation, comparable regions in mutant hypertrophic and proliferating chondrocyte (Figure 3F), perichondrium (Figure 3G), trabecular bone area (Figure 3H), and bone lining cell (Figure 3J) showed very week staining result. We further performed Q-PCR to quantify the *Zdhhc13* level in the WT and

mutant mice. Interestingly, Zdhhc13 gene expression increased post-natally and correlated with age after birth in WT (Figure 3L). In contrast, in mutant mice gene expression of *Zdhhc13*, quantified by Q-PCR, was decreased to 40% of WT at P7 and to less than 25% after P14 (Figure 3L).

ZDHHC13 interacts and palmitoylates MT1-MMP

Previous studies reported a phenotype for MT1-MMP (membrane type 1- matrix metalloproteinase, also known as MMP14)-deficient mice [19,20] that was remarkably similar to that of the *Zdhhc13* mutant, namely, impaired endochondral ossification,

Table 1. Quantitative μCT results of WT and mutant femur trabecular bone at P28.

	WT	Mutant
BV/TV (%)	6.60±2.15	0.89±0.63**
Tb.Th (mm)	0.07±0.004	0.05±0.004**
Tb.Sp (mm)	0.39±0.09	0.62±0.04**
Tb.N (1/mm)	0.99±0.27	0.17±0.17**
SMI	2.31±0.13	2.68±0.17**
BMD (g/cm³)	0.50±0.01	0.44±0.03**

3 WT and mutant mice littermates were analyzed. BV/TV: bone volume/ tissue volume; Tb.Th: trabecular bone thickness; Tb.Sp: trabecular seperation; Tb.N: trabecular bone number; SMI: structure model index; BMD: bone mineral density.

defective angiogenesis, and osteopenia. We hypothesized that MT1-MMP might be a direct palmitoylation substrate of ZDHHC13 and the palmitoylation of MT1-MMP may play a regulatory role in the skeletal system. For this reason we examined the expression and palmitoylation of MT1-MMP in the *Zdhhc13* mutant mice. By immunohistochemistry (IHC) (Figure S4A-F) and Western blot (Figure S4G), WT and mutant Zdhhcc13 epiphyseal tissue had similar levels of MT1-MMP protein expression.

Finally, co-immunoprecipitation (Co-IP) was performed using ZDHHC13-myc (ZDWT-myc) and MT1-MMP-V5 co-overex-

pressing HEK293 cells to examine whether ZDHHC13 interacted with MT1-MMP. MT1-MMP-V5 was successfully immunoprecipitated with anti-myc antibodies (Figure 4A left) and conversely, ZDHHC13-myc was successfully immunoprecipitated by anti-V5 antibodies (Figure 4A right). In support of the specificity of the interaction between ZDHHC13 and MT1-MMP, the vector immunoprecipitation controls had no signal.

We used acyl-biotin exchange (ABE) to evaluate the palmitoylation level of MT1-MMP. A ZDHHC13-mutant-Flag (ZDK) expression vector, without the DHHC domain, was constructed

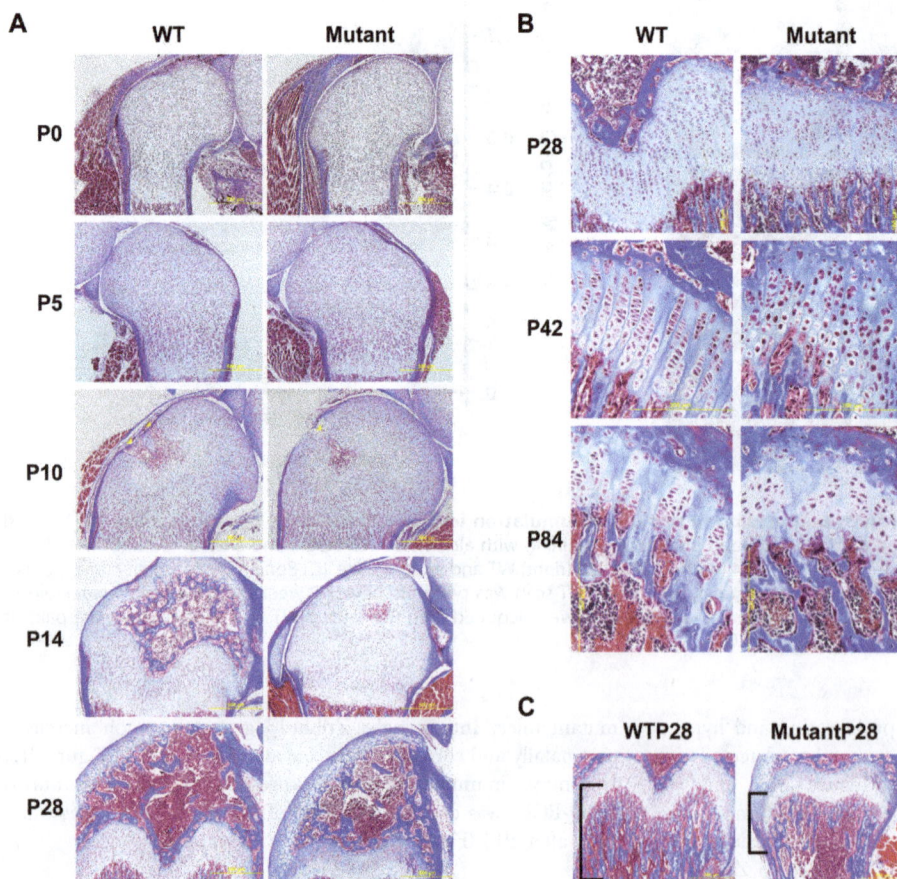

Figure 2. Delayed epiphysis maturation, growth plate disorganization, and diminished endochondral bone in *Zdhc13* deficiency mutation mice. (A) WT and mutant distal femoral epiphysis at age of P0, P5, P10, P14, and P28. Yellow arrows: canals invaded from perichondrium. (B) WT and mutant femoral growth plate at age P28, P42, and P84. (C) Endochondral bone of WT and mutant at P28. Square brackets: the region of trabecular bone. 3 WT and mutant littermate pairs were analyzed by Masson's trichrome stain at each time point.

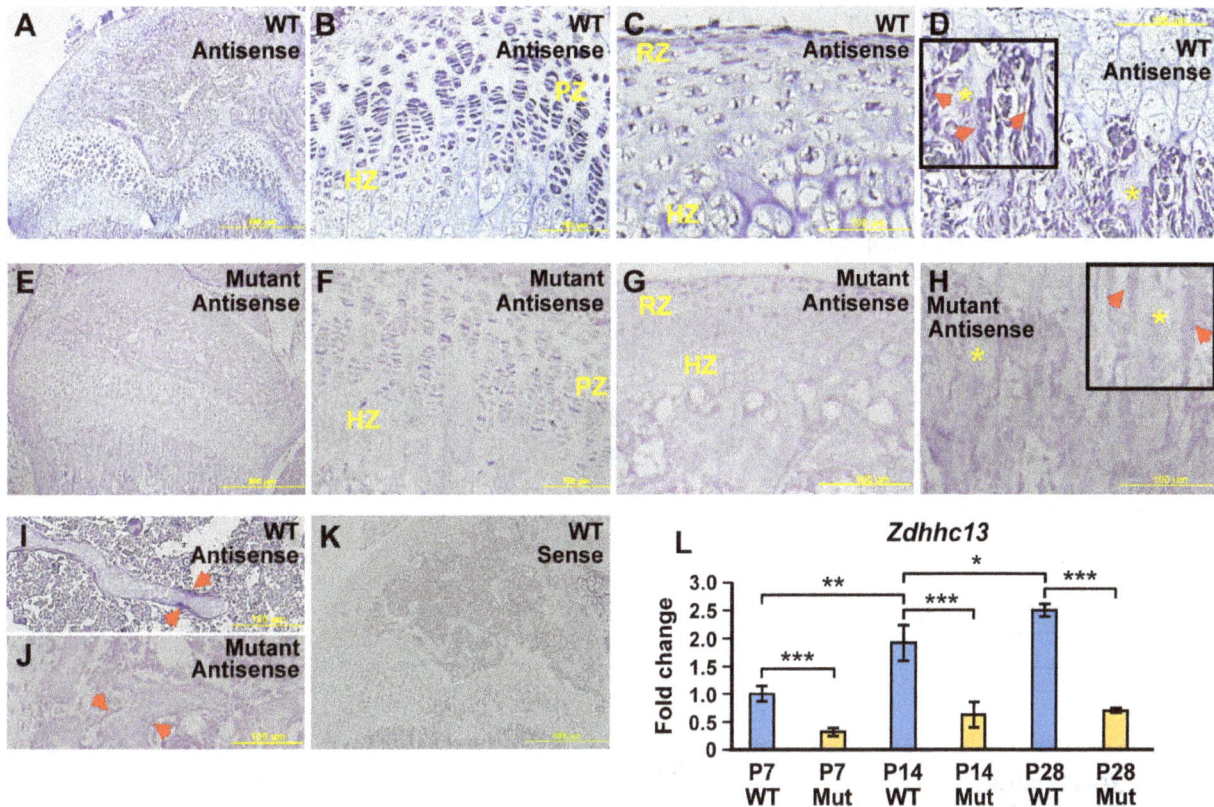

Figure 3. Expression pattern of *Zdhhc13* expression in bone cells. The mRNA expression of Zdhhc13 gene was determined by in situ hybridization using Zdhhc13-specific antisense probes. Expression of *Zdhhc13* in P14 (**A-D, I**) WT distal femur and (**E-F, J**) mutant proximal tibia. Higher power images of (**B**) WT (**F**) mutant hypertrophic and proliferating chondrocytes in the growth plate (**C**) WT (**G**) mutant resting and hypertrophic chondrocytes adjacent to perichondrium (**D**) WT (**H**) mutant osteoblasts (red arrow) surrounding trabecular bone (yellow star) (**I**) WT (**J**) mutant bone lining cells (red arrow). (**K**) Sense probe was used as negative control. (**L**) Postnatal *Zdhhc13* expression pattern in P7, P14, and P28 epiphysis tissue by Q-PCR. 5 WT and mutant littermate pairs were analyzed for each age. HZ: hypertrophic zone; RZ: resting zone; PZ: proliferating zone. Mut: mutant. *$P<0.05$; **$P<0.01$; ***$P<0.001$.

to mimic the *Zdhhc13* mutation in our mouse model. MT1-MMP-V5 was co-overexpressed with Flag vector, ZDHHC13-Flag-WT (ZDWT) or ZDHHC13-mutant-Flag (ZDK) in HEK293 cells. Results of ZDWT and ZDK were compared to Flag vector control which indicating basal palmitoylation level. The palmitoylation level of MT1-MMP-V5 was quantified to be nearly 2 fold higher in the ZDWT co-expressing group than in the vector control or ZDK (mutant mimicking construct) co-expressing groups (Figure 4B). Protein expression of transfected MT1-MMP was comparable with the exception of ZDWT for which it was slightly less (Figure 4C). Abolishment of the palmitoylation signal by palmitoylation inhibitor, 2-bromopalmitate (2-BP), evidenced the MT1-MMP palmitoylation and the cysteine 574 of MT1-MMP was confirmed to be the palmitoylation site by mutagenesis (Figure S5). Finally, we confirmed the ability of Zdhhc13 to palmitoylate MT1-MMP *in vivo* using ABE with direct immunoprecipitation of MT1-MMP protein from P14 epiphyses of WT and mutant mice. MT1-MMP in WT mice was 70% palmitoylated compared with only 40% in mutant mice (Figure 4D). These results confirm that ZDHHC13 is a PAT responsible for a substantial amount (30%) of MT1-MMP palmitoylation.

Palmitoylation affects the subcellular distribution of MT1-MMP

As palmitoylation is highly involved in regulating protein subcellular trafficking, we further explored the subcellular localization of MT1-MMP in primary osteoblasts and chondrocytes. While MT1-MMP actively formed cytoplasmic speckles in WT primary osteoblasts, a significantly 60% fewer speckles with 50% increased nuclear localization were observed in mutant primary osteoblasts (Figure 5A). The reduction in MT1-MMP cytoplasmic speckles was also observed and quantified to similar degree in mutant primary epiphyseal chondrocytes when compared to WT (Figure 5B). To further confirm the importance of this palmitoylation on MT1-MMP distribution, MT1-MMP WT and the C574S construct were overexpressed in the chondrocytic ATDC5 cells. WT MT1-MMT formed a cytoplasmic speckled pattern but C574S showed a more condensed pattern in the perinuclear region (Figure 5C). Palmitoylation was known to affect clathrin-mediated MT1-MMP trafficking [21]. We observed 15% reduction of MT1-MMP-clathrin co-localization in *Zdhhc13* mutant primary osteoblasts (Figure S6). These results suggested that cysteine 574 palmitoylation was important for the subcellular localization of MT1-MMP.

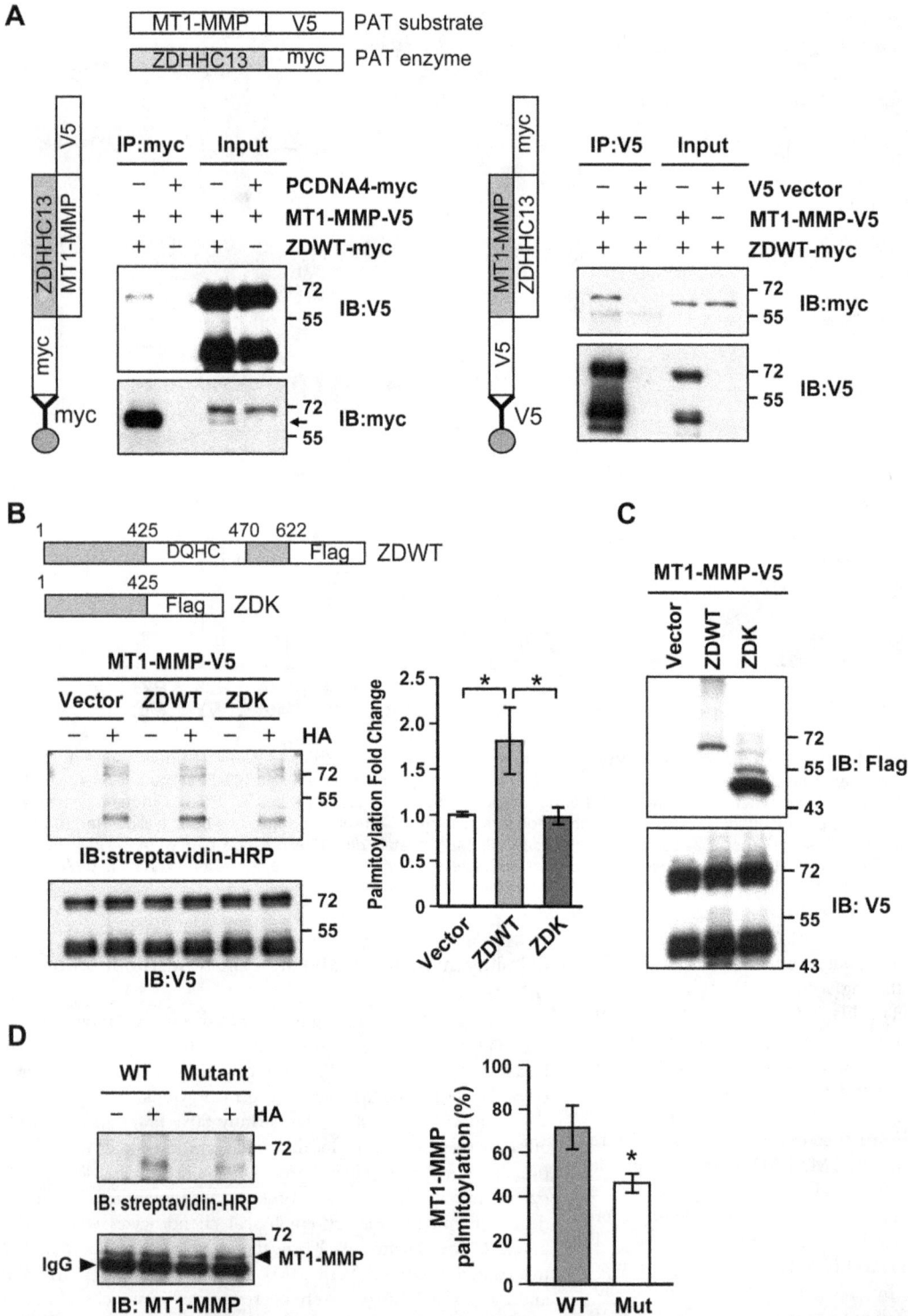

Figure 4. Interaction and direct palmitoylation of MT1-MMP by ZDHHC13. HEK293 cells were co-transfected with ZDHHC13-myc (ZDWT-myc) and MT1-MMP-V5. Co-Immunoprecipitation (IP) were performed to determine interaction between ZDHHC13 and MT1-MMP (**A**) IP using myc antibody (IP: myc) pulled down both ZDWT-myc and MT1-MMP-V5 (left). Arrow indicates the band of ZDWT. Anti-V5 antibody IP (IP: V5) pulled down both MT1-MMP-V5 and ZDWT-myc (right). Vector (PCDNA4-myc) IP group was used as control. Protein lysate before IP was used as input. The cartoon illustrated the constructs and grouping of co-IP experiments. PAT: palmitoyl acyltransferase. (**B**) Palmitoylation level of MT1-MMP examined by acyl-biotin exchange (ABE). ZDHHC13-flag (ZDWT) or ZDK-flag (mimic mutation in our mice) were co-transfected with MT1-MMP-V5 in HEK293 cells. Streptavisdin-HRP signal represented palmitoylation level. Purified MT1-MMP was analyzed by V5 antibody and used as input normalization control. The quantitative palmitoylation level from three independent repeats was shown as fold change to vector (right). MT1-MMP-V5 has multiple molecular weights of ~66 KDa and ~45 KDa (self-processed form). The cartoon illustrated the construct of ZDWT and ZDK. Number represented the amino acid position. DQHC is the domain with PAT activity. (**C**) WB examination of ZDWT, ZDK (enzyme), and MT1-MMP-V5 (substrate) expression using flag and V5 antibody respectively. (**D**) Palmitoylation of MT1-MMP in WT and mutant distal femur epiphysis. MT1-MMP was directly purified

from P14 WT and mutant epiphysis protein lysate to perform ABE. Streptavidin-HRP signal represented palmitoylation level. Purified MT1-MMP was analyzed by specific antibody. Quantitative result from three independent experiments of three P14 littermate pairs was shown as palmitoylation percentage (right). *P<0.05.

MT1-MMP palmitoylation is associated with VEGF expression in chondrocytes and osteocalcin level in osteoblasts

To determine the effects of ZDHHC13-mediated MT1-MMP palmitoylation in the skeletal system, mutagenesis was performed to disrupt cysteine 574 (C574) palmitoylation. The C574 was converted to alanine (MT1-MMP C574A-V5) or serine (MT1-MMP C574S-V5). MT1-MMP WT, C574A, C574S and V5 vector control were transfected into a mouse chondrocyte cell line, ATDC5. VEGF expression was analysed using Western blot. VEGF level was significantly elevated 1.5 fold in the WT MT1-MMP overexpressing group comparing to vector control. The elevation was abolished in C574A and C574S overexpressing groups. Palmitoylation of MT1-MMP WT was inhibited using 4-hour 25 μM of 2-BP treatment. 2B-P inhibition of MT1-MMP WT palmitoylation resulted in greater inhibition of VEGF expression (Figure 6A). To mimic the condition in our mutant mice and confirm the involvement of ZDHHC13, ATDC5 cells were co-transfected with ZDWT and MT1-MMP WT or ZDK and MT1-MMP WT. Western blot showed that, with comparable MT1-MMP expression, the ZDWT but not ZDK group was able to elevate VEGF level (Figure 6B). In addition to chondrocytes, we also explored the effects of MT1-MMP palmitoylation in osteoblasts. The mouse osteoblastic cell line, MC3T3E1, was transfected with MT1-MMP WT, C574A, or C574S construct. The maturation and ossification marker osteocalcin was analysed by Western blot. The expression of osteocalcin increased 2 fold when overexpressing WT MT1-MMP. The incensement was significantly attenuated by C574 mutation (Figure 6C). Likewise, MC3T3E1 cells were co-transfected with ZDWT and MT1-MMP WT or ZDK and MT1-MMP WT to mimic our mouse model. Western blot demonstrated that, under similar MT1MMP expression level, ZDWT but not ZDK expression was able to significantly increase osteocalcin level (Figure 6D). Collectively, these results indicated that ZDHHC13-mediated MT1-MMP palmitoylation positively associated with VEGF expression in chondrocytes and osteocalcin expression in osteoblasts.

Reduced VEGF level associated with less vascularity in Zdhhc13 mutant epiphysis and the reduced osteocalcin expression at hypertrophic cartilage and bone surface in Zdhhc13 mutant mice

To evaluate the effects of ZDHHC13- mediated MT1-MMP palmitoylation on VEGF and osteocalcin in vivo, VEGF and osteocalcin IHC was performed on WT and mutant epiphyses. Reduced VEGF level was observed in mutant hypertrophic chondrocytes near cartilage canals (Figure 7A upper panel) and in growth plate (Figure 7A lower panel). Reduced osteocalcin expression was also detected at the hypertrophic zone cartilage (calcified region) and cells on trabecular bone surface of the mutant (Figure 7B). We finally examined whether the reduced VEGF expression was associated with changes in the vascularity of the epiphysis. Staining with the endothelial marker PECAM was performed. Significantly fewer PECAM positive cells were shown in mutant SOC (Figure 7C) and hypertrophic zone- trabecular bone region (Figure 7D). The IHC quantification results (Figure 7E) demonstrated that mutant VEGF level decreased to 50% and 60% of WT in P10 and P14, respectively. The osteocalcin also

reduced significantly to half of WT in mutant bone surface area. The vascularized area of mutant epiphysis and hypertrophic-trabeculae region were only 25% and 50% of WT, respectively. These results suggested that ZDHHC13- mediated MT1-MMP palmitoylation is a candidate to cause delayed SOC formation and reduced endochondral bone formation through regulating VEGF and osteocalcin expression in the skeletal system.

Discussion

Osteoporosis is the most common metabolic bone disorder in elders [22]. Bone density acquired during childhood development and early adult age impacts the incidence of osteoporosis in later life [23,24]. Recent genome-wide association studies have shown that osteoporosis and BMD are associated with genes participating in skeletal development, bone cell differentiation, and endochondral ossification [25]. In this study we newly identified a molecule, Zdhhc13, as critical for endochondral bone synthesis and normal bone structure.

In the present study, using histology and microCT, Zdhhc13 mutant mice clearly demonstrated a delay in SOC formation with disorganized growth plate structure, short long bone and diminished endochondral bone formation with poor postnatal bone mass accumulation and a bone phenotype compatible with severe osteoporosis. While our experiments were carried out in the ENU-generated Zdhhc13 nonsense mutation mouse model which had reduced expression of Zdhhc13, we have also validated the osteoporosis phenotype in our gene-trap mice (Figure S3). Although a recent study of the Zdhhc13 gene-trap mouse model reported a Huntington's disease phenotype [26], we did not observe this phenotype in our Zdhcc13 deficient mouse model.

To investigate the possible function of Zdhhc13 in the skeletal system, we explored the expression of Zdhhc13 in bone cells. We determined that Zdhhc13 mRNA was detected in a variety of cells, importantly, in osteoblasts and at especially high levels in proliferating and hypertrophic chondrocytes. The expression level of Zdhhc13 mRNA increased from the first week after birth in WT but was dramatically degraded in mutant due to the nonsense mutation (Figure 3). These data suggested the critical function of Zdhhc13 in postnatal bone growth.

Since ZDHHC13 is a PAT, we speculated that its substrates might mediate regulation of bone growth and development. MT1-MMP is an important factor that governs skeletal development. A previous study reported that MT1-MMP is palmitoylated at cysteine 574 (C574) [21]. Further, MT1-MMP-deficient mice had defects in SOC maturation and endochondral bone formation, as well as kyphosis, osteopenia, dwarfism, and short lifespan [19,20]. Although, our Zdhhc13 mutant mice were not MT1-MMP deficient, we demonstrated for the fist time that MT1-MMP is a direct substrate of ZDHHC13. The palmitoylation was evidenced by 2-BP treatment and MT1-MMP C574 mutation. MT1-MMP was confirmed to be under palmitoylated in mutant mice (Figure 4). Clathrin-mediated MT1-MMP endocytosis has been shown to be regulated by palmitoylation of MT1-MMP [32]. However, the Zdhhc13 deficiency mutation had only a minor effect (~15% reduction) on clathrin-mediated MT1-MMP endocytosis in osteoblasts (Figure S6). We did however find an altered subcellular distribution of MT1-MMP based on palmitoylated state - less cytoplasmic speckle with more nuclear localization- in the Zdhhc13

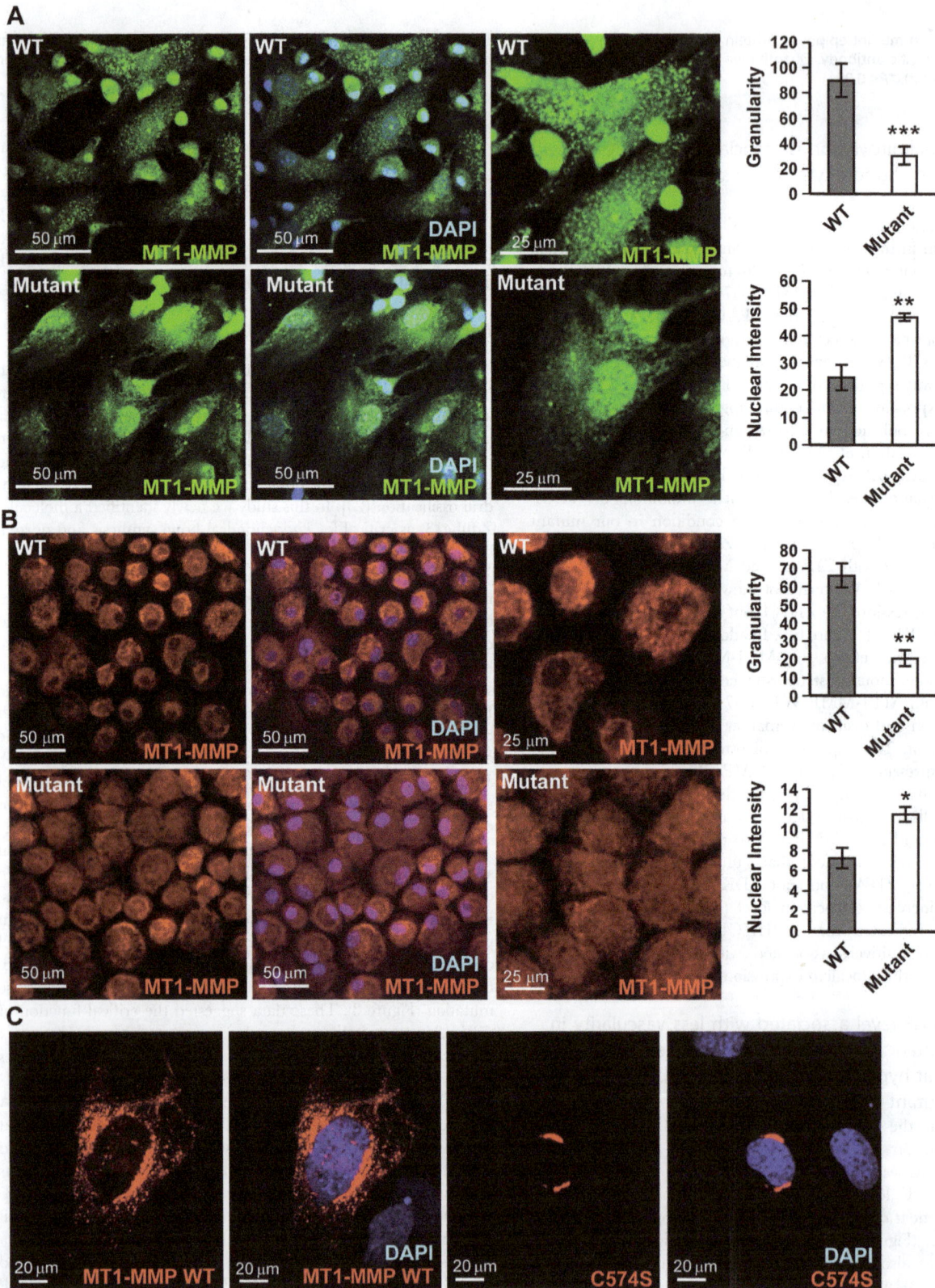

Figure 5. Effect of palmitoylation on MT1-MMP subcellular distribution. (A) Immunofluorescence (IF) microscopy of primary osteoblasts from P14 WT (upper panel) and mutant (lower panel) long bone showing MT1-MMP subcellular localization. The granularity (average speckle number per cell) and nuclear intensity quantification results were shown (right). MT1-MMP: Alexa Fluor 488 (green); nucleus: DAPI (blue). **(B)** IF microscopy of primary chondrocytes from P10 WT (upper panel) and mutant (lower panel) epiphysis showing MT1-MMP cellular localization. The granularity (average speckle number per cell) and nuclear intensity quantification results were shown (right). MT1-MMP: Alexa Fluor 594 (red); nucleus: DAPI (blue). **(C)** IF microscopy of ATDC5 cells transfected with WT MT1-MMP-V5 (upper panel) and C574S MT1-MMP-V5 (lower panel). MT1-MMP distribution was analyzed by V5 primary antibody and visualized with Alexa Fluor 594 (red). Nucleus: DAPI (blue). *$P<0.05$;**$P<0.01$; ***$P<0.001$.

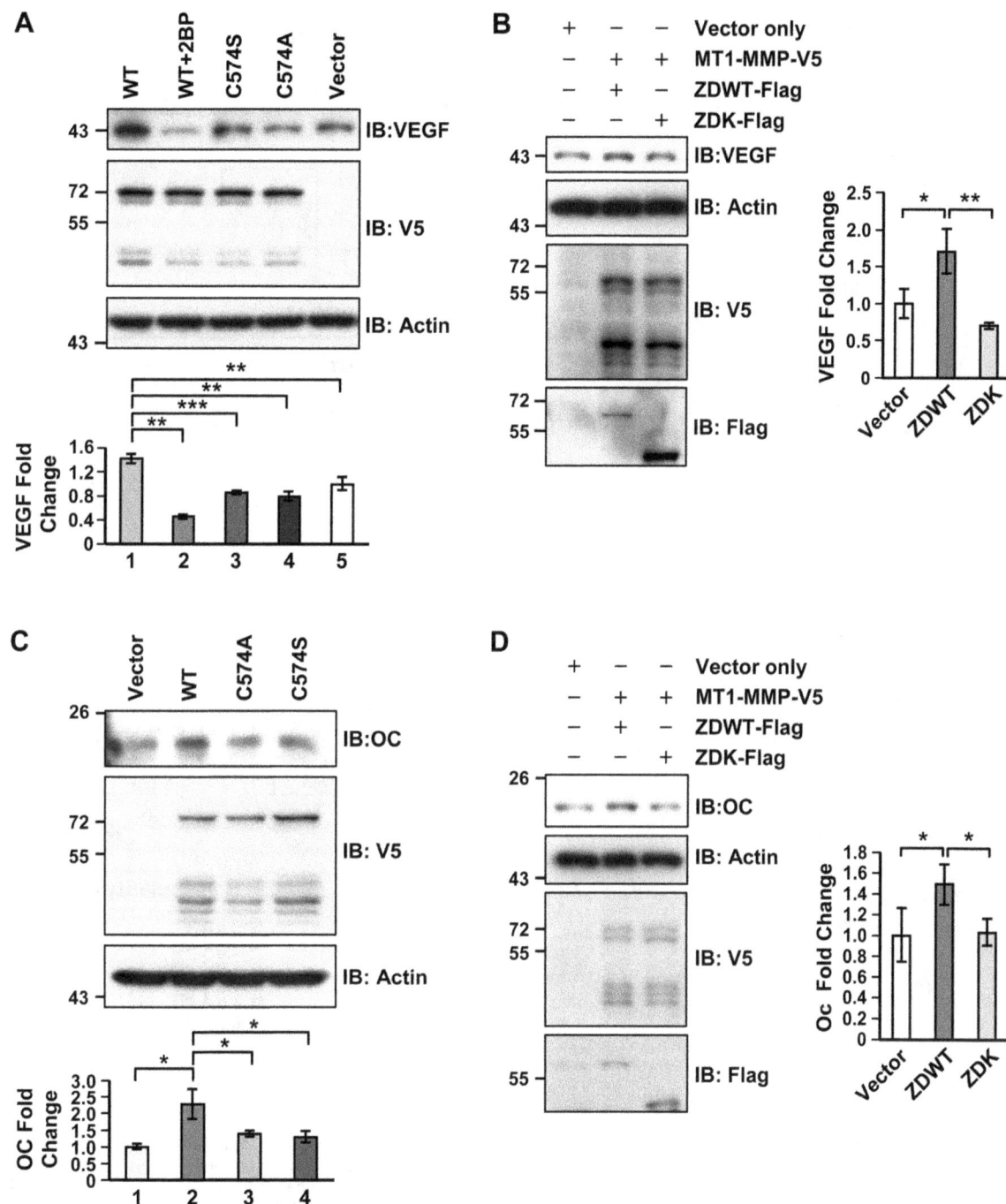

Figure 6. ZDHHC13- mediated MT1-MMP palmitoylation is associated with VEGF expression in chondrocytes and osteocalcin expression in osteoblast. (A) WB of VEGF in ATDC5 cells transfected with WT MT1-MMP or blocking it's palmitoylation by either 2-BP treatment or cysteine 574 mutagenesis (C574A/S). Quantitative fold change to vector was shown below the blot. The number represents lane number from left to right. **(B)** WB of VEGF in ATDC5 cells co-overexpressing WT ZDHHC13 (ZDWT) or mutant ZDHHC13 (ZDK) with WT MT1-MMP. Quantitative fold change to vector was shown (right). **(C)** Osteocalcin (OC) level in MC3T3E1 cells overexpressed with WT MT1-MMP and blocking MT1-MMP palmitoylation by mutant construct (C574A/S). Quantitative fold change to vector was shown below the blot. The number represents lane number from left to right. **(D)** OC level in MC3T3E1 cells co-overexpressing WT ZDHHC13 (ZDWT) or mutant ZDHHC13 (ZDK) with WT MT1-MMP. Quantitative fold change to vector was shown (right). 2BP: 2-bromopalmitate. *$P<0.05$;**$P<0.01$; ***$P<0.001$.

mutant in both primary osteoblasts and chondrocytes. Mutation of MT1-MMP C574 also certified our finding of palmitoylation on MT1-MMP subcellular distribution. Since protein interactions can be regulated by palmitoylation [27], we speculated that the altered

subcellular speckle localization of under palmitoylated MT1-MMP adversely impacted key regulatory bone functions by MT1-MMP.

MT1-MMP regulates the skeletal system in diverse ways. Manduca, et al. reported the critical temporal regulation of MT1-MMP in governing osteogenesis and mineralization in osteoblasts

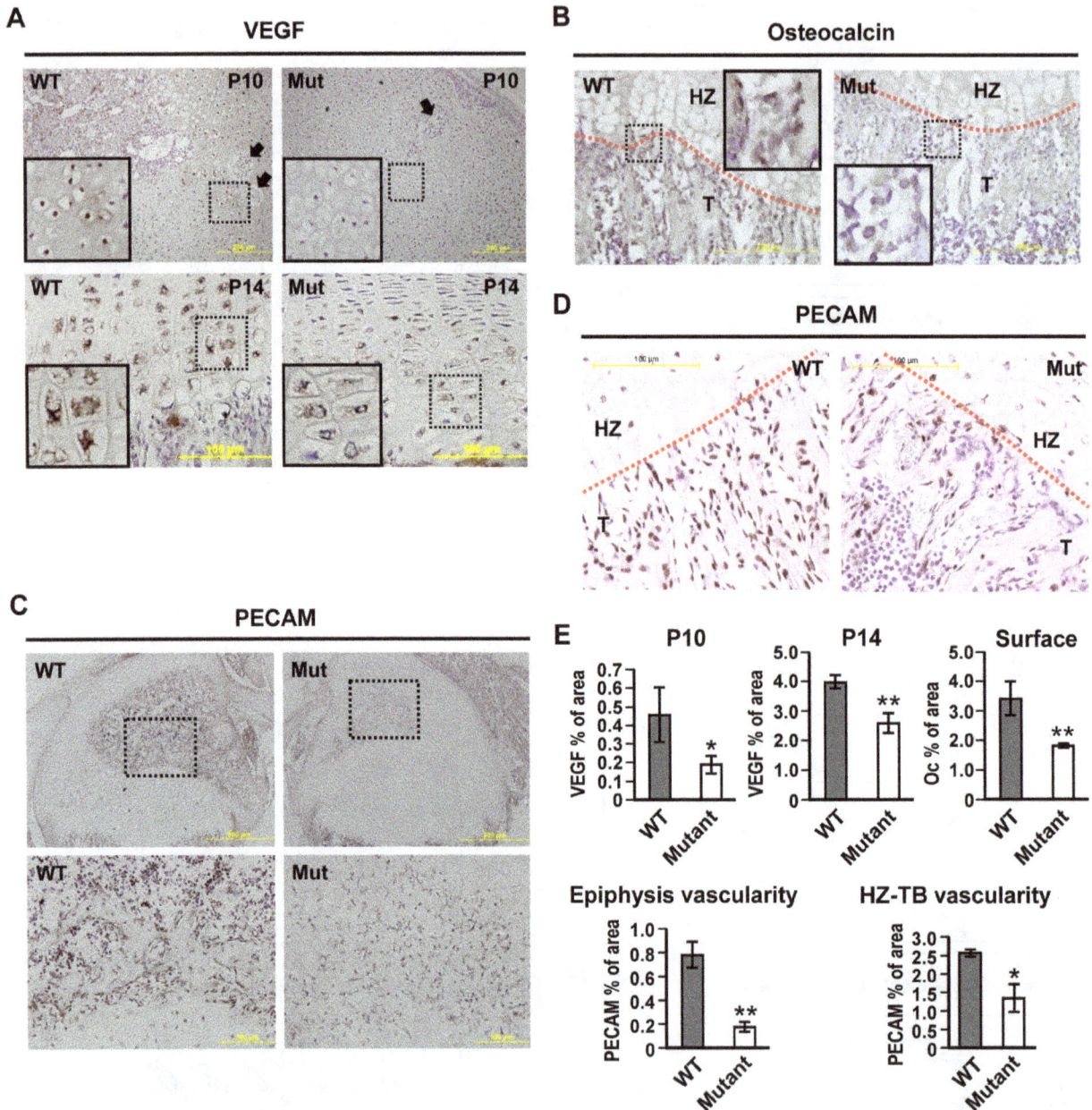

Figure 7. Reduced VEGF and osteocalcin expression with reduced vascularity in *Zdhhc13* deficiency mutation mice. Immunohistochemistry (IHC) of (**A**) VEGF in P10 (upper panel) and P14 (lower panel) WT and mutant distal femoral epiphysis. Black arrows indicate the cartilage canals surrounded by hypertrophic chondrocytes. Dashed-squares indicated the emphasized area shown in bottom left. (**B**) Osteocalcin in P14 WT and mutant epiphysis growth plate. Dashed-squares indicate the emphasized area. (**C**) Endothelial marker PECAM in P14 epiphysis SOC (upper panel) and higher magnification of dashed-area showing PECAM positive cells aligned cartilage canals and SOC cavity (lower panel). (**D**) PECAM in P14 WT and mutant epiphysis growth plate. (**E**) Quantitative results of VEGF, Oc and PECAM IHC. The results were demonstrated as % of area. VEGF staining was quantified as positive stained area among HZ region (represents panel A). Oc staining was quantified as positive stained area on trabecular bone surface (represents panel B). PECAM quantification was separated in to positive stained area within epiphysis (epiphysis vascularity, represents panel C) and positive area among HZ and trabecular bone (HZ-TB vascularity, represents panel D). The statistic comparison was performed using three WT and three mutants IHC in each group. Mut: mutant; HZ: hypertrophic zone; T: trabecular bone; red dash lines: interface of cartilage and bone. *$P<0.05$;**$P<0.01$.

[28]. MT1-MMP was also shown to be an essential factor in osteocytogenesis through its proteolytic activity [29]. The ability to shed RANKL and ADAM9 makes it both a negative regulator in local osteoclastogenesis [30] and a positive modulator in calvarial osteogenesis [31]. Tang et al. reported recently that MT1-MMP-dependent extracellular matrix remodelling is able to mediate integrin signalling and determine skeletal stem cell differentiation

[32]. Independent of its catalytic activity, the cytoplasmic tail (where the palmitoylation site locates) of MT1-MMP is required for myeloid cell nuclear fusion to form osteoclasts [33]. The cytoplasmic tail of MT1-MMP is also able to induce VEGF expression in cancer cells [34]. VEGF is one of the essential factors in bone formation [35]. For long bones to grow, endochondral ossification consistently deposits new bone by replacing cartilage.

Cartilage is unique in its avascular nature. Thus, penetration of a well-functioning vascular system is the foundation for the establishment of the growth plate and endochondral ossification [36]. Mice lacking VEGF showed impaired SOC maturation and endochondral ossification due to lack of vascularity [35,37]. Here we demonstrated that ZDHHC13-mediated MT1-MMP palmitoylation was associated with facilitating VEGF expression in *in vitro* chondrocytic ATDC5 cell system. The reduction of VEGF was also observed and quantified to be 50%- 60% of WT in *Zdhhc13* mutant hypertrophic chondrocytes. A 75% less vascularity was further shown by PECAM IHC in mutant epiphysis. The vascularity also revealed to be only 50% of WT in HZ-TB region of *Zdhhc13* mutant mice. Besides, osteocalcin expression was found to be associated with ZDHHC13-mediated MT1-MMP palmitoylation in MC3T3 cells and in cartilage-bone interface. Collectively, these suggested that *Zdhhc13*-mediated MT1-MMP palmitoylation was a novel regulator in skeletal vascularity and endochondral ossification. These also highlighted the potential diverse roles of ZDHHC13-mediated MT1-MMP palmitoylation in modulating bone homeostasis.

A PAT enzyme, Zdhhc13, may have numerous downstream substrates. A matrix metalloproteinase, MT1-MMP, may also have diverse substrates or interacting molecules. In this complex regulatory network we revealed a novel potential pathway involving regulation of bone formation, development and structure by palmitoylation. The involvement of other ZDHHC13 palmitoylation targets or MT1-MMP substrates is worthy of further investigation.

Conclusions

To the best of our knowledge, this is the first report showing involvement of a DHHC PAT enzyme, *Zdhhc13*, in epiphyseal maturation and endochondral bone formation. This study revealed a novel pathogenic mechanism of osteoporosis governed by palmitoylation.

Supporting Information

Figure S1 Postnatal growth retardation of *Zdhhc13* deficient mutation mice. Appearance of WT and mutant mice at age P10, P14, P28, and P70.

Figure S2 Bone length of P0, P14 and P28 *Zdhhc13* WT and mutant mice. Femurs were dissected and their lengths were measured. The values from 3 WT and 3 mutant were shown as mean±SD. The square is in 1 mm×1 mm of size. Statistical significance was determined by two-tailed Student's t-test. A *P*-value <0.05 was considered statistically significant (**P-value < 0.05, **P-value <0.01). The yellow color of P0 femurs was resulted from fixation in Bouin's solution.

Figure S3 Bone phenotype in *Zdhhc13* gene-trap mice. MicroCT (**A**) 3D images and (**B**) bone volume/ tissue volume (BV/TV) ratio of trabecular bone in *Zdhhc13* WT and gene-trap (Gt) (5 month of age). The method for generation of this gene-trap model was described in our previous paper [15].

Figure S4 Comparable MT1-MMP expression in WT and mutant epiphysis and primary chondrocytes. MT1-MMP IHC of P10 (**A-C**) WT and (**D-F**) mutant distal femoral epiphyseal sections. High power view of (**B**) WT and (**E**) mutant mice MT1-MMP expression in chondrocytes around cartilage canal. MT1-MMP expression in (**C**) WT and (**F**) mutant growth plate chondrocytes. Yellow star indicted the canal that will contribute to future SOC formation. (**G**) Expression of MT1-MMP in P14 epiphysis tissue by WB and quantitative results from three WT and mutant littermate pairs (below).

Figure S5 Abolishment of palmitoylation of mutant MT1-MMP (C574A, C574S) and 25 μM, 50 μM, 100 μM 2-Bromopalmitate treatment. Palmitoylation level was examined by acyl-biotin exchange. MT1-MMP-V5 WT or C574A or C574S were overexpressed in HEK293 cells. Palmitate was switched to biotin and detected by streptavidin-HRP. Purified MT1-MMP was analyzed by V5 antibody. Red arrows indicate the palmitoylation signals of WT MT1-MMP which was not detected in C574 mutation constructs and 2-BP treatment groups. The 2-BP concentration of 25 μM was used in further experiment. HA: hydroxylamine; 2BP: 2-bromopalmitate.

Figure S6 Clathrin-mediated MT1-MMP trafficking in WT and *Zdhhc13* mutant primary osteoblast. (**A**) Localization patterns of MT1-MMP in primary osteoblast (OB) from P14 WT and mutant femur. MT1-MMP staining (green), Clathrin staining (red), and merge of MT1-MMP and Clathrin (yellow shows the colocalization of two proteins) in WT (upper panel) and mutant (lower panel) primary OB. White arrows indicated non-clathrin colocalized speckles. (**B**) Colocalization MT1-MMP and clathrin quantitative data. **P*-value <0.05, t-test.

Table S1 Quantitative microCT results of WT and mutant femur trabecular bone and bone mineral density (BMD) at P10 and P14. 3 WT and 3 mutants were analyzed at each time point. Data was presented as average ± standard deviation. Statistical significance was determined by two-tailed Student's t-test. A P-value <0.05 was considered statistically significant (**P* <0.05, **P <0.01). BV/TV: bone volume/ tissue volume; Tb.Th: trabecular bone thickness; Tb.Sp: trabecular separation; Tb.N: trabecular bone number; SMI: structure model index.

Acknowledgments

We thank the Sequencing Core Facility, Scientific Instrument Center at Academia Sinica for DNA sequencing, and the Taiwan Mouse Clinic funded by the National Research Program for Biopharmaceuticals (NRPB) at the National Science Council (NSC) of Taiwan, for technical support in microCT.

Author Contributions

Conceived and designed the experiments: IWS LFS KML. Performed the experiments: IWS WRL LYC. Analyzed the data: IWS Yi-Ju Chen. Contributed reagents/materials/analysis tools: JJYY Yu-Ju Chen JYW YTC. Wrote the paper: IWS WRL VK MTML JYW YTC.

References

1. Schmidt MF, Schlesinger MJ (1979) Fatty acid binding to vesicular stomatitis virus glycoprotein: a new type of post-translational modification of the viral glycoprotein. Cell 17: 813–819.

2. Linder ME, Deschenes RJ (2007) Palmitoylation: policing protein stability and traffic. Nat Rev Mol Cell Biol 8: 74–84.

3. Iwanaga T, Tsutsumi R, Noritake J, Fukata Y, Fukata M (2009) Dynamic protein palmitoylation in cellular signaling. Prog Lipid Res 48: 117–127.

4. Charollais J, Van Der Goot FG (2009) Palmitoylation of membrane proteins (Review). Mol Membr Biol 26: 55–66.
5. Zhao L, Lobo S, Dong X, Ault AD, Deschenes RJ (2002) Erf4p and Erf2p form an endoplasmic reticulum-associated complex involved in the plasma membrane localization of yeast Ras proteins. J Biol Chem 277: 49352–49359.
6. Lobo S, Greentree WK, Linder ME, Deschenes RJ (2002) Identification of a Ras palmitoyltransferase in Saccharomyces cerevisiae. J Biol Chem 277: 41268–41273.
7. Linder ME, Deschenes RJ (2004) Model organisms lead the way to protein palmitoyltransferases. J Cell Sci 117: 521–526.
8. Kang JU, Koo SH, Kwon KC, Park JW, Kim JM (2008) Gain at chromosomal region 5p15.33, containing TERT, is the most frequent genetic event in early stages of non-small cell lung cancer. Cancer Genet Cytogenet 182: 1–11.
9. Oyama T, Miyoshi Y, Koyama K, Nakagawa H, Yamori T, et al. (2000) Isolation of a novel gene on 8p21.3-22 whose expression is reduced significantly in human colorectal cancers with liver metastasis. Genes Chromosomes Cancer 29: 9–15.
10. Yamamoto Y, Chochi Y, Matsuyama H, Eguchi S, Kawauchi S, et al. (2007) Gain of 5p15.33 is associated with progression of bladder cancer. Oncology 72: 132–138.
11. Fukata Y, Fukata M (2010) Protein palmitoylation in neuronal development and synaptic plasticity. Nat Rev Neurosci 11: 161–175.
12. Li Y, Hu J, Hofer K, Wong AM, Cooper JD, et al. (2010) DHHC5 interacts with PDZ domain 3 of post-synaptic density-95 (PSD-95) protein and plays a role in learning and memory. J Biol Chem 285: 13022–13031.
13. Mukai J, Liu H, Burt RA, Swor DE, Lai WS, et al. (2004) Evidence that the gene encoding ZDHHC8 contributes to the risk of schizophrenia. Nat Genet 36: 725–731.
14. Mill P, Lee AW, Fukata Y, Tsutsumi R, Fukata M, et al. (2009) Palmitoylation regulates epidermal homeostasis and hair follicle differentiation. PLoS Genet 5: e1000748.
15. Saleem AN, Chen YH, Baek HJ, Hsiao YW, Huang HW, et al. (2010) Mice with alopecia, osteoporosis, and systemic amyloidosis due to mutation in Zdhhc13, a gene coding for palmitoyl acyltransferase. PLoS Genet 6: e1000985.
16. Watanabe K, Yamada H, Yamaguchi Y (1995) K-glypican: a novel GPI-anchored heparan sulfate proteoglycan that is highly expressed in developing brain and kidney. J Cell Biol 130: 1207–1218.
17. Bakker AD, Klein-Nulend J (2012) Osteoblast isolation from murine calvaria and long bones. Methods Mol Biol 816: 19–29.
18. Gosset M, Berenbaum F, Thirion S, Jacques C (2008) Primary culture and phenotyping of murine chondrocytes. Nat Protoc 3: 1253–1260.
19. Holmbeck K, Bianco P, Caterina J, Yamada S, Kromer M, et al. (1999) MT1-MMP-deficient mice develop dwarfism, osteopenia, arthritis, and connective tissue disease due to inadequate collagen turnover. Cell 99: 81–92.
20. Zhou Z, Apte SS, Soininen R, Cao R, Baaklini GY, et al. (2000) Impaired endochondral ossification and angiogenesis in mice deficient in membrane-type matrix metalloproteinase I. Proc Natl Acad Sci U S A 97: 4052–4057.
21. Anilkumar N, Uekita T, Couchman JR, Nagase H, Seiki M, et al. (2005) Palmitoylation at Cys574 is essential for MT1-MMP to promote cell migration. FASEB J 19: 1326–1328.
22. Rachner TD, Khosla S, Hofbauer LC (2011) Osteoporosis: now and the future. Lancet 377: 1276–1287.
23. Javaid MK, Cooper C (2002) Prenatal and childhood influences on osteoporosis. Best Pract Res Clin Endocrinol Metab 16: 349–367.
24. Loro ML, Sayre J, Roe TF, Goran MI, Kaufman FR, et al. (2000) Early identification of children predisposed to low peak bone mass and osteoporosis later in life. J Clin Endocrinol Metab 85: 3908–3918.
25. Richards JB, Rivadeneira F, Inouye M, Pastinen TM, Soranzo N, et al. (2008) Bone mineral density, osteoporosis, and osteoporotic fractures: a genome-wide association study. Lancet 371: 1505–1512.
26. Sutton LM, Sanders SS, Butland SL, Singaraja RR, Franciosi S, et al. (2013) Hip14l-deficient mice develop neuropathological and behavioural features of Huntington disease. Hum Mol Genet 22: 452–465.
27. Resh MD (2006) Trafficking and signaling by fatty-acylated and prenylated proteins. Nat Chem Biol 2: 584–590.
28. Manduca P, Castagnino A, Lombardini D, Marchisio S, Soldano S, et al. (2009) Role of MT1-MMP in the osteogenic differentiation. Bone 44: 251–265.
29. Holmbeck K, Bianco P, Pidoux I, Inoue S, Billinghurst RC, et al. (2005) The metalloproteinase MT1-MMP is required for normal development and maintenance of osteocyte processes in bone. J Cell Sci 118: 147–156.
30. Hikita A, Yana I, Wakeyama H, Nakamura M, Kadono Y, et al. (2006) Negative regulation of osteoclastogenesis by ectodomain shedding of receptor activator of NF-kappaB ligand. J Biol Chem 281: 36846–36855.
31. Chan KM, Wong HL, Jin G, Liu B, Cao R, et al. (2012) MT1-MMP inactivates ADAM9 to regulate FGFR2 signaling and calvarial osteogenesis. Dev Cell 22: 1176–1190.
32. Tang Y, Rowe RG, Botvinick EL, Kurup A, Putnam AJ, et al. (2013) MT1-MMP-Dependent Control of Skeletal Stem Cell Commitment via a beta1-Integrin/YAP/TAZ Signaling Axis. Dev Cell.
33. Gonzalo P, Guadamillas MC, Hernandez-Riquer MV, Pollan A, Grande-Garcia A, et al. (2010) MT1-MMP is required for myeloid cell fusion via regulation of Rac1 signaling. Dev Cell 18: 77–89.
34. Eisenach PA, Roghi C, Fogarasi M, Murphy G, English WR (2010) MT1-MMP regulates VEGF-A expression through a complex with VEGFR-2 and Src. J Cell Sci 123: 4182–4193.
35. Maes C, Carmeliet P, Moermans K, Stockmans I, Smets N, et al. (2002) Impaired angiogenesis and endochondral bone formation in mice lacking the vascular endothelial growth factor isoforms VEGF164 and VEGF188. Mech Dev 111: 61–73.
36. Blumer MJ, Longato S, Fritsch H (2008) Structure, formation and role of cartilage canals in the developing bone. Ann Anat 190: 305–315.
37. Maes C, Stockmans I, Moermans K, Van Looveren R, Smets N, et al. (2004) Soluble VEGF isoforms are essential for establishing epiphyseal vascularization and regulating chondrocyte development and survival. J Clin Invest 113: 188–199.

21

Chinese Bone Turnover Marker Study: Reference Ranges for C-Terminal Telopeptide of Type I Collagen and Procollagen I N-Terminal Peptide by Age and Gender

Mei Li[1], Yan Li[2], Weimin Deng[3], Zhenlin Zhang[4], Zhongliang Deng[5], Yingying Hu[1], Weibo Xia[1]*, Ling Xu[6]*

1 Department of Endocrinology, Key Laboratory of Endocrinology of Ministry of Health, Peking Union Medical College Hospital, Peking Union Medical College, Chinese Academy of Medical Sciences, Beijing, China, 2 Department of Laboratory, People's Hospital, Hubei Province, Wuhan, China, 3 Department of Geriatrics, General Hospital of Guangzhou Military Command, Guangzhou, China, 4 Department of Osteoporosis, Sixth People's Hospital, Shanghai Jiaotong University, Shanghai, China, 5 Department of Orthopedics, Second Affiliated Hospital of Chongqing Medical University, Chongqing, China, 6 Department of Obstetrics and Gynecology, Chinese Academy of Medical Sciences, Peking Union Medical College, Peking Union Medical College Hospital, Beijing, China

Abstract

Background: Bone formation marker procollagen I N-terminal peptide (PINP) and resorption marker C-terminal telopeptide of type I collagen (β-CTX) are useful biomarkers for differential diagnosis and therapeutic evaluation of osteoporosis, but reference values are required.

Methods: The multi-center, cross-sectional Chinese Bone Turnover Marker Study included 3800 healthy volunteers in 5 Chinese cities. Serum PINP, β-CTX, parathyroid hormone (PTH) and 25OHD levels were measured by chemiluminescence assay. Lumbar spine and proximal femur BMD were measured by dual-energy X-ray absorptiometry. Serum PINP and β-CTX levels were assessed by age, gender, weight, recruitment latitude, levels of PTH and 25OHD.

Results: Subjects ($n = 1436$, M:F, 500:936; mean age 50.6 ± 19.6 years) exhibited non-normally distributed PINP and β-CTX peaking between 15–19 years, gradually declining throughout adulthood, elevating within 10 years of postmenopause, and then declining by age 70. In women between the age of 30 and menopause, median PINP and β-CTX levels were 40.42 (95% CI: 17.10–102.15) and 0.26 (95% CI: 0.08–0.72) ng/mL, respectively. β-CTX and PINP were positively linearly correlated ($r = 0.599$, $P < 0.001$). β-CTX correlated positively ($r = 0.054$ and 0.093) and PINP correlated negatively ($r = -0.012$ and -0.053) with 25OHD and PTH ($P < 0.05$).

Conclusions: We established Chinese reference ranges for PINP and CTX. Chinese individuals exhibited high serum PINP and β-CTX levels between 15 and 19 years of age and at menopause, which gradually declined after 70 years of age.

Editor: Dimitrios Zeugolis, National University of Ireland, Galway (NUI Galway), Ireland

Funding: This study was supported by national natural science foundation of China (No. 81100623) and the Beijing Natural Science Foundation (No. 7121012). The funders had no role in study design, data collection and analysis, decision to publish, or preparation of the manuscript.

Competing Interests: The authors have declared that no competing interests exist.

* Email: xiaweibo@medmail.com.cn (WX); xuling@pumch.cn (LX)

Introduction

Osteoporosis is characterized by decreased bone mineral density (BMD) and increased risk of bone fracture, affecting over 10% of men and nearly 20% of women in China [1]. In China and other developing countries, osteoporosis has reached epidemic proportions, with the occurrence of the disease increasing by nearly 300% over the last three decades [2]. The pathology of osteoporosis is diverse and linked with many risk factors for impaired bone remodeling; however, a critical risk factor for age-related osteoporosis is baseline BMD and age related bone loss, which has alarmingly been reported to be lower in Chinese-born individuals than those born in developed countries [3,4]. Recently, biochemical bone turnover markers (BTM) have been employed to accurately and non-invasively assess decomposition and anabolism of bone tissues, thus providing an indication of osteoblast and osteoclast activities in bone remodeling critical to differential

diagnosis of osteoporosis, assessment of bone fracture risk and effect evaluation of anti-osteoporosis therapy [5]. Reliable reference ranges for acceptable BTM, however, have not been developed for Chinese patients.

Bone remodeling is a dynamic process of spatiotemporal coupling that involves bone resorption mediated by osteoclasts and bone formation induced by osteoblasts [5]. Conventionally, osteoporosis diagnosis and treatment are assessed by BMD, measured by double-energy X-ray absorptiometry (DEXA) [6]. However, changes in BMD may not be immediately apparent after treatment, which need to take 12–24 months to indicate moderate efficacy [7]. As an alternative, serum BTM can be used to much more rapidly indicate the condition of bone loss or formation [7]. Furthermore, it has also been suggested that BTM may be useful in predicting bone fracture risk [8], potentially useful in osteoporosis and fracture prevention. Notably, Vasikaran *et al.* [7] highlighted in his review of BMD versus BTM utilities for osteoporosis management that the major limitation of wide employment of BTM was the lack of internationally agreed-upon standards for bone resorption and formation assessment, highlighting the need for precise and accurate standard reference ranges for normal BTM, as well as standards for osteoporosis and metabolic bone disease-associated BTM abnormalities.

Over the past two decades, numerous potential candidate markers of bone remodeling and their variability had been extensively examined [9]. Procollagen I N-terminal peptide (PINP) is a well-accepted marker of bone formation, produced by formation of type I collagen, a major component of bone matrix, by amino-terminal and carboxy-terminal splicing of type I procollagen in osteoblasts [10]. Conversely, C-terminal telopeptide of type I collagen (β-CTX) is considered as a marker of bone resorption, reflecting the degradation of type I collagen by osteoclasts to produce amino-terminal and carboxy-terminal fragments [11]. Recently, PINP and β-CTX have been recommended by the International Osteoporosis Foundation (IOF) and International Federation of Clinical Chemistry and Laboratory Medicine (IFCC) as the standard bone formation and resorption markers in the management of osteoporosis [12]. Furthermore, parathyroid hormone (PTH) and 25-hydroxyvitamin D (25OHD) have been suggested to be important hormones in the regulation of calcium and phosphorus metabolism, and thus play major roles in osteoporosis, though their relationship with BTMs remains unclear [10,13]. Because PINP and β-CTX are key markers for differential diagnosis and therapeutic evaluation of osteoporosis, establishment of standard reference ranges for these BTMs is of great clinical importance.

This study was conducted in order to establish a set of comprehensive standard reference ranges for PINP and β-CTX levels in Chinese populations based on age and gender. Furthermore, the effect of location and latitude, body weight and circulating levels of PTH and 25OHD were assessed. These studies would provide a key preliminary step to establishment of internationally recognized standards for BTMs for use in Chinese osteoporosis prevention and treatment strategies.

Subjects and Methods

Study design

A total of 3800 age- and gender-stratified randomly selected healthy volunteers (capped at 100 subjects/strata) were recruited by the outpatient department of participating hospitals for a multi-center, parallel-group, cross-sectional study named the Chinese Bone Turnover Marker Study (CHBTM) between May 2011 and May 2012. Due to the higher prevalence of osteoporosis in females, females were recruited at a 2:1 ratio to males. Subjects were recruited from hospitals in 5 cities located in different geographic regions of China (Beijing, Wuhan, Guangzhou, Shanghai, and Chongqing). Subjects were divided into subgroups according to age: 15–19 years, 20–29 years, 30–39 years, 40 years to menopause (40–49 years for men), menopause to 54 years (50–54 years for men), 55–59 years, 60–64 years, 65–69 years, 70–80 years, and >80 years. The Ethics Committees of all participating hospitals approved the study protocol (Peking Union Medical College Hospital, approval No. 2010-05-12; Hubei Province Hospital, approval No. 2010-05-18; General Hospital of Guangzhou Military Command, approval No. 2010-05-21; the Sixth People's Hospital of Shanghai Jiaotong University, approval No. 2010-05-22; the Second Affiliated Hospital of Chongqing Medical University, approval No. 2010-05-25). All participations were voluntary, and provided written informed consents. Written informed consents of children were obtained from guardians.

Subjects

Subjects were included that (1) were aged ≥15 years; (2) were in good health according to medical history and current physical and laboratorial examinations; (3) exhibited body mass index (BMI) between 18 and 30 kg/m^2; and (4) had normal anatomical structure of the lumbar vertebra suitable for DEXA assessment of BMD, with ≥three measurable vertebrae. Subjects were excluded that (1) had used bisphosphonates within the year directly preceding the study; (2) had used estrogen, strontium ranelate, raloxifene, parathyroid hormone preparations, or calcitonin in the three months directly preceding the study; (3) had undergone any therapy affecting bone metabolism for more than two weeks in the three months directly preceding the study, including therapy of androgen-stimulating, glucocorticoid or progestin; (4) had experienced bone fracture in the six months directly preceding the study; (5) had a history of metabolic bone disease other than postmenopausal bone loss, including hyperparathyroidism, hypoparathyroidism, Paget's disease and osteomalacia; (6) were pregnant or lactating in the two years directly preceding the study; (7) had abnormal thyroid function in the year directly preceding the study, identified as abnormal thyroid-stimulating hormone levels detected by super-sensitive thyroid function test; (8) had type 1 or type 2 diabetes; or (9) had severe liver and kidney damage, indicated by serum alanine aminotransferase more than two fold of the upper limit of normal values and serum creatinine level ≥150 μmol/L.

Clinical assessments

For each subject clinical symptoms of osteoporosis, previous history of chronic disease, history of combined medication, menstrual, marital and child-bearing status, age at menopause, and family history were recorded. All subjects completed routine physical examination, including measurements of height and body weight.

Blood sample collection

Fasting venous blood samples were collected from each subject between 8:00 and 9:00 AM local time and transferred to serum separation tubes (Covance, Indianapolis, IN, USA) supplied by the Department of Endocrinology, Peking Union Medical College Hospital (Beijing, China). Blood samples were placed at room temperature for 30 min to coagulate, and then centrifuged at $2500 \times$ g for 10 min to separate serum, which was stored at $-70°C$. Frozen serum was sent to the laboratory of the Department of Endocrinology, Peking Union Medical College Hospital (Beijing, China), and serum levels of PINP, β-CTX, PTH, and 25OHD were determined.

Biochemical index determination

Unified detection of serum levels of β-CTX, PINP, PTH, and 25OHD was conducted in the laboratory of the Department of Endocrinology, Peking Union Medical College Hospital (Beijing, China) using a computer-controlled automatic analyzer (Roche cobas e 601) for chemiluminescence workstation with β-Crosslaps, total PINP, PTH and 25OHD with Elecsys reagent kits supplied by Roche Diagnostics (Basel, Switzerland). Detection of these parameters within each batch was completed simultaneously using the same reagent kits by the same technician, conducted according to the manufacturer-provided operating processes and special laboratory quality control procedures. Intra- and inter-assay coefficients of variation (CV) for detection of serum levels and minimum measureable values (MMV), respectively, were: PINP CVs = 1.2%–4.9% and 4.3%–6.5%, MMV = 5.0 ng/ml; β-CTX CV = 1.6%–3.0% and 1.3%–4.3%, MMV = 0.01 ng/ml; PTH

CV = 1.5%–4.1% and 2.6%–6.2%, MMV = 1.2 pg/ml; 25OHD CV = 1.7%–7.8% and 2.2%–10.7%, MMV = 3.0 ng/ml. Liver and kidney functions, serum calcium, phosphorus, and alkaline phosphatase levels were detected using automated analyzers in each local hospital. Vitamin D deficiency, insufficiency and sufficiency were defined as serum 25OHD levels <20 ng/ml, ≥ 20 but <30 ng/ml, and ≥30 ng/ml, respectively [14].

Bone density measurement

Bone density of the lumbar vertebra (postero-anterior projection, L1–4), left-sided proximal hip were measured using a Lunar Prodigy (GE Healthcare, Madison WI, USA) or Hologic QDR2000 (Hologic Inc., Bedford MA, USA) dual energy X-ray absorptiometry (DEXA) scanner. Bone density measurement, quality control, and data analyses were performed by a trained radiologist for each center blind to patient clinical data that analyzed each region of interest of bone density scanning. Bone density of the lumbar vertebra and proximal hip was automatically calculated by DEXA with an accuracy of 0.8–2.0%.

Statistical analysis

Quantitative parameters were expressed as means ± standard deviation (SD), median, and 95% confidence interval, while qualitative variables were described as numbers and percentage values. All statistical analyses were performed using SPSS v.20 (SPSS Inc., Chicago, IL, USA). In order to investigate the characters of biomarkers of BTM, all parameters were described after age-, gender-, and site-based stratifications, and latitude of the sites of recruitment was in analyses. Distributions were described by scatter plot. Pearson's correlation analysis was used for normally distributed data, and Spearman's correlation analysis was used for non-normally distributed data, as well as multivariate analysis was performed, thus evaluating associations between BTMs with the age, body weight, height, recruitment location latitude, PTH and 25OHD levels. After base 10 logarithmic transformations, non-normally distributed data were fitted by linear regression. BTMs were compared among regions by Kruskal-Wallis test with Mann-Whitney U test for posthoc analysis. P-values less than 0.05 indicated statistical significance ($P<0.05$).

Results

Characteristics of the study population

Of the total 3800 subjects screened, 805 (21.2%) were excluded for taking medications affecting bone densities, 489 (12.9%) were excluded for recent fracture or pregnancy, and 411 (10.8%) did not consent to participation. Of the remaining 2095 (55.1%) subjects, 659 (17.3%) were excluded due to medication use affecting bone turnover, and the remaining 1436 subjects were included in the study (Fig. 1). The study population included 936 women (65.2%) and 500 men (34.8%). We enrolled 189 (13.16%) participants from Beijing, 320 (22.28%) from Shanghai, 334 (23.26%) from Guangzhou, 217 (15.11%) from Chongqing, and 376 (26.18%) from Wuhan. The mean age of participants was 50.6±19.6 (range, 15–110) years, with mean body weight of 61.6±3.5 (range, 41.0–80.0) kg, and mean BMI of 23.1±5.3 (18.8–29.5) kg/m^2. For the included postmenopausal women ($n = 601$), the mean age at menopause was 49.5±2.8 (age range of menopause, 40.0–56.0) years. Demographic and clinical characteristics for each age group were shown in Table 1.

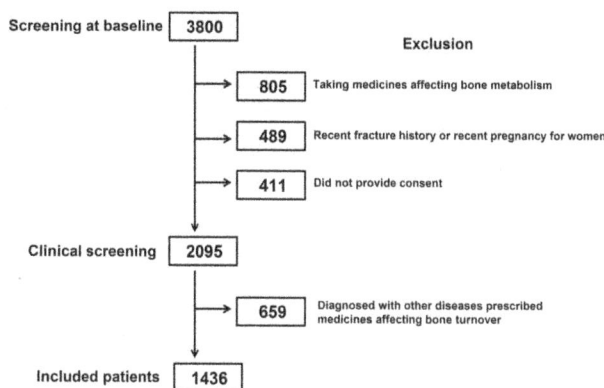

Figure 1. Subject screening and recruitment.

Serum β-CTX, PINP, PTH, 25OHD levels and stratified analysis

PINP and β-CTX levels were non-normally distributed, with median levels of 49.36 (95% CI: 18.79–155.55) and 0.37 (95% CI: 0.11–0.90) ng/ml, respectively. Median PTH and 25OHD levels were 28.41 (95% CI: 8.62–71.08) and 18.39 (95% CI: 7.37–38.68) ng/ml, respectively. The mean serum 25OHD level was 17.9±8.1 ng/ml in the 936 female participants and 22.2±8.6 ng/ml in the 500 male participants. 68.6%, 19.2% and 12.2% of the female participants met the criteria for vitamin D deficiency, vitamin D insufficiency, and vitamin D sufficiency, respectively. 44.5%, 37.9% and 17.6% of the male participants met the criteria for vitamin D deficiency, vitamin D insufficiency, and vitamin D sufficiency, respectively.

Age-stratified analysis revealed relatively high levels of PINP and β-CTX in women between 15 and 19 years of age, thereafter gradually declining with age. Significantly elevated levels of PINP and β-CTX were observed again in women from menopause to 60 years of age; however, PINP and β-CTX levels slowly declined in women beyond ages of 70 and 65 years, respectively (Fig. 2A and 2C). Similarly, PINP and β-CTX peaked in men between 15 and 19 years of age, thereafter, levels of both markers gradually declined. PINP and β-CTX remained at low levels in men from 40 to 69 years of age, declining further after age 70 (Fig. 2B and 2D). PINP and β-CTX levels in men between the age of 15 and 19 years were significantly higher than in women in the same age bracket ($P<0.001$, Fig. 2A and 2C). PINP and β-CTX levels in postmenopausal women aged <64 years were significantly higher than those in men aged 50–64 years ($P<0.001$, Fig. 2B and 2D).

Correlations among β-CTX, PINP, PTH, and 25OHD

Spearman's correlation analysis revealed a significant positive correlation between PINP and β-CTX levels in the whole study population ($r = 0.599$, $P<0.001$) (Fig. 2E). After base 10 logarithmic transformations, a simple linear equation ($y = 1.869+0.191x$, $R^2 = 0.362$) was fitted, indicating the close coupling relationship between bone resorption and bone formation. PINP levels negatively correlated with 25OHD and PTH levels, with low correlation coefficients ($r = -0.012$ and -0.053, both $P<0.05$) (Fig. 2E). β-CTX positively correlated with PTH and 25OHD levels, though correlation coefficients were relatively low ($r = 0.054$ and 0.093, $P<0.05$ and 0.001) (Fig. 2E).

Table 1. Characteristics and age distribution of the study population.

Characteristic	Female (*n*=936)	Male (*n*=500)	Total (*n*=1436)
Age (years)	52.71±18.22(17–110)	46.45±21.33(15–105)	50.56±19.57(15–110)
Age group (years)			
15–19	17 (1.82%)	32 (6.40%)	49 (3.41%)
20–29	142 (15.17%)	122 (24.40%)	264 (18.38%)
30–39	88 (9.40%)	69 (13.80%)	157 (10.93%)
40–49	102 (10.9%)	54 (10.80%)	156 (10.86%)
50–54	92 (9.83%)	34 (6.80%)	126 (8.77%)
55–59	120 (12.82%)	35 (7.00%)	155 (10.79%)
60–64	123 (13.14)	33 (6.60%)	156 (10.86%)
65–69	92 (9.83%)	29 (5.80%)	121 (8.43%)
70–80	117 (12.5%)	58 (11.6%)	175 (12.19%)
>80	43 (4.59%)	34 (6.80%)	77 (5.36%)
Body weight (kg)	56.55±8.08 (41.0–84.0)	68.80±10.25 (43.0–98.5)	61.59±3.54 (41.0–80.0)
BMI (kg/m^2)	22.96±3.30(18.90–29.50)	23.81±3.29 (18.8–29.03)	23.06±5.28 18.80–29.50)
BMD of L2–4 (g/cm^2)	0.94±0.27 (0.40–1.98)	1.05±0.31 (0.66–1.64)	0.98±0.29 (0.4–1.98)
BMD of femoral neck (g/cm^2)	0.81±0.40 (0.13–1.26)	0.95±0.65 (0.51–1.57)	0.86±0.51 (0.13–1.57)
Total hip BMD (g/cm^2)	0.67±0.18 (0.20–1.86)	0.79±0.23 (0.27–1.59)	0.71±0.21 (0.20–1.86)

Correlations of β-CTX and PINP levels with recruitment location latitude and body weight

No significant differences were observed in PINP and β-CTX levels in either men or women among the 5 cities with different latitudes (all $P>0.05$) after the age, body weight and height were adjusted (Table 2). PINP and β-CTX levels did, however, positively correlated with body weight, exhibiting low correlation coefficients ($r=0.097$ and 0.19, both $P<0.001$).

Discussion

As the first comprehensive, multi-center, age- and gender-stratified report of standard reference ranges for BTMs PINP and β-CTX in five geographically distant Chinese cities, this study is uniquely capable of describing the BTM characteristics of the Chinese populace. This study provides novel indications of high levels of bone turnover in both men and women during late adolescence and in women during menopause. Bone turnover levels also gradually declined in both men and women throughout adulthood and, more dramatically, above 70 years of age. As the age range in our study was very wide (15–110 years old), we were able to study BTMs in an elderly population. Furthermore, PINP and β-CTX levels correlated with each other and with body weight. Additionally, β-CTX level correlated positively ($r=0.054$ and 0.093, $P<0.05$ and 0.001) and PINP level correlated negatively ($r=-0.012$ and -0.053, both $P<0.05$) with serum 25OHD and PTH levels. However, the correlation coefficients between β-CTX, PINP and 25OHD, PTH levels were extremely low ($r<0.1$), so the clinical significance of this correlations was limited. This study provides reference interval values for PINP and CTX in healthy Chinese adults, which will contribute to appropriate assessment of bone turnover and suggest appropriate treatment targets.

Significant overlap had been reported between PINP and β-CTX levels in both healthy individuals and subjects with osteoporosis, suggesting that BTMs such as PINP and β-CTX

had variant utilities for diagnosis of osteoporosis, prediction of bone turnover, and prevention of fracture, though these relationships were not fully understood [15,16]. As a result, primary diagnosis of osteoporosis may not be the most notable use of BTMs. Notably, elevation of PINP and β-CTX did, however, reliably predict the presence of bone diseases associated with malignant tumors, including breast cancer, prostate cancer, and lung cancer and early signs of metabolic bone diseases [17–20]. Therefore, standard reference ranges for PINP and β-CTX would make these markers much more useful for differential diagnosis of osteoporosis. Furthermore, establishment of standard reference ranges for PINP and β-CTX would facilitate the development of improved treatment strategies for osteoporosis by allowing dynamic assessment of changes in bone metabolism in the immediate period following treatment [21–23]. However, reference ranges for PINP and β-CTX may be different between age groups, duration of disease, and physiological status. As the present study was a cross-sectional one, it did not allow dynamic assessment of changes in bone metabolism during biological variation. Therefore, more prospective studies are needed to clarify these issues.

As in North American and European populations [24–26], in this study BTM levels changed predictably with age and gender in the Chinese population. The highest rate of bone turnover in both genders occurred in late adolescence and thereafter declined, consistent with a previous study of 1541 Chinese youths by Guo *et al.* [27] indicating that Chinese adolescents aged 16 to 19 exhibited the greatest BMD changes, most notably in males. Furthermore, significantly higher levels of PINP and β-CTX were detected in postmenopausal women (between menopause and 64 years of age) than in men between 50 and 64 years of age, consistent with previous reports indicating that significant bone density loss was associated with a rapid reduction in estrogen of menopausal women [28]. Notably, bone turnover level gradually reduced in both men and women aged over 70 years, potentially associated with the dysfunction of osteoblasts and osteoclasts and

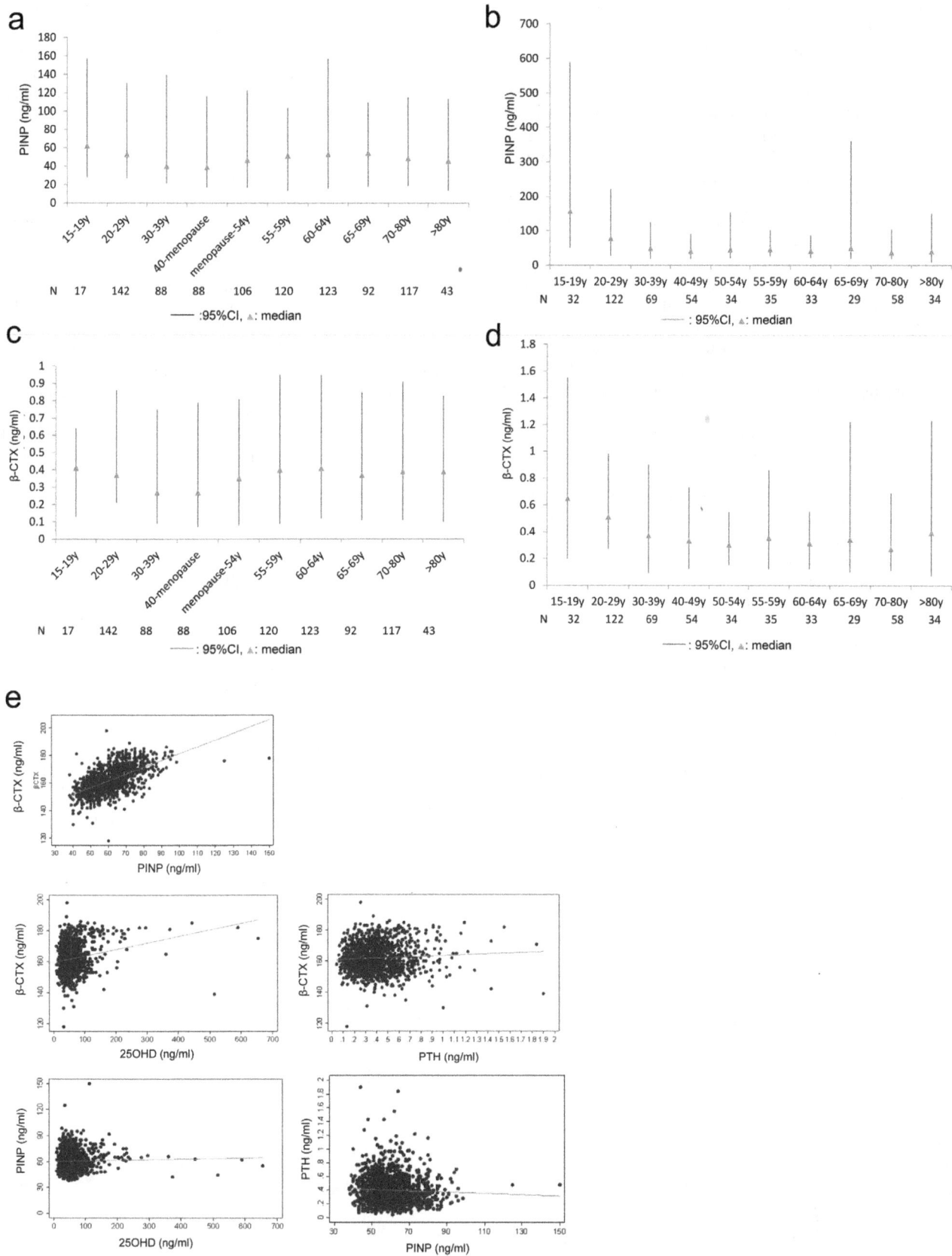

Figure 2. PINP and β-CTX levels in different groups and the results of correlation analysis. a PINP levels in female age groups. b PINP levels in male age groups. c β-CTX levels in female age groups. d β-CTX levels in male age groups. e The correlation between β-CTX, PINP, PTH and 25OHD levels in participants.

altered calcium metabolism in the oldest-old [29]. Thus, the current results were generally consistent with those found in other populations and previous reports of Chinese patients.

Notably, we observed a significant positive and linear correlation between PINP and β-CTX levels and between these BTMs and body weight, suggesting that bone turnover closely reflected coupling processes of bone resorption and bone formation. In a study of 87 healthy Brazilian males aged 10–18 years, similar positive correlations were observed between body weight and serum carboxyterminal telopeptide ($r = 0.40$) and osteocalcin levels ($r = 0.21$) that may have resulted from adipokine effects on the skeletal bone targets, altering sympathetic impulses and exerting paracrine effects bone tissues [30]. Correlations between BTM levels and geographic locations were poor in the present study, which remained controversial, perhaps due to nutritional and lifestyle variations more than the nature of the location itself [4]. In a study of 637 healthy premenopausal women from the United Kingdom, France, Belgium, and the United States, β-CTX was significantly higher in France relative to the United Kingdom, and PINP was higher in France and Belgium relative to the United Kingdom, with researchers similarly concluded that these variations were predominantly due to lifestyle rather than genetic or geographic variations [31]. This was further confirmed by the limited variation exhibited among 5 European centers in a report by Blumsohn *et al.* [32], and higher bone turnover levels in North America than those in German and Spanish women [33]. Thus, further work would be required to determine the precise lifestyle and nutritional factors responsible for raised osteoporosis risk; however, implementation of BTM measurements would be certain to improve the feasibility of such research.

BTMs ranges in healthy premenopausal women had garnered increasing recent research attention, potentially due to therapeutic goals of restoring normal BTM levels in patients with osteoporosis and metabolic bone diseases [34]. Interestingly, the median levels of PINP and β-CTX in the 176 premenopausal women from 30 years old to menopause in the current study (40.42 and 0.26 ng/mL, respectively) were very similar to those reported in 194 premenopausal European women aged 35–39 years reported by Eastell *et al.* in 2012 [9], 153 women aged 35–45 years reported by Glover *et al.* in 2008 [35], 637 premenopausal women aged 35–39 years reported by Glover *et al.* in 2009 [31], and in premenopausal women aged 28–45 years reported by de Papp *et al.* in 2007 [36],

suggesting that the range of PINP and β-CTX levels in premenopausal women, as the normal reference range, had no apparent racial variation. We studied a wide range of Chinese women from five cities, and found that the BTM characteristics of these participants were not very different from the results reported by similar studies of European and American women in studies using similar techniques [9,30,34,35]. However, we cannot exclude the possibility that these studies enrolled non equivalent populations based on inclusion and exclusion criteria different to that we employed in participant screening.

The current study, however, was limited by the failure to record dietary calcium intake and daily exercise, thus we could not assess the impact of lifestyle on BTMs. Furthermore, the smaller numbers of participants in certain subgroups (e.g., 17 women and 32 men aged 15–19; 13 men from Shanghai) had limited the significance and applicability of these analyses. We also did not record serum estrogen and androgen levels, and bone density was measured using Lunar or Hologic dual-energy X-ray bone absorptiometry scanners, which may exhibit some variation due to equipment types or calibration. Additionally, all study subjects were urban residents, which avoided the effect of variations of living environments and habits on BTMs levels but may limited broad applicability to rural populations due to lifestyle and nutritional variations, meriting further investigation.

Conclusions

This large-scale, multi-center, cross-sectional study provided a novel, comprehensive determination of standard reference ranges for the bone formation marker PINP and bone resorption marker β-CTX in Chinese men and women by age. High bone turnover levels were detected in both men and women during late adolescence and in women at menopause, and bone turnover gradually declined in both men and women after age 70.

Acknowledgments

We would like to thank the Shanghai Roche Pharmaceutical Co., Ltd. for the free providing reagent kits of biochemical markers detection and technical support. We thank the support by a grant from The Ministry of Science and Technology of the People's Republic of China (National Science and Technology Major Projects for "Major New Drugs Innovation and Development 2008ZX09312-016"). We thank the support of the

Table 2. PINP and β-CTX levels in male and female subjects by sites of recruitment latitude.

City (Latitude)	PINP (ng/ml)		β-CTX (ng/ml)	
	Female	Male	Female	Male
Beijing	43.01(15.27,96.96)	40.40(18.23,94.15)	0.28(0.09,0.79)	0.28(0.10,0.68)
(39°54′27″N)	(n = 93)	(n = 96)	(n = 93)	(n = 96)
Shanghai	53.08(14.92,135.43)	29.74(17.31,56.74)	0.41(0.11,0.88)	0.25(0.10,0.39)
(31°13′56″N)	(n = 307)	(n = 13)	(n = 307)	(n = 13)
Wuhan	46.02(20.95,105.18)	47.85(24.10,163.43)	0.35(0.12,0.75)	0.39(0.17,1.01)
(29°58′20″N)	(n = 207)	(n = 169)	(n = 207)	(n = 169)
Chongqing	53.07(20.66,120.34)	47.07(20.08,125.11)	0.42(0.12,0.91)	0.39(0.12,1.21)
(29°36′21″N)	(n = 134)	(n = 83)	(n = 134)	(n = 83)
Guangzhou	48.33(19.77,116.69)	76.46(29.41,402.45)	0.33(0.08,0.82)	0.45(0.15,1.14)
(23°06′32″N)	(n = 195)	(n = 139)	(n = 195)	(n = 139)

There were no significant differences in the β-CTX and PINP concentrations among different cities after the age, body weight and height were adjusted.

National Natural Science Foundation of China (No. 81100623), (No. 7121012) and National Key Program of Clinical Science (WBYZ2011-873).

Author Contributions

Conceived and designed the experiments: WX LX. Performed the experiments: ML YL WD ZZ ZD YH. Analyzed the data: ML. Contributed reagents/materials/analysis tools: ML WX. Wrote the paper: ML.

References

1. Li N, Ou P, Zhu H, Yang D, Zheng P (2002) Prevalence rate of osteoporosis in the mid - aged and elderly in selected parts of China. Chin Med J (Engl) 115: 773–775.
2. Heo HD, Cho YJ, Sheen SH, Kuh SU, Cho SM, et al. (2009) Morphological changes of injected calcium phosphate cement in osteoporotic compressed vertebral bodies. Osteoporos Int 20: 2063–2070.
3. Shen C, Deng J, Zhou R, Chen J, Fan S, et al. (2012) Relation between bone mineral density, bone loss and the risk of cardiovascular disease in a Chinese cohort. Am J Cardiol 110: 1138–1142.
4. Lauderdale DS, Kuohung V, Chang SL, Chin MH (2003) Identifying older Chinese immigrants at high risk for osteoporosis. J Gen Intern Med 18: 508–515.
5. Naylor K, Eastell R (2012) Bone turnover markers: use in osteoporosis. Nature Reviews Rheumatology 8: 379–389.
6. Anastasopoulou C, Rude RK (2002) Bone mineral density screening: assessment of influence on prevention and treatment of osteoporosis. Endocr Pract 8: 199–201.
7. Vasikaran SD (2008) Utility of biochemical markers of bone turnover and bone mineral density in management of osteoporosis. Crit Rev Clin Lab Sci 45: 221–258.
8. Vasikaran SD, Glendenning P, Morris HA (2006) The role of biochemical markers of bone turnover in osteoporosis management in clinical practice. Clin Biochem Rev 27: 119–121.
9. Eastell R, Baumann M (2001) Bone Markers: Biochemical and Clinical Perspectives. London: Martin Dunitz Ltd.
10. Lee J, Vasikaran S (2012) Current recommendations for laboratory testing and use of bone turnover markers in management of osteoporosis. Ann Lab Med 32: 105–112.
11. Seibel MJ (2005) Biochemical markers of bone turnover: part I: biochemistry and variability. Clin Biochem Rev 26: 97–122.
12. Vasikaran S, Cooper C, Eastell R, Griesmacher A, Morris HA, et al. (2011) International Osteoporosis Foundation and International Federation of Clinical Chemistry and Laboratory Medicine position on bone marker standards in osteoporosis. Clin Chem Lab Med 49: 1271–1274.
13. Silva BC, Camargos BM, Fujii JB, Dias EP, Soares MM (2008) [Prevalence of vitamin D deficiency and its correlation with PTH, biochemical bone turnover markers and bone mineral density, among patients from ambulatories]. Arq Bras Endocrinol Metabol 52: 482–488.
14. Holick MF, Binkley NC, Bischoff-Ferrari HA, Gordon CM, Hanley DA, et al. (2011) Evaluation, treatment, and prevention of vitamin D deficiency: an Endocrine Society clinical practice guideline. J Clin Endocrinol Metab 96: 1911–1930.
15. Garnero P (2008) Biomarkers for osteoporosis management: utility in diagnosis, fracture risk prediction and therapy monitoring. Mol Diagn Ther 12: 157–170.
16. Bauer DC, Garnero P, Harrison SL, Cauley JA, Eastell R, et al. (2009) Biochemical markers of bone turnover, hip bone loss, and fracture in older men: the MrOS study. J Bone Miner Res 24: 2032–2038.
17. Dean-Colomb W, Hess KR, Young E, Gornet TG, Handy BC, et al. (2013) Elevated serum P1NP predicts development of bone metastasis and survival in early-stage breast cancer. Breast Cancer Res Treat 137: 631–636.
18. Som A, Tu SM, Liu J, Wang X, Qiao W, et al. (2012) Response in bone turnover markers during therapy predicts overall survival in patients with metastatic prostate cancer: analysis of three clinical trials. Br J Cancer 107: 1547–1553.
19. Valencia K, Martin-Fernandez M, Zandueta C, Ormazabal C, Martinez-Canarias S, et al. (2013) miR-326 associates with biochemical markers of bone turnover in lung cancer bone metastasis. Bone 52: 532–539.
20. Alonso S, Ferrero E, Donat M, Martinez G, Vargas C, et al. (2012) The usefulness of high pre-operative levels of serum type I collagen markers for the prediction of changes in bone mineral density after parathyroidectomy. J Endocrinol Invest 35: 640–644.
21. McClung MR, Lewiecki EM, Geller ML, Bolognese MA, Peacock M, et al. (2013) Effect of denosumab on bone mineral density and biochemical markers of bone turnover: 8-year results of a phase 2 clinical trial. Osteoporos Int 24: 227–235.
22. Eastell R, Reid DM, Vukicevic S, Ensrud KE, LaCroix AZ, et al. (2012) Effects of 3 years of lasofoxifene treatment on bone turnover markers in women with postmenopausal osteoporosis. Bone 50: 1135–1140.
23. Brixen K, Chapurlat R, Cheung AM, Keaveny TM, Fuerst T, et al. (2013) Bone density, turnover, and estimated strength in postmenopausal women treated with odanacatib: a randomized trial. J Clin Endocrinol Metab 98: 571–580.
24. Jurimae J, Maestu J, Jurimae T (2010) Bone turnover markers during pubertal development: relationships with growth factors and adipocytokines. Med Sport Sci 55: 114–127.
25. Fares JE, Choucair M, Nabulsi M, Salamoun M, Shahine CH, et al. (2003) Effect of gender, puberty, and vitamin D status on biochemical markers of bone remodedeling. Bone 33: 242–247.
26. Valimaki VV, Alfthan H, Ivaska KK, Loyttyniemi E, Pettersson K, et al. (2004) Serum estradiol, testosterone, and sex hormone-binding globulin as regulators of peak bone mass and bone turnover rate in young Finnish men. J Clin Endocrinol Metab 89: 3785–3789.
27. Guo B, Xu Y, Gong J, Tang Y, Xu H (2013) Age trends of bone mineral density and percentile curves in healthy Chinese children and adolescents. J Bone Miner Metab 31: 304–314.
28. Seifert-Klauss V, Fillenberg S, Schneider H, Luppa P, Mueller D, et al. (2012) Bone loss in premenopausal, perimenopausal and postmenopausal women: results of a prospective observational study over 9 years. Climacteric 15: 433–440.
29. Passeri G, Vescovini R, Sansoni P, Galli C, Franceschi C, et al. (2008) Calcium metabolism and vitamin D in the extreme longevity. Exp Gerontol 43: 79–87.
30. Kawai M, de Paula FJ, Rosen CJ (2012) New insights into osteoporosis: the bone-fat connection. J Intern Med 272: 317–329.
31. Glover SJ, Gall M, Schoenborn-Kellenberger O, Wagener M, Garnero P, et al. (2009) Establishing a reference interval for bone turnover markers in 637 healthy, young, premenopausal women from the United Kingdom, France, Belgium, and the United States. J Bone Miner Res 24: 389–397.
32. Blumsohn A, Naylor KE, Timm W, Eagleton AC, Hannon RA, et al. (2003) Absence of marked seasonal change in bone turnover: a longitudinal and multicenter cross-sectional study. J Bone Miner Res 18: 1274–1281.
33. Cohen FJ, Eckert S, Mitlak BH (1998) Geographic differences in bone turnover: data from a multinational study in healthy postmenopausal women. Calcif Tissue Int 63: 277–282.
34. Eastell R, Barton I, Hannon RA, Chines A, Garnero P, et al. (2003) Relationship of early changes in bone resorption to the reduction in fracture risk with risedronate. J Bone Miner Res 18: 1051–1056.
35. Glover SJ, Garnero P, Naylor K, Rogers A, Eastell R (2008) Establishing a reference range for bone turnover markers in young, healthy women. Bone 42: 623–630.
36. de Papp AE, Bone HG, Caulfield MP, Kagan R, Buinewicz A, et al. (2007) A cross-sectional study of bone turnover markers in healthy premenopausal women. Bone 40: 1222–1230.

22

Abandoned Acid? Understanding Adherence to Bisphosphonate Medications for the Prevention of Osteoporosis among Older Women

Charlotte Salter[1]*, **Lisa McDaid**[1], **Debi Bhattacharya**[2], **Richard Holland**[1], **Tarnya Marshall**[3], **Amanda Howe**[1]

1 Norwich Medical School, Faculty of Medicine & Health Science, University of East Anglia, Norwich, Norfolk, United Kingdom, 2 School of Chemistry and Pharmacy, University of East Anglia, Norwich, Norfolk. United Kingdom, 3 Rheumatology Department, Norfolk & Norwich University Foundation Trust Hospital. Norwich, Norfolk. United Kingdom

Abstract

Background: There is significant morbidity and mortality caused by the complications of osteoporosis, for which ageing is the greatest epidemiological risk factor. Preventive medications to delay osteoporosis are available, but little is known about motivators to adhere to these in the context of a symptomless condition with evidence based on screening results.

Aim: To describe key perceptions that influence older women's adherence and persistence with prescribed medication when identified to be at a higher than average risk of fracture.

Design of Study: A longitudinal qualitative study embedded within a multi-centre trial exploring the effectiveness of screening for prevention of fractures.

Setting: Primary care, Norfolk. United Kingdom

Methods: Thirty older women aged 70–85 years of age who were offered preventive medication for osteoporosis and agreed to undertake two interviews at 6 and 24 months post-first prescription.

Results: There were no overall predictors of adherence which varied markedly over time. Participants' perceptions and motivations to persist with medication were influenced by six core themes: understanding adherence and non-adherence, motivations and self-care, appraising and prioritising risk, anticipating and managing side effects, problems of understanding, and decision making around medication. Those engaged with supportive professionals could better tolerate and overcome barriers such as side-effects.

Conclusions: Many issues are raised following screening in a cohort of women who have not previously sought advice about their bone health. Adherence to preventive medication for osteoporosis is complex and multifaceted. Individual participant understanding, choice, risk and perceived need all interact to produce unpredictable patterns of usage and acceptability. There are clear implications for practice and health professionals should not assume adherence in any older women prescribed medication for the prevention of osteoporosis. The beliefs and motivations of participants and their healthcare providers regarding the need to establish acceptable medication regimes is key to promoting and sustaining adherence.

Editor: Christy Elizabeth Newman, The University of New South Wales, Australia

Funding: Funding came from Research for Patient Benefit Programme National Institute for Health Research PG-PB-0807-14068. The funder had no role in study design, data collection and analysis, decision to publish, or preparation of the manuscript.

Competing Interests: The authors have declared that no competing interests exist.

* E-mail: c.salter@uea.ac.uk

Introduction

There is significant morbidity and mortality caused by the complications of osteoporosis, for which ageing is the greatest epidemiological risk factor. While other risks such as immobility, persistent low body weight, early menopause and corticosteroid use may lead to early onset of osteoporosis, around 40% of women aged 70 will have osteoporosis, and as many as 90% will have a significantly increased risk of fracturing a bone in a fall or accident [1], [2]. This has led to a major research focus on the prevention of osteoporosis which has established that osteoporotic fractures can be significantly reduced by a combination of pharmacological (bisphosphonates with calcium and vitamin D supplements) and behavioural interventions (dietary intake, smoking cessation, and weight bearing exercise).

More recent initiatives include the development of treatment algorithms and encouragement for primary care practitioners to identify patients who may be at 'risk' of fracturing and may benefit from preventive options [3],[4]. However, as the National Institute for Clinical Excellence (NICE) acknowledge, *"identifying who will benefit from preventative treatment is imprecise"* [5]. No population screening programme currently exists for osteoporosis risk, and individuals are identified clinically on a case by case basis. Predictive risk of fracture compared to the norm for age and sex can now be calculated using clinical risk factors in conjunction with bone mineral density (BMD) measurements using Dual energy X-ray Absorbtiometry (DXA) scans [6], [7], creating new opportunities to identify individuals yet to sustain a fracture.

For screening to be effective, participants identified as high risk must be receptive to the intervention. Achieving long-term adherence to prescribed medications is more complex than just providing sufficient information or an acceptable medication regimen. The literature suggests adherence is highly variable in osteoporosis prevention with age and co-morbidity explaining relatively little of the variability [8], [9]. Attempts to reduce complexity in dosing regimens do not necessarily improve adherence [10], [11]. Patients are recommended to take their bisphosphonates first thing in the morning before eating or drinking and with a glass of water. There is a requirement for them to remain upright for 30 minutes to avoid irritation to the oesophagus. Calcium supplements are frequently provided in the form of chewy tablets. Patients may understand the potential for osteoporosis to have a negative effect on their lives, and express strong motivation to protect their health, but this does not always align with taking medications [12], [13]. This therefore makes the motivations and decision making of older women around uptake of preventive medication of primary importance to the public health impact of any potential screening programme as well as to the individual patient.

It is also known that patterns of adherence to osteoporosis medications vary over time [14], [15]. However, a survey of patients and physicians showed that poor adherence reflected patient scepticism about the risks and values of treatment, rather than a lack of factual knowledge. A qualitative synthesis of studies on lay experience of medicine taking found widespread caution about taking medication with many participants 'testing' pre-scribed medicines for efficacy and adverse side effects [14]. Our pilot study found as many as 50% of women at 'high risk' of fracture in the 70–85 age group were not receiving treatment four months later [16]. We therefore undertook this study to explore the factors that influence older women's adherence to prescribed prophylactic medication when assessed to have higher than average risk of fracture following screening. This paper describes the perceptions and motivations to which participants attributed their willingness and ability to adhere to osteoporosis prevention regimes, and considers implications for practice.

Methods

Participants and procedure

The Adherence To Osteoporosis Medication (ATOM Study) was established as a longitudinal qualitative study embedded within the Medical Research Council funded UK multi-centre randomised control trial on Screening for Osteoporosis in Older Women for the Prevention of Fractures (SCOOP). SCOOP [17] aims to explore the effectiveness of screening women aged 70–85

for the prevention of fractures using a risk-prediction algorithm. The qualitative study took place in Norfolk, United Kingdom.

Ethics Statement

We secured approval from North West National Health Service Research Ethics Committee (Ref: 07/H1010/70). Written in-formed consent was obtained from participants. Two participants with mild cognitive impairment were supported in the consenting and interview process by their husbands.

The research comprised a longitudinal design with two in-depth interviews conducted 18 months apart, the first at around 6 months post-randomisation. The sample was drawn from those found to be at 'higher than average' risk of a subsequent fracture and whose prescribing data showed they had started medications for the prevention of osteoporosis. Participants were purposively sampled from demographic and adherence data already collected by the SCOOP trial (see Table 1). As the focus of our study was to explore why older women were adherent, we constructed our sample to include more women self-reporting they were adherent when contacted by phone than reporting they were non-adherent to their osteoporosis medication.

For the purpose of this study 'adherent' included both women stating they were taking bisphosphonate medication as instructed, and those stating they were intentionally or unintentionally missing doses but no more than 1 in 5 (i.e. 80% adherence or more). Non-adherent' included all those who had discontinued bisphosphonate medication, or were taking them <80% of the time, but who might still be taking prescribed supplements (calcium and vitamin D).

The interviews

Interviews took place at participants' homes and lasted an average of 74 minutes. They were based on a topic guide developed to explore women's understanding of osteoporosis, responses to screening results, current usage of preventive medicine, motivators and detractors from taking medication and follow up with healthcare professionals. Interview recordings were transcribed verbatim and anonymised. Familiarisation, data management, coding and categorisation were carried out by the interdisciplinary research team including CS, LM and AH. Iteration between both data sets and the research literature helped inform the analysis at the explanatory level. The principles of Framework Analysis [18] were used to order, chart and search the data both manually and supported by relevant software (NVivo 9 Software, MSWord and Framework). Illustrative quotations are selected to elucidate the study findings. Extracts are labelled using participant number, age at interview and summary adherence status to both bisphosphonates and calcium supplements.

Results

Ninety women in the 'higher than average' risk group recruited to the Norwich arm of the SCOOP Trial indicated they would be willing to take part in the qualitative sub-study. From these we recruited a sample of 30 (33%) women, age range 73–85 years (Table 1). Five participants were unable to participate in the follow-up interview due to death or withdrawal from the study.

Understanding adherence and non-adherence

All 30 participants were prescribed bisphosphonates and all except one commenced their first course. Of the 10 participants shown in Table 2 who reported being non-adherent at Phase 1 Interviews, nine made this decision without discussion with their

Table 1. Sample characteristics using pre-collected trial data.

Sample Characteristic	Category	Number (%)
Self-reported adherence status given on phone at recruitment	Adherent	19 (63)
	Non-adherent	11 (37)
Age	70–74	9 (30)
	75–79	10 (33)
	80+	11 (37)
GP practice	Urban	14 (47)
	Rural	16 (53)
Social class	I	3 (10)
	II	6 (20)
	IIIN	6 (20)
	IIIM	10 (33)
	IV	5 (17)
	V	0

general practitioner. All bar one said they had done this within a month of collecting their first prescription. The combination of bisphosphonate and calcium: vitamin D supplements was reported to be taken by 12 participants.

Of the 25 participants who took part in Phase 2 Interviews, thirteen had remained adherent to bisphosphonate medication and one previously non-adherent participant reported she had started taking her medication as prescribed. Eleven were non-adherent including three women that had given up their bisphosphonate medicine between interviews. Thus, a significant proportion of our sample were taking *no medication* for the prevention of fracture and osteoporosis at 18 months (44%). Even within the 'adherent' group, many women admitted deficits in their adherence; sometimes this was deliberate, to avoid inconvenience, sometimes it was because they forgot one day, but took it the next.

We found no obvious pattern or factors linking with adherence. Responses to screening, acceptance of risk status, existing medical history, previous experience of falls, fractures and family history did not appear to predict womens' adherence status.

Some participants complained about the complexity of the regimen, many had experienced side effects, some said their general practitioner had stopped the medication, and some had

misunderstood the reasons for taking them long-term. However, many adherent women reported similar issues. Few cited 'forgetting' as a key cause of non-adherence. Almost all respondents declared a willingness to 'in principle' do what their general practitioner advised, but some non-adherent women cited medical permission or support for their choice to stop:

He was quite happy, he said alright just stop. He said we've had no broken bones in your family, he said you'll probably be quite alright. (Participant 12, age 84 – became Non-Adherent to Bisphosphonates by Phase 2. Refused Calcium)

Personal scepticism about the value of the treatments did not seem to link clearly with non-adherence. For example, the following participant was adherent to her medications, but demonstrated very little belief that she needed them at her age:

I thought well yes I am 80, so I probably have anyway (thinning bones) and I also thought it is a bit *late* to start treating me now I honestly did. That was my sort of attitude but the letter said 'go and see your doctor', so I went and saw my doctor and he gave me those. (Participant 24, age 80

Table 2. Summary of Patterns of Adherence.

	Bisphosphonates	Calcium Supplements	Bisphosphonates & Calcium Supplements
	N (%)	N (%)	N (%)
Phase 1			
Adherent	20 (67)	15 (50)	12 (40)
Non-adherent	10 (33)	10 (33)	13 (43)
Not prescribed	-	5 (17)	5 (17)
Total	30 (100)	30 (100)	30 (100)
Phase 2			
Adherent	14 (56)	12 (48)	9 (36)
Non-adherent	11 (44)	9 (36)	12 (48)
Not prescribed	-	4 (16)	4 (16)
Total	25 (100)	25 (100)	25 (100)

- Adherent to both Bisphosphonates & Calcium Phase 1, subsequently withdrew)

By contrast Participant 22 was non-adherent. She felt anyone could break a bone in the next 10 years and would have expected to fracture by now if she was really at risk. She described how her own mother had fallen and broken her hip yet appeared to remain personally unconcerned:

When they said well look 'a higher risk of breaking a bone over the next 10 years' and I thought well *I'm over 80 so it's not surprising* (laughs). (Participant 22, age 84 – Continually Non-Adherent to both Bisphosphonates & Calcium)

Motivations, self-care and adherence

All the respondents regardless of adherence status seemed to have accepted the need for better self-care and an altered lifestyle in order to prevent fractures. Many believed they had been doing this all their lives through a good diet, plenty of physical activity and exercise:

Because I've always taken calcium you know. I've always had a lot of cheese, a lot of yoghurt and I drink a certain amount of milk I have calcium and I have a lot of vegetables. (Participant 10, age 73 - Continually adherent bisphosphonates. Calcium not prescribed)

I take a cod liver oil pill every day, winter and summer. I'm sure that's a help. (Participant 09, age 85 - Continually non-adherent bisphosphonates & calcium)

In addition, many participants had adjusted their daily routines to enhance their capacity to take their regimens as prescribed. Weekly doses were linked with memorable events, and chores such as ironing utilised to fulfil the half hour required in remaining upright:

So I try and get up early, take it with this load of water and find something to do standing up, whether it's ironing for an hour which I did this week (laughs) or going round the garden seeing what's in flower. You have just got to find something to do which takes your mind off it. (Participant 06, age 80 – Continually Adherent to Bisphosphonates. Non-adherent to Calcium)

Market day is a Wednesday and I always used to go down to buy plants every Wednesday. I always used to think I can't go down and get any plants, so I always remember Wednesday. That was my day. (Participant 30, age 75 – Continually Non-Adherent to Bisphosphonates. Took Calcium supplements at Phase 2)

Carers played a role in aiding adherence for two participants with cognitive impairments by bringing the medication to them and altering the routine to ensure no food or cup of tea at the same time:

He'd put it on his computer to remind me (and) he puts them in front of me and lets me get on with it. (Participant

17, age 75 – Continually Adherent Bisphosphonates. Calcium not prescribed).

Autonomy was also a powerful motivator, characterised by the need to be independent and responsible in order to be able to care for self and others:

Well it is just the independence. I don't want to be a nuisance to the family at all if I can help it, and if I haven't done something that might have helped I'd feel a bit guilty. If you can do anything to prevent that happening it does help a little bit. (Participant 03, age 83 – Continually Adherent Bisphosphonates. Calcium not prescribed)

I like to protect myself as much as possible for my husband, well for me (too) for me I mean obviously. (Participant 18, age 80 – Non-Adherent Bisphosphonates by Phase 2. Non-adherent to Calcium)

Appraising and prioritising risk

Phase 1 interviews specifically asked participants about their reaction to their recent risk assessment. Risk perceptions at this phase were mostly expressed in 'sense making' comments regarding the context of ageing. There was added complexity for participants who had been given a risk status of 'higher than average' but had no visible signs or experience of symptoms:

Not in a million years. I thought oh they'll come back and say oh you're fine. And they wrote back and said I wasn't. Yes I thought I couldn't believe it because I've always had a balanced diet. (Participant 29, age 75 – Continually Adherent to both Bisphosphonates & Calcium)

Many of those who had initially questioned their risk status and expressed negative reactions had adjusted to their status and cited measures taken to be self-protective such as not climbing ladders and prioritising a calcium rich diet:

Oh yeah it's made me *more* careful since I had that density scan and had the letter to say that um (pause) you know on average, if I fell over I would more easily break a bone than you know than normal. So that was a *good* thing because it has made me more (careful) and as you notice, I've got no rugs. (Participant 24, age 80 - Adherent to both Bisphosphonates & Calcium Phase 1, subsequently withdrew)

We explored the data for links between positive self-caring attitudes (as exemplified by women in the first interviews giving examples of longstanding commitment to weight bearing exercise and good nutrition) and active embracing of pharmacological options for preventing fractures. We also looked for an interrelationship between women's 'accepting' versus 'questioning' of their risk assessment and adherence to prescribed medication, including their reported participation in the decision making process and recourse to other support and information. Neither state appeared to be linked with long-term adherence with equal numbers of women remaining adherent to their medication who were 'questioning' (n = 7) as 'accepting' (n = 7). Furthermore, there was no link to adherence from either an initial strong emotive reaction or passive acceptance. For example, the following initially adherent participant had moved from a state of shock to positive acceptance, and yet gave up on her medication within a year:

> Well in a way when I got over the shock I thought well I know something more about my body. (Participant 07, age 74 - Became Non- Adherent to Bisphosphonates by Phase 2. Adherent to Calcium)

However, the long-term and hidden changes of bones which 'thin' or 'crumble' seemed a lower priority than other illnesses. Participants' recall of medication reviews mirrored this, with most women reporting that their osteoporosis medications was rarely reviewed or mentioned in consultations.

Anticipating and managing side effects

Eighteen women experienced side effects from mild to very severe. These ranged from unsettled stomach problems to violent nausea, vomiting bile, and burning:

> They're *horrible* they really were. Well I mean honestly I got a really sore stomach and then on Monday my stomach was really bad and honestly it just felt full of air and I'd touch it and it was sore. (Participant 24, age 80 - Adherent to both Bisphosphonates & Calcium Phase 1, subsequently withdrew)

While severe side effects were linked to non-adherence, there was no simple relationship between side effects and persisting with medication, some trying up to 3 different medications. In fact, the anticipation of side effects seemed to be enough to put off some participants, with three in particular reporting that they were put off by the possible side effects described in the medicines information leaflet. Even the name 'alendronic acid' was cause for concern for some:

> Because it says *acid* (laughs). It isn't a natural thing. I just don't like the idea of taking an acid and not lying down. (Participant 13, age 75 – became adherent by Phase 2. Adherent to Calcium)

The need for support concerning side effects was also highlighted by a number of non-adherent women who anticipated side effects that might aggravate existing problems:

> To me it seemed more important that I, you know, (avoid) this reflux than breaking my hip because I thought I can be *careful*. (Participant 23, age 81 – tried one Bisphosphonate tablet only. Non-starter Calcium)

> The tablets that he gave me when I read the side effects it was like a *horror film* really. And I thought well I'm better off chancing, sort of breaking a bone, than all the horrible things it said on there about (how) you could get these stomach ulcers and all things like that. And I do suffer sort of with heartburn and things like that. You have to sort of keep upright for so long after taking the tablets. I thought well I'm better off as I am than more things wrong really. (Participant 21, age 75 – non-starter Bisphosphonates and Calcium)

Problems of understanding

A number of problems of understanding were evident in the interviews regarding osteoporosis risk, prevention and management in older women. Although there was fear and concern about developing osteoporosis, there was also a perception that falling and fracturing were normal in old age. Others debated the magnitude of risk, especially when compared to problems such as diabetes and heart disease. Some women questioned why the Dual energy X-ray Absorbtiometry screening had not been repeated to monitor the effectiveness of the medication. Nine patients adherent at Phase 1 mentioned this specifically, and 3 of these had become non-adherent by Phase 2:

> I really would like to have another scan to see how my body is now, if it's any worse or still the same or whatever. I'd like to do that but apparently they don't, they like to leave it a certain amount of years don't they? I've read that. (Participant 24, age 80 - Adherent to both Bisphosphonates & Calcium Phase 1, subsequently withdrew)

> I mean if you're going through all that performance, well it was for me with the lack of being able to swallow, but if you think you are doing that to no avail, you think well what's the point. (Participant 25, age 77 - became Non-adherent to Bisphosphonates & Calcium Phase 2)

A number of women in both groups expressed significant confusion about the nature and importance of the risk portrayed by the positive screening result. There was also confusion between falls and fractures, with some participants talking about their fracture risk in terms of instability rather than fragility:

> As I say, I would have thought somebody with osteoporosis would have fallen over and broken their bones. (Participant 07, age 74 - Non adherent to Bisphosphonates by Phase 2. Adherent to Calcium)

> I was surprised because I felt that I'd not had a lot of falls or tottery or anything. I thought people that were at higher risk were inclined to fall. (Participant 01, age 75 - Continually Adherent to Bisphosphonates. Took Calcium intermittently)

> So I thought well that (bisphosphonate medication) will prevent me falling cos the main reason was if my bones got stronger I could do more in the garden and things like that and get on the steps more often. I can't anyway cos I get dizzy (but) that was my thoughts. (Participant 30, age 75 - Continually Non adherent to Bisphosphonates. Took Calcium at Phase 2)

Confusion about the effectiveness of the medication was common and participants frequently reflected on 'not knowing' if they were getting any benefit from taking the medication or not. Participant 16 was fully adherent with no side effects, but felt it was 'discouraging not knowing if it works', as did others:

> I suppose the fact of never having broken anything coupled with the fact there's no signal in your body is there? There's nothing that tells you that there is anything wrong, so you

don't feel that there's anything wrong. (Participant 08, age 75 – Continually Adherence Bisphosphonates and Calcium)

Decision making around medication

Overall we found clear if unpredictable narratives around medication choice, with key factors being the initial result, side effects and subsequent health service intervention of medication prescription. Decisions were reviewed in a number of situations and personal costs weighed up against perceived benefits of taking the medication. Participant 09 described how she made the decision in the light of her own understanding of her needs and the relative benefit of taking the medication. She made her final decision in consultation with her doctor:

There is no bone disease or any sign of it in our family but I said I would take it and see what happened. It didn't suit me and I said I'm not taking them anymore and he (doctor) agreed. He said 'it's no good taking them if they upset you because your diabetes is more important'. (Participant 09, age 85 – became non adherent by Phase 2 to Bisphosphonates and Calcium)

Many of those non-adherent to bisphosphonate medication at Phase 2 had not asked for, or been offered, a change of medication (n = 10). However, five women still adherent to their medications and experiencing side effects had been back to their doctor at least once for an alternative prescription by Phase 2 (Table 3).

Although most participants cited encouragement by doctors, pharmacists, family, friends and the media, only three participants specifically mentioned any sort of formal follow-up (one at a diabetic review, one with a pharmacist and one with a nurse). Many felt specific follow-up would have given them more confidence:

I mean I'm all for taking it if I know what it's doing and if it's doing you good, but there's no follow up on these things. I have to go and get my blood pressure taken every six months. I feel like they know what's going on cos they have changed the different strengths at different times you know depending on how my blood pressure is. But you don't get any follow up with this…. I think they need to have more follow up on this. I'm taking it because it's doing me what it's supposed to be doing, but it's the not knowing and it's the not having the follow up to see whether you need to be taking it or not. (Participant 11, age 77 – Continually Adherent Bisphosphonates. Calcium not prescribed)

Table 3. Summary of Bisphosphonate medication changes and adherence for participants that experienced side effects at Phase 2 (n = 18).

	Adherent	Non-adherent
No change	2 (11)	10 (56)
Changed once	4 (22)	0
Changed twice	1 (6)	1 (6)
Total	**7 (39)**	**11 (61)**

One participant explicitly changed her mind and became adherent by Phase 2 having previously rejected the medication because of her doctor's insistence:

I didn't used to take that but then once I had this polymyalgia and I had to take the steroids. As I walked out of the doctors' room she said 'now look you must take that acid tablet because if not your bones will just crumble'. So whether I like it or not I'm taking it. (Participant 13, age 75 – became adherent by Phase 2. Adherent to Calcium)

In summary, many participants saw the medication as an adjunct to their own efforts to remain healthy and ward off the impacts of ageing. Additional convenience of medication dosing, a less off-putting name, and ways to reduce side effects would be likely to positively influence people's decisions to remain adherent to these medications.

Discussion

The data overall show a group of resilient older women doing their best to make sense of a particular set of health opportunities in their lives, and keen to manage the impacts of ageing and minimise increasing frailty and dependence. There was evidence that those who had engaged with professionals to establish and maintain regimens could tolerate and overcome barriers to adherence which had defeated others. The variation of adherence over time suggests that health professionals should not assume adherence in any older women who has relevant medication on their repeat medication list, and that the uncertainty of risk and desire not to worry participants must not confuse messages that these drugs can have a real positive health gain.

To our knowledge, no previous studies have undertaken longitudinal in depth interviews to identify factors which influence adherence to osteoporosis regimens in women who have been identified at high risk of fracture. Thus, the strength of this study is the repeat in depth interviews with older women that enabled follow up and discussion of change overtime. The limitations include potential sample bias: women who are keen to help research are potentially more motivated to self-care and take an active part in their own health.

However the context of this work is multifaceted and reflects the issues that arise following screening in a cohort of women who have not previously sought advice about their bone health. Overtime many medications that are routinely prescribed become objects embedded within everyday life and invested with particular meanings, values and identities [19]. However, our findings underline the fact that medications are complex social phenomena that may take time to embed and become routinized and acceptable to patients and healthcare professionals alike [20]. Medications, particularly medication prescribed prophylactically, have many levels of meaning [21]. Bisphosphonate medication for the prevention of osteoporosis and fracture is currently framed by a more complex social context where understanding, choice, risk and perceived need all interact to produce unpredictable patterns of usage and acceptability [22].

This study did not record consultation data or the perspective of general practitioners on their interactions around decision making on bisphosphonates. In depth sociolinguistic research has highlighted that patients talk and deploy different discourses and narratives depending on both the context and on the interactional resources available to them [23], [24], [25], [26]. Although most patients and their health care providers are likely to be keen to ensure that they utilise the outputs of modern medical advances, this is in the context of the increasing biomedicalisation of life, especially as people in developed countries are living longer [27]. Whether this is framed as a sophisticated commercial exploitation of societal fears of frailty and death, or as an unpredicted consequence of applying multiple disease related guidelines without considering the overall impact, there are consequences for individuals in making choices about their health-related practices each day. For example, recent authors have pointed out the likelihood of older people routinely being in receipt of multiple medications, even if they have not yet developed any specific disease [28], [29]. The cumulative costs of screenings, follow-ups, treatments and personal sequelae in terms of time, side effects, and perceived vulnerability or risk all need to be set against the potential benefits. The impacts of knowing that they are deemed to be at risk can move people from a narrative of their self as a healthy empowered person to one who is frail and in need of help, which can also have unexpected consequences [27].

Within this complex context, each patient and their doctor or nurse has to make individual decisions as to whether a risk factor should be prioritised or treated once detected. General practitioners are probably the medical professionals who are most aware of the extent to which the uptake of any new test or treatment is dependent on the beliefs, understanding, needs and expectations of the individual in front of them. It is a tenet of their discipline and training that any new health issue needs to be debated in the context of the person's whole life context, while maximising health gain and minimising adverse consequences of any intervention. It is the skill of a general practitioner to enable patients to make considered judgements in the face of these multiple choices. However, both the literature and our interviews suggest that

preventive health measures often pose a challenge in time limited appointments, which may have influenced the decision made in some clinical encounters [30], [31], [32]. Furthermore, the fact that this was a research study may also have influenced overall uptake and follow-up in clinical practice. More research is needed on the effectiveness and efficacy of secondary prevention and the role of healthcare providers in this field.

Acknowledgments

We would like to acknowledge the staff and researchers of the Screening for Osteoporosis in Older women for the Prevention of fracture Trial from which this study grew, and the patients who were willing to undertake both studies. We also wish to thank our patient and public involvement leads from the NHS Norfolk 'PPIRes' panel, for their excellent guidance and input.

Disclaimer

This paper outlines independent research funded by the National Institute for Health Research (NIHR) under its Research for Patient Benefit Programme (RfPB) RfPB PB-PG-0807-14068. The views expressed are those of the authors and not necessarily those of the NHS, the NIHR or the Department of Health. The funders had no role in study design, data collection and analysis, decision to publish, or preparation of the manuscript.

Author Contributions

Conceived and designed the experiments: CS RH TM AH. Performed the experiments: CS LM. Analyzed the data: CS LM AH. Contributed reagents/materials/analysis tools: CS LM DB RH TM AH. Wrote the paper: CS LM DB RH TM AH.

References

1. Kanis JA (2002) Diagnosis of osteoporosis and assessment of fracture risk. Lancet 359: 1929–1936.
2. WHO (2003) Prevention and Management of osteoporosis. Geneva: WHO.
3. Verdijk NA, Romeijnders AC, Ruskus JJ, Van Der Sluijs C, Pop VJ (2009) Validation of the Dutch guidelines for dual X-ray absorptiometry measurement. The British Journal of General Practice 59: 256–260.
4. (SIGN) SIGN (2003) Management of osteoporosis risk.
5. NICE (2012) Osteoporosis: Assessing the risk of fragility fracture London: NICE.
6. WHO Fracture Risk Assessment Tool.
7. Kanis J, Glüer CC (2000) An update on the diagnosis and assessment of osteoporosis with densitometry. Osteoporosis International 11: 192–202.
8. Marshall IJ WC, McKevitt C (2012) Lay perspectives on hypertension and drug adherence: systematic review of qualitative research British Medical Journal 345.
9. Solomon DH AJ, Katz JN, Finklestein JS, Arnold M, Polinski JM, et al. (2005) Compliance with osteoporosis medications Arch Intern Med 165: 2414–2419.
10. Recker RR GR, MacCosbe PE (2005) Effect of dosing frequency on bisphosphonate medication adherence in a large longitudinal cohort of women Mayo Clin Proc 80: 856–861.
11. Rossini M BG, Di Munno O, Giannini S, Minisula S, Sinigaglia L, et al (2006) Determinants of adherence to osteoporosis treatment in clinical practice Osteoporosis International 17: 941-921.
12. (IOF) IOF (2005) The adherence gap: Why osteoporosis patients don't continue with treatment Nyon: IOF.
13. Pound P BN, Morgan M, Yardley L, Pope C, Daker-White G, et al. (2005) Resisting medicines: A synthesis of qualitative studies of medicine taking. Social Science & Medicine 61: 133–155.
14. Brookhart MA AJ, Katz JN, Finklestein JS, Arnold M, Polinski JM, et al. (2007) Gaps in treatment among users of osteoporosis medications: the dynamics of noncompliance Am J Med 120: 251–260.
15. Pickney CS AJ (2005) Correlation between patient recall of bone densitometry results and subsequent treatment adherence Osteoporosis International 16: 1156–1160.
16. L. S A Pragmatic Randomised Clinical Trail of the Effectiveness and Cost Effectiveness of Targeted Population Screening for Low Bone Mineral Density in the Prevention of next of Femur Fractures: ISRCTN 11021925.
17. Shepstone L FR, Lenaghan E, Harvey I, Cooper C, Gittoes N, et al. (2012) A pragmatic randomised controlled trial of the effectiveness and cost-effectiveness of screening older women for the prevention of fractures: Rationale, design and methods for the SCOOP study Osteoporosis International 23: 2507–2515.
18. Ritchie J LJ (2003) Qualitative research practice: A guide for social science students and researchers. London: Sage Publications.
19. Hodgetts D, Chamberlain K, Gabe J, Dew K, Radley A, et al. (2011) Emplacement and everyday use of medications in domestic dwellings. Health & Place 17: 353–360.
20. Cohen D, McCubbin M, Collin J, Pérodeau G (2001) Medications as social phenomena. Health: 5: 441–469.
21. Shoemaker SJ, Ramalho de Oliveira D, Alves M, Ekstrand M (2011) The medication experience: Preliminary evidence of its value for patient education and counseling on chronic medications. Patient education and counseling 83: 443–450.
22. Brown P, Calnan M (2012) Braving a faceless new world? Conceptualizing trust in the pharmaceutical industry and its products. Health: 16: 57–75.
23. Murdoch J, Salter C, Cross J, Smith J, Poland F (2013) Resisting medications: moral discourses and performances in illness narratives. Sociology of Health & Illness 35: 449–464.
24. Salter C, Holland R, Harvey I, Henwood K (2007) "I haven't even phoned my doctor yet." The advice giving role of the pharmacist during consultations for medication review with patients aged 80 or more: qualitative discourse analysis. BMJ 334: 1101.
25. Britten N, Stevenson F, Gafaranga J, Barry C, Bradley C (2004) The expression of aversion to medicines in general practice consultations. Social science & medicine 59: 1495–1503.
26. Murdoch J, Salter, C., Cross, J., & Poland, F. Misunderstandings, communicative expectations and resources in illness narratives: Insights from beyond interview transcripts.
27. Salter CI HA, Howe A, McDaid L, Lenaghan E, Blacklock J, et al (2011) Risk, significance and biomedicalisation of a new population: Older women's experience of osteoporosis screening Social Science & Medicine 73: 808–815.
28. Moynihan R DJ, Henry D (2012) Preventing overdiagnosis: How to stop harming the healthy British Medical Journal 244.
29. Moynihan R HI, Henry D (2002) Selling sickness: The pharmaceutical industry and disease mongering. British Medical Journal 324: 886–891.
30. Mirand AL BG, Kuo CL, Mahoney MC. (2003) Explaining the de-prioritization of primary prevention: Physicians' perceptions of their role in the delivery of primary care. BMC Public Health 3: 1–15.
31. Williams SJ CM (2008) Perspectives on prevention: The views of general practitioners. Sociol Health Ill 16: 372.393.
32. Poole KES CJ (2006) Osteoporosis and its management. BMJ 333.

23

Autoreactivity to Glucose Regulated Protein 78 Links Emphysema and Osteoporosis in Smokers

Jessica Bon[1⑤], Rehan Kahloon[1⑤], Yingze Zhang[1*], Jianmin Xue[1], Carl R. Fuhrman[2], Jiangning Tan[1], Mathew Burger[1], Daniel J. Kass[1], Eva Csizmadia[3], Leo Otterbein[3], Divay Chandra[1], Arpit Bhargava[1], Joseph M. Pilewski[1], G. David Roodman[4], Frank C. Sciurba[1], Steven R. Duncan[1*¤]

1 Department of Medicine, University of Pittsburgh, Pittsburgh, Pennsylvania, United States of America, 2 Department of Radiology, University of Pittsburgh, Pittsburgh, Pennsylvania, United States of America, 3 Department of Surgery, Beth Israel Deaconess Medical Center, Harvard Medical School, Boston, Massachusetts, United States of America, 4 Department of Medicine, Indiana School of Medicine, Indianapolis, Indiana, United States of America

Abstract

Rationale: Emphysema and osteoporosis are epidemiologically associated diseases of cigarette smokers. The causal mechanism(s) linking these illnesses is unknown. We hypothesized autoimmune responses may be involved in both disorders.

Objectives: To discover an antigen-specific autoimmune response associated with both emphysema and osteoporosis among smokers.

Methods: Replicate nonbiased discovery assays indicated that autoimmunity to glucose regulated protein 78 (GRP78), an endoplasmic reticulum chaperone and cell surface signaling receptor, is present in many smokers. Subject assessments included spirometry, chest CT scans, dual x-ray absorptiometry, and immunoblots for anti-GRP78 IgG. Anti-GRP78 autoantibodies were isolated from patient plasma by affinity chromatography, leukocyte functions assessed by flow cytometry, and soluble metabolites and mediators measured by immunoassays.

Measurements and Main Results: Circulating anti-GRP78 IgG autoantibodies were detected in plasma specimens from 86 (32%) of the 265 smoking subjects. Anti-GRP78 autoantibodies were singularly prevalent among subjects with radiographic emphysema (OR 3.1, 95%CI 1.7–5.7, p = 0.003). Anti-GRP78 autoantibodies were also associated with osteoporosis (OR 4.7, 95%CI 1.7–13.3, p = 0.002), and increased circulating bone metabolites (p = 0.006). Among emphysematous subjects, GRP78 protein was an autoantigen of CD4 T-cells, stimulating lymphocyte proliferation (p = 0.0002) and IFN-gamma production (p = 0.03). Patient-derived anti-GRP78 autoantibodies had avidities for osteoclasts and macrophages, and increased macrophage NFkB phosphorylation (p = 0.005) and productions of IL-8, CCL-2, and MMP9 (p = 0.005, 0.007, 0.03, respectively).

Conclusions: Humoral and cellular GRP78 autoimmune responses in smokers have numerous biologically-relevant pro-inflammatory and other deleterious actions, and are associated with emphysema and osteoporosis. These findings may have relevance for the pathogenesis of smoking-associated diseases, and development of biomarker immunoassays and/or novel treatments for these disorders.

Editor: Mark Allen Pershouse, University of Montana, United States of America

Funding: This work was supported by U.S. NIH grants HL084948, HL107172, AR57308, and HL007563. The funders had no role in study design, data collection and analysis, decision to publish, or preparation of the manuscript.

Competing Interests: The authors have declared that no competing interests exist.

* Email: duncsr@upmc.edu; duncsr@upmc.edu

⑤ These authors contributed equally to this work.

¤ Current address: Department of Medicine, University of Alabama, Birmingham, Alabama, United States of America.

Introduction

Emphysema, defined as radiologic and/or histological evidence of lung parenchymal destruction, accounts for enormous world-wide morbidity and mortality [1]. Emphysema among tobacco smokers often occurs in association with chronic obstructive pulmonary disease (COPD), a complex syndrome typified by airway narrowing and inflammation, and diagnosed by the presence of expiratory airflow obstruction on spirometric testing [1–4]. Nonetheless, emphysema and COPD are by no means invariably concordant, and many patients severely afflicted by one of these lung abnormalities may have little or no evidence of the other [2–4]. In addition to directly attributable disability and premature deaths, smoking-associated lung diseases are also linked to many systemic abnormalities, including vasculopathies [5], lung cancer [6], renal dysfunction [7], and osteoporosis [8]. The abnormal and often pathological bone demineralization that occurs in smokers is particularly notable for being highly related to the presence and severity of emphysema, and is independent of the co-existence or magnitude of COPD *per se* [8].

While tobacco smoking is the single greatest risk factor for the development of lung disease in industrialized societies, additional mechanisms are also important, since only a fraction of heavy smokers have severe clinical manifestations [1]. Moreover, symptomatic, pathologic, and radiographic features are highly variable among afflicted individuals, familial clustering of cases is evident, and the disorders often progress despite smoking cessation [1,4,9,10]. The pathophysiological processes that cause or promote emphysema and its co-morbidities remain enigmatic, although systemic immunological responses, including the actions of activated monocyte-lineage phagocytes, have been implicated in these disorders [11,12].

Adaptive immune responses against a variety of autoantigens appear to be common among patients with lung disease attributable to smoking [13–15]. Unspecified autoantibodies from smokers have been shown to induce pulmonary epithelial cell cytotoxicity *in vitro*. [13] Immune complex and complement depositions are important mediators of autoantibody-induced tissue injury, and these abnormalities are also prevalent in the diseased lungs of smokers [13,14]. Nonetheless, most reports of autoimmunity in patients with smoking-related lung disease to date are correlative rather than mechanistic. To our knowledge, moreover, no antigen-specific immune response has yet been implicated in the systemic co-morbidities of these pulmonary disorders [5–8].

Given the systemic nature of many immunological processes [16–19], we hypothesized autoimmune responses that could contribute to lung parenchyma destruction may also be involved in pathogenesis of one or more extrapulmonary co-morbidities that are associated with the emphysema. Accordingly, we conducted investigations to identify antigen-specific autoimmune responses relevant to both emphysema and osteoporosis in smoke-exposed subjects.

Methods

Subjects

Clinical and immunological correlation studies were performed in consecutive subjects with $\geq$10 pack-years of cigarette smoking, ages 40–79 years old, who were recruited under auspices of the Specialized Center for Clinically Oriented Research (SCCOR) registry at the University of Pittsburgh Medical Center. Subjects with unstable cardiovascular disease, malignancies, chronic oral steroid use, or BMI >35 were excluded. Each subject completed demographic and medical history questionnaires, and chest CT scans [6–8,13]. Spirometry, lung volumes, and diffusion capacity (DLCO) were measured using standardized methods and reference equations. Healthy, never-smoked control subjects were recruited by solicitation of hospital personnel.

Ethics Statement

The protocol was approved by the University of Pittsburgh Investigational Review Board. Each subject provided written informed consent.

Emphysema Assessments

Chest CT examinations were performed with a General Electric (GE) LightSpeed VCT (64-detector) scanner at a radiation exposure of 100 mAs [6,8]. A single expert radiologist, blinded to subject identities and other characteristics, interpreted the CT images using a validated [6]. 6-point semi-quantitative visual scoring system to define emphysema severity (0 = none, 1 = trace/

minimal, 2 = mild, 3 = moderate, 4 = severe, 5 = very severe), corresponding to 0%, <10%, 10–25%, 26–50%, 51–75%, and >75% visual emphysema [6–8]. Our group has previously shown these visual emphysema scores are associated with clinically important outcomes in smokers [6–8], and the validity and comparability of these assessments with other radiographic measures of emphysema has also been established [2,3].

Blood Specimens

Plasma was obtained by centrifugation of heparinized phlebotomy specimens. Peripheral blood mononuclear cells (PBMNC) were isolated by density-gradient centrifugation [20]. Serum was obtained as the supernatant of clotted (non-heparinized) blood.

Dual X-Ray Absorptiometry (DXA)

DXA measurements of bone mineral density (BMD) at the hip and lumbar spine were added to subject assessments after the initiation of enrollments in the SCCOR, and were available in the last 200 smoking subjects who provided plasma for immunological studies. Bone mineral density (BMD) was measured at the hip and lumbar spine using a Hologic 4500A Discovery bone densitometer and previously detailed methods [8]. BMD is reported as a T score, the number of standard deviations from young, gender and ethnic-specific reference means. T scores $\leq -2 \cdot 5$ defined osteoporosis [8].

Macrophages and Osteoclasts

$CD14^+$ cells were isolated from PBMNC of normal, nonsmoking humans using anti-CD14 immunomagnetic beads (Miltenyi Biotec, Auburn, CA), and differentiated in the presence of M-CSF. In brief, cells were cultured for 7–10 days in complete RPMI with 10% FCS that was also supplemented with 50 ng/ml M-CSF (R&D Systems, Minneapolis, MN), and changed every 2–3 days. Flow cytometry confirmed >98% of the cells harvested $\geq$day seven expressed intracellular $CD68^+$ and were $CD3^-$ and $CD19^-$.

Osteoclasts were derived from two healthy bone marrow donor volunteers. Mononuclear cells within the bone marrow aspirates were isolated by density gradient centrifugation and incubated in α-MEM with 20% FCS overnight at 37°C. Non-adherent cells were collected and cultured for 28 days in the same media supplemented with 25 ng/ml M-CSF and 30 ng/ml RANKL (R&D Systems), with frequent replenishment.

Autoantigen Discovery

The nonbiased discovery assays that resulted in identification of autoreactivity to glucose regulated protein 78 (GRP78) among smokers with lung disease parallel those reported previously [21].

In brief, we hypothesized *a priori* that autoantigens associated with smoking-related emphysema could be identified by using patient-derived IgG antibodies to immunoprecipitate these autoantigens from cell lysates. The biologic validity of the putative autoimmunity could then be substantiated by demonstrating correlations between the presence of humoral autoreactivity to these self-proteins and disease prevalences. Additional evidence could be provided by finding concurrent T-cell autoreactivity, HLA bias, and discovering disease-relevant functional effects of the autoantibody(ies) [15–21].

Pooled circulating IgG antibodies isolated from six emphysematous subjects, known to have autoantibodies on previous study [13], were used to immunoprecipitate autoantigens from cell lysates. IgG from these subjects and another preparation from six normal control specimens were isolated by protein G, and then adhered to and covalently cross-linked to protein A columns (HP

SpinTrap, GE Healthcare, Piscataway, New Jersey), per the manufacturer's protocol.

The cell lysates were preadsorbed with the normal IgG-protein A columns, and then applied to the emphysema IgG-protein A columns. After extensive washing, the putative IgG-bound autoantigens were eluted by acidification, pH neutralized, concentrated by centrifugal size-filtration (Millipore, Bellerica, MA), and identified by two dimension 10.5% sodium dodecyl sulfate polyacrylamide gel electrophoresis (SDS-PAGE). Gels were imaged by Typhoon TRIO (GE Healthcare) and analyzed by Image QuantTL software (GE Healthcare). Individual proteins were harvested by spot picking (Ettan Spot Picker, GE Healthcare), trypsin digested, and sequenced by matrix-assisted laser adsorption/ionization tandem time of flight mass spectrometry (MALDI-TOF/TOF) (Applied Biosystems, Carlsbad, CA).

Unpublished findings of previous investigations [13] had indicated the presence of an autoantibody with specificity for a then cryptic ~75 kDa cell antigen tended to be associated with disease manifestations among smokers, and hence discovery of potential autoantigens of this ~size was a particular interest.

Glucose regulated protein 78 (GRP78), a member of the heat shock protein 70 family, was identified in two sequential discovery assays. In addition to having an appropriate size, GRP78 seemed worthy of focus for additional study as a potential autoantigen in smokers given its myriad cellular functions [22–24] and role as an known autoantigen in other immunologic disorders [25,26].

Circulating Anti-GRP78 IgG

Immunoblots are a highly specific ("Gold Standard") method for detection of antibodies [21]. These assays were performed using modifications of previously described methods. [21]

In brief, recombinant GRP78 (rGRP78) was purchased from Prospec (Rehovot, Israel). rGRP78 was prepared as a bulk solution and aliquots were frozen at −80°C until use. Volumes corresponding to two hundred and fifty (250) ng rGRP78 were concurrently added to multiple lanes of running gels (NuPage 4–12% Bis–Tris, Invitrogen, Carlsbad, CA) and electrophoresed. The proteins were transferred to nitrocellulose membranes and blocked with 5% dry milk in TTBS (50 mM Tris HCl [pH 7.4], 150 mM NaCl, 0.1% Tween 20). Membrane strips were separated by sectioning and each of these was individually incubated overnight at 4° with a particular subject plasma specimen (@ 1:20 dilution). All of the laboratory investigators performing these assays (RAK, JX, AB) concurrently incubated multiple subject plasma specimens, each with one of the individual membrane strips available from gels (plus positive and negative controls), as well as molecular weight markers, and were completely oblivious to subject identities or disease manifestations. Pilot study had shown that 1:20 dilutions optimally distinguished emphysematous from normal populations, whereas more dilute specimens were too seldom positive in the disease subject specimens (and never positive among normal specimens). The strips were washed in TTBS, and then incubated for one hour with 1:8000 dilutions of chicken anti-human IgG conjugated to horseradish peroxidase (HRP) (Thermo Scientific, Rockfort, IL). After another washing, HRP was detected by addition of Super Signal West Pico Chemiluminescent Substrate (Thermo Scientific), instantaneous exposure to radiographic film, and scored (positive or negative) by unanimous consensus of three investigators who were blinded to subject identities and clinical characteristics (Figure S1 in File S1). The few equivocal specimens (n<5) were repeated until all blinded judges were in agreement.

Lung Specimens

Tissue (~0.5–1 cm³) was dissected from emphysematous lungs explanted during therapeutic transplantations and cadaveric normal lungs that were not used as donor organs [20]. These specimens were fixed in neutral buffer Zn-formalin, paraffin embedded, and sectioned for immunohistochemistry (IHC) assays.

Bronchoalveolar lavage fluid (BALF) was obtained from lung explants by wedging sterile 5 mm plastic tubing in segmental bronchi, and successively infusing and aspirating 30 ml PBS aliquots using a syringe. BALF was centrifuged (400 g), and the supernatant was filtered (0.4 μm), concentrated using 3 kDa centrifugation-size filters (Millipore, Billerica, MA), and quantified by bicinchoninic acid (BCA) assay (Thermo Scientific). Alveolar macrophages within BALF were isolated by plastic adherence.

Detection of GRP78 in Lung Specimens

Immunohistochemistry was used to assess in situ GRP78 expression in paraffin-embedded lung tissue sections [13,21]. In brief, immunostaining was performed with a rabbit monoclonal antibody directed against Grp78 (Cell Signaling Technology, Danvers, MA) employing citrate antigen retrieval, as per the manufacturer's recommendation, biotinylated goat anti-rabbit IgG Jackson Immunoresearch West Grove, PA), and AB Complex HRP (Vector Laboratories, Burlingame, CA). Imaging methods have been previously detailed [13,21].

GRP78 in BALF was detected by immunoblotting. Concentrated BALF (12 mcg protein) specimens were electrophoresed and processed as described above. Membranes were incubated with 1:1000 dilutions of mouse anti-human GRP78 mAb (R&D Systems) at 4°C, followed by 1:4000 dilutions of chicken anti-mouse IgG-HRP (Santa Cruz Biotechnology, Santa Cruz, CA). This immunoblotting method was validated using both commercial rGRP78 and lysates of normal human CD14⁺-derived macrophages (Figure S2 in File S1).

Patient-Derived Anti-GRP78 Autoantibodies

IgG from pooled plasma specimens of six emphysema patients known to have anti-GRP78 autoantibodies (by prior immunoblot assays) was isolated by adherence to protein G. The IgG was applied to rGRP cross-linked to an AminoLink Plus Gel Spin column (Thermo Scientific), following manufacturer protocols. After extensive washing, anti-GRP78 was eluted by acidification, pH neutralized, concentrated using 5 kDa centrifugation filters and validated for IgG characteristics and specific avidity (Figure S3 in File S1). Eleven (11) ml plasma yielded 120 mcg of anti-GRP78 IgG. The endotoxin concentration within this autoantibody preparation was below the detection threshold of the limulus amebocyte lysate assay (LAL Chromogenic Endotoxin Quantitation Kit, Thermo Scientific), i.e., <0.1 EU/2 mcg of autoantibody.

Indirect Immunofluorescence Assays (IFA)

Plate-bound normal alveolar macrophages from BALF (n = 3) and bone marrow osteoclasts (n = 2) were pre-incubated with 0.1 bovine serum albumin and azide-free Fc receptor blocker (Innovex Biosciences, Richmond, CA). After washing, the cells were incubated for 30 minutes with 0.5 mcg/ml of patient-derived anti-GRP78 IgG or the same concentration of pooled normal human IgG. After another washing, cells were incubated with FITC-conjugated anti-human IgG antibody (ImmunoConcepts, Sacramento, CA) and assessed by fluorescence microscopy, as detailed previously [13,21].

Macrophage Stimulation Assays

Media was removed from concurrent, autologous macrophage cultures, and the cells were incubated with 2 mcg/ml of either anti-GRP78 or normal human IgG for 30 minutes at 37°C. Media was then replaced, and both cells and supernatant were harvested after 18 hours.

Macrophages were suspended, fixed and permiabilized, and stained with anti-NFkB AlexFluor 647 (Cell Signaling Technologies, Danvers, MA), which has specificity for phosphorylated (Ser536) NFkB p65 subunits. Mean fluorescence intensities of the anti-GRP78-treated and normal IgG-treated macrophages were compared in ≥10,000 live cells, and analyzed using a BD FACSCalibur (BD Bioscience, San Jose, CA). Flow cytometry gates were established using control fluorochrome positive and negative macrophages (including isotype controls), as detailed elsewhere [20,21].

Macrophage supernatants were analyzed for mediator productions using protein-suspended bead array platform multiplex kits (Bio-Rad, Hercules, CA), following the manufacturer's protocols [21].

Bone Metabolites

Collagen type 1 C-telopeptide (CTX) was measured in sera by sandwich immunoassays using CTX reagents in an Elecsys 2010 (Roche, Indianapolis, IN), according to manufacturer protocols. Type 1 (N-terminal) Procollagen (P1NP) in plasma specimens was measured using a radioimmunoassay kit (Orion Diagnostica, Espoo, Finland).

Human Leukocyte Antigen (HLA) Class II *DRB1*15*

Allele prevalence was determined by leukocyte DNA PCR-SSP [21]. Assessment of this particular allele was prompted by recent findings it is over-represented among idiopathic pulmonary fibrosis (IPF) patients with clinically-relevant autoimmunity [21].

T-cell Functional Studies

PBMNC collected from consecutive SCCOR subjects were cultured for five days in complete media[13,20,21] in the presence of no added protein (baseline controls), or test antigens (i.e., rGRP78 or elastin split products [ESP]). ESP was purchased from Elastin Products Company (Owensville, MO). Both test antigens were boiled for 20 minutes and cooled on ice immediately prior to use, to obviate nonspecific mitogen effects, and added to cultures at final concentrations of 1 μg/ml. Pilot studies had shown there were no consistent relationships between test antigen concentrations ranging from 0.3 mcg-to-30 mcg/ml and assay results.

Proliferation was determined by incorporation of bromodeoxyuridine (BrdU), added two days prior to cell harvest, with measurements in gated CD4 T-cells established by flow cytometry, as detailed previously [20,21]. Specific indices (SI) of proliferation were calculated as %CD4 T-cells that incorporated BrdU in cultures supplemented with the respective test antigen *minus* incorporation in concurrent unstimulated (control) cultures [20].

Intracellular IFN-gamma production in the last cohort of these culture specimens were also assessed by flow cytometry, using methods fully detailed previously [20,21]. Specific indices (SI) of IFN-gamma production were calculated as %CD4 T-cells that produced this cytokine in cultures with added test antigen(s) *minus* cytokine production in concurrent unstimulated (control) cultures.

Statistical Analysis

Ordered and continuous data were compared by Mann-Whitney tests. Wilcoxon signed rank tests compared results of two or more assays in the same specimen, with Bonferroni corrections for multiple comparisons. Dichotomous outcomes were analyzed by chi-square. Odds ratios (OR) and confidence intervals (CI) were calculated with univariate logistic regression. Multivariate logistic regression analysis was used to adjust for confounding factors. Alpha levels <0.05 were considered significant. All data was analyzed using SAS 9.2.

Results

Subjects

Characteristics of the smoke-exposure cohort are detailed in Table 1. The majority (79%, n = 209) of the 265 smoking subjects had one or more lung abnormalities (i.e., COPD and/or emphysema). One-hundred thirty-three (133), or 80%, of the 167 subjects who had expiratory airflow obstruction on spirometry (i.e., those who had COPD) also had emphysema. Conversely, forty-two (42), or 24%, of the 175 emphysematous subjects had normal spirometry. Another distinct cohort of healthy controls who had never smoked (n = 27) were 59±5 years old and 63% were male.

Circulating Anti-GRP78 Antibodies

The prevalence of autoantibodies to GRP78 was greater in smokers (32.2%) than in the healthy, never-smoked controls (7.4%) (p = 0.007). The latter prevalence is similar to "false positive" rates of other disease-associated autoantibodies in healthy populations [13,16,20,21].

Females were over-represented among the smokers who had anti-GRP78 autoantibodies (Table 1). Those who had anti-GRP78 autoantibodies also had decreased diffusion capacities, although their other pulmonary function tests, as well as medication use, were comparable to the autoantibody negative subjects.

HLA Class II *DRB1*15* was under-represented among smokers with anti-GRP78 autoantibodies (22.4%) compared to the subjects who were autoantibody negative (34.7%) (OR 0.54, 95%CI = 0.3–0.99, p = 0.04). *DRB1*15* prevalence in a local normal population was previously found to be 23% [21].

Clinical Associations of Anti-GRP78 Antibodies

There were no significant differences of anti-GRP78 autoantibody prevalences in the smokers with COPD (35.9%) compared to those with normal spirometry (26.5%, p = 0.11), nor a significant correlation of this autoreactivity with the severity of airflow obstruction (Figure 1A).

However, the presence of anti-GRP78 autoantibodies was significantly associated with the prevalence (Figure 1B) and severity of emphysema (Figure 1C). Multivariate analyses showed that adjustment for gender and severity of expiratory airflow obstruction did not alter the relationship between anti-GRP78 positivity and emphysema (OR 3.1, 95%CI = 1.6–6.1, p = 0.001).

The presence of anti-GRP78 autoantibodies was also highly associated with decreased bone mineral density and osteoporosis (Figure 2A), and remained significant after multivariate adjustment for gender, airflow obstruction severity, tobacco burden, and steroid use (OR 4.2, 95%CI = 1.5–12.2, p = 0.008). Circulating metabolites of bone turnover were also greatest in the subjects with anti-GRP78 autoantibodies (Figures 2B,2C).

Given the associations of anti-GRP78 autoreactivity with emphysema and abnormalities of bone mineralization, a *post hoc* analysis was performed to compare autoantibody prevalence in those subjects who have **concurrent** emphysema and low BMD *vs*. the remaining smoking cohort. Anti-GRP78 autoantibody

Table 1. Demographic and Clinical Characteristics of the Study Cohort.

	Aggregate	GRP78 Ab⁻	GRP78 Ab⁺	p value
Number	265	179	86	
Age (years old)*	67±0.4	67±0.5	67±0.7	NS
% male	58	63	47	0.01
Still smoking (%)	42	41	43	NS
Pack-years*	63±2	65±2	59±3	NS
ICS (%)	22	20	28	NS
Past oral steroids (%)	7	7	7	NS
FEV$_1$% predicted*	77±1	78±2	74±3	NS
FEV$_1$/FVC*	0.63±0.01	0.64±0.1	0.60±0.2	NS
DLCO% predicted*	68±2	71±2	64±2	0.02
Obstructed (%)	63	60	70	NS
Emphysema (%)	66	59	81	0.0003
Low Bone Density (%)	51	46	62	0.03
Osteoporosis (%)	9	4	18	0.002

All these subjects had ≥10 pack yr smoking histories. ICS = inhaled corticosteroid use; past oral steroids = oral steroid use within the preceding six months (none were currently taking oral steroids); FEV$_1$% predicted = forced expiratory volume in the first second of expiration as percentages of predicted values; FEV$_1$/FVC = ratio of FEV$_1$ to forced vital capacity; DLCO% predicted = diffusing capacity for carbon monoxide as percentages of predicted values; Obstructed = subjects with spirometric findings of expiratory airflow obstruction (i.e., COPD); Emphysema = subjects with emphysema on CT scan; p values are for nonparametric comparisons of smokers who do not have anti-GRP78 IgG autoantibodies (GRP78⁻) vs. subjects who have these autoantibodies (GRP78⁺); NS = not significant. * denotes data are depicted as mean ± standard errors.

prevalence was significantly greater in the subjects who had **both** emphysema and osteopenia (50.7% *vs.* 25%, OR 3.1, 95%CI = 1.8–5.4, p<0.0001), and even more so among those with **both** emphysema and osteoporosis (80.0% *vs.* 29.6%, OR 9.5, 95%CI = 2.6–34.7, p<0.0001). A gender stratified analysis showed this relationship is strongest in males (Figure 2D).

Intrapulmonary GRP78 Expression

GRP78 protein was and increased in emphysema specimens and predominantly localized in alveolar epithelial cells and macrophages (Figure 3A). GRP78 concentrations were also much greater in BALF from diseased lungs compared to the normal control preparations (Figure 3B).

Anti-GRP78 Binding

In order to explore the possibility that anti-GRP78 autoantibodies have actions relevant to emphysema and osteoporosis, we first examined macrophage and osteoclast binding of anti-GRP78 IgG isolated from patient plasma. IFA showed the anti-GRP78 autoantibodies have avidity for these cells (Figure 3C).

Cellular Effects of Anti-GRP78 Autoantibodies

To test for direct function-altering effects, patient-derived anti-GRP78 autoantibodies were incubated overnight with macrophages. These treatments resulted in increased macrophage NFkB activation (Figure 4A) and augmented productions of IL-8 (Figure 4B), CCL-2 (Figure 4C), and MMP9 (Figure 4D).

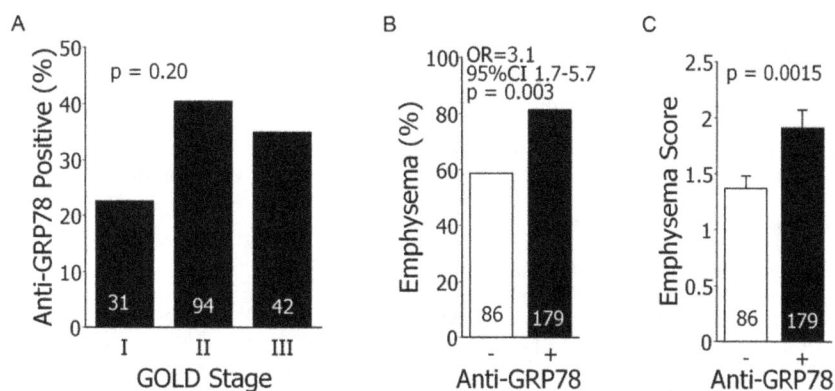

Figure 1. Anti-GRP78 autoantibodies, airflow obstruction, and emphysema. *A.*) Anti-GRP78 autoantibody prevalence was not significantly associated with COPD severity (GOLD stages) [40]. Numbers within columns denote subject n. *B.*) Anti-GRP78 autoantibodies are significantly associated with emphysema prevalence (%) in the smoking subjects. OR = odds ratio; CI = confidence interval. *C.*) Emphysema scores per CT were also significantly greater among those subjects with anti-GRP78 autoantibodies.

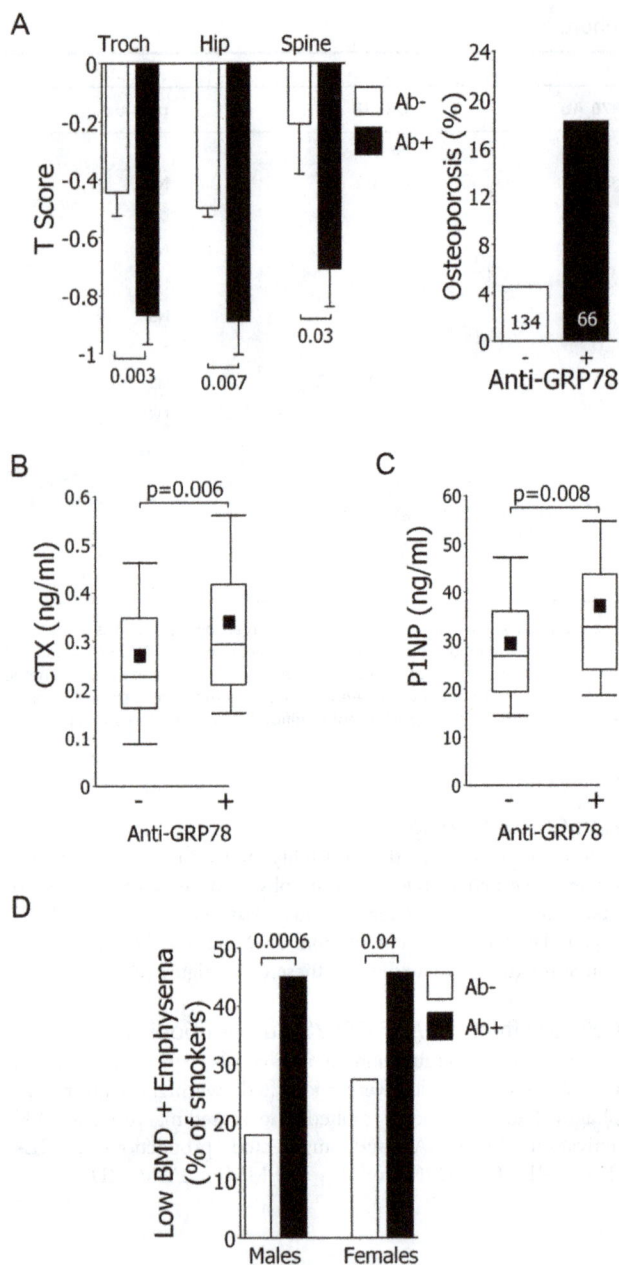

Figure 2. Anti-GRP78 autoantibody association with osteoporosis, bone metabolism markers, and concurrent low bone density and emphysema. A.) T scores (left panel) and osteoporosis prevalence (at either/both hip or spine) (right panel) among the smoking cohort. B.) Serum levels of bone turnover metabolite collagen type 1 cross-linked C-telopeptide (CTX) were greatest among smokers with anti-GRP78 autoantibodies. The lowest, second lowest, middle, second highest, and highest lines represent 10th, 25th, median, 75th, and 90th percentiles, respectively. Means are denoted by solid squares. C.) Serum levels of bone turnover metabolite type 1 (N-terminal) procollagen (P1NP) were greatest among smokers with anti-GRP78 autoantibodies. D.) The relationship between GRP78 autoantibody positivity and the concurrent co-existences of low BMD and emphysema in smokers is significant in both genders, but greatest in males.

CD4 T-cell Autoreactivity

Disease-associated autoantibody responses are also accompanied by concurrent T-cell responses to the autoantigen(s)

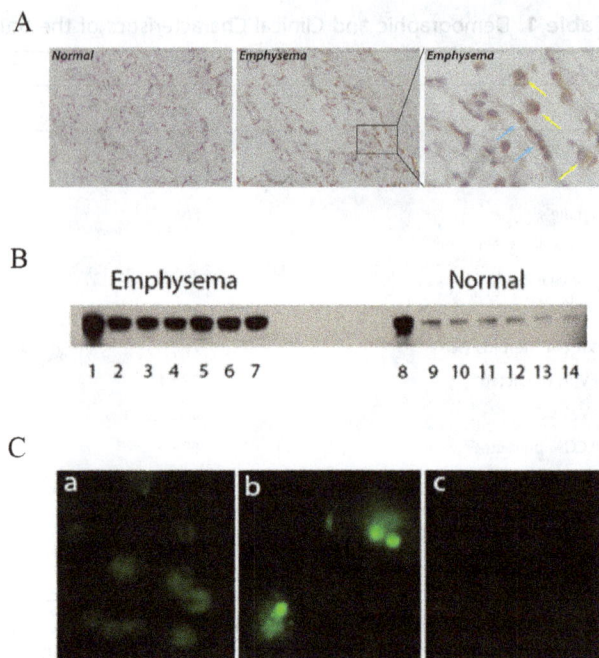

Figure 3. GRP78 expression in lung, bronchoalveolar lavage fluid, alveolar macrophages, and bone marrow derived osteoclasts. A.) Compared to normal lung (Left panel), emphysematous lungs (middle and right panels) demonstrated increased immunostaining in macrophages (yellow arrows) and alveolar epithelial cells (blue arrows). Magnification x100 left and middle panels, and magnification x400 in the right panel, n = 3. B.) GRP78 was also greater in bronchoalveolar lavage fluid (BALF) from emphysematous lungs compared to normal preparations. Lanes 1 and 8 are rGRP78 standards. Lanes 2–7 are BALF from individual emphysematous lung explants; lanes 9–14 are BALF from normal lung explants. All specimen lanes were loaded with equal amounts of BALF proteins. C.) Indirect immunofluorescent assays showed anti-GRP78 IgG isolated from patients bind to alveolar macrophages from normal lung explants (panel a), and osteoclasts derived from bone marrow (panel b). Normal human IgG control is illustrated in panel c.

[15,16,20,21]. Addition of heat-denatured rGRP78 protein to PBMNC cultures from smokers induced proliferations of their CD4 T-cells, unlike effects of denatured ESP (Figure 5A). Moreover, the magnitude of the GRP78-triggered proliferative responses was greatest among the CD4 T-cells from emphysematous smokers (Figure 5B). CD4 T-cell IFN-gamma production was also uniquely increased in rGRP78-supplemented cultures (Figure 5C) and, again, especially so in the preparations from subjects with emphysema (Figure 5D). rGRP78 does not induce proliferation or IFN-gamma production in CD4 T-cells from normal nonsmoking subjects (data not shown) nor IPF patients [21].

Discussion

Autoimmunity is a frequent complication of numerous, varied, primary injury responses [15–18]. The microbiome within smoke-damaged lungs is postulated to be highly immunogenic and, hence, a likely predisposition for the development of autoimmunity [13–15]. Neoantigens generated by reactive constituents within tobacco smoke can also provoke autoimmune responses [14]. Most "secondary" autoimmune responses are benign and clinically irrelevant. In some cases they are highly pathogenic and injurious, however, as exampled by carditis associated with microbial

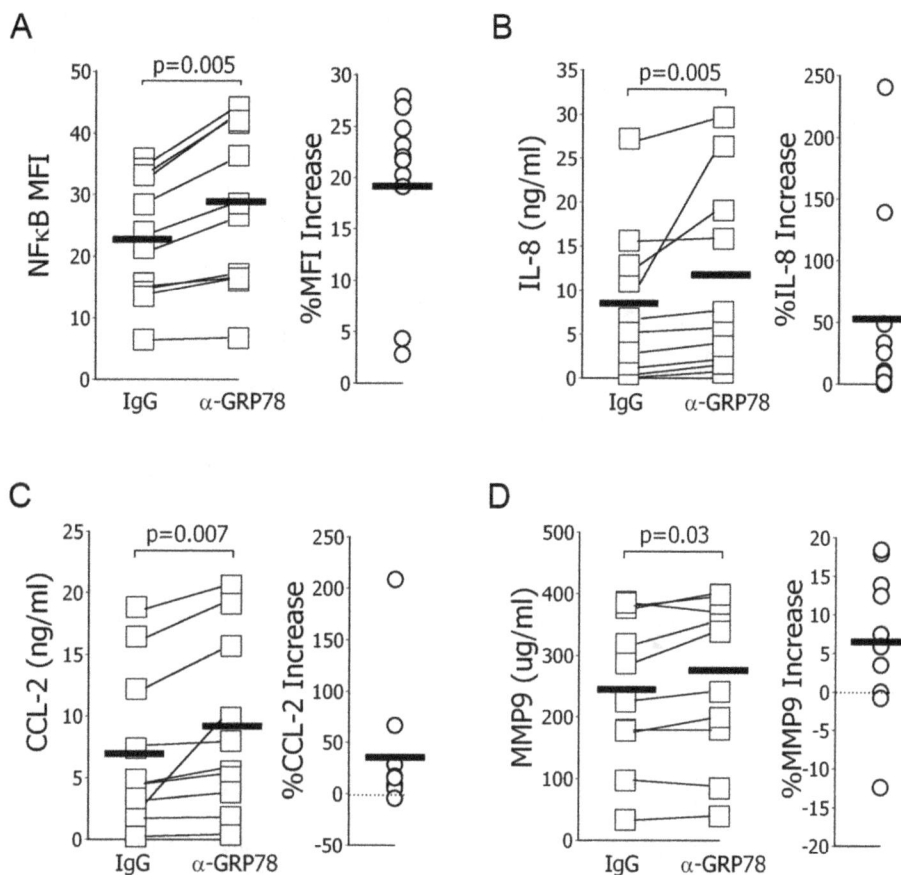

Figure 4. Cellular effects of autoantibodies to GRP78 on macrophages. *A.*) Mean fluorescence intensity (MFI) for phosphorylated NFkB among paired, concurrent autologous CD14$^+$ derived macrophages was increased in all 10 normal specimens after incubation with patient-derived autoantibodies to GRP78 (α-GRP78), relative to control cells treated with normal human IgG. Patient derived anti-GRP78 autoantibodies also increased macrophage production of IL-8 (*B.*), CCL-2 (*C.*) and MMP9 (*C.*). Population means are denoted with a horizontal line.

infections, neurological syndromes linked to malignancies, and myriad other tissue-specific autoimmune disorders [16–18,26].

The adaptive immune responses to GRP78 in smokers have several features of classical autoimmunity [15–20]. The biological plausibility of a particular autoimmune response is conditional on the presence of the corresponding autoantigen in the target organ(s), and GRP78 is highly expressed in lungs, especially in the disease specimens (Figures 3A,3B). HLA haplotypes are major (and often the strongest) known genetic determinants of autoimmune susceptibilities. Finding distinct HLA alleles are over- or under-represented (conferring predilection or protection, respectively) within a defined disease population is a hallmark of autoimmune disorders [16,21]. *DRB1*15* appears to "protect" smokers against the production of disease-associated anti-GRP78 autoantibodies. This result is the obverse of analogous studies in IPF patients, in whom *DRB1*15* is over-represented among those with autoantibodies against heat shock protein 70 (HSP70), a stress response protein with considerable sequence homology to GRP78 [21]. These disparate findings are thus indicative of biologically-distinct, antigen- and disease-specific autoimmune responses, rather than being a generalized epiphenomenon of "lung disease".

Most compellingly, the increased prevalence of anti-GRP78 autoantibodies in emphysematous smokers is a defining criteria of "abnormal" autoreactivity [15–20]. The pathogenicity of anti-GRP78 IgG in smokers is at least implied by the stringent, independent, and overlapping associations of this specific autoan-

tibody with concurrent emphysema, osteoporosis, and increased bone turnover. Furthermore, other findings here showing that patient-derived anti-GRP78 autoantibodies activate monocyte-lineage phagocytes, and enhance their productions of injurious mediators that are implicated in the genesis of emphysema and osteoporosis are direct evidences of deleterious autoantibody effects [11,12,27–29].

In particular, anti-GRP78 IgG treatments increased cellular elaborations of IL-8 and CCL2 (aka MCP-1), which are potent pro-inflammatory chemoattractants of neutrophils and mono-cytes/macrophages, respectively. Both of these mediators also stimulate osteoclastogenesis, and are increased among patients with osteoporosis and emphysema [11,12]. Incubations with anti-GRP78 also increased macrophage production of MMP9, a Type IV collagenase produced by macrophages and osteoclasts that promotes enzymatic breakdown of extracellular matrix. MMP9 has an imputed causal or contributing role in lung parenchyma destruction, pulmonary metastases, and bone resorption [27–29].

Moreover, these varied effects occurred after only limited (18 hour) macrophage exposures to subphysiological concentrations (2 µg/ml) of the anti-GRP78 autoantibody. It seems possible that even greater effects might result from incubations with autoantibody concentrations found *in vivo* (~11 µg/ml), and for longer periods. The cumulative effects of increased inflammation and protease activity in target tissues over many months-to-years may be especially deleterious, and emphysema and osteoporosis

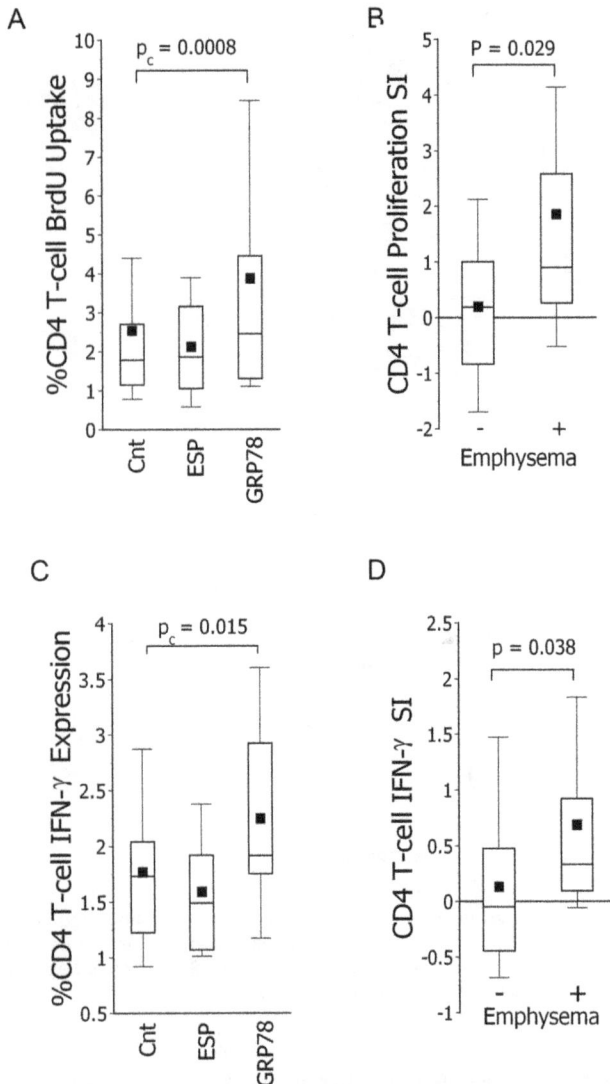

Figure 5. CD4 T-cell autoreactivity to GRP78. *A.*) Addition of GRP78 to PBMNC cultures increased CD4 T-cell proliferation (BrdU uptake) relative to media controls (no added protein) (n = 47), unlike addition of elastin split products (ESP). P$_c$ denotes alpha level corrected for multiple comparisons. *B.*) GRP78-induced CD4 T-cell proliferation was greatest among cultures from smokers with emphysema (n = 34). Specific indices (SI) of proliferation were calculated as %CD4 T-cells incorporating BrdU in GRP78-supplemented cultures *minus* incorporation in concurrent media controls. *C.*) GRP78 also increased percentages of CD4 T-cells that produced IFN-gamma again, unlike effects of ESP. *D.*) IFN-gamma production was also greatest in the CD4 T-cells from the emphysematous smokers. Specific indices (SI) were calculated as %CD4 T-cells producing IFN-gamma production in GRP78-supplemented cultures *minus* that of concurrent controls.

are typically most prominent among middle-aged or elderly smokers [1].

The *in situ* pathogenicity of GRP78 autoimmunity in smokers is also strongly supported by finding this stress response protein is an autoantigen of CD4 T-cells in these subjects, especially among those with emphysema. T-cells are inert to anatomically accessible self-constituents in healthy subjects, whereas overt reactivity of these lymphocytes to a protein that is abundant in diseased organs (Figures 3A,3B) is a "Gold Standard" of autoimmune disease [16,19]. Antigen- (or autoantigen-) stimulated CD4 T-cells have

protean and typically very injurious actions, including elaboration of numerous mediators that recruit and activate diverse leukocyte and somatic effector cells [21]. A finding of T-cell autoreactivity is very unlikely to be a benign epiphenomenon [16,19]. Increased production of IFN-gamma in particular (Figures 5C,5D) is believed to be an important factor in the pathogenesis of smoking-associated lung disease [11]. Furthermore, the GRP78 reactivity of CD4 T-cells in emphysematous subjects cannot be simply attributable to global, nonspecific hyperactivity, since elastin split products (ESP) were inert (Figures 5A and 5C). Although ESP was previously reported to be an autoantigen of emphysema [30], we have been unable to replicate those findings, and similarly negative studies have been reported by other investigators [31–33].

GRP78 is also a frequent antigen of other autoimmune syndromes [25,26]. GRP78 expression and extracellular export are up-regulated by varied stresses, including viral infections and smoke inhalation [22–24]. Ongoing immunologic responses that were initially directed at other antigenic peptides may generalize to co-associated chaperone proteins, such as GRP78, by a bystander mechanism and/or by epitope spread [25]. Subsequent injury (or infection) could cause further up-regulation of the newly antigenic GRP78, potentially creating a positive feedback loop that promotes immune responses and disease progression.

The specific mechanism(s) by which anti-GRP78 autoantibodies affect phagocytes is yet unknown, and is a focus of ongoing investigations in our laboratories. In addition to intracellular actions as an endoplasmic reticulum protein transporter and scavenger, and importance in the unfolded protein response, cell surface and extracellular GRP78 mediate anti-inflammatory and pro-resolutory effects [22–24]. Anti-GRP78 might counter these actions by decreasing the concentrations or bioavailability of immunomodulatory extracellular GRP78, and/or by activating signal transduction pathways after cross-linking cell surface GRP78. Anti-GRP78 autoreactivity is notably prevalent among subjects with rheumatoid arthritis, another smoking-associated disease, and the autoantibodies from these patients also enhance macrophage pro-inflammatory functions, again, by mechanisms still unknown [26].

The findings of GRP78 autoreactivity here lend support to an evolving paradigm of autoimmune pathogenesis in smoking-associated lung diseases [13–15]. The present studies show anti-GRP78 responses in smokers are manifest by activation of autoantigen-specific T-cells, a process that leads to numerous deleterious consequences [19], and anti-GRP78 IgG autoantibodies directly exert pro-inflammatory effects. Even if these pathogenic actions are completely discounted, the multiple strong clinical-immunological associations here indicate assays for specific autoimmune responses may be useful to identify smokers who are most at-risk for these interrelated disorders. Nonetheless, these findings need additional corroboration and refinement before the adoption of autoimmune assays into the clinical management of smoking patients.

In addition, many immune diseases, and antibody-mediated lung disorders in particular, are refractory to treatment with nonspecific immunosuppressive regimens (e.g., glucocorticoids). Conversely, however, specific therapies that directly target pathological autoimmune processes, including autoantibody removal or interruption of autoantibody production *per se*, more often have clinical efficacy [34–39]. The most important ultimate result of the present study and related reports may be to draw attention to the potential for novel treatments, mechanistically-focused at critical stages of autoimmune cascades, to prevent or slow progression of the morbid and refractory syndromes associated with smoking [15,34–39].

Supporting Information

File S1 Contains Figure S1, Immunoblot Detection of Anti-GRP78 Autoantibodies. Detection of circulating anti-GRP78 IgG. Immunoblots were used to detect circulating anti-GRP78 autoantibodies in plasma specimens See manuscript text for methodological details. *Left panel*: 75 kDa molecular weight marker (MW) and adjacent plasma specimen negative for anti-GRP78 (Lane A). *Right panel*: 75 kDa molecular weight marker (MW) and subject plasma specimen positive for anti-GRP78 IgG (Lane B). Note: GRP78 migrates on 12% Bis–Tris gels as though it were slightly smaller than its expected 78 kDa size. Figure S2, Detection of GRP78 Protein in Lung Specimens. Control immunoblots. *Lane A.*) rGRP detected with mouse anti-human GRP78 monoclonal antibody (R and D Systems) at 1:500 dilution. The secondary antibody was chicken anti-mouse human IgG at 1:4000 dilution. *Lane B.*) GRP78 in a human CD14⁺-derived

macrophage lysate (29 µg total protein) was also detected using this anti-human GRP78 monoclonal antibody. MW.) 75 kDa molecular weight marker. Figure S3, Patient-Derived Anti-GRP78 Autoantibody Characterizations. Validations of patient-derived anti-GRP78 autoantibodies. *Left panel*: Evaluations of the patient-derived anti-GRP78 on SDS gels showed protein bands typical for IgG, i.e., 25 kDa light chains and 50 kDa heavy chains. *Right panel*: The avidity of the isolated, patient-derived autoantibody for GRP78 was confirmed by rGRP78 immunoblot. Lane A.) 75 kDa molecular weight marker; Lane B.) rGRP78. The patient-derived anti-GRP78 IgG was used here at a concentration of 1 µg/ml.

Author Contributions

Conceived and designed the experiments: JB SRD. Performed the experiments: RK YZ JX CF EC LO AB GDR SRD JT MB DJK. Analyzed the data: JB DC SRD. Contributed reagents/materials/analysis tools: JP FS DJK. Wrote the paper: JB SRD. Rdited the manuscript: JB DC FS RK YZ JX CF EC LO AB GDR SRD JT MB DJK.

References

1. Mannino DM (2002) COPD: epidemiology, prevalence, morbidity and mortality, and disease heterogeneity. Chest 121: 121S–26S.
2. Washko GR, Criner GJ, Mohsenifar Z, Sciurba FC, Sharafkhaneh A, et al. (2008) Computed tomographic-based quantification of emphysema and correlation to pulmonary function and mechanics. COPD 5: 177–86.
3. COPDGene CT Workshop Group (2012) A combined pulmonary-radiology workshop for visual evaluation of COPD: study design, chest CT findings and concordance with quantitative evaluation. COPD 9: 151–9.
4. Han MK, Agusti A, Calverley PM, Celli BR, Criner G, et al. (2010) Chronic obstructive pulmonary disease phenotypes: The future of COPD. Am J Respir Crit Care Med 182: 598–604.
5. Sin DD, Man SF (2005) Chronic obstructive pulmonary disease as a risk factor for cardiovascular morbidity and mortality. Proc Amer Thorac Soc 2: 8–11.
6. Wilson DO, Weissfeld JL, Balkan A, Schragin JG, Fuhrman CR, et al. (2008) Association of radiographic emphysema and airflow obstruction with lung cancer. Am J Respir Crit Care Med 178: 738–44.
7. Chandra D, Stamm JA, Palevsky PM, Leader JK, Fuhrman CR, et al. (2012) The relationship between pulmonary emphysema and kidney function in smokers. Chest 142: 655–62.
8. Bon JM, Fuhrman CR, Weissfeld JL, Duncan SR, Branch RA, et al. (2011) Radiographic emphysema predicts low bone mineral density in a tobacco exposed cohort. Am J Respir Crit Care Med 103. 885–90.
9. Retamales I, Elliott WM, Meshi B, Coxson HO, Pare PD, et al. (2001) Amplification of inflammation in emphysema and its association with latent adenoviral infection. Am J Respir Crit Care Med 164: 469–73.
10. Kurzius-Spencer M, Sherrill DL, Holberg CJ, Martinez FD, Lebowitz MD (2001) Familial correlation in the decline of forced expiratory volume in one second. Am J Respir Crit Care Med 164: 1261–5.
11. Kim V, Rogers TJ, Criner GJ (2008) New concepts in the pathobiology of chronic obstructive pulmonary disease. Proc Am Thorac Soc 5: 478–85.
12. Lorenzo J, Horowitz M, Choi Y (2008) Osteoimmunology: interactions of the bone and immune system. Endocr Rev 29: 403–40.
13. Feghali-Bostwick CA, Gadgil AS, Otterbein LE, Pilewski JM, Stoner MW, et al. (2008) Autoantibodies in patients with chronic obstructive pulmonary disease. Am J Resp Critical Care Med 177: 156–63.
14. Kirkham PA, Caramori G, Casolari P, Papi AA, Edwards M, et al. (2011) Oxidative stress-induced antibodies to carbonyl-modified proteins correlate with severity of COPD. Am J Respir Crit Care Med 184: 796–802.
15. Duncan SR (2012) Clues, Not Conclusions. Nature 489: S15.
16. Fu SM, Deshmukh US, Gaskin F (2011) Pathogenesis of systemic lupus erythematosus revisited 2011: end organ resistance to damage, autoantibody initiation and diversification, and HLA-DR. J Autoimmun 37: 140–47.
17. Franks AL, Slansky JE (2012) Multiple associations between a broad spectrum of autoimmune diseases, chronic inflammatory diseases and cancer. Anticancer Res 32: 1119–36.
18. Pordeus V, Szyper-Kravitz M, Levy RA, Vaz NM, Shoenfeld Y (2008) Infections and autoimmunity: a panorama. Clin Rev Allergy Immunol 34: 283–99.
19. Monaco C, Andreakos E, Kiriakidis S, Feldmann M, Paleolog E (2004) T-cell-mediated signaling in immune, inflammatory and angiogenic processes: the cascade of events leading to inflammatory diseases. Curr Drug Targets Inflamm Allergy 3: 35–42.
20. Feghali-Bostwick CA, Tsai CG, Valentine VG, Kantrow S, Stoner MW, et al. (2007) Cellular and humoral autoreactivity in idiopathic pulmonary fibrosis. J Immunol 179: 2592–9.
21. Kahloon RA, Xue J, Bhargava A, Csizmadia E, Otterbein L, et al. (2013) Idiopathic pulmonary fibrosis patients with antibodies to heat shock protein 70 have poor prognoses. Am J Respir Crit Care Med 187: 768–75.
22. Kelsen SG, Duan X, Rong J, Perez O, Liu C, et al. (2008) Cigarette smoke induces an unfolded protein response in the human lung. Am J Respir Cell Mol Bio 38: 541–50.
23. Chan C-P, Siu K-L, Chin K-T, Yuen K-Y, Zheng B, et al. (2006) Modulation of the unfolded protein response by the severe acute respiratory syndrome coronavirus spike protein. J Virol 80: 9279–87.
24. Shields AM, Panayi GS, Corrigall VM (2011) Resolution-associated molecular patterns (RAMP): RAMParts defending immunological homeostasis. Clin Exp Immunol 165: 292–300.
25. Purcell AW, Todd A, Kinoshita G, Lynch TA, Keech CL, et al. (2003) Association of stress proteins with autoantigens: a possible mechanism for triggering autoimmunity. Clin Exp Immunol 132: 193–200.
26. Lu M-C, Lai N-S, Yu H-C, Huang H-B, Hsieh S-C, et al. (2010) Anticitrullinated protein antibodies bind surface-expressed citrullinated Grp78 on monocyte/macrophages and stimulate tumor necrosis factor alpha production. Arthritis Rheum 62: 1213–23.
27. Gosselink JV, Hayashi S, Elliot WM, Xing L, Chan B, et al. (2010) Differential expression of tissue repair genes in the pathogenesis of chronic obstructive pulmonary disease. Am J Respir Crit Care Med 181: 1329–35.
28. Van Kempen LCL, Coussens LM (2002) MMP9 potentiates pulmonary metastasis formation. Cancer Cell 2: 251–2.
29. Sundaram K, Nishimura R, Senn J, Youssef RF, London SD, et al. (2007) RANK ligand signaling modulates the matrix metalloproteinase-9 gene expression during osteoclast differentiation. Exp Cell Res 313: 168–78.
30. Lee S-H, Goswami S, Grudo A, Song L-Z, Bandi V, et al. (2007) Antielastin autoimmunity in tobacco smoking-induced emphysema. Nat Med 13: 567–69.
31. Greene CM, Low TB, O'Neill SJ, McElvaney NG (2010) Anti-proline-glycine-proline or antielastin autoantibodies are not evident in chronic inflammatory lung disease. Am J Respir Crit Care Med 181: 31–5.
32. Brandsma CA, Kerstjens A, Geerlings M (2011) The search for autoantibodies against elastin, collagen and decorin in COPD. Eur Respir J 37: 1289–92.
33. Rinaldi MA, Lehouck N, Heulens R, Lavend'homme R, Carlier V, et al. (2012) Antielastin B-cell and T-cell immunity in patients with chronic obstructive pulmonary disease. Thorax 67: 694–700.
34. Erickson SB, Kurtz SB, Donadio JV, Holley KE, Wilson CB, et al. (1979). Use of combined plasmapharesis and immunosuppression in the treatment of Goodpasture's syndrome. Mayo Clin Proc 54: 714–20.
35. Sem M, Molberg O, Lund MB, Gran JT (2009). Rituximab treatment of the anti-synthetase syndrome: a retrospective case series. Rheumatology (Oxford) 48: 968–71
36. Borie R, Debray MP, Laine C, Aubier M, Crestani B (2009) Rituximab therapy in autoimmune pulmonary alveolar proteinosis. Eur Respir J 33,1503–06.
37. Keir GJ, Maher TM, Hansell DM, Denton CP, Ong VH, et al. (2012) Severe interstitial lung disease in connective tissue disease: rituximab as rescue therapy. Eur Resp J 40: 641–8.
38. Stone JH, Merkel PA, Spiera R, Seo P, Langford CA, et al. (2010) Rituximab versus cyclophosphamide for ANCA-associated vasculitis. N Engl J Med 363: 221–32.

39. Furie R, Petri M, Zamani O, Cervera R, Wallace DJ, et al. (2011) A phase III, randomized, placebo-controlled study of belimumab, a monoclonal antibody that inhibits B lymphocyte stimulator, in patients with systemic lupus erythematosus. Arthritis Rheum 63: 3918–30.

40. Vestbo J, Hurd SS, Agusti AG, Jones PW, Vogelmeier C., et al. (2013). Global strategy for the diagnosis, management, and prevention of chronic obstructive pulmonary disease: GOLD executive summary. Am J Respir Crit Care Med 187; 347–65

24

Delphinidin, One of the Major Anthocyanidins, Prevents Bone Loss through the Inhibition of Excessive Osteoclastogenesis in Osteoporosis Model Mice

Sawako Moriwaki[1,2]9, **Keiko Suzuki**[3]9, **Masashi Muramatsu**[1]¤, **Atsushi Nomura**[4], **Fumihide Inoue**[4], **Takeshi Into**[5], **Yuji Yoshiko**[6], **Shumpei Niida**[1,2]*

1 Laboratory of Genomics and Proteomics, National Center for Geriatrics and Gerontology (NCGG), Aichi, Japan, **2** Biobank Omics Unit, National Center for Geriatrics and Gerontology (NCGG), Aichi, Japan, **3** Department of Pharmacology, School of Dentistry, Showa University, Tokyo, Japan, **4** Nihon Seiyaku Kogyo, Co., Ltd., Aichi, Japan, **5** Department of Oral Bacteriology, Division of Oral Infections and Health Sciences, Asahi University School of Dentistry, Gifu, Japan, **6** Department of Oral Growth and Developmental Biology, Hiroshima University Graduate School of Biomedical Sciences, Hiroshima, Japan

Abstract

Anthocyanins, one of the flavonoid subtypes, are a large family of water-soluble phytopigments and have a wide range of health-promoting benefits. Recently, an anthocyanin-rich compound from blueberries was reported to possess protective property against bone loss in ovariectomized (OVX) animal models. However, the active ingredients in the anthocyanin compound have not been identified. Here we show that delphinidin, one of the major anthocyanidins in berries, is a potent active ingredient in anti-osteoporotic bone resorption through the suppression of osteoclast formation. In vitro examinations revealed that delphinidin treatment markedly inhibited the differentiation of RAW264.7 cells into osteoclasts compared with other anthocyanidins, cyanidin and peonidin. Oral administration of delphinidin significantly prevented bone loss in both RANKL-induced osteoporosis model mice and OVX model mice. We further provide evidence that delphinidin suppressed the activity of NF-κB, c-fos, and Nfatc1, master transcriptional factors for osteoclastogenesis. These results strongly suggest that delphinidin is the most potent inhibitor of osteoclast differentiation and will be an effective agent for preventing bone loss in postmenopausal osteoporosis.

Editor: Mohan R. Wani, National Center for Cell Science, India

Funding: This work has been supported by Japan Society for the Promotion of Science (KAKENHI Grant No. 20390469 to SN and No. 21791802 to SM) and by Ministry of Health Labour and Welfare (Health Labour Sciences Research Grant No. H24-Choju-007 to SN). The funders had no role in study design, data collection and analysis, decision to publish, or preparation of the manuscript.

Competing Interests: AN and FI are employees of Nihon Seiyaku Kogyo Co., Ltd. Tama Biochemical Co. Ltd., who donated experimental material Cassis-extract-35, also declared that no competing interests exist. This does not alter adherence to all PLOS ONE policies on sharing data and materials.

* E-mail: sniida@ncgg.go.jp

¤ Current address: Department of Cancer Genetics, Roswell Park Cancer Institute, Elm and Carlton Streets, Buffalo, New York, United States of America

9 These authors contributed equally to this work.

Introduction

Osteoporosis, characterized by low bone mineral density (BMD) and fragility of the bone matrix, is a complex bone disease with various causes, including aging, estrogen deficiency and genetics, and leads to increased fracture risk, especially in the elderly population. Current anti-osteoporosis drugs such as bisphosphonates have been widely used and their bone protective effects are well established. However, many individuals with osteoporosis remain undiagnosed, untreated and at risk of fracture because of the lack of symptoms and public awareness [1]. Hence, a dietary nutritional approach is important for primary prevention of bone loss.

Natural compounds in fruits and vegetables such as polyphenols have a wide range of biological and pharmacological effects [2–5]. Several flavonoids, a subgroup of polyphenols including hesperidin, quercetin and luteolin, have been shown to possess preventive efficacy for bone loss in ovariectomized (OVX) animal models [6–8]. Most showed potent suppressive effects on the differentiation

and/or function of osteoclasts, bone resorbing multinucleated giant cells [7–10]. Osteoclasts are formed by the fusion of mononuclear preosteoclasts derived from monocyte-macrophage linage cells. Osteoclast differentiation is tightly regulated by two key molecules, receptor activator of NF-κB ligand (RANKL), a TNF super-family cytokine, produced by osteoblasts, and its receptor RANK, which are expressed on osteoclast precursors [11]. Several flavonoids seem to be inhibitors of RANKL-RANK signaling-related molecules, including NF-κB and nuclear factor for activated T cells (NFATc1), master osteoclastogenic molecules located downstream of NF-κB [7–10].

In this study, we focused on delphinidin, one of the aglycone nuclei of anthocyanins, as an active agent for anti-bone loss in vivo. Anthocyanins are a large family of water-soluble red/blue/purple flavonoid pigments in fruits and vegetables, and have a wide range of health-promoting benefits, for example, as anti-oxidants. Many studies have demonstrated the pharmacological effects of anthocyanidins on human diseases, including night blindness, cancer, obesity and heart diseases [12–16]. Recently, a blueberry extract,

A

B

C

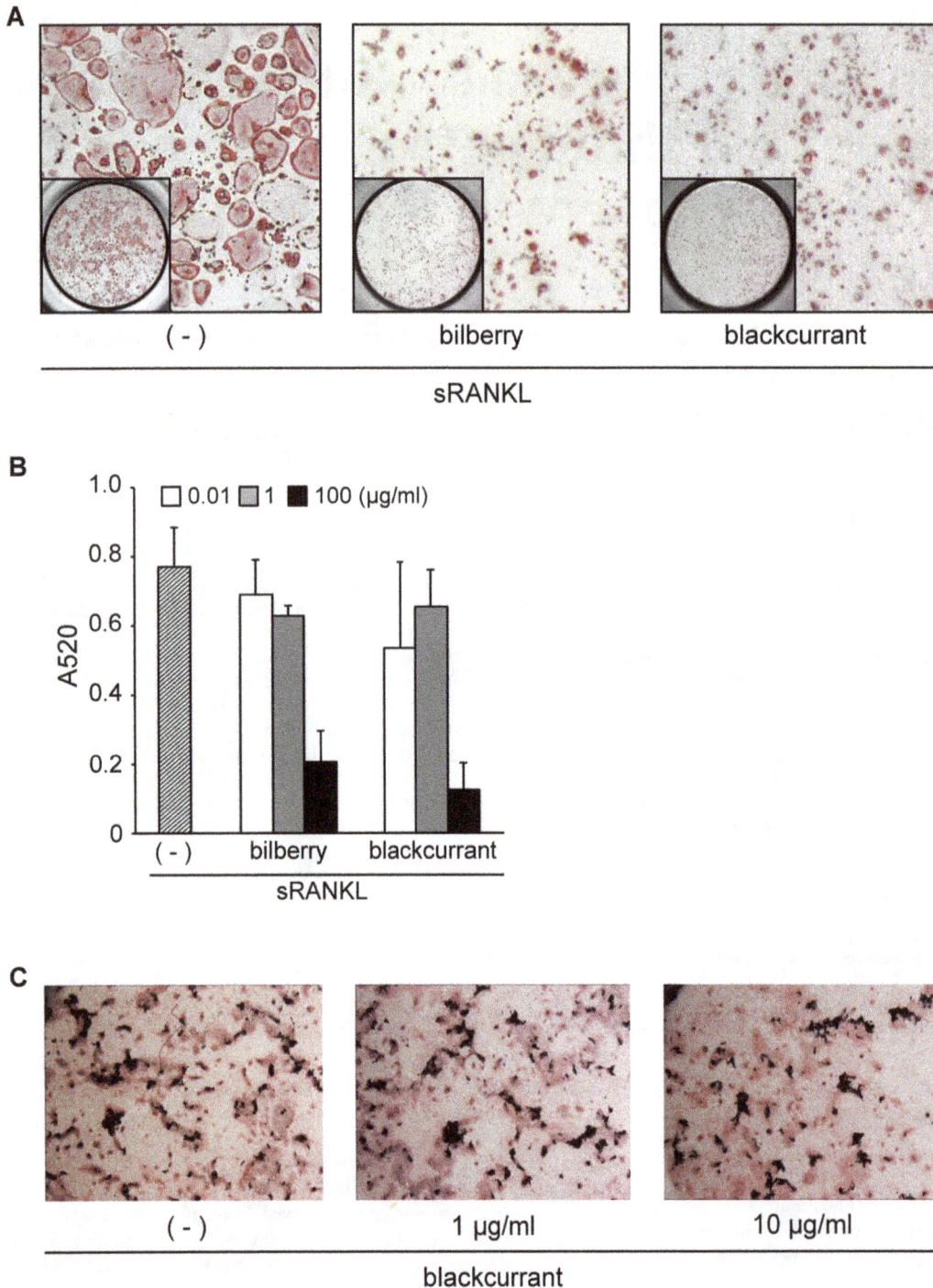

Figure 1. Anthocyanin-rich compounds extracted from bilberry and blackcurrants inhibit *in vitro* osteoclastogenesis, but not osteogenesis. RAW264.7 cells were pre-incubated for 1 h in the presence of various concentrations of anthocyanin compounds, and subsequently cultured for 4 days in the presence of 100 ng/ml RANKL. Cells were fixed and stained with TRAP. A: Numerous TRAP-positive multinucleated giant cells, osteoclasts, were induced by RANKL treatment (left panel). In contrast, large osteoclasts were significantly decreased by addition of anthocyanin compounds (middle and right panels). B: Anti-osteoclastogenic activity of anthocyanin compound was evaluated by the absorption ratio of the red-stained area per well at 520 nm on a spectrometer. C: Primary osteoblastic cells were cultured in the medium containing 50 µg AA, 10 µM Dex and 10 mM β-GP with or without anthocyanin compound for 2 weeks. No significant effect was observed on the osteoblast differentiation and mineral apposition.

an anthocyanin-rich compound, was reported to possess protective properties against bone loss in OVX rats [17]. Moreover, it has been reported that anthocyanins extracted from bilberry and blackcurrant exerted potent inhibitory effects on NF-κB activation in activated monocytes, and consequently led to the downregulation of pro-inflammatory mediators [18]. The NF-κB signaling pathway is well established to be critical for osteoclastogenesis. Commonly, extracted anthocyanin compounds consist of several kinds of anthocyanins derived from plural aglycone bases such as cyanidin, delphinidin and peonidin, major anthocyanidins in extracts of berries, including blueberry. However, to our knowledge, the active ingredients for bone metabolism have not been identified. To address this question is useful for not only developing the high efficient dietary supplements but also finding novel drug seeds. Here we show that delphinidin is the most potent inhibitor of osteoclastogenesis and will be an effective agent for preventing *in vivo* bone degradation.

Materials and Methods

Anthocyanins and Anthocyanidins

Bilberon-25, a concentrated extract of bilberry, was purchased from Tokiwa Phytochemical Co., Ltd. (Chiba, Japan). Cassis extract-35, a concentrated extract of blackcurrant, was generously donated by Tama Biochemical Co., Ltd. (Tokyo, Japan). Cyanidin chloride ($C_{15}H_{11}ClO_6$), delphinidin chloride ($C_{15}H_{11}ClO_7$) and peonidin chloride ($C_{16}H_{13}ClO_6$) were from Extrasynthése (Lyon, France) and Sigma-Aldrich (St Louis, MO, USA), respectively. Epicatechin ($C_{15}H_{14}O_6$) was purchased from Kurita Analysis Service Co., Ltd. (Ibaraki, Japan).

Cell Culture

RAW264.7 cells, a mouse macrophage cell line, were used as osteoclast precursor cells and maintained in α modified essential medium (α-MEM) supplemented with 10% fetal bovine serum (FBS) at 37°C and 5% CO_2. For osteoclast induction, cells were plated in a 96-well plate at a density of 4×10^3 cells/well and stimulated with 100 ng/ml RANKL for 4 days. For the inhibition study, cells were pre-incubated in α-MEM supplemented with vehicle or with various concentrations of anthocyanin-rich extracts and anthocyanidins, 1 h before the addition of RANKL. To confirm multinucleated osteoclast formation, the cultured cells were fixed in 10% formalin for 3 minutes, and then stained with an osteoclast marker enzyme, tartrate-resistant acid phosphatase (TRAP). Effects of anthocyanins and anthocyanidins on osteoclast formation were evaluated by morphological observations and the intensity of TRAP staining was measured at 520 nm using a spectrophotometer (SpectraMax M5; Molecular Devices, Sunnyvale, CA, USA).

Osteoblasts were isolated from newborn calvariae of C57BL/6J mice, as described previously with slight modifications [19]. Briefly, calvariae were minced and sequentially digested with collagenase solution at 37°C. Cells retrieved from the osteogenic cell fractions were separately cultured in α-MEM supplemented with 10% FBS and antibiotics. After 24 h, cells were pooled and grown in multi-well plates in the same medium containing 50 μg/ml of ascorbic acid (AA), 10 μM dexamethasone (Dex) and 10 mM β-glycerophosphate (β-GP) with or without anthocyanin-rich extracts. After two weeks culture, cells were stained with *von Kossa' s* staining to determine the matrix mineralization, as described previously [19].

Animals and Treatments

To assess the protective effect of delphinidin on *in vivo* bone loss, we created soluble RANKL (sRANKL)-induced osteoporosis model mice, which were established by Yasuda and his colleagues [20]. Seven-week-old female C57BL/6 mice (n = 17) were purchased from CLEA Japan (Tokyo, Japan). Mice were divided into three groups: control mice (cont, n = 5), osteoporosis model mice (vehicle, n = 6) and delphinidin-treated osteoporosis mice

(Del, n = 6). Twelve mice were intraperitoneally injected with GST-RANKL (1 mg/kg; Oriental Yeast Co., Ltd., Kyoto, Japan) twice at interval of 3 days. First injection was performed at 3 days after starting of delphinidin-treatment. For six mice, delphinidin treatment (10 mg/kg/day) via gavage started 3 days before the first injection of GST-RANKL, and continued for 14 days. Another six mice received the same volume of vehicle, a mixture of dimethyl sulfoxide (DMSO) and water.

We further assessed the effect of delphinidin using OVX mice. Eight-week-old female C57BL/6 mice were purchased from Charles River Laboratory Japan (Kanagawa, Japan). Thirty mice were either sham-operated (n = 6) or OVX (n = 24). OVX mice were divided into four groups (n = 6×4): OVX control, low-dose delphinidin (1 mg/kg), intermediate-dose delphinidin (3 mg/kg), and high-dose delphinidin (10 mg/kg) groups. After OVX, delphinidin was administrated orally, as mentioned above, for 28 days. OVX-control mice received the same volume of vehicle, a mixture of DMSO and water.

All mice were housed in an animal room (temp, $22 \pm 2°C$; humidity, 50%; light/dark cycle, 12 h) with free access to food and water. At the end of treatment, the mice were sacrificed. Femora were removed and fixed with 3.7% formaldehyde in phosphate-buffered saline solution (pH7.4) for 16 h. After rinsing, bones were immersed in 80% ethanol and stored at 4°C in a refrigerator. These experiments were approved by the Animal Experimental Committees of Showa University and NCGG, respectively.

Microcomputed Tomography

Bone morphometric parameters and microarchitectual properties of the femur were determined using a microcomputed tomography (μCT) system (inspeXio SMX-90CT; Shimadzu Co., Kyoto, Japan) with X-ray tube settings of 90 kV and 108 μA. The femur was placed in a microcentrifuge tube filled with PBS and scanned at a voxel size of 15.0 μm. TRI/3D-BON software (RATOC System Engineering Co., Tokyo, Japan) was used to generate 3D models from 272 2D-transverse slices, and bone morphometry was performed in the distal metaphyseal region (500 μm in length) of femora. For quantitative analysis, BV/TV, trabecular thickness, trabecular number, trabecular separation and trabecular spacing were determined using TRI/3D-BON software.

Histomorphometric Analysis of Bone

Femora were fixed in 70% ethanol and embedded in glycolmethacrylate (GMA) without decalcification. Serial sections were cut and stained with Villanueva bone stain for bone histomorphometry, as previously reported [21]. The histomorphometorical analysis was performed at the Ito Bone Science Institute (Niigata, Japan).

Extraction of Nuclear Protein and Assessment of NF-κB Activation

Nuclear cell lysates were prepared using a Nuclear Extract Kit (Active Motif, Tokyo, Japan) following the manufacturer's instructions. We examined the inhibitory effect of delphinidin on NF-κB activation in RAW264.7 cells. Briefly, cells were pretreated with delphinidin or vehicle for 1 h, and subsequently stimulated with sRANKL. After 3 h of stimulation, cells were washed with ice-cold PBS(−) and hypotonic buffer added from the kit to explore the nucleus. To dissolve the nuclear protein, complete lysis buffer containing 1 mM DTT and protease inhibitor cocktail were added to the cell lysate precipitation and the concentration of protein was measured using Prostain (Active Motif). Cell lysates

A

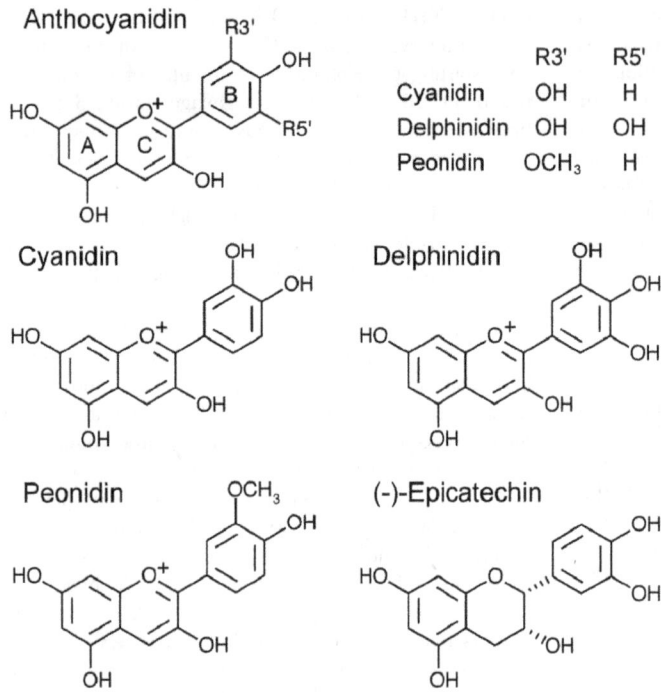

B

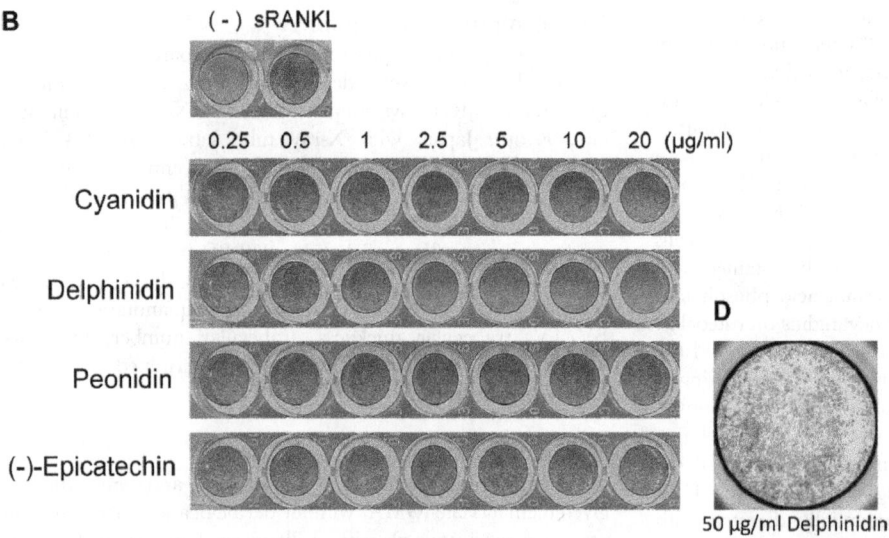

C

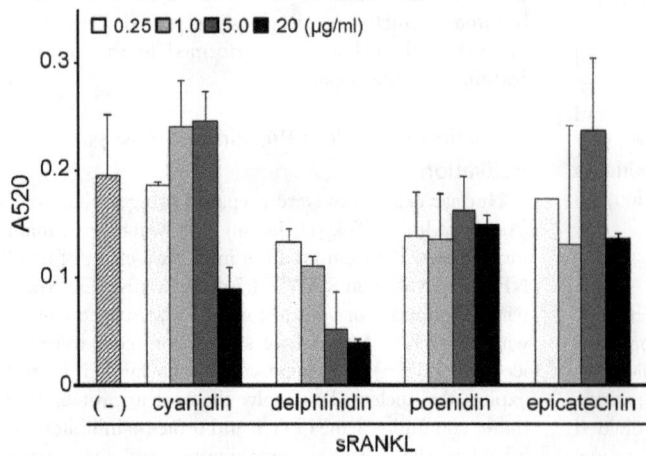

Figure 2. Effects of various anthocyanidins on *in vitro* osteoclastogenesis. A: The structure of tested three anthocyanidins and (−)-epicatechin as a negative control. B: RAW264.7 cells were pretreated for 1 h with increasing concentrations (0.25–20 μg/ml) of three anthocyanidins and epicatechin, and cultured for 4 days in the presence of RANKL (100 ng/ml). Red-stained area in each well indicates osteoclast population. Delphinidin strongly inhibited RANKL-induced osteoclastogenesis at >1 μg/ml. Cyanidin showed moderate inhibition at 20 μg/ml. C: Absorption ratio also supported the results of TRAP-staining observation. D: RAW264.7 cells were cultured with delphinidin alone for 4 days. No cytotoxic effect of delphinidin was found. Cells were stained by crystal violet.

equal to the concentration were measured by TransAM NF-κB p65 Chemiluminescence (Active Motif), which is a high-throughput assay to quantify NF-κB activation, that is, binding activity to DNA-binding fragments fixed to the plate bottom.

Reverse Transcriptase-polymerase Chain Reaction Analysis

For reverse transcriptase-polymerase chain reaction (RT-PCR) assays, total RNA was prepared using an AurumTotal RNA Mini Kit (Bio-Rad, Richmond, CA, USA) according to the manufacturer's instructions. One microgram of total RNA from each sample was reverse-transcribed with Ready-To-Go You-Prime First-Strand Beads (GE Healthcare, Piscataway, NJ, USA). cDNA was amplified by PCR. The PCR products were electrophoresed on a 1.2% agarose gel.

Quantitative Real-time PCR Analysis

Quantitative real-time PCR (qPCR) assays were performed with the CFX96 Real-Time system (Bio-Rad) using the Thunderbird SYBR qPCR Mix (Toyobo, Osaka, Japan). Expression levels were normalized to glyceraldehyde-3-phosphate dehydrogenase (GAPDH).

Statistical Analysis

All data are the mean ± standard deviation (SD). Statistical analyses were performed using unpaired Student t tests. $P < 0.05$ was considered significant.

Results

Effects of Anthocyanin on Osteoclastogenesis and Osteogenesis

Initially, we tested the effects of anthocyanin compound extracted from bilberry (*Vaccinium myrtillus* L.) and blackcurrant (*Ribes nigrum*) on osteoclast formation using RAW264.7 cells as osteoclast precursors. The number of TRAP-positive multinucleated giant cells, osteoclasts, differentiated from sRANKL-stimulated RAW246.7 cells, was markedly decreased by pretreatment with both extracts, suggesting that both anthocyanin compounds contain active ingredients to suppress osteoclast formation (Figure 1A and 1B). In contrast, no significant effect of anthocyanin compound (blackcurrant) was found on mineral apposition (Figure 1C). These results indicated that target cell of anthocyanin may be osteoclasts in bone metabolism.

Effects of Anthocyanidins on Osteoclastogenesis

Next, to identify the active ingredients (aglycone bases) as anti-osteoclastogenic factors, we investigated three major anthocyanidins, cyanidin, delphinidin and peonidin, which are commonly contained in many purple berries, including bilberry and blackcurrant (Figure 2A). RAW264.7 cell cultures containing various concentrations of these anthocyanidins were incubated with sRANKL (100 ng/ml) for 4 days. As shown in Figure 2, delphinidin treatment caused a dose-dependent inhibition of osteoclastogenesis. Although cyanidin treatment showed a mild suppressive effect on osteoclastogenesis at a concentration of

20 μg/ml, doses ≤10 μg/ml did not affect osteoclastogenesis. In contrast, peonidin treatment showed no significant effect on osteoclastogenesis, similar to the control compound, (−)-epicatechin. Similar results were also obtained at a higher concentration (50 μg/ml) of anthocyanidins (data not shown). Additionally, we confirmed that delphinidin did not induce cell death in RAW264.7 cell cultures without RANKL (Figure 2D).

Inhibitory Effects of Dietary Delphinidin on Bone Loss *in vivo*

To determine the relevance of our *in vitro* findings of delphinidin bioactivity to the *in vivo* situation, we investigated the anti-osteoporotic effect of delphinidin on sRANKL-induced osteoporosis model mice. 3D-images and morphometric parameters clearly demonstrated that the cancellous bone volume of femoral distal metaphysis was markedly decreased by sRANKL treatment, compared with intact control mice. In contrast, delphinidin treatment significantly inhibited cancellous bone degradation in sRANKL-treated mice (Figure 3A, B).

All animals were weighed daily for 17 days, and there was no significant change among the experimental groups (Figure 3C). Although liver and kidney weights were slightly decreased in sRANKL-treated mice compared with control mice, these differences were not significant (Figure 3D). Also, there was no significance between sRANKL-treated mice and sRANKL/delphinidin-treated mice (Figure 3C).

We further performed histomorphometrical observation of bone tissues. Microscopic observation demonstrated that the number of bone trabeculare obviously decreased in sRANKL-treated osteoporotic mice. In contrast, many bone trabeculae remained in the bones of delphinidin-treated mice (Figure 4A). Despite the limited number of bone trabeulare, osteoclast number was significantly decreased ($p = 0.03$) in delphinidin-treated mice than non-treated osteoporotic mice (Figure 4B). Other major two resorption-parameters were also downregulated in the mice administrated delphinidin, although there were no statistically significant differences between these two groups (Figure 4B). Consistent with the *in vitro* examinations, these results suggested that delphinidin acts, at least, on the osteoclast differentiation directly.

We further assessed the anti-bone resorption effect of delphinidin using OVX mice, a standard model of osteoporosis. OVX mice were orally administered delphinidin at three different doses. A significant anti-osteoporotic effect was confirmed in over half the mice treated with not only high-dose (10 mg/kg) but also intermediate-dose (3 mg/kg) delphinidin (Figure 5). In this examination, uterus weight did not change in delphinidin-treated OVX mice (data not shown), suggesting that delphinidin did not act on the uterus like SERMs (selective estrogen receptor modulators) such as isoflavons [22]. Together, our results demonstrated that ingestion of delphinidin acts as a potent anti-osteoporotic agent for preventing osteoporosis.

Mechanism of Delphinidin-mediated Inhibition of Osteoclastogenesis

Since previous work indicated that anthocyanin extract inhibited NF-κB activation in activated monocytes, we first

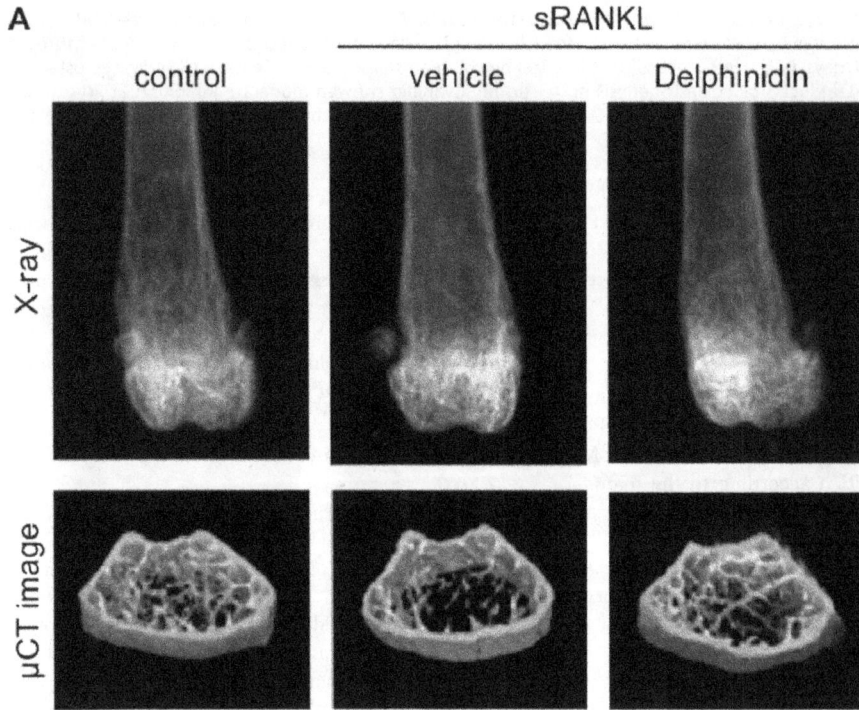

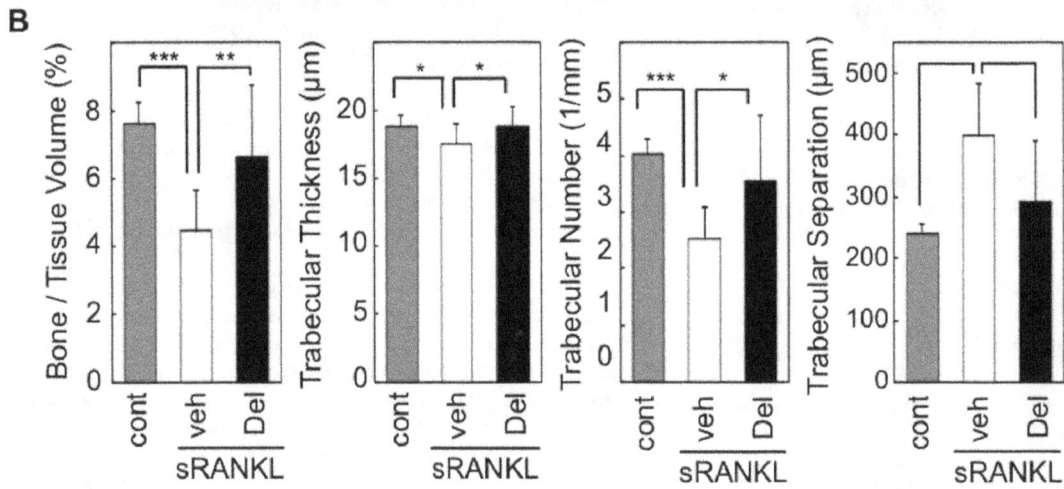

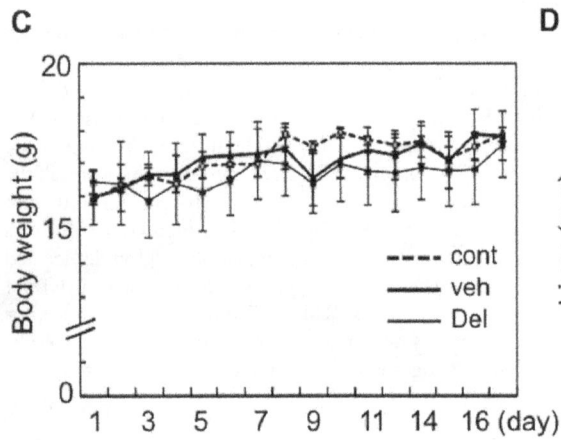

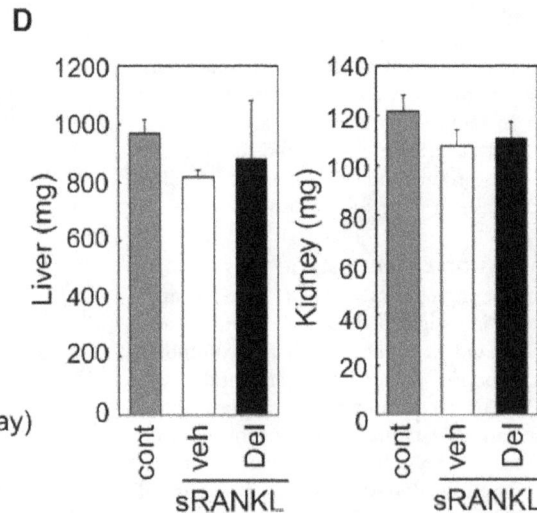

Figure 3. Effect of delphinidin on bone loss in RANKL-induced osteoporosis mice. A: Representative X-ray and microcomputed tomography images of the distal femurs of intact mice (control), RANKL-induced osteoporosis mice (vehicle), and delphinidin-treated RANKL-induced osteoporosis mice (Delphinidin). B: Effect of RANKL injection and delphinidin treatment on trabecular microarchitectural parameters. Values are expressed as the mean ± SD. *$p < 0.05$, **$p < 0.01$, ***$p < 0.001$. C: Comparison of body weight between each experimental group. Values are expressed as the mean ± SD. D: Comparison of weights of liver and kidney in each experimental group. Values are expressed as the mean ± SD.

examined the activation of NF-κB in RAW264.7 cells using the TransAM assay. When the cells were stimulated by sRANKL, the activation of NF-κB p65 subunit was upregulated promptly. In contrast, RANKL-mediated NF-κB activation was markedly downregulated in cells treated by delphinidin, suggesting its effect at a transcriptional level (Figure 6A).

RANKL-induced *c-fos* activation is another pivotal event in the early phase of osteoclastogenesis [11], [23]. NFATc1 is a master transcriptional factor located at the downstream cross-point of both NF-κB and c-Fos pathways in osteoclastogenesis [11], [23]. We therefore investigated whether delphinidin affects the activation of *c-fos* and *Nfatc1* genes. Additionally, we examined the alteration of the expression levels of osteoclast marker genes in delphinidin-treated RAW264.7 cells. Our results demonstrate that RANKL-induced *c-fos* activation was attenuated by delphinidin treatment. Furthermore, expression levels of the *Nfatc1* gene were

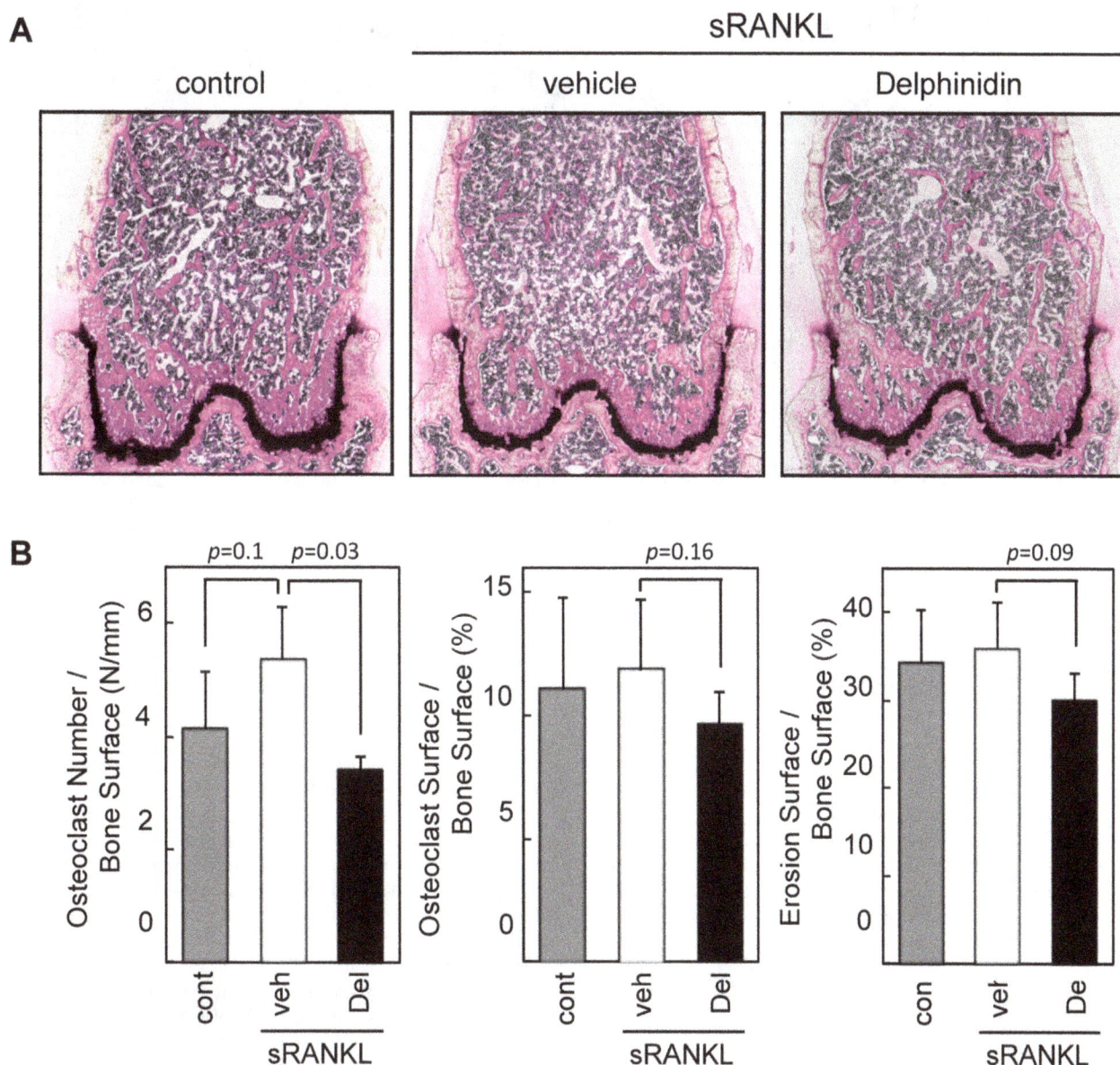

Figure 4. Histomorphometric analysis of anti-bone resorption effect of delphinidin. A: Histological images of distal femurs of intact mice (control), RANKL-induced osteoporosis mice (vehicle), and delphinidin (10 mg/Kg)-treated RANKL-induced osteoporosis mice (Delphinidin). Sections were stained by Villanueva staining. B: Bone-resorption parameters were determined by histomorphometric analysis. Values are expressed as the mean ± SD.

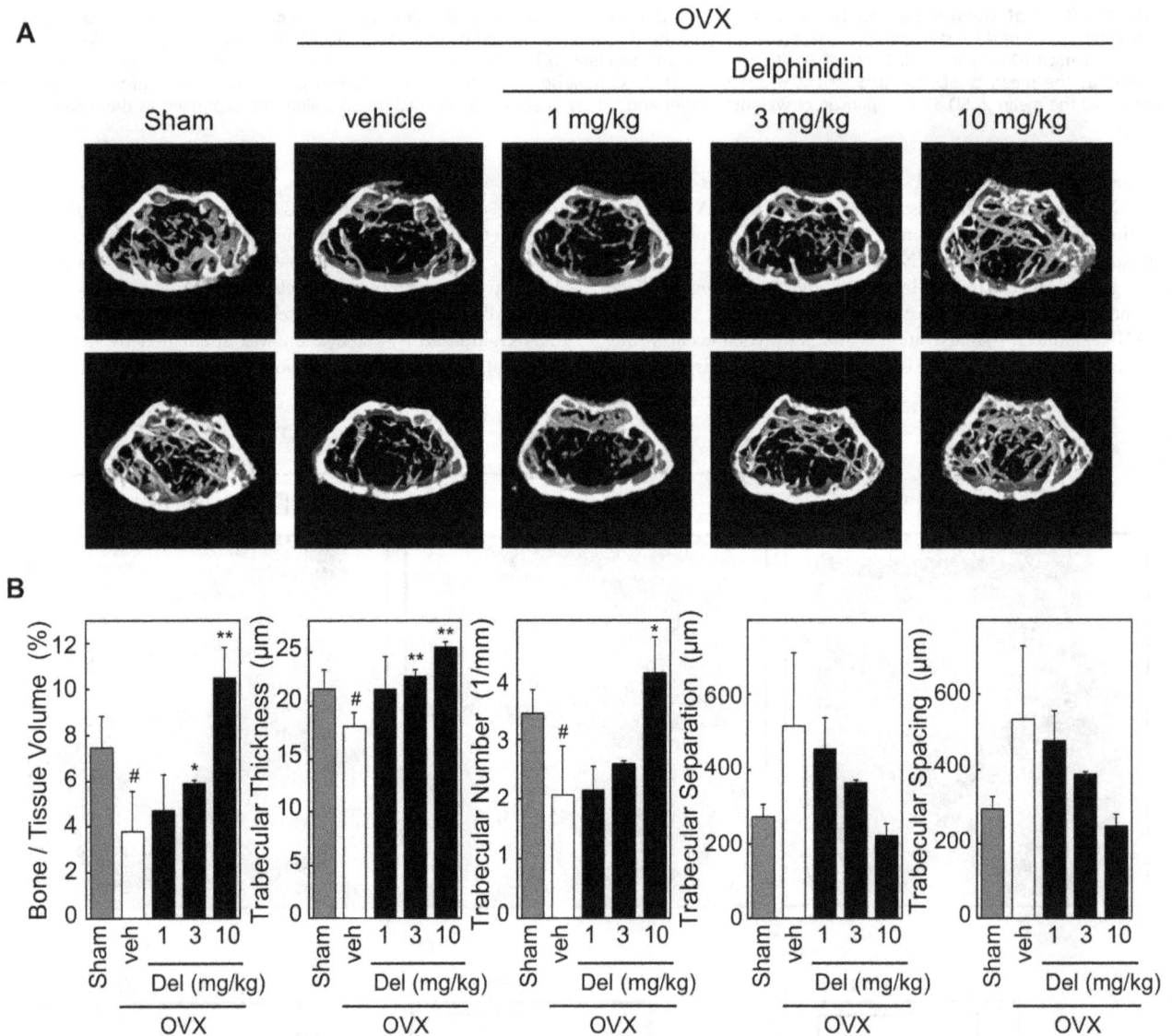

Figure 5. Effect of delphinidin on bone loss in OVX mice. A: Microcomputed tomography images of the distal femurs (axial view of the metaphyseal region) of sham-operated mice, OVX mice (vehicle), and delphinidin-treated OVX mice (Delphinidin). B: Effect of delphinidin on trabecular microarchitectural parameters. Values are expressed as the mean $\pm$ SD. *$p<0.05$, **$p<0.01$ (vs vehicle), #$p<0.05$ (vs sham).

markedly decreased in delphinidin-treated cells (Figure 6B, C). Consequently, expression levels of osteoclast marker genes, especially *Mmp9* and *Trap*, were reduced by delphinidin treatment (Figure 6B, C). In addition, expression levels of *Dc-stamp*, a fusion protein gene for multinucleation, were significantly decreased in delphinidin-treated cells (Figure 6B, C). Together, these results suggest that the anti-osteoclastogenic effect of delphinidin is clearly associated with alteration of the signaling cascade triggered by RANKL.

Discussion

Last year, an interesting epidemiological report was published in the Journal of Bone Mineral Research. Welch and his colleagues investigated the association between habitual flavonoid intake with bone mineral density in 3,160 women, and concluded that flavonoid intake, especially anthocyanin (median intake: 13.7 mg/day), was beneficial for bone-protective effects in women [24].

Devareddy *et al.* previously reported that the extracted anthocyanin compound showed a protective property against bone loss in OVX rats [17]. However, the active ingredients in the anthocyanin compound still have not been identified. In the present study, we provide evidence that delphinidin, one of the major anthocyanidins, is a potent preventive natural agent for osteoporosis and might support the conclusion of the epidemiological investigation experimentally.

We evaluated the inhibitory effects of three major anthocyanidins contained in berries on *in vitro* osteoclast formation, and consequently identified that delphinidin was the most potent active ingredient. In our preliminary tests using their glycosides, similar results in terms of potency were obtained (data not shown), suggesting that anti-osteoclastogenic activity depends on the structure of aglycone form. Since anthocyanins are much more stable than other hydrophilic flavonoid glycosides, they are rapidly absorbed into blood as glycosides without changing to aglycones after consumption [25], [26]. Then, we directly administrated

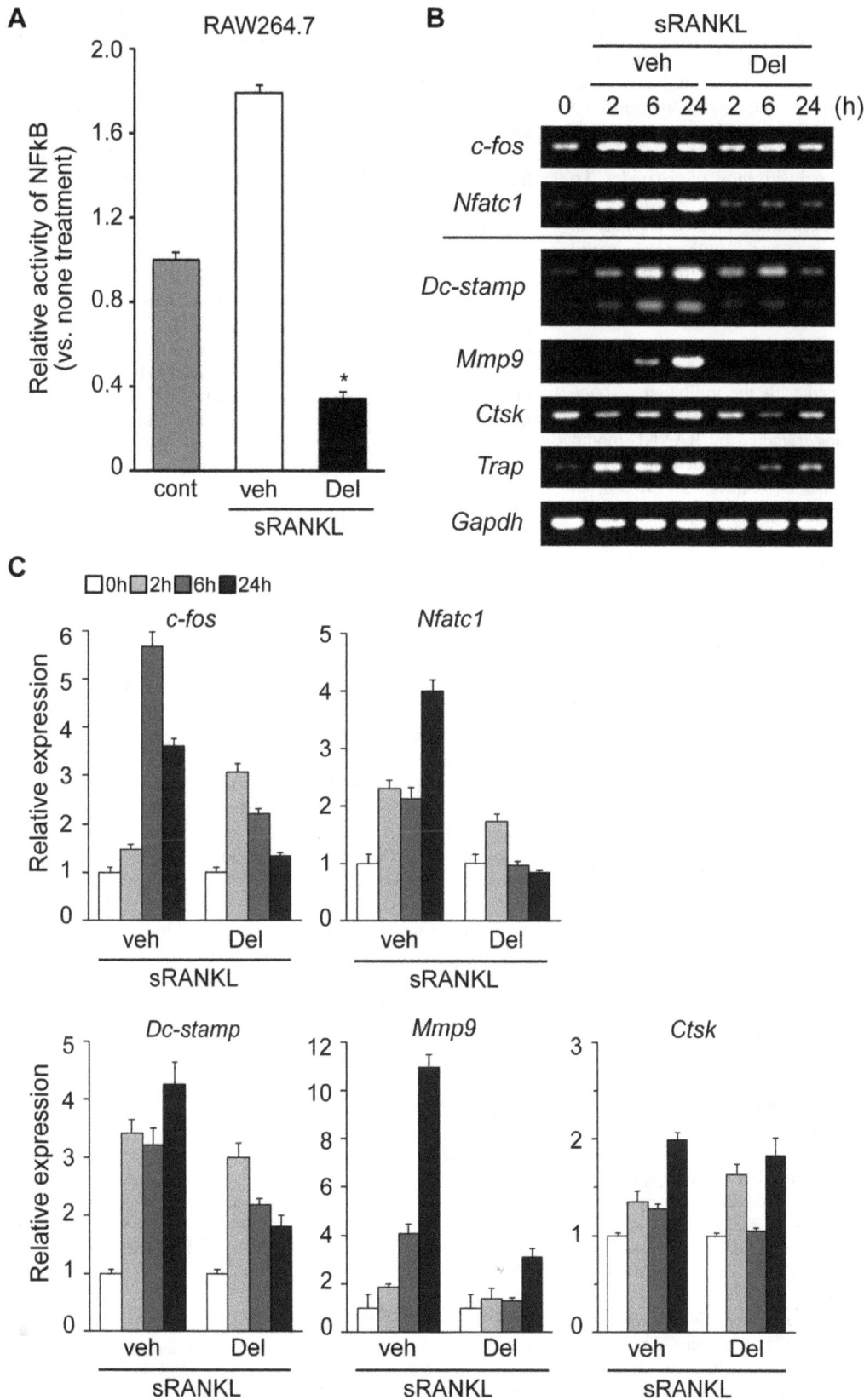

Figure 6. Delphinidin suppresses the expression of major osteoclastogenic molecules in osteoclast precursor cells. (A) Quantification of NF-κB DNA-binding activity in control cells, agent stimulated cells and delphinidin-treated cells. RANKL-stimulated NF-κB DNA-binding activity was significantly inhibited by delphinidin treatment (*$p<0.001$). (B) RT-PCR and (C) qPCR analysis of the expression of osteoclastogenic transcriptional genes, *c-fos* and *Nfatc1*, and osteoclast marker genes, *Dc-stamp, Mmp9, Ctsk* and *Trap,* in RAW264.7 cells.

delphinidin into the osteoporosis mice, and consequently obtained significant results that delphinidin acts as an inhibitor of bone loss. Generally, aglycones of flavonoids are absorbed more rapidly and in greater amounts than their glycoside forms in human and animals [27], [28]. It is supposed that delphinidin administrated orally was quickly absorbed and delivered to bone tissue. However, *in vivo* kinetics of anthocyanidins (aglycones) have not been much investigated as compared with those of glycosides. To elucidate the mechanisms of absorption and metabolism of the aglycones are important for understanding of bioavailability of anthocyanidins. The results obtained from this study may be useful to investigate the *in vivo* circulation of anthocyanidins in the future.

Consistent with *in vitro* examinations, the increased number of osteoclasts under osteoporotic conditions was significantly decreased by delphinidin treatment, resulting in prevention of bone loss. Delphinidin-mediated suppression of osteoclast formation is likely to be a key event associated with the inhibition of bone resorption in osteoporosis mice, as well as anti-osteoporosis drugs, bisphosphonates. RANK signaling triggered by RANKL modulates the activation of various signal pathways including NF-κB and mitogen-activated protein kinases (MAPKs) via TRAF6, an essential mediator of RANK signaling. Previous studies revealed that anthocyanin compounds or anthocyanidins were involved in several signal pathways in various cell types. Karlsen and his colleagues revealed that anthocyanin inhibited LPS-induced NF-κB activation in monocytes [18]. Hafeez *et al.* indicated that delphinidin inhibited NF-κB signaling at multiple levels in prostate cancer cells, and induced apoptosis [29]. These reports have important implications for our understanding of the mechanism of delphinidin in osteoclastogenesis. Consistent with previous work from other groups, our results demonstrate that delphinidin strongly suppressed the activation of NF-κB in RANKL-stimulated osteoclast precursors, RAW264.7 cells. We also found the downregulation of *c-fos* and *Nfatc1*, pivotal regulators of osteoclastogenesis, in delphinidin-treated cells (Figure 6). It is recognized that the induction of NFATc1 depends on NF-κB and AP-1 containing c-Fos. Karlsen *et al.* further demonstrated that plasma levels of NF-κB-related pro-inflammatory mediators were downregulated in participants receiving anthocyanin supplementation compared with the placebo group [18]. In this context, it is plausible that delphinidin administration limits the number of osteoclasts through the downregulation of osteoclastogenic genes in osteoporotic mice. However, details of the molecular mechanism whereby delphinidin attenuates the activation of these osteoclastogenic regulators are still unclear. For example, the anti-oxidant property of anthocyanidins including delphinidin is one of the possible mechanisms underlying the limited gene expression, as in other cell types [14–16]. Reactive oxygen species (ROS) act as second messengers in signal transduction and gene expression in various cell types. In osteoclast precursors, intracellular levels of ROS are transiently increased in response to RANKL, and modulate the activity of the RANKL signaling pathway [30,31]. Since NF-κB is an oxidative stress-sensitive molecule [32], downregulation of NF-κB might depend on the anti-oxidant activity of delphinidin.

The finding that peonidin failed to suppress *in vitro* osteoclastogenesis is important to clarify the mechanism. This result suggests that anthocyanidins cannot always inhibit osteoclastogenesis. Peonidin is another representative anthocyanidin and is the principal ingredient in, for example, cranberry anthocyanin extracts. Previous work using mouse epidermal cells (JB6 cells) suggested that peonidin exhibited chemopreventive activity through inhibition of the phosphorylation of extracellular signal-regulated kinases (ERKs) in the cells [33]. If so, peonidin possibly alters the phenotype of osteoclast formation because RANKL-mediated activation of MAPKs, including ERKs, would be implicated in osteoclastogenesis [11], [30], [34]. However, there was no influence of peonidin on osteoclast differentiation in our experiments. Another investigation using JB6 cells also mentioned that peonidin treatment could not attenuate MAPK activity, including ERKs, in activated cells [35]. By contrast, cyanidin exhibited a mild suppressive effect on osteoclastogenesis at high concentration (≥ 20 μg/ml). Bioactivity of anthocyanidins may be characterized according to different substituent groups on the B-ring. As shown in Figure 2A, the C3' positions (R3') of the B-ring of cyanidin and delphinidin are hydroxyl (–OH) groups, while that of peonidin is a methoxy (–OCH$_3$) group. The ortho-dihydroxyphenyl structure seems to be critical for triggering anti-osteoclastogenic activity among the anthocyanidins. In addition, to clarify the difference whereby delphinidin induces more potent anti-osteoclastogenic activity compared with cyanidin, further studies will be required.

Meanwhile, the bone histomorphometry revealed that delphinidin treatment caused not only decrease of bone resorption but also a slight increase in number of osteoblasts and osteoid volume (no statistical significance). However, in our preliminary tests using the mouse primary osteoblasts, anthocyanin treatment did not stimulate calcification nodule formation (data not shown). Delphinidin consumption may have stimulated concomitantly upregulation of osteogenic potential through the in vivo network. It is desirable that delphinidin induces bone formation simultaneously in osteoporosis. In OVX rats, blueberry diet altered bone formation markers [17]. To investigate regarding the effect of delphinidin on the bone formation may be needed in future.

In summary, this study demonstrated for the first time that delphinidin possesses a potent inhibitory effect against RANKL-mediated osteoclastogenesis via downregulation of osteoclastogenic factors such as *Nfkb*, *c-fos* and *Nfatc1*. Oral administration of delphinidin showed a preventive effect on bone loss in osteoporosis model mice. Our results suggest that dietary delphinidin or anthocyanin supplements containing delphinidin may be useful for the prevention of RANKL-mediated bone loss such as postmenopausal osteoporosis.

Acknowledgments

We are grateful to M. Etoh and T. Ishizuya at Asahi Kasei Phama Corporation for assessment of OVX mice. We thank T. Oki at NARO Kyushu Okinawa Agricultural Research Center for preliminary experiments related to the current study and suggestions, respectively. We also thank S-I. Yasutake for his encouragement of this work. We had native speakers of English (Medical English Service, Kyoto, Japan) proofread our manuscript before resubmission.

Author Contributions

Conceived and designed the experiments: SN. Performed the experiments: SM KS MM YY. Analyzed the data: KS TI YY. Contributed reagents/materials/analysis tools: AN FI. Wrote the paper: SN.

References

1. Gehlbach SH, Fournier M, Bigelow C (2002) Recognition of osteoporosis by primary care physicians. Am J Public Health 92: 271–273.

2. Havsteen B (1983) Flavonoids, a class of natural products of high pharmacological potency. Biochem Pharmacol 32: 1141–1148.

3. Middleton E Jr, Kandaswami C (1992) Effects of flavonoids on immune and inflammatory cell functions. Biochem Pharmacol 43: 1167–1179.
4. Ueda H, Yamazaki C, Yamazaki M (2002) Luteolin as an anti-inflammatory and anti-allergic constituent of Perilla frutescens. Biol Pharm Bull 25: 1197–1202.
5. Gryglewski RJ, Korbut R, Robak J, Swies J (1987) On the mechanism of antithrombotic action of flavonoids. Biochem Pharmacol 36: 317–322.
6. Chiba H, Uehara M, Wu J, Wang X, Masuyama R, et al. (2003) Hesperidin, a citrus flavonoid, inhibits bone loss and decreases serum and hepatic lipids in ovariectomized mice. J Nutr 133: 1892–1897.
7. Tsuji M, Yamamoto H, Sato T, Mizuha Y, Kawai Y, et al. (2009) Dietary quercetin inhibits bone loss without effect on the uterus in ovariectomized mice. J Bone Miner Metab 27: 673–681.
8. Kim TH, Jung JW, Ha BG, Hong JM, Park EK, et al. (2011) The effects of luteolin on osteoclast differentiation, function in vitro and ovariectomy-induced bone loss. J Nutr Biochem 22: 8–15.
9. Wattel A, Kamel S, Prouillet C, Petit JP, Lorget F, et al. (2004) Flavonoid quercetin decreases osteoclastic differentiation induced by RANKL via a mechanism involving NF kappa B and AP-1. J Cell Biochem 92: 285–295.
10. Bu SY, Lerner M, Stoecker BJ, Boldrin E, Brackett DJ, et al. (2008) Dried plum polyphenols inhibit osteoclastogenesis by downregulating NFATc1 and inflammatory mediators. Calcif Tissue Int 82: 475–488.
11. Wada T, Nakashima T, Hiroshi N, Penninger JM (2006) RANKL-RANK signaling in osteoclastogenesis and bone disease. Trends Mol Med 12: 17–25.
12. Matsumoto H, Nakamura Y, Tachibanaki S, Kawamura S, Hirayama M (2003) Stimulatory effect of cyanidin 3-glycosides on the regeneration of rhodopsin. J Agric Food Chem 51: 3560–2563.
13. Einbond LS, Reynertson KA, Luo XD, Basile MJ, Kennelly EJ (2004) Anthocyanin antioxidants from edible fruits. Food Chem 84: 23–28.
14. Mazza G, Kay CD, Cottrell T, Holub BJ (2002) Absorption of anthocyanins from blueberries and serum antioxidant status in human subjects. J Agric Food Chem 50: 7731–7737.
15. Meydani M, Hasan ST (2010) Dietary polyphenols and obesity. Nutrients 2: 737–751.
16. Wallace TC (2011) Anthocyanins in cardiovascular disease. Adv Nutr 2: 1–7.
17. Devareddy L, Hooshmand S, Collins JK, Lucas EA, Chai SC, et al. (2008) Blueberry prevents bone loss in ovariectomized rat model of postmenopausal osteoporosis. J Nutr Biochem 19: 694–699.
18. Karlsen A, Retterstøl L, Laake P, Paur I, Bøhn SK, et al. (2007) Anthocyanins inhibit nuclear factor-kappaB activation in monocytes and reduce plasma concentrations of pro-inflammatory mediators in healthy adults. J Nutr 137: 1951–1954.
19. Yoshiko Y, Maeda N, Aubin JE (2003) Stanniocalcin 1 stimulates osteoblast differentiation in rat calvaria cell cultures. Endocrinology 144: 4134–4143.
20. Tomimori Y, Mori K, Koide M, Nakamichi Y, Ninomiya T, et al. (2009) Evaluation of pharmaceuticals with a novel 50-hour animal model of bone loss. J Bone Miner Res 24: 1194–1205.
21. Kawamori Y, Katayama Y, Asada N, Minagawa K, Sato M, et al. (2010) Role for vitamin D receptor in the neuronal control of the hematopoietic stem cell niche. Blood 116: 5528–5535.
22. Diel P, Geis RB, Caldarelli A, Schmidt S, Leschowsky UL, et al. (2004) The differential ability of the phytoestrogen genistein and of estradiol to induce uterine weight and proliferation in the rat is associated with a substance specific modulation of uterine gene expression. Mol Cell Endocrinol 221: 21–32.
23. Takayanagi H, Kim S, Koga T, Nishina H, Isshiki M, et al. (2002) Induction and activation of the transcription factor NFATc1 (NFAT2) integrate RANKL signaling in terminal differentiation of osteoclasts. Dev Cell 3: 889–901.
24. Welch A, MacGregor A, Jennings A, Fairweather-Tait S, Spector T, et al. (2012) Habitual flavonoid intakes are positively associated with bone mineral density in women. J Bone Miner Res 27: 1872–1878.
25. Matsumoto H, Inaba H, Kishi M, Tominaga S, Hirayama M, et al. (2001) Orally administered delphinidin 3-rutinoside and cyanidin 3-rutinoside are directly absorbed in rats and humans and appear in the blood as the intact forms. J Agric Food Chem 49: 1546–1551.
26. McGhie TK, Walton MC (2007) The bioavailability and absorption of anthocyanins: towards a better understanding. Mol Nutr Food Res 51: 702–713.
27. Manacha C, Moranda C, Demignéa C, Texierb O, Régérat F, et al. (1997) Bioavailability of rutin and quercetin in rats. FEBS Lett 409: 12–16.
28. Hollman PCH (2004) Absorption, bioavailability, and metabolism of flavonoids. Pharm Biol, 42(s1): 74–83.
29. Bin Hafeez B, Asim M, Siddiqui IA, Adhami VM, Murtaza I, et al. (2008) Delphinidin, a dietary anthocyanin in pigmented fruits and vegetables: a new weapon to blunt prostate cancer growth. Cell Cycle 7: 3320–3326.
30. Lee NK, Choi YG, Baik JY, Han SY, Jeong DW, et al. (2005) A crucial role for reactive oxygen species in RANKL-induced osteoclast differentiation. Blood 106: 852–859.
31. Srinivasan S, Koenigstein A, Joseph J, Sun L, Kalyanaraman B, et al. (2010) Role of mitochondrial reactive oxygen species in osteoclast differentiation. Ann N Y Acad Sci 1192: 245–52.
32. Sen CK, Packer L (1996) Antioxidant and redox regulation of gene transcription. FASEB J 10: 709–20.
33. Kwon JY, Lee KW, Hur HJ, Lee HJ (2007) Peonidin inhibits phorbol-ester-induced COX-2 expression and transformation in JB6 P+ cells by blocking phosphorylation of ERK-1 and -2. Ann NY Acad Sci 1095: 513–520.
34. Inami K, Sawai H, Yakushiji K, Katao Y, Matsumoto N, et al. (2008) Augmentation of TNF-induced osteoclast differentiation by inhibition of ERK and activation of p38: Similar intracellular signaling between RANKL- and TNF-induced osteoclast differentiation. Orthodontic Waves 67: 150–156.
35. Hou DX, Kai K, Li JJ, Lin S, Terahara N, et al. (2004) Anthocyanidins inhibit activator protein 1 activity and cell transformation: structure-activity relationship and molecular mechanisms. Carcinogenesis 25: 29–36.

25

External Validation of the Garvan Nomograms for Predicting Absolute Fracture Risk: The Tromsø Study

Luai A. Ahmed[1]*, Nguyen D. Nguyen[2], Åshild Bjørnerem[1], Ragnar M. Joakimsen[3,4], Lone Jørgensen[1], Jan Størmer[5], Dana Bliuc[2], Jacqueline R. Center[2,6,8], John A. Eisman[2,6,7,8], Tuan V. Nguyen[2,8,9,10], Nina Emaus[1]

1 Department of Health and Care Sciences, Faculty of Health Sciences, UiT – The Arctic University of Norway, Tromsø, Norway, 2 Osteoporosis & Bone Biology Program, Garvan Institute of Medical Research, Sydney, Australia, 3 Department of Clinical Medicine, Faculty of Health Sciences, UiT – The Arctic University of Norway, Tromsø, Norway, 4 Medical Clinic, University Hospital of Northern Norway, Tromsø, Norway, 5 Department of Radiology, University Hospital of Northern Norway, Tromsø, Norway, 6 Department of Endocrinology, St Vincent's Hospital, Sydney, Australia, 7 School of Medicine Sydney, University of Notre Dame Australia, Sydney, Australia, 8 St. Vincent's Clinical School, UNSW Australia, Sydney, Australia, 9 School of Public Health and Community Medicine, University of New South Wales, Sydney, Australia, 10 Centre for Health Technologies, University of Technology, Sydney, Australia

Abstract

Background: Absolute risk estimation is a preferred approach for assessing fracture risk and treatment decision making. This study aimed to evaluate and validate the predictive performance of the Garvan Fracture Risk Calculator in a Norwegian cohort.

Methods: The analysis included 1637 women and 1355 aged 60+ years from the Tromsø study. All incident fragility fractures between 2001 and 2009 were registered. The predicted probabilities of non-vertebral osteoporotic and hip fractures were determined using models with and without BMD. The discrimination and calibration of the models were assessed. Reclassification analysis was used to compare the models performance.

Results: The incidence of osteoporotic and hip fracture was 31.5 and 8.6 per 1000 population in women, respectively; in men the corresponding incidence was 12.2 and 5.1. The predicted 5-year and 10-year probability of fractures was consistently higher in the fracture group than the non-fracture group for all models. The 10-year predicted probabilities of hip fracture in those with fracture was 2.8 (women) to 3.1 times (men) higher than those without fracture. There was a close agreement between predicted and observed risk in both sexes and up to the fifth quintile. Among those in the highest quintile of risk, the models over-estimated the risk of fracture. Models with BMD performed better than models with body weight in correct classification of risk in individuals with and without fracture. The overall net decrease in reclassification of the model with weight compared to the model with BMD was 10.6% ($p = 0.008$) in women and 17.2% ($p = 0.001$) in men for osteoporotic fractures, and 13.3% ($p = 0.07$) in women and 17.5% ($p = 0.09$) in men for hip fracture.

Conclusions: The Garvan Fracture Risk Calculator is valid and clinically useful in identifying individuals at high risk of fracture. The models with BMD performed better than those with body weight in fracture risk prediction.

Editor: Yi-Hsiang Hsu, Harvard Medical School, United States of America

Funding: This work was supported by an internal grant from the UiT – The Arctic University of Norway. The funder had no role in study design, data collection and analysis, decision to publish, or preparation of the manuscript.

Competing Interests: NDN, JRC, TVN, and JAE are the developers of the Garvan Fracture Risk Calculator. There is no patent for this calculator and it is freely available at <http://fractureriskcalculator.com.au/>.

* Email: luai.ahmed@uit.no

Introduction

Osteoporotic fractures are an important public health problem. With increasing aging populations, their number will increase placing an additional burden on individuals and society in terms of functional limitations, morbidity, mortality, and costs [1–3]. Individuals with high fracture risk are those who can effectively benefit from preventive measures and pharmaceutical interventions and therefore need to be identified in clinical settings. The tools used to identify persons with increased fracture risk have been expanded to rely not only on bone mineral density (BMD) measurements but also to include informative clinical risk factors.

Absolute risk or individualized prognosis is considered to be a preferred approach in the assessment of fracture risk and treatment decision making. Several prediction models and tools have been developed to calculate absolute fracture risk. These tools vary according to the number and type of fracture risk factors included, and on the complexity of fracture risk computation [4,5]. Systematic reviews highlighted that simple tools performed as well as complex tools [5–7]. The Garvan Fracture Risk Calculator (www.fractureriskcalculator.com) was stated as one of the simplest tools for fracture prediction developed in a population-based setting applying proper methodology [5]. It is based on data from the Dubbo Osteoporosis Epidemiology Study (DOES) and integrates sex, age, BMD (or body weight), and history of prior fracture and falls into the nomograms. It includes two nomograms; one for prediction of absolute risk for hip fracture and another for any fragility fracture [8,9]. These nomograms predict the individualized 5-year or 10-year absolute fracture risk for both women and men.

Assessment of the performance of prognostic models in different populations is necessary [4,10,11]. The Garvan Fracture Risk Calculator was examined in independent cohorts [11–15] and performed well in predicting fracture. However, these validation studies compared the nomograms with other prediction tools, and did not compare the predictive performance between the model with BMD and the model with body weight.

Norway has the highest incidence of hip fractures in the world [16]. Therefore, identification of those at high risk of fracture is warranted, and tools that can be used readily in clinical settings are definitely needed. The present study was designed to evaluate and validate the performance of the Garvan nomograms for predicting 5-year and 10-year risk of fragility fracture in an independent Norwegian cohort of women and men.

Methods

Study population

The Tromsø Study [17] is a longitudinal population-based multipurpose study focusing on lifestyle-related diseases. The first survey was conducted in 1974, with repeated surveys in 1979/80, 1986/87, 1994/95, 2001/02 and 2007/08. The fifth survey in 2001/02 (Tromsø 5) invited all persons living in Tromsø between 55–74 years of age and a randomly selected (5–10%) sub-set of women and men in the age groups 25–54 and 75–84 years, who had participated in the second visit of the fourth survey (Tromsø 4) in 1994/95. Of 10,353 persons invited to the first visit of Tromsø 5, 8,130 (79%) attended, and among them, a preselected random sample of 6,969 persons were invited for a second visit one month later, and 5,939 (85%) attended. At the second visit, hip BMD was measured in 3,094 women and 2,132 men, all of whom had one or both hips without nails or prostheses.

Women (n = 2256) and men (n = 1702) aged 60 years or older were selected in order to examine the nomograms performance in a population of similar age as the population in which the nomograms were developed. Of these, 1637 women and 1355 men (aged 60+ years) were included in this analysis. Subjects with missing data were excluded; 603 subjects with missing history of fall and/or previous fracture, 98 subjects with invalid BMD measurements, 8 subjects with pathological fractures, 85 subjects using bisphosphonates, and 184 women using hormone therapy (numbers are overlapping).

The Regional Committee of Medical Research Ethics and the Norwegian Data Inspectorate approved the study. All participants gave written informed consent.

Questionnaires and measurements

Two self-administered questionnaires were completed by the participants, one before entering the survey, and the other between the two visits of the survey. The questionnaires covered, among others, history of previous fractures, history of falls in the last 12 months, and use of medications. Height and weight were measured to the nearest centimetre/half kilogram whilst wearing light clothing and no shoes.

Dual hip BMD expressed as g/cm^2 was measured by DXA (GE Lunar Prodigy, LUNAR Corporation, Madison, WI, USA). The scans were performed by specially trained technicians according to

the manufacturer provided protocol. The short term in vivo precision error was 1.7% and 1.2% for femoral neck and total hip measurement, respectively, and daily phantom measurements were stable throughout the survey. All scans were reviewed and reanalysed if necessary [18]. Technically incorrect scans and scans of hips with severe deformities were excluded. Scans of the left hip were used for analyses but, if the left hip measurement was ineligible, the right hip scan was used.

Fracture registration

The fracture registry covered the 15-year period from the date of examination in Tromsø 4 (1994/95) through December 31st 2009 with respect to all non-vertebral fractures. Vertebral fractures were excluded, as date of occurrence for vertebral fractures are not reliable. The fracture registry is based on the radiological archives at the University Hospital of North Norway in Tromsø. The nearest alternative radiology service or fracture treatment facility is located 250 km from Tromsø. The only fractures that would be missed are those, for which no radiology was performed or where such investigations occurred while the subject was travelling and without any subsequent local follow-up examination. The computerized records in the radiological archives of the University Hospital contain the national personal identification number (unique for each resident of Norway), time of investigation, fracture codes and descriptions. All abnormal radiological examinations were reviewed to ascertain the fracture code, to identify exact fracture type and anatomical location, to distinguish consecutive fracture occasions in the same person, and to capture fractures that had not been coded correctly as fractures. In addition, the hospital discharge records were checked with respect to hip fractures. A similar registration has previously been described and validated [19].

Statistical analysis

Fractures were classified as hip or non-vertebral osteoporotic fractures. The latter included all non-vertebral fractures except fractures of the finger, toe, or skull. Descriptive statistics of the study cohort are presented by sex and fracture status. Comparison of women and men with and without fracture were performed using T-test for continuous variables and chi-square test for categorical variables. Follow-up time was assigned from the date of the BMD measurement at Tromsø 5 (in 2001/02) for each participant, to date of first fracture, migration, death, or to December 31st 2009. Incidence rates (per 1000 person-years) were calculated by dividing the total number of first incident fractures by the sum of person-years during the follow-up period.

The Garvan Fracture Risk Calculator (Appendix S1) estimates the 5-year and 10-year risks of fracture for an individual based on the individual's risk profile which includes gender, age, bone mineral density (or body weight), frequency of falls during the past 12 months, and the frequency of prior fractures [8,9]. Two models were used; the first model included BMD, age, prior fracture and fall; the second model replaced BMD with body weight. The prognostic discrimination - between those who suffered a fracture and those who did not - of the models was assessed by the area under the receiver operating characteristics curve (AUC). The predictive accuracy (calibration) of the two models was assessed by the concordance index [20], where the concordance between quintiles of observed and predicted risk of fracture was used as a measure of fit. Moreover, ratios of the predicted fracture risk between those with and without fracture were calculated as back transformation of the log values of the predicted risk difference. Reclassification analysis [21] was used to compare the prognostic performance between the two models. In this analysis, the net

Table 1. Baseline characteristics of women and men. The Tromsø Study.

| Variables | Non-fracture | Non-vertebral osteoporotic fractures | | | |
		Any	p-value*	Hip	p-value*
Women	**(n = 1281)**	**(n = 356)**		**(n = 88)**	
Age (y)	69.0 (6.3)	70.3 (6.3)	0.001	74.1 (6.3)	<0.001
Height (cm)	160.3 (6.0)	160.9 (5.9)	0.09	160.6 (6.1)	0.74
Weight (kg)	69.5 (11.9)	67.9 (11.3)	0.03	66.1 (11.9)	0.01
Femoral neck BMD (g/cm^2)	0.83 (0.12)	0.79 (0.11)	<0.001	0.75 (0.11)	<0.001
Femoral neck T-scores	−1.46 (1.19)	−1.89 (1.10)	<0.001	−2.30 (1.06)	<0.001
Prior fracture, n (%)			0.004		0.11
0	972 (75.9)	242 (68.0)		60 (68.2)	
1	185 (14.4)	68 (19.1)		16 (18.2)	
2	89 (7.0)	26 (7.3)		6 (6.8)	
3	35 (2.7)	20 (5.6)		6 (6.8)	
Fall in the last 12 month, n (%)			0.03		0.02
0	903 (70.5)	228 (64.0)		52 (59.1)	
1	360 (28.1)	125 (35.1)		36 (40.9)	
2	18 (1.4)	3 (0.8)		0 (0)	
Men	**(n = 1238)**	**(n = 117)**		**(n = 47)**	
Age (y)	69.6 (5.6)	71.1 (6.5)	0.006	72.8 (5.9)	<0.001
Height (cm)	174.2 (6.6)	176.1 (6.4)	0.002	176.7 (6.8)	0.008
Weight (kg)	80.5 (11.5)	83.0 (13.8)	0.02	82.4 (14.6)	0.26
Femoral neck BMD (g/cm^2)	0.94 (0.13)	0.88 (0.13)	<0.001	0.84 (0.1)	<0.001
Femoral neck T-scores	−0.91 (1.22)	−1.40 (1.18)	<0.001	−1.74 (0.88)	<0.001
Prior fracture, n (%)			0.057		0.12
0	1119 (90.4)	101 (86.3)		38 (80.9)	
1	90 (7.3)	10 (8.6)		7 (14.9)	
2	21 (1.7)	6 (5.1)		2 (4.2)	
3	8 (0.7)	0 (0)		0 (0)	
Fall in the last 12 month, n (%)			0.16		0.63
0	856 (69.1)	71 (60.7)		32 (68.1)	
1	361 (29.2)	44 (37.6)		15 (31.9)	
2	21 (1.7)	2 (1.7)		0 (0)	

Values are mean (SD), unless otherwise specified.
* Compared with non-fracture group.

reclassification improvement (NRI) for fracture prediction was calculated as the sum of differences in proportions of subjects with fracture and proportions of subjects without fracture who were correctly reclassified with higher/lower risk, between the model with BMD and the model with weight, where positive values would indicate better performance of the model with weight or vice versa. The quartiles of the predicted risk from both models were used as thresholds for the risk groups in the reclassification analysis.

The analyses were performed using the SAS statistical package, v9.2 (SAS Institute Inc., Cary, NC, USA), STATA 12.0 (StataCorp. 2011. Stata Statistical Software: Release 12. College Station, TX: StataCorp LP), and R (R core team 2012). The criterion for statistical significance was set at $p<0.05$.

Results

Among 1637 women, 356 suffered non-vertebral osteoporotic fractures including 88 hip fractures (mean follow-up 6.9 years).

Among 1355 men, 117 suffered non-vertebral osteoporotic fractures where 47 of them were hip fractures (mean follow-up 7.1 years). During the first 5 years of follow-up, 210 women suffered non-vertebral fractures (42 hip) and 68 men suffered non-vertebral fractures (24 hip). The incidences per 1000 person-years of non-vertebral osteoporotic and hip fractures during the follow-up were, respectively, 31.5 (95% Confidence Interval (CI) 28.3–34.9) and 8.6 (95% CI 7.0–10.6) in women, and 12.2 (95% CI 10.2–14.6) and 5.1 (95% CI 3.8–6.7) in men. The baseline characteristics of the study cohort are shown in Table 1.

The area under receiver operating characteristics curve (AUC) illustrates the prognostic discrimination for non-vertebral osteoporotic and hip fractures of both models (Figure 1A and 1B). The AUCs for both models were higher for hip (ranging from 0.73 to 0.79) than non-vertebral osteoporotic fractures (AUC 0.61–0.67) with the highest AUC in the 5-year risk analyses. Moreover, the AUCs for the model with BMD were significantly higher than the

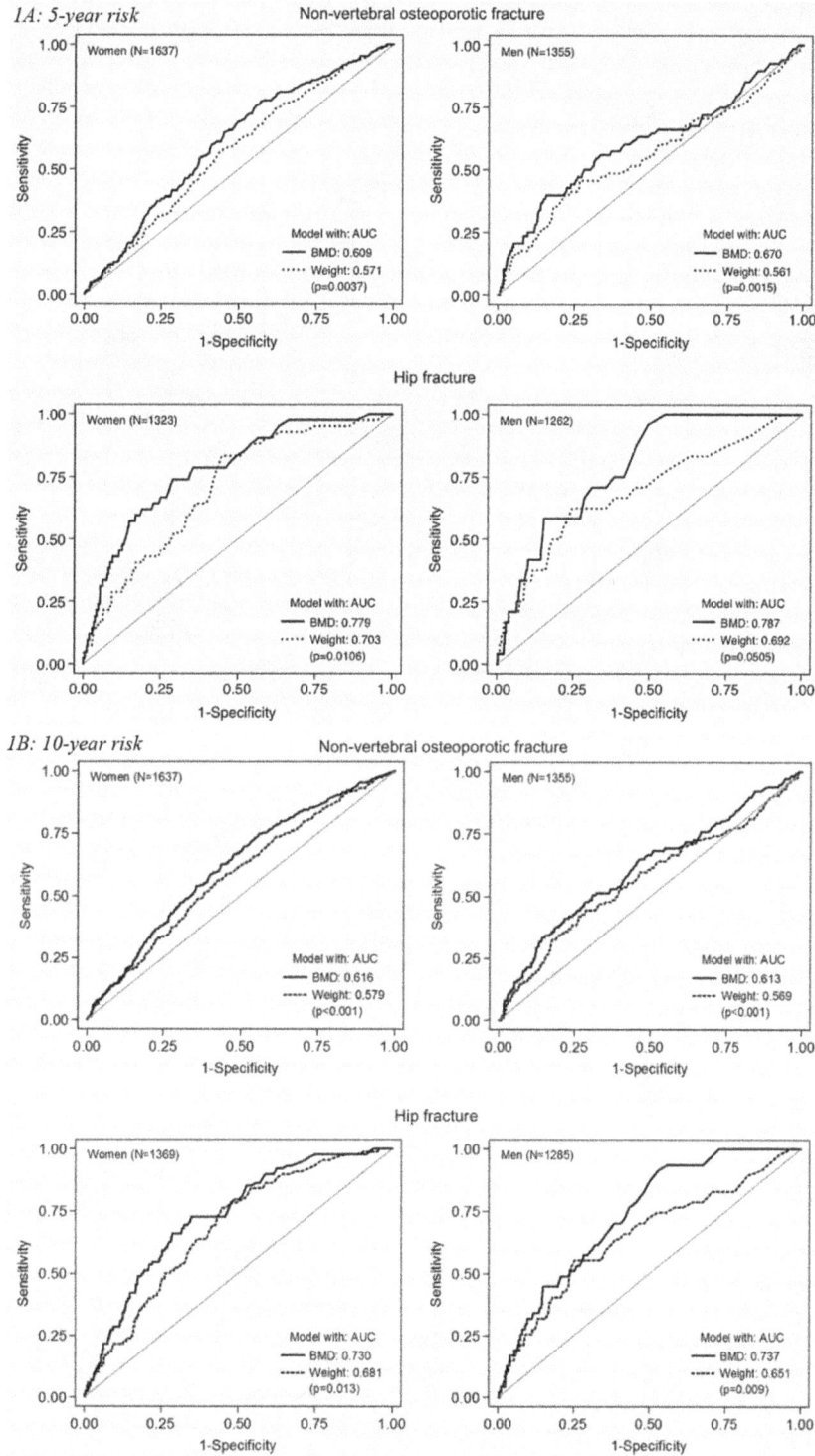

Figure 1. Receiver Operating Characteristic (ROC) curves for model with BMD (continuous line) and model with weight (dashed line) for non-vertebral osteoporotic fracture (upper panel) and hip fracture (lower panel) in women and men based on (1A): 5-year predicted risk, and (1B): 10-year predicted risk.

model with weight for both fracture types among both women and men (all $p<0.05$).

With respect to predictive accuracy of the two models (Figure 2A and 2B), there was a close agreement between predicted and observed risk of fracture, with higher concordance between predicted and observed risk in general for women than for men. In women and men with fracture risk in the highest quintile, both BMD and weight models over-estimated the 5-year and 10-year risks of fracture. Moreover, both the 5-year and the 10-year probability of fracture in those with fracture were on

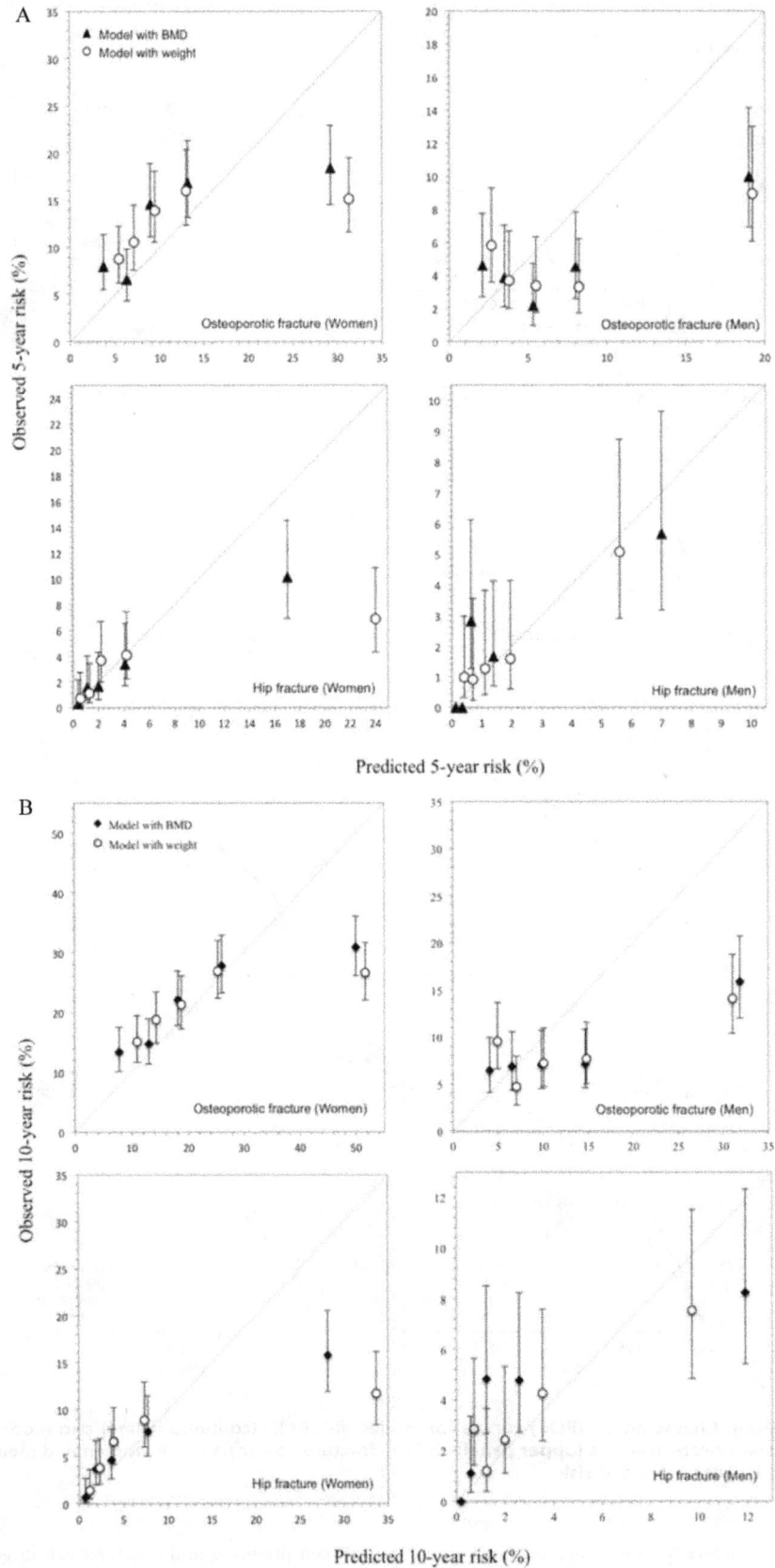

Figure 2. Concordance between the predicted and observed risk of non-vertebral osteoporotic fracture (upper panel) and hip fracture (lower panel) in the Tromsø Study cohort, according to the Garvan nomograms. (A): Quintile cut-offs for the predicted 10-year risk (%) of non-vertebral osteoporotic fracture in women were: 10.8, 15.3, 21.2 and 31.9 for model with BMD (M1); and 12.5, 16.3, 21.3 and 31.5 for

model with weight (M2). Corresponding cut-offs in men were 5.3, 8.0, 11.7 and 18.3 for M1; and 5.9, 8.3, 12.1, 17.9 for M2. Quartile cut-offs for the predicted 10-year risk (%) of hip fracture in women were: 1.3, 2.6, 4.9 and 11.2 for M1 and 1.7, 2.9, 5.0 and 11.1 for M2; In men, 0.3, 0.8, 1.6 and 3.9 for M1; and 0.9, 1.5, 2.6 and 4.8 for M2. (B): Quintile cut-offs for the predicted 5-year risk (%) of non-vertebral osteoporotic fracture in women were: 5.2, 7.4, 10.5 and 16.4 for model with BMD (M1); and 6.2, 8.1, 10.8 and 16.5 for model with weight (M2). Corresponding cut-offs in men were 2.8, 4.2, 6.3 and 10.0 for M1; and 3.2, 4.5, 6.6, 10.1 for M2. Quartile cut-offs for the predicted 5-year risk (%) of hip fracture in women were: 0.7, 1.4, 2.7 and 5.8 for M1 and 0.9, 1.6, 2.8 and 6.3 for M2; In men, 0.2, 0.4, 0.8 and 2.1 for M1; and 0.5, 0.8, 1.4 and 2.7 for M2.

average consistently higher than in those without fracture for both models. The 10-year probability analyses showed that in women, the ratios of predicted risk of non-vertebral osteoporotic fracture between fracture and non-fracture groups were 1.30 (95% CI 1.20–1.40) and 1.16 (1.09–1.24) for BMD and weight models, respectively. The corresponding ratios for hip fracture were, respectively, 2.80 (2.12–3.70) and 2.02 (1.58–2.59). Similar results were obtained in men; for non-vertebral osteoporotic fracture 1.36 (1.19–1. 56) and 1.19 (1.05–1.34) for BMD and weight models, respectively and for hip fracture 3.10 (2.08–4.62) and 1.67 (1.17–2.28).

Models with BMD performed better than models with weight in terms of correct reclassification of fracture and non-fracture subjects in their risk groups in women and in men (Table 2). Compared to the model with BMD, the model with weight showed a net decrease of 9.6% in women and 17.1% in men, in reclassifying non-vertebral osteoporotic fracture cases as "high risk" group, and a decrease of 1.1% in women and 0.1% in men in reclassifying non-fracture subjects as "low risk" group. The overall net decrease in reclassification of the model with weight was 10.6% ($p = 0.008$) in women and 17.2% ($p = 0.001$) in men. For hip fracture, there was no significant difference between the two models. The overall reclassification index showed a net decrease of 13.3% ($p = 0.07$) in women and 17.5% ($p = 0.09$) in men for the model with weight compared to the model with BMD.

Discussion

This study validated the Garvan nomograms in a new population with a substantially higher fracture risk. The nomograms were valid and reasonably accurate in identifying individuals at high risk of fracture in this population. The models with BMD performed better than those with body weight in fracture prediction.

The assessment of fracture risk is moving toward the absolute risk approach, in which an individual's risk is estimated based on the individual's unique risk profile. The individualization of risk

can help make decision concerning treatment for a patient. A number of fracture risk assessment tools have been developed, and among the most popular algorithms are the World Health Organization's FRAX and Garvan Fracture Risk Calculator. These algorithms have been widely validated in independent populations. A recent review of 13 tools for prediction of fractures found that the Garvan model performed as good as or better than more complex models [5]. Compared to other tools, the Garvan nomogram is easy to use without complex computation or the need of computer software which can be impractical or inaccessible in primary care settings [9]. Although the nomograms incorporate fewer number of risk factors compared to other prediction tools, their good predictive performance might be attributed to the strong contribution of the cumulative effect of history of previous fracture and falls on fracture risk [12].

Our findings of moderate discriminative performance of the nomograms with BMD are similar to those reported earlier on the 10-year prediction model. In New Zealand postmenopausal women followed more than 8 years, the Garvan nomograms had AUC values of 0.64 for osteoporotic fractures and 0.67 for hip fractures [14]. In the Global Longitudinal Study of Osteoporosis in Women (GLOW) study (including 60+ years old women from 10 countries with 2 years follow-up), the AUC was 0.64 for osteoporotic fractures and 0.61 for hip fractures [15]. In a Canadian cohort of women and men followed more than 8 years, the discrimination was assessed using the Harrell's C statistics (analogous to AUC) and found to be 0.69 in women and 0.70 in men for low-trauma fractures, and 0.80 in women and 0.85 in men for hip fractures [13]. In addition to previous validations, the current validation also tested the performance of a model with body weight instead of BMD. Overall, the discrimination values for the model with weight were lower than the model with BMD for both fracture types in women and in men. Nonetheless, the model with weight showed a modest performance for hip fractures.

The discriminative value (AUC) of a model does not reflect its clinical value, however evaluation of calibration of prediction models is important for the translation to clinical practice [22].

Table 2. Net Reclassification Improvement (NRI) of model with body weight compared to model with BMD.

	Women			Men		
	Index	(SE)	p-value	Index	(SE)	p-value
Osteoporotic fracture						
NRI for fracture	−0.096	0.036	0.008	−0.171	0.049	0.0009
NRI for non-fracture	−0.011	0.018	0.536	−0.001	0.017	0.961
NRI overall	−0.106	0.040	0.008	−0.172	0.052	0.001
Hip fracture						
NRI for fracture	−0.125	0.070	0.078	−0.191	0.098	0.061
NRI for non-fracture	−0.008	0.019	0.676	0.016	0.021	0.450
NRI overall	−0.133	0.072	0.070	−0.175	0.100	0.093

Values are differences in proportion of correct classification between the models with weight and BMD in each category. Negative values showed that the model with BMD performed better than the model with weight and vice versa.

Similar to previous validations [13,14], this study showed very good calibration of the nomograms, particularly in women in the four lower quintiles of risk. Although the nomograms (with BMD or body weight) over-estimated the risk of fracture in high risk individuals, these individuals would be candidates for intervention in any case. In fact their outcomes may have been modified by treatment received. However, data on treatment were not available in the present study. Compared to women and men in the lower risk quintiles, those in the highest risk quintile were older and had shorter mean follow-up, indicating an increased competing risk of death and thus potentially lower observed risk. In addition, the predicted 10-year risk was compared with an observed risk of shorter duration (mean follow-up 6.9–7.1 years), although similar effects were observed in the 5-year risk analyses. However, possibility of starting osteoporosis treatment during follow-up or model shrinkage – models' tendency to overestimate when using independent data– could contribute to the over-estimates [10,13]. Nonetheless, the nomograms overall predictive ability at the individual level can potentially be useful in clinical practice and as a measure of severity of osteoporosis for the identification of patients in need to be on anti-osteoporosis treatment, and even can be used for selecting patients for clinical trials [9].

This study provides the first external evaluation of performance of the model with body weight compared to model with BMD. The model with BMD performed better in reclassifying both those with and without fracture. The decrease in reclassification for the model with weight is attributed to the overall better sensitivity and specificity of the model with BMD. The reclassification analysis is useful for comparison of the two models in the same group of patients, but not for necessarily for assessment of the models' clinical utility [23]. However, the high predictive accuracy of the model with weight demonstrated by the calibration performance indicates its validity in clinical settings where BMD measurements may not be readily available.

Strengths of this validation analysis include the prospective population-based design with a long follow-up of a large cohort of women and men, with a validated fracture registry capturing all non-vertebral fractures in the cohort. This gave the opportunity to

examine the nomograms performance in a similar study design as the one in which the nomograms were developed but in a distinct independent cohort in a distinct geographic location. Limitations of the study included the lack of vertebral fracture registration, the identification of the energy involved (i.e. low versus higher trauma) in all of the fractures, and data on treatment during follow-up, which would have strengthened the validation. Furthermore, the results cannot be extrapolated to younger women and men, and because of lack of certain data, it was not possible to make performance comparisons between the nomograms and the widely used FRAX tool [4,5].

In conclusion, the Garvan nomograms were valid and clinically accurate in discriminating between fracture and non-fracture subjects in an independent Norwegian cohort of women and men supporting the robustness of the algorithms. Models with BMD performed better than those with body weight in fracture prognosis. Although the nomograms somewhat over-estimated the risk of fracture in high risk individuals, their predictive ability would be useful in clinical practice.

Acknowledgments

The authors thank the participants of the Tromsø Study for their continuing cooperation and the leaders of the Tromsø Study for providing access to the data.

Author Contributions

Conceived and designed the experiments: LAA NDN JRC JAE NE. Analyzed the data: LAA NDN. Contributed reagents/materials/analysis tools: LAA ÅB RMJ LJ JS NE NDN TVN. Wrote the paper: LAA NDN NE. Revised manuscript content: LAA NDN ÅB RMJ LJ JS DB JRC JAE TVN NE. Approved final version of manuscript: LAA NDN ÅB RMJ LJ JS DB JRC JAE TVN NE.

References

1. Cooper C (2010) Osteoporosis: disease severity and consequent fracture management. Osteoporos Int 21 Suppl 2: S425–429.
2. Cummings SR, Melton LJ (2002) Epidemiology and outcomes of osteoporotic fractures.[see comment]. Lancet 359: 1761–1767.
3. Melton LJ 3rd (2003) Adverse outcomes of osteoporotic fractures in the general population. J Bone Miner Res 18: 1139–1141.
4. Leslie WD, Lix LM (2014) Comparison between various fracture risk assessment tools. Osteoporosis International 25: 1–21.
5. Rubin KH, Friis-Holmberg T, Hermann AP, Abrahamsen B, Brixen K (2013) Risk assessment tools to identify women with increased risk of osteoporotic fracture: complexity or simplicity? A systematic review. J Bone Miner Res 28: 1701–1717.
6. Nelson HD, Haney EM, Dana T, Bougatsos C, Chou R (2010) Screening for Osteoporosis: An Update for the U.S. Preventive Services Task Force. Annals of Internal Medicine 153: 99–111.
7. Nayak S, Edwards DL, Saleh AA, Greenspan SL (2014) Performance of risk assessment instruments for predicting osteoporotic fracture risk: a systematic review. Osteoporosis International 25: 23–49.
8. Nguyen ND, Frost SA, Center JR, Eisman JA, Nguyen TV (2007) Development of a nomogram for individualizing hip fracture risk in men and women. Osteoporos Int 18: 1109–1117.
9. Nguyen ND, Frost SA, Center JR, Eisman JA, Nguyen TV (2008) Development of prognostic nomograms for individualizing 5-year and 10-year fracture risks. Osteoporos Int 19: 1431–1444.
10. Altman DG, Vergouwe Y, Royston P, Moons KG (2009) Prognosis and prognostic research: validating a prognostic model. BMJ 338: b605.
11. Sandhu SK, Nguyen ND, Center JR, Pocock NA, Eisman JA, et al. (2010) Prognosis of fracture: evaluation of predictive accuracy of the FRAX algorithm and Garvan nomogram. Osteoporosis International 21: 863–871.
12. Pluskiewicz W, Adamczyk P, Franek E, Leszczynski P, Sewerynek E, et al. (2010) Ten-year probability of osteoporotic fracture in 2012 Polish women assessed by FRAX and nomogram by Nguyen et al.-Conformity between methods and their clinical utility. Bone 46: 1661–1667.
13. Langsetmo L, Nguyen TV, Nguyen ND, Kovacs CS, Prior JC, et al. (2011) Independent external validation of nomograms for predicting risk of low-trauma fracture and hip fracture. CMAJ : Canadian Medical Association journal = journal de l'Association medicale canadienne 183: E107–114.
14. Bolland MJ, Siu ATY, Mason BH, Horne AM, Ames RW, et al. (2011) Evaluation of the FRAX and Garvan fracture risk calculators in older women. Journal of Bone and Mineral Research 26: 420–427.
15. Sambrook PN, Flahive J, Hooven FH, Boonen S, Chapurlat R, et al. (2011) Predicting fractures in an international cohort using risk factor algorithms without BMD. Journal of Bone and Mineral Research 26: 2770–2777.
16. Cheng SY, Levy AR, Lefaivre KA, Guy P, Kuramoto L, et al. (2011) Geographic trends in incidence of hip fractures: a comprehensive literature review. Osteoporos Int 22: 2575–2586.
17. Jacobsen BK, Eggen AE, Mathiesen EB, Wilsgaard T, Njølstad I (2012) Cohort profile: The Tromsø Study. International Journal of Epidemiology 41: 961–967.
18. Emaus N, Omsland TK, Ahmed LA, Grimnes G, Sneve M, et al. (2009) Bone mineral density at the hip in Norwegian women and men–prevalence of osteoporosis depends on chosen references: the Tromsø Study. Eur J Epidemiol 24: 321–328.
19. Joakimsen RM, Fønnebø V, Søgaard AJ, Tollan A, Størmer J, et al. (2001) The Tromsø Study: Registration of fractures, how good are self-reports, a computerized radiographic register and a discharge register? Osteoporos Int 12: 1001–1005.

20. Harrell FE Jr, Lee KL, Mark DB (1996) Multivariable prognostic models: issues in developing models, evaluating assumptions and adequacy, and measuring and reducing errors. Stat Med 15: 361–387.

21. Pencina MJ, D'Agostino RB Sr, D'Agostino RB Jr, Vasan RS (2008) Evaluating the added predictive ability of a new marker: from area under the ROC curve to reclassification and beyond. Stat Med 27: 157–172; discussion 207–112.

22. Steyerberg EW, Vickers AJ, Cook NR, Gerds T, Gonen M, et al. (2010) Assessing the performance of prediction models: a framework for traditional and novel measures. Epidemiology 21: 128–138.

23. Premaor M, Parker RA, Cummings S, Ensrud K, Cauley JA, et al. (2013) Predictive value of FRAX for fracture in obese older women. J Bone Miner Res 28: 188–195.

26

Japanese Medaka: A Non-Mammalian Vertebrate Model for Studying Sex and Age-Related Bone Metabolism *In Vivo*

Admane H. Shanthanagouda[1◑], **Bao-Sheng Guo**[2◑], **Rui R. Ye**[1], **Liang Chao**[2], **Michael W. L. Chiang**[1], **Gopalakrishnan Singaram**[1], **Napo K. M. Cheung**[1], **Ge Zhang**[2]*, **Doris W. T. Au**[1]*

1 State Key Laboratory in Marine Pollution, Department of Biology and Chemistry, City University of Hong Kong, Hong Kong, **2** Institute for Advancing Translational Medicine in Bone & Joint Diseases, School of Chinese Medicine, Hong Kong Baptist University, Hong Kong

Abstract

Background: In human, a reduction in estrogen has been proposed as one of the key contributing factors for postmenopausal osteoporosis. Rodents are conventional models for studying postmenopausal osteoporosis, but the major limitation is that ovariectomy is needed to mimic the estrogen decline after menopause. Interestingly, in medaka fish (*Oryzias latipes*), we observed a natural drop in plasma estrogen profile in females during aging and abnormal spinal curvature was apparent in old fish, which are similar to postmenopausal women. It is hypothesized that estrogen associated disorders in bone metabolism might be predicted and prevented by estrogen supplement in aging *O. latipes*, which could be corresponding to postmenopausal osteoporosis in women.

Principal findings: In *O. latipes*, plasma estrogen was peaked at 8 months old and significantly declined after 10, 11 and 22 months in females. Spinal bone mineral density (BMD) and micro-architecture by microCT measurement progressively decreased and deteriorated from 8 to 10, 12 and 14 months old, which was more apparent in females than the male counterparts. After 10 months old, *O. latipes* were supplemented with 17α-ethinylestradiol (EE2, a potent estrogen mimic) at 6 and 60 ng/mg fish weight/day for 4 weeks, both reduction in spinal BMD and deterioration in bone micro-architecture were significantly prevented. The estrogenic effect of EE2 in *O. latipes* was confirmed by significant up-regulation of four key estrogen responsive genes in the liver. In general, bone histomorphometric analyses indicated significantly lowered osteoblasts and osteoclasts numbers and surfaces on vertebrae of EE2-fed medaka.

Significance: We demonstrate osteoporosis development associated with natural drop in estrogen level during aging in female medaka, which could be attenuated by estrogen treatment. This small size fish is a unique alternative non-mammalian vertebrate model for studying estrogen-related molecular regulation in postmenopausal skeletal disorders *in vivo* without ovariectomy.

Editor: Christoph Winkler, National University of Singapore, Singapore

Funding: The work described in this paper was supported by grants from the CityU Seed Grant (Project No. 7003024), the University Grants Committee, Area of Excellence Grant (AoE/P-04/04), the State Key Laboratory in Marine Pollution and Hong Kong General Research Fund (HKBU479111). The funders had no role in study design, data collection and analysis, decision to publish, or preparation of the manuscript.

Competing Interests: The authors have declared that no competing interests exist.

* E-mail: bhdwtau@cityu.edu.hk (DWTA); zhangge@hkbu.edu.hk (GZ)

◑ These authors contributed equally to this work.

Introduction

Osteoporosis is a systemic skeletal disease characterized by low bone mass and architectural deterioration with a consequential increase in bone fragility, decrease in biomechanical properties and susceptibility to fractures [1,2]. Postmenopausal osteoporosis (PMO) commonly occurs in women approximately 10 years after the onset of menopause. In human, depletion of estrogen has been shown as a key factor in pathogenesis of PMO [3,4,5,6]. Supplement with estrogen in postmenopausal women can prevent or attenuate bone loss in postmenopausal women [7].

Rodent models have long been used for studying PMO for R & D of anti-osteoporosis drugs. However, female rodents have no menopausal drop in estrogen level during aging (Fig. 1) [8].

Therefore, ovariectomy (OVX) has to be conducted in rodents to mimic a natural estrogen decline after menopause in women (Fig. 1) [9,10]. The imbalanced body homeostasis associated with a sudden loss of estrogen in the artificial OVX animals, which is different from a natural drop of estrogen in postmenopausal women, may influence the precise interpretation of *in vivo* data. Therefore, an alternative vertebrate model with a natural decline of estrogen in females during aging and with similar bone metabolism and therapeutic response as that of the humans would be desirable for R & D for PMO (Fig. 1).

Recently, we reported a natural drop of estrogen level in the small sized laboratory fish, Japanese medaka *Oryzias latipes*, in females during aging, which is akin to "menopause" in women

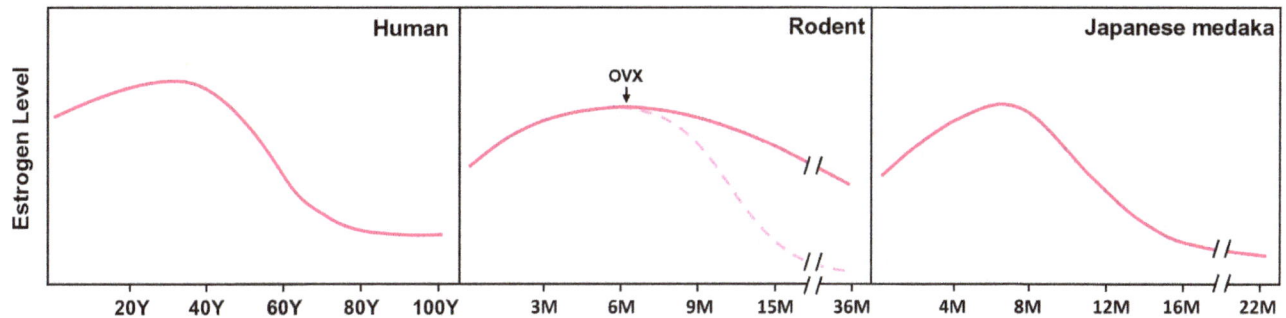

Figure 1. A comparison of estrogen (E2) profiles among aging women, female rodent and female *Oryzias latipes*. Human age is presented in years, and that for both rodent and *Oryzias latipes* is presented in months. Dashed line in rodent panel indicates estrogen level after overiectomy (OVX). Sources: E2 in women by Riggs et al. [34]; E2 in female rodents by Steger and Peluso [8]; E2 in female *Oryzias latipes* by Gopalakrishnan et al. [11] and present study.

[11]. In addition, *O. latipes* has been well studied for bone cell biology, which is similar to that of the humans [12,13,14]. Osteoclasts (OCs) in *O. latipes* are multinucleated, bearing a mammal OC like ruffled border [15,16]. Our preliminary study of *O. latipes* bone specimen also demonstrated that mammal like osteoblasts (OBs) in cubic or lining forms located on osteoid surfaces as indicated by Trichrome staining. Furthermore, high genomic homology of twist, core binding factor-a1 (*cbfa1*) and osteoprotegerin (*opg*) of OBs were found between *O. latipes* and other vertebrates [17,18,19]. Moreover, abnormal hunchback profile is a hallmark of aging in *O. latipes* [20]. The above evidence strongly supported that *O. latipes* could be developed toward an alternative vertebrate model for osteoporosis research, *e.g.* PMO.

Thus far, there is a lack of information on bone metabolism and osteoporosis development in aging *O. latipes*. Our earlier studies have established the *O. latipes* an alternative vertebrate model for sex and aging research [11,21,22]. It is hypothesized that estrogen associated disorders in bone metabolism might be predicted and prevented by estrogen supplement in aging *O. latipes*, which could be corresponding to postmenopausal osteoporosis in women. In this study, we first investigated age-related changes in spinal bone mineral density (BMD), bone micro-architecture and plasma estrogen levels in both sexes of *O. latipes*, with an attempt to corroborate plasma estrogen levels and spinal BMD *in vivo*. Subsequently, synthetic 17α-ethinylestradiol (a potent estrogen mimic) was administered as estrogen supplement to study the changes of BMD, bone micro-architecture and histomorphology

induced by estrogen in both sexes of 10-month old *O. latipes* (shortly after estrogen decline in the females).

Materials and Methods

Ethics Statement

European Union directive 86/609/EEC are strictly adhered throughout the study. Ethics committee specifically approved this study and all animal handling procedures mentioned in this study were accepted by the Animal Ethics Committee, City University of Hong Kong.

Japanese Medaka Culture

The orange-red line medaka *Oryzias latipes* was originated from the Molecular Aquatic Toxicology Laboratory, Duke University, USA. Fish were transferred to the City University of Hong Kong in 2008. Briefly, 15 pairs of male and female medaka of the same age group were housed in aquaria of dimensions: 39.5L×23.5W×27.5H (cm) and kept under static conditions at 26±1°C, 7.2±0.2 ppm O_2 under 14 h:10 h light:dark cycle. Fifty percent of tank water was replaced daily with dechlorinated tap water. Fish were fed twice daily with estrogen free diet Otohime β1 (Nisshin Co, Japan), and supplemented with hatched brine shrimp *Artemia nauplii* (Lucky Brand, O.S.I. USA) for 3 days per week. Under the stated husbandry conditions, the fish reach sexual maturity at three months-post-hatch and lay eggs daily. Japanese medaka at different ages: 4 months (young), 8 months (mature), 10–14 months (senior) and 22 months (very old) were sampled for measurement of plasma estrogen by ELISA analysis and bone mass and micro-architecture by microCT analysis.

EE2 Exposure Experiment: Food Preparation and Administration

17α-ethinylestradiol [EE2] (Cat. No. E4876, Sigma-Aldrich Pty. Ltd), a potent estrogen agonist [23] and more stable in water as compared to the synthetic 17β-estradiol (E2) [24], was used as an estrogen supplement in this study. Two EE2 stock solutions were prepared by dissolving 2.592 and 25.92 mg of EE2 each in 10 mL of absolute ethanol. Dissolved EE2 was mixed with 4.32 g fish feed (Otohime β1) and ethanol was evaporated by nitrogen. The EE2 infused feed was homogenized in distilled water, making two EE2 stock concentrations at 0.012 and 0.12 mg EE2/mL water. The EE2 solutions were aliquot in tubes, stored at −20°C. Control feed was prepared by the same way, except with the omission of EE2.

For the EE2 experiment, fourteen pairs of 10 months old male and female fish (showing a natural drop of estrogen) were used.

Table 1. Gene specific primers used for quantification by qPCR.

Primers	Sequence	Accession number
ChgHF	TACTTTCCCGTCACTTATTGC	D89609
ChgHR	TTCCACGACCAGAGTTTCAAC	D89609
ERαF	GAGGAGGAGGAGGAGGAGGAG	D28954
ERαR	GTGTACGGTCGGCTCAACTTC	D28954
Vtg1F	AGTGCTCGTCGTTCAATGC	NM001104677
Vtg1R	AGTCGCTGCTTCTGCTTCTA	NM001104677
Vtg2F	CACCTGACTACTCCTCTGTTG	NM001104840
Vtg2R	GTAATGGAATGCTCTGCTGAAG	NM001104840

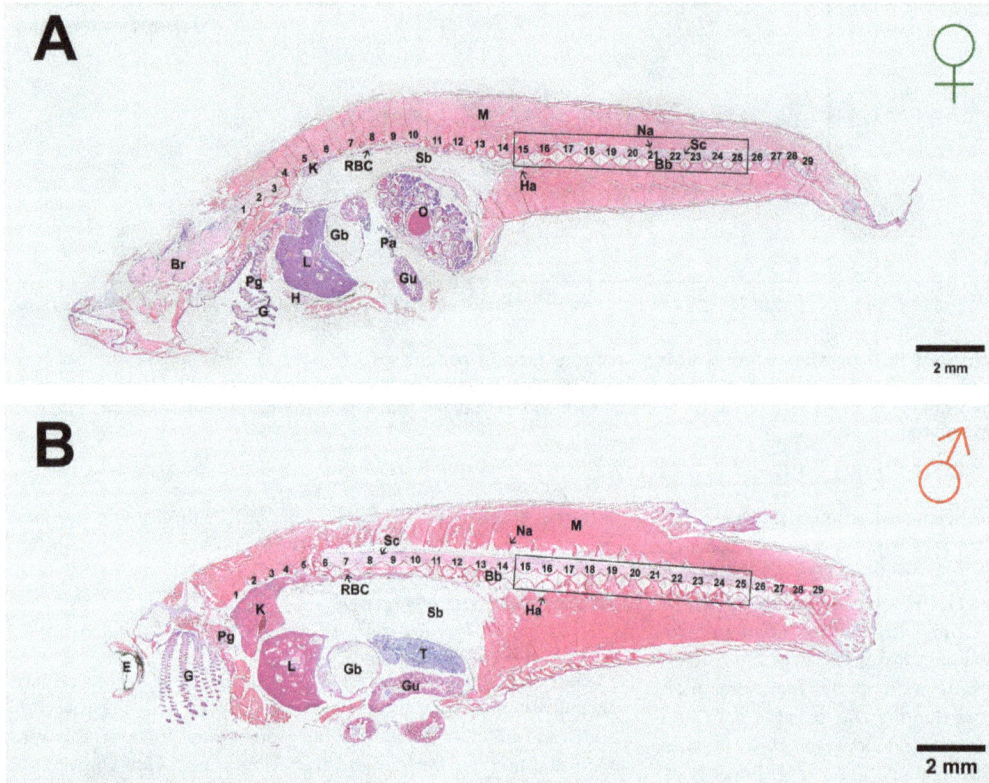

Figure 2. Haematoxylin and Eosin (H and E) staining of sagittal sections from whole adult Japanese medaka *Oryzias latipes* **in (A) female and (B) male at 13 months old.** Fish anterior is to the left. Spinal vertebrae are numbered. The rectangular box showing the vertebrae 15th–25th was used for both microCT scanning and histomorphometry. Letters on the sections indicate Br, Brain; Bb, Backbone; E, Eye; G, Gill; Gb, Gall bladder; Gu, Gut; H, Heart; Ha, Hemal arch; K, Kidney; L, Liver; M, Muscle; Na, Neural arch; O, Ovary; Pa, Pancreas; Pg, Pharyngeal gill; RBC, Red Blood Cells, Sb, Swim bladder; Sc, Spinal cord; T, Testis.

Each pair of fish was kept in a glass tank having dimensions of 15 cm^3. Fish was fed daily with EE2 diet or control diet for 4 weeks. EE2 diet was prepared by spiking a 100 μL of high or low EE2 stock solution into 2 mg of fish feed (ca. 1% of body weight). This was equivalent to 6 and 60 ng EE2/mg fish wt./day for low and high dose EE2 treatments, respectively. To avoid uneven consumption of EE2/solvent diet, a glass divider was gently inserted at each tank to separate the fish pair prior to feeding. Upon completion of feed, the glass plate divider was removed.

During the experiment, fish were also fed approximately 4 mg of Otohime β1 once daily for growth purpose.

Fish Sampling

After 4 weeks of EE2 feeding, all fish were anaesthetized by immersing in ice-cold aquarium water for 30 sec. Immediately after anaesthesia, blood sample was collected from individual fish by cutting the tail between 28th and 29th vertebra (i.e. at caudal peduncle). Blood samples were stored at −80°C for estrogen

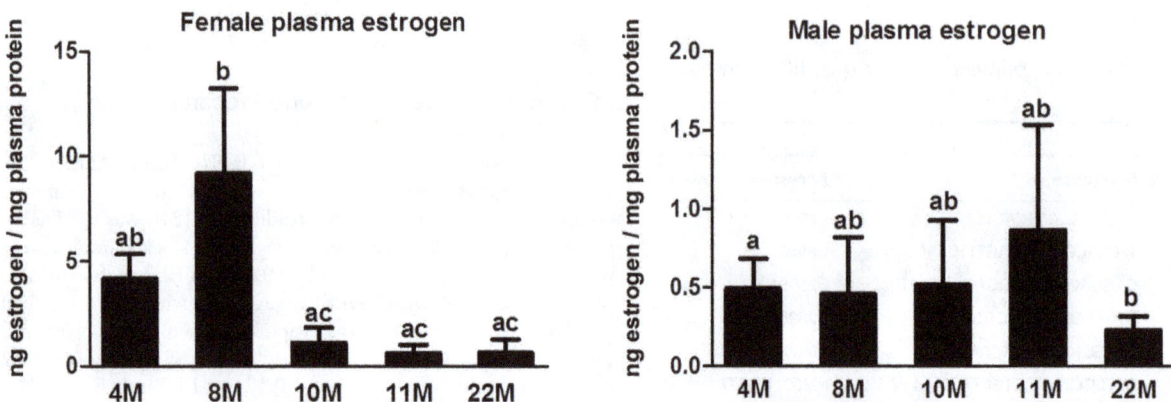

Figure 3. Plasma estrogen levels in aging female (left) and male (right) Japanese medaka *Oryzias latipes*. Bars labeled by the same letter (a, b, c) on the graph are not significantly different from each other (p<0.05) by one-way ANOVA followed by Tukey's post hoc test.

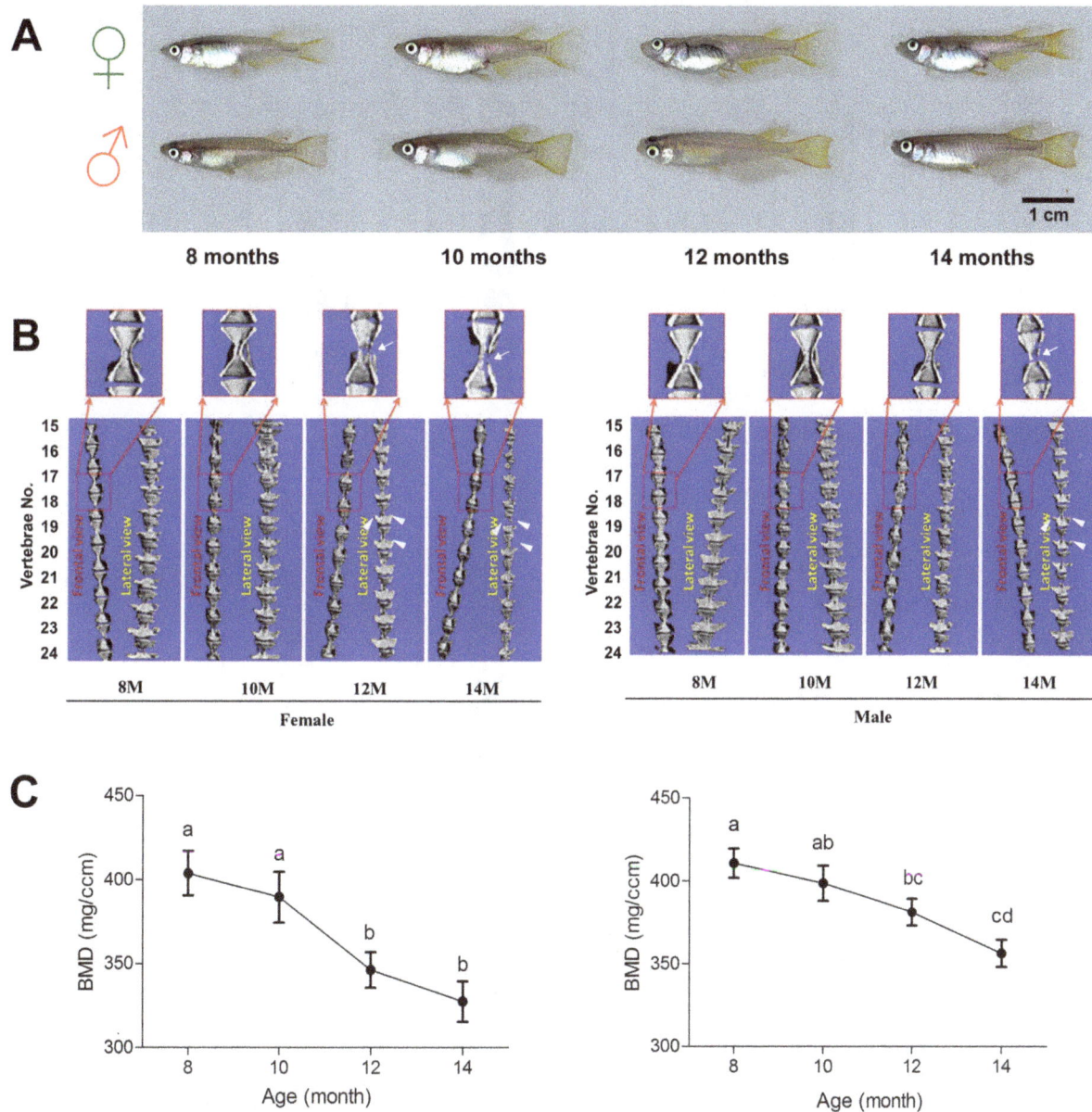

Figure 4. Representative appearance of female (top) and male (bottom) Japanese medaka *Oryzias latipes* at 8, 10, 12 and 14 months old (Fig. A). (B) Representative micro-architecture of vertebrae bodies at 8, 10, 12 and 14 months in females (left) and males (right) by 3-dimensional microCT reconstruction. (C) Age-related changes in bone mineral density (BMD) from 8 to 14 months in females (left) and males (right) by microCT analysis. White arrows and arrowheads indicate micro-cracks and thinner arches found in 10–14 months old fish. BMD values labeled by the same letter (a, b, c, d) on the graph are not significantly different from each other (p<0.05).

analysis. Fish liver was immediately isolated, snap-frozen in liquid nitrogen and stored at −80°C for qRT-PCR. The remaining fish body was fixed in 4% paraformaldehyde in phosphate buffered saline (PBS) overnight at 4°C, then transferred to 70% ethanol for subsequent microCT scanning and quantitative histomorphometry (n = 6 per sex for each treatment).

Plasma Estrogen Assay

To extract the plasma estrogen, 5 mL diethyl ether was added to the blood sample, then vortexed and centrifuged at 3000 rpm for 10 min at room temperature. After centrifugation, the organic phase was retrieved using a glass pipette. The extraction procedure was repeated 3 more times for each sample. The level of plasma

estrogen was measured using commercially available ELISA Kits (Cat#582251, Cayman Chemical Pty. Ltd.) according to the manufacturer's instructions. Note that this procedure only detects endogenous plasma estrogen, but not the exogenously added EE2.

Estrogen Responsive Marker Genes Expression

To confirm the estrogenic effect of EE2 treatment in fish, hepatic expression of estrogen responsive genes including choriogeninH (*ChgH*), estrogen receptor alpha (*ERα*) and vitellogenins (*Vtg1* and *Vtg2*) were measured by qRT-PCR. Isolated liver was homogenized by sterilized micropestle (n = 6 per sex for each treatment). Total RNAs were extracted by RNeasy mini Kit (Qiagen, Germany) and cDNA templates were generated using

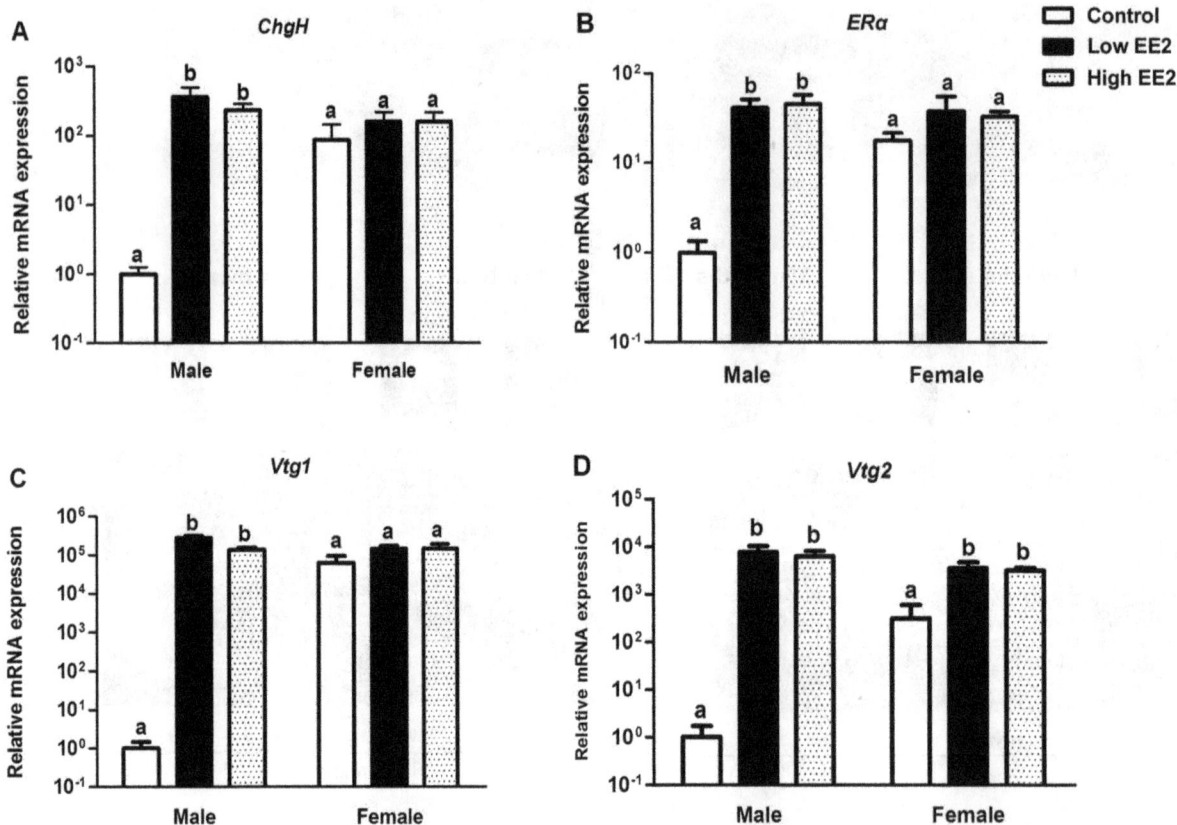

Figure 5. Hepatic expression of estrogen responsive genes in male and female *Oryzias latipes* **treated with low and high EE2 for 4 weeks.** (A) Choriogenin H (*ChgH*), (B) Estrogen Receptor α (*ERα*), (C) Vitellogenin1 (*Vtg1*), (D) Vitellogenin2 (*Vtg2*). Bars labeled by the same letter on the graphs are not significantly different from each other (p<0.05).

TaKaRa Primescript™ RT (TaKaRa, China). Briefly, the assay was performed using Master Mix (2x) Universal (KAPA, USA) in ABI 7500 fast system. The primer sets used for qPCR are given in Table 1. The relative mRNA expression level was calculated by the classical $2^{-\Delta\Delta CT}$ method using 18 s rRNA as an endogenous control to normalize the data.

Bone Mass and Micro-architecture Quantified by microCT Analysis

The bone mass and micro-architecture was measured by microCT (µCT40, SCANCO MEDICAL, Switzerland). Briefly, the whole body of medaka was fixed in a plastic tube (SCANCO MEDICAL, Switzerland) of 5 mm diameter and scanned for scout view. The 15th to 25th vertebrae region (Fig. 2) were selected for scanning with a voxel size of 6 µm. Totally, 900 continuous slices (each slice with a thickness of 6 µm) were selected and all the

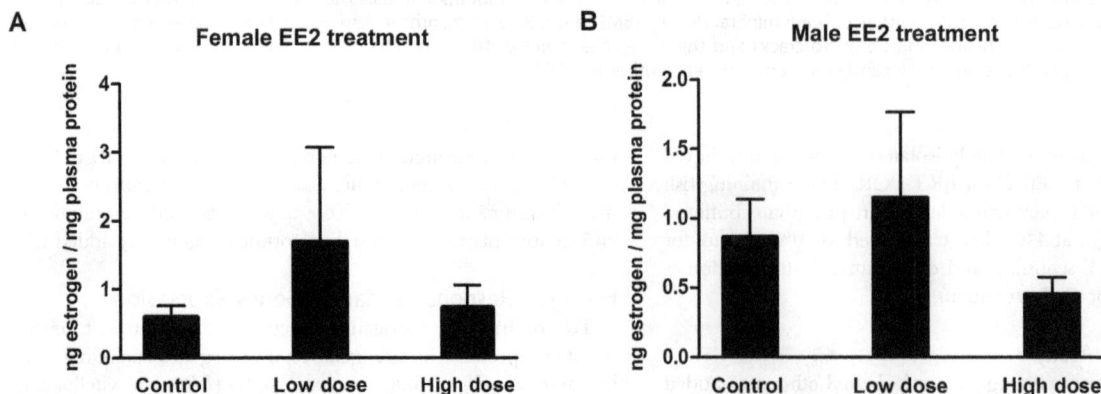

Figure 6. Plasma estrogen in 10 months old female (A) and male (B) Japanese medaka *Oryzias latipes* **treated with low and high EE2 for 4 weeks.** No significance at P<0.05.

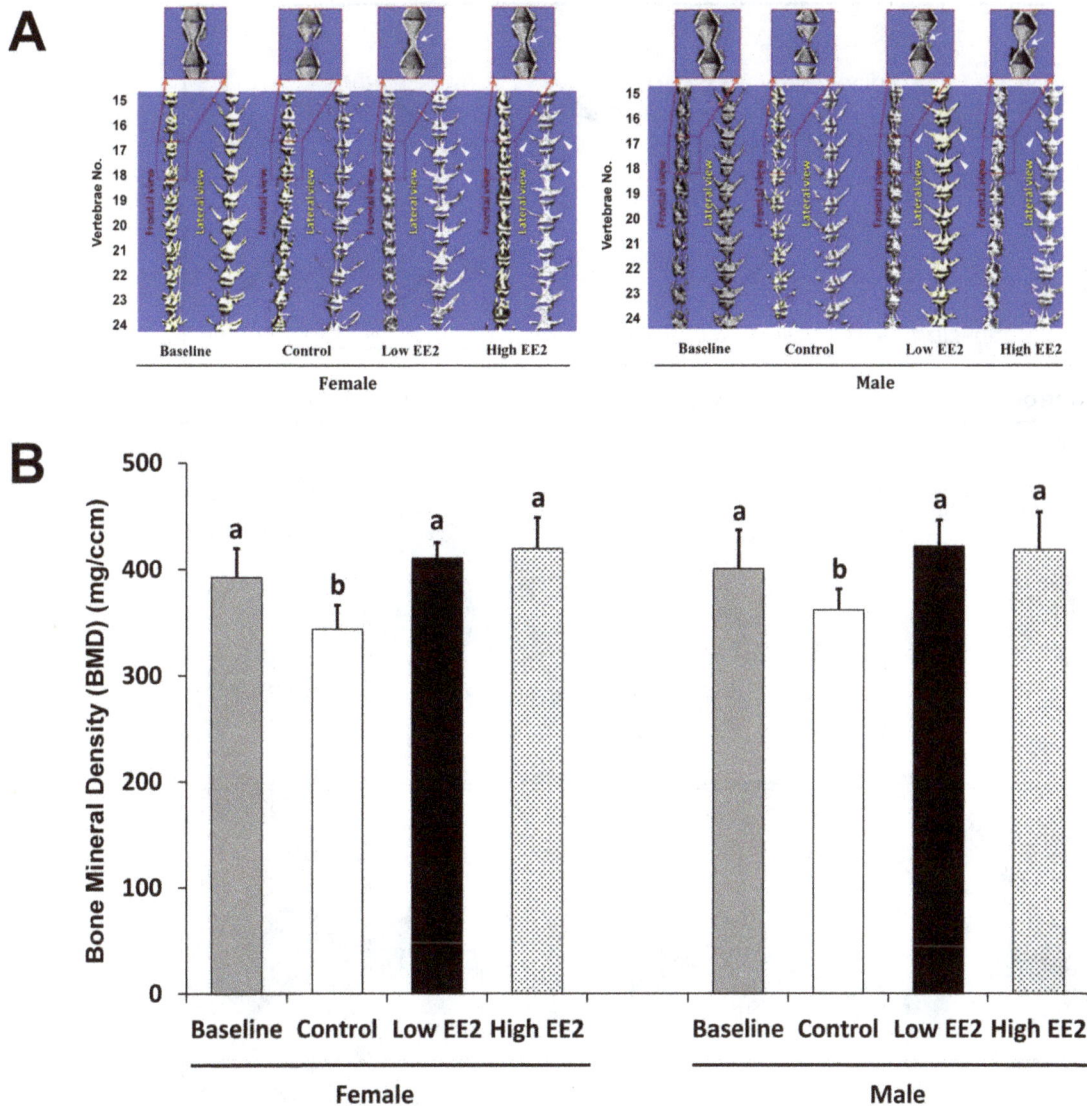

Figure 7. Changes in micro-architecture (A) and bone mineral density (BMD) (B) of vertebrae bodies from 10 months old (baseline) to 11 months old female and male Japanese medaka *Oryzias latipes* after low and high EE2 treatment for 4 weeks. White arrows and arrowheads indicate improved micro-architecture and arches in EE2 treated fish. Bars labeled by the same letter (a, b) on the graph are not significantly different from each other (P<0.05).

mineralized bone from each selected slice was segmented for three-dimensional reconstruction of micro-architecture and analysis of volumetric bone mineral density (BMD) (Sigma = 1.2, Supports = 2 and Threshold = 160).

Bone Histology

Whole medaka fish were fixed and processed according to the protocol described by Kong et al. [25], which allows bone histology without decalcification. Briefly, adult medaka were anaesthetized and dissected, hard substances including skull, otoliths and fins removed, and fixed in GPHS [0.05% glutaraldehyde, 2% paraformaldehyde, 80% histochoice MB fixative (Cat# 64115-04, Electron Microscopy Sciences, USA), 1% sucrose and 1% $CaCl_2$] fixative for 48 h. Fixed fish were dehydrated in series of methanol and chloroform and embedded in paraffin. Serial sections of a single fish were cut (7 μm) using rotary microtome (Leica RM2125RT, Germany). Sections were

mounted onto SuperFrost® Plus slides (Menzel-Gläser, Germany) and dried at 33°C overnight. Whole fish sections were observed under compound microscope, sections showing vertebral columns were chosen for staining. Solvent control and EE2 treated sections were collected and number coded for quantitative histochemical staining of OBs and OCs.

Identification and Localization of OBs and OCs by Goldner's Trichrome and TRAP Staining, Respectively

Osteoblasts (bone forming cells) were detected and localized by Alkaline Phosphatase (ALPase) activity using the Goldner's Trichrome modified staining protocol. Briefly, deparaffinized medaka tissue sections were placed in Weigert's haematoxylin for nuclei staining (15 min). The tissue sections were put in Ponceau/acid fuchsin/azaphloxine for 5 minutes, followed by differentiation with 0.5% acid alcohol for 20 sec. The stained sections were subject to phosphomolybdic acid and light green

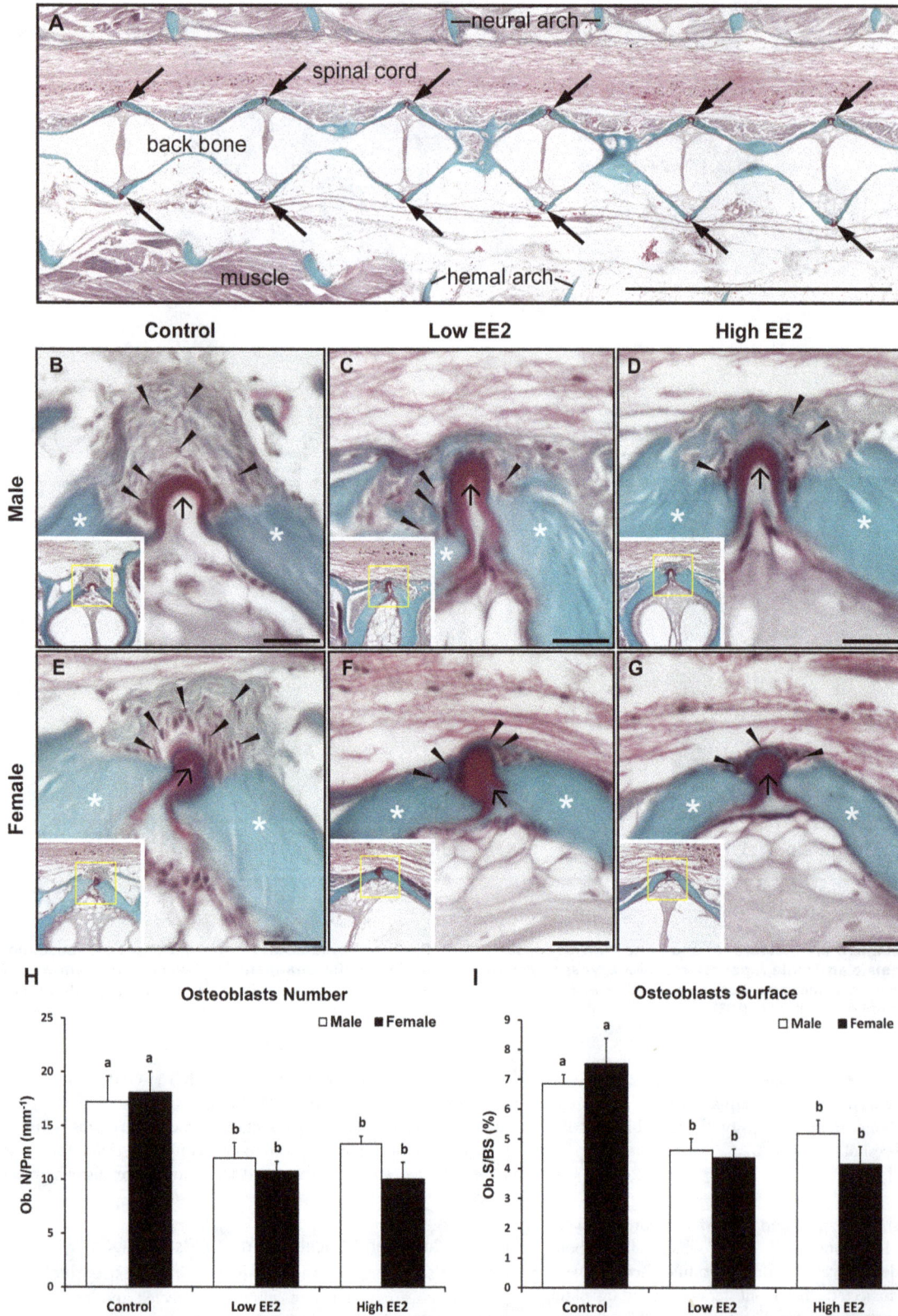

Figure 8. Representative histology pictures of Goldner's Trichrome staining for detection of osteoblasts (black arrowheads), osteoid (black arrows) and mineralized bone (asterisks) in both sexes of Japanese medaka *O. latipes* after 4 weeks of EE2 treatment (Control = no EE2 fed; Low = 6 ng EE2/mg body wt./day and High = 60 ng EE2/mg body wt./day) (Fig. A–G). (A) The location of the corresponding cells on the serial tissue sections is indicated by arrows (scale bar 1000 μm). (B) Male untreated/Control, (C) Male with low EE2 treatment, (D) Male with high EE2 treatment, (E) Female untreated/Control, (F) Female with low EE2 treatment and (G) Female with high EE2 treatment. Scale bars 20 μm. Figure 8 H and I. Bone histomorphometric parameters in both sexes of *O. latipes* upon EE2 treatment (H) Osteoblasts

Number/Bone Perimeter (mm)(Ob.N/B. Pm), (I) Osteoblasts Surface/Bone surface (Ob.S/BS). Bars labeled by the same letter on the graphs are not significantly different from each other (At significant level p<0.05).

treatment for 5 and 20 minutes, respectively, prior to dehydration in series of ethanol and xylene.

Osteoclasts (bone resorbing cells) were localized by Tartrate Resistant Acid Phosphatase (TRAP) enzyme activity using acid phosphatase, leucocyte (387A, Sigma-Aldrich) staining protocol according to the manufacturer's instructions (Sigma-Aldrich). The stained sections were briefly air dried and mounted in permount (SP15-500, Fisher scientific) for further analyses.

All stained sections were examined under light microscopy [40x objective magnification] (Axioplan 2 Imaging, Germany) and images were captured using a color viewII camera (Soft Imaging Solutions, GmbH, Germany) for identification of OBs and OCs.

Quantification of Number and Surface of OBs and OCs by Bone Histomorphometric Analyses

Four bone histomorphometric parameters (i) osteoblasts number/mm of bone perimeter (Ob.N/B.Pm), (ii) osteoclasts number/mm of bone perimeter (Oc.N/B.Pm), (iii) osteoblasts surface/bone surface (Ob.S/BS) and (iv) osteoclasts surface/bone surface (Oc.S/BS) were quantified by Bioquant Osteo v13.1.60 image analysis software (BIOQUANT Image Analysis Corporation, USA). The above parameters were measured and expressed according to the standardized nomenclature for bone histomorphometry [26].

Statistical Analyses

The data of estrogen levels was analyzed by Kruskal-Wallis test using the Graphpad prism 6.01 v package. The data for estrogen responsive gene expressions, microCT and bone histomorphometric parameters in aging/EE2 treatment studies were analyzed among groups by one-way ANOVA and followed by Tukey's posthoc test to determine the sex and treatment effect using SPSS package (SPSS Inc. 2008) at P<0.05 significance.

Results

Declined Estrogen Level in Aging *O. latipes*

Plasma estrogen levels in 4, 8, 10, 11, and 22 months old *O. latipes* were analyzed for both sexes. In females, the estrogen level was peaked at 8 months old, declined rapidly at 10–11 months old (P<0.05 and P<0.001, respectively) and remained low at 22 months old (P<0.0001) (Fig. 3A). In males, the estrogen level was lower than the females and declined gradually from 4 to 22 months old (Fig. 3B).

Decreased Bone Mass in Aging *O. latipes*

The BMD and micro-architecture of 15th~25th vertebrae bodies were measured by microCT for both genders at four different age groups (8, 10, 12 and 14 months old) (Fig. 4A). As revealed by three dimensional reconstruction images using microCT, the micro-architecture of the vertebrae bodies deteriorated, including the formation of micro-cracks (white arrows), thinner arches (hemal and neural) (white arrowheads) and progressively curved vertebral column (Fig. 4B), which was obvious in females at 12 months old onwards and in males at 14 months. The BMD in females declined from 8 to 10 months old and reached significantly lower level at 12 and 14 months (P<0.05) (Fig. 4C, left). In males, the BMD declined gradually with age and towards significantly lower level at 12 months onwards compared to 8 and 10 months (Fig. 4C, right). Age-associated

decline of BMD was faster in females than males after 10 months old (Fig. 4C).

Estrogenic Effects in *O. latipes* after EE2 Treatment

The estrogenic effect of EE2 was confirmed by significant up-regulation of estrogen responsive marker genes in liver of EE2 treated fish (Fig. 5 A to D). In males, *Vtg1* was the most sensitive marker (ca. 1.4–2.9×10^5 folds), followed by *Vtg2* (ca. 7×10^3 folds), *ChgH* (ca. 400 folds) and *ERα* (ca. 40 folds) for both EE2 treatments. In females, probably due to high endogenous expressions of all four estrogen responsive genes, only *Vtg2* expression was significantly up-regulated upon EE2 treatment (ca. 10 folds) (Fig. 5D).

We also tested the effect of EE2 addition on the endogenous plasma estrogen levels. While these levels varied among fish within each EE2 treatment group, no significant change observed (Fig. 6 A, B).

Improved Micro-architecture and Prevented BMD Decline after EE2 Treatment

A better organized micro-architecture, including less micro-cracks (white arrows), thicker arches (hemal and neural) (white arrowheads) and also no abnormal vertebral column curvature, was found in EE2 treated fish for both genders (Fig. 7A).

EE2 treatment could prevent bone loss in aging *O. latipes*. Under normal condition, between the 10 months old "Baseline" and the 11 months old "Control", the spinal BMD declined from an average of 392 to 344 mg/ccm (12.2%) and 401 to 362 mg/ccm (9.7%) in females and males, respectively (n = 6 per group) (Fig. 7B). Upon EE2 treatment for 4 weeks, BMD in both low and high EE2 treated females was significantly higher than the control females and showed no difference to the "Baseline" (P< 0.05, n = 6 per group) (Fig. 7B). Similar trend was found in males (P<0.05) (Fig. 7B).

Changes in Bone Turnover (Bone Formation and Resorption) after EE2 Treatment in *O. latipes*

Bone histomorphometry results by Goldner's Trichrome staining indicate changes in OBs numbers (arrowheads) on the bone surfaces around the osteoid (black arrows) and OBs surface (asterisks on green surface indicate mineralized bone) were quantified between 15th–25th vertebrae in all EE2 experimental male and female *O. latipes* (Fig. 8 B–G). In males, low and high EE2 treatments induced significantly lower OBs numbers and surfaces as compared to control (Fig. 8 H, I). Similarly, in females, OBs numbers and surfaces were significantly lower in both low and high EE2 treatments compared to controls (Fig. 8 H, I). Further, no sex differences for OBs numbers and surfaces were observed in the controls and EE2 treatment groups (Fig. 8 H, I).

Bone histomorphometry results by TRAP staining showed that EE2 treatment lowered OCs numbers (red arrows) in both sexes of *O. latipes* as compared to their respective controls (Fig. 9 B–G). The OCs numbers were quantified on hemal and neural arches of the vertebrae between 15th–25th vertebrae. In males, the OCs numbers and surfaces were significantly lower only in the low EE2 treatment as compared to the control (Fig. 9 H, I). Whereas, in females, OCs numbers and surfaces were significantly lower in both low and high EE2 treatment as compared to the control

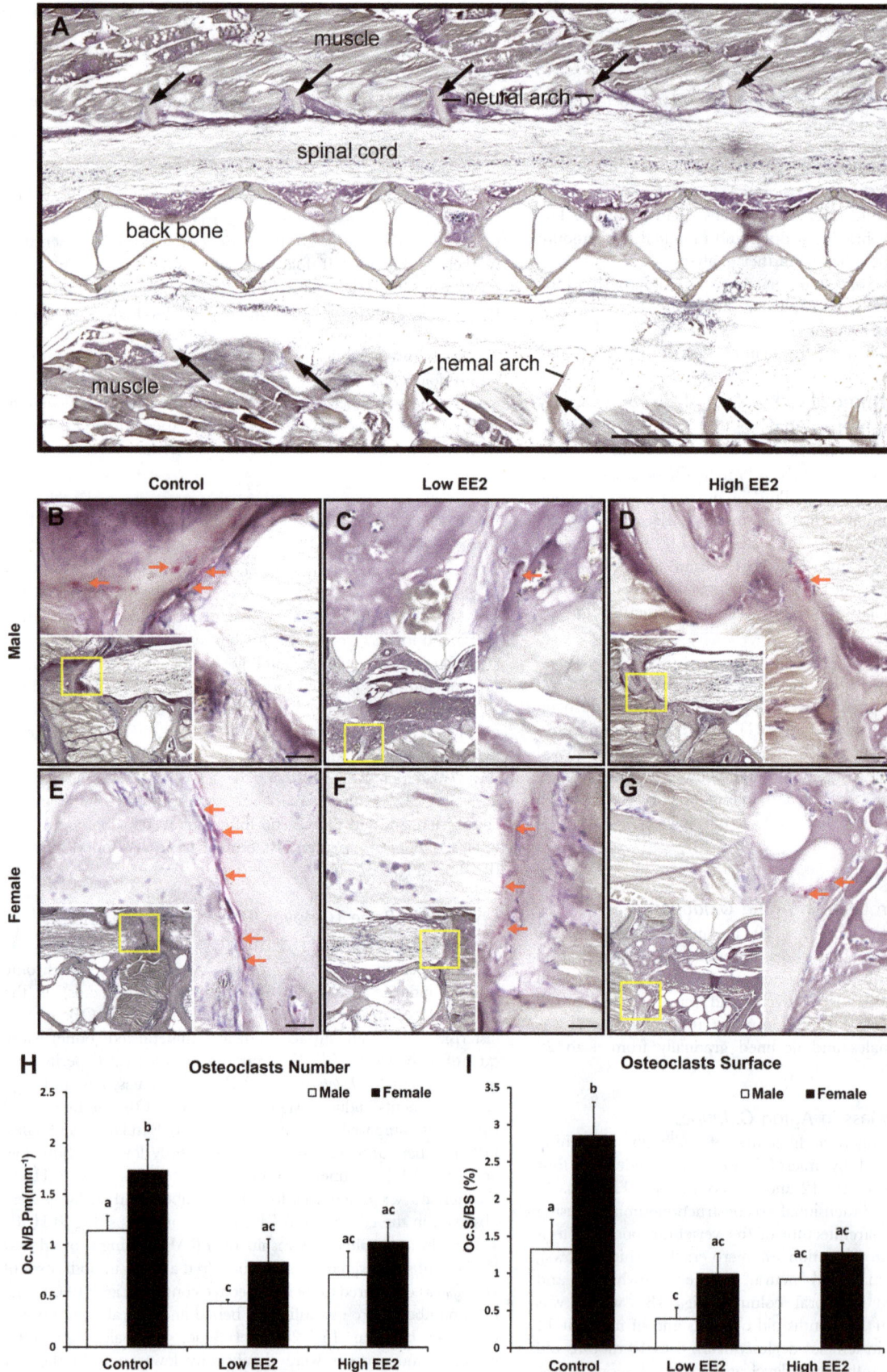

Figure 9. Representative histology pictures of TRAP staining for detection of osteoclasts in both sexes of Japanese medaka *O. latipes* after 4 weeks of EE2 treatment (Control = no EE2 fed; Low = 6 ng EE2/mg body wt./day; High = 60 ng EE2/mg body wt./day)

(Fig. A–G). (A) The location of the corresponding cells on the serial tissue sections is indicated by arrows (scale bar 1000 μm). (B) Male untreated/ Control, (C) Male with low EE2 treatment, (D) Male with high EE2 treatment, (E) Female untreated/Control, (F) Female with low EE2 treatment and (G) Female with high EE2 treatment. Red arrows on histology sections indicate TRAP signals. Scale bars 20 μm. Figure 9 H and I. Bone histomorphometric parameters on vertebrae in both sexes of *O. latipes* upon EE2 treatment (H) Osteoclasts Number/Bone Perimeter (mm) (Oc.N/B. Pm) and (I) Osteoclasts Surface/Bone Surface (Oc.S/BS). Bars labeled by the same letter on the graphs are not significantly different from each other (At significant level p<0.05).

(Fig. 9 H, I). Sex differences in OCs numbers and surfaces were only observed in the controls, where female >male (Fig. 9 H, I).

Overall, a concomitantly lowered bone formation and resorption indicates reduction in bone turnover in *O. latipes* after 4 weeks of EE2 treatment.

Discussion

In the current study, for the first time we demonstrate osteoporosis development associated with natural drop in estrogen level during aging in female medaka, which could be attenuated by estrogen treatment.

Osteoporosis Development Associated with Natural Drop in Estrogen Level in Medaka

Here we report striking similarities between female *O. latipes* and women in age-dependent natural drop of estrogen [11], and subsequent deterioration of bone metabolism including decreased BMD, poor organized bone micro-architecture and high bone turnover. Such changes were also observed in male medaka, but gradually occurred.

Using the medaka-human age conversion model developed by our team [11], females at 8- and 10- months old, showing a drastic decline in plasma estrogen level after the peak level at 8-month, could be corresponding to women at 46- and 55- years old (postmenopausal age) [3]. Further study should be conducted using a wide spectrum of teleosts to ascertain whether estrogen decline associated osteoporosis is a general phenomenon in bony fish during aging. Perhaps this could shed light on such conserved fundamental mechanism during evolution from lower vertebrates to human.

We also observed gender difference in bone mass and micro-architecture deterioration in medaka, which occurred later in the males (Fig. 4B, see arrows in 14 months panel) as compared to the

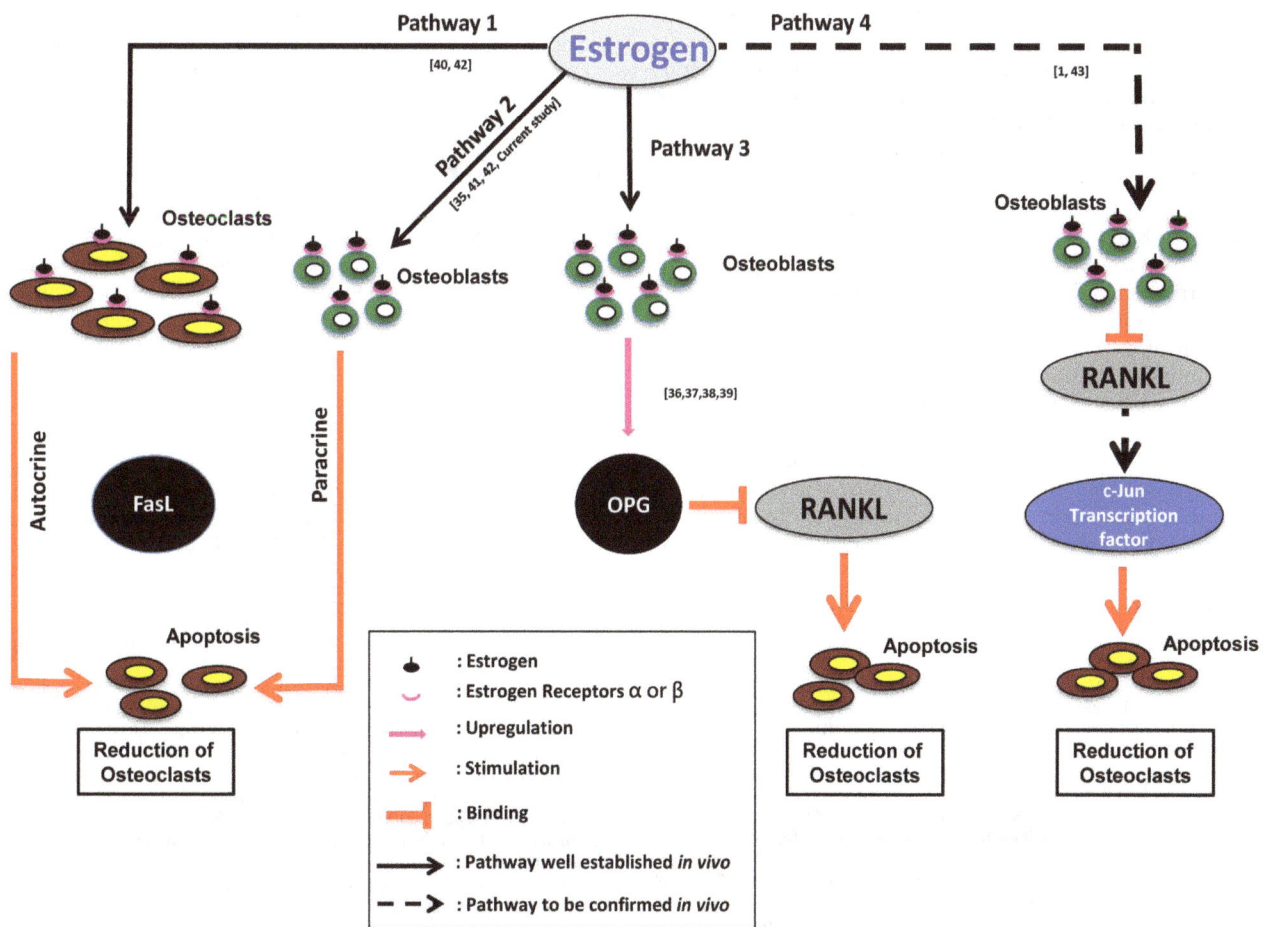

Figure 10. Schematic diagram showing estrogen mediated regulation of bone metabolism based on *in vitro* and *in vivo* findings in mammals. FasL: Fatty acid synthatase Ligand, RANKL: Receptor Activator of Nuclear factor Kappa-B Ligand, OPG: Osteoprotegerin. Dark arrows indicate up-regulation; Red arrows indicate down-regulation/apoptosis of osteoclasts. Please refer to the details in Text S1.

females (Fig. 4B, see arrows in 12 and 14 months panel). A two months difference in medaka age (12 months vs 14 months) is equivalent to a 10 years difference of human age (60 vs 70 years old) [11]. In another study, a significant decrease in estrogen level was observed after 11 months in males [11]. Therefore, it is clear that the osteoporosis prevalence in medaka is delayed in males compared to females. The prevalence of osteoporosis in male medaka also corresponded with a significant decline in estrogen level in males after 12 months of age [11]. The present study further illustrates a gender difference (female>male) in OCs numbers and surfaces (Fig. 9G, H), not OBs (Fig. 8G, H), which could explain a higher bone mass in males as compared to the female.

Our results are in agreement with earlier reports that OCs were only found on hemal and neural arches, but not on the main vertebrae in *O. latipes*, unlike those reported findings in other mammalian studies [14,27].

Estrogen Treatment Attenuated Osteoporosis Development in Medaka

The numerical values of plasma estrogen in females were higher than controls after EE2 treatment, but no statistical significance was observed due to large variation. This response is not surprising due to the very complex feedback mechanisms in regulation of estrogen level *in vivo* [28]. Nevertheless, the estrogenic effect due to supplementation of exogenous EE2 in *O. latipes* was confirmed by up-regulation of four key estrogen responsive genes (*ERα*, *Vtg1*, *Vtg2* and *ChgH*) in the liver.

EE2 treatment could attenuate decreased BMD and deteriorated bone micro-architecture observed in the spine during aging (between the 10 months old "Baseline" vs the 11 months old "Control") in both sexes. This could be explained by multiple levels of evidence, at the molecular (estrogen responsive gene expressions), cellular (quantitative bone histomorphometry) and organ level (BMD and micro-architecture by microCT scanning) obtained in the current study. Mechanistically, quantitative histomorphometry analyses clearly evidenced a concomitant reduction in OBs and OCs numbers and surfaces on vertebrae of EE2 treated *O. latipes*, suggesting EE2-induced slowdown in bone turnover. The above findings were consistent with observations in postmenopausal women with osteoporosis after estrogen replacement therapy (ERT) [7,29,30,31]. Overall, a concomitantly lowered bone formation and resorption in *O. latipes* indicates a lowered 'Bone turnover' after 4 weeks of EE2 treatment.

This is the first report that EE2 treatment could be effective in inducing improvement on estrogen declined associated bone

disorders in teleost. However, it is still prudent to understand the prolonged treatment effect on bone metabolism in bony fish.

Estrogen Mediated Regulation of Bone Metabolism based on *in vitro* and *in vivo* Findings in Mammals

Several molecular mechanisms have been postulated on estrogen-mediated modulation of bone metabolism, based on *in vivo* and *in vitro* evidence using mammals, which are summarized in Figure 10 [35,36,37,38,39,40,41,42,43]. These mechanisms may be conserved in vertebrates from fish to mammals, which warrant further investigations.

The Translational Significance of the Findings

This work provides a unique, non-mammalian vertebrate model with natural estrogen decline for biomedical research on postmenopausal osteoporosis *in vivo* without the need of invasive overiectomy. Further, findings of the present study support the development of small sized *O. latipes* as an alternative, cost-effective vertebrate model for not only studying disorders in bone metabolism, but also R & D for drugs screening.

On the other hand, *O. latipes* has been a well-established *in vivo* laboratory model for toxicological research [32]. From the perspectives of environmental toxicology, the understandings of bone biology in *O. latipes* will contribute greatly to unravel the mechanisms underlying the high incidences of fish skeletal deformation in polluted waters [33]. We anticipate the current findings on estrogen and bone metabolism in fish will also facilitate exploring future research on evolutionary biology in vertebrates.

Acknowledgments

The authors greatly appreciated Jun Bo, Andy C.K. Cheung and Hong-Lin Ren for their assistance on fish sampling. The assistance of Wong K.L in fish husbandry is greatly appreciated. Authors also thank the academic editor and the two anonymous reviewers for their valuable comments and suggestions that have assisted us in improving the quality of the manuscript.

Author Contributions

Conceived and designed the experiments: DWTA. Performed the experiments: AHS BSG RRY LC MWLC GS NKMC. Analyzed the data: AHS BSG RRY. Contributed reagents/materials/analysis tools: DWTA GZ. Wrote the paper: AHS BSG GZ DWTA.

References

1. Rodan GA, Martin TJ (2000) Therapeutic approaches to bone diseases. Science 289: 1508–1514.
2. Kraenzlin M (2007) Biochemical markers of bone turnover and osteoporosis management. Bonekey Osteovision 4: 191–203.
3. Khosla S, Melton LJ, Atkinson EJ, O'Fallon WM, Klee GG, et al. (1998) Relationship of serum sex steroid levels and bone turnover markers with bone mineral density in men and women: a key role for bioavailable estrogen. J Clin Endocrinol Met 83: 2266–2274.
4. Faienza MF, Ventura A, Marzano F, Cavallo L (2005) Postmenopausal osteoporosis: The role of immune system cells. Clinical Dev Immunol doi: 10.1155/2013/575936.
5. Weitzmann MN, Pacifici R (2006) Estrogen deficiency and bone loss: an inflammatory tale. J Clinical Investigat 116: 1186–1194.
6. Zhao R (2012) Immune regulation of osteoclast function in postmenopausal osteoporosis: A critical interdisciplinary perspective. Inter J Medical Sci 9: 825–832.
7. Delmas PD (2002) Treatment of postmenopausal osteoporosis. Lancet 359: 2018–2026.
8. Steger RW, Peluso JJ (1982) Effects of age on hormone levels and in vitro steroidogenesis by rat ovary and adrenal. Exp Aging Res 8: 203–208.
9. Thompson DD, Simmons HA, Pirie CM, Ke HZ (1995) FDA guidelines and animal models for osteoporosis. Bone 17: 25S–133S.
10. Khajuria DK, Razdan R, Mahapatra DR, Bhat MR (2013) Osteoprotective effect of propranolol in ovariectomized rats: a comparison with zoledronic acid and alfacalcidol. J Orthop Sci doi:10.1007/s00776-013-0433-y.
11. Gopalakrishnan S, Cheung NKM, Yip BWP, Au DWT (2013) Medaka fish exhibits longevity gender gap, a natural drop in estrogen and telomere shortening during aging: A unique model for studying sex dependent longevity. Front Zool 10: 78. doi:10.1186/1742-9994-10-78.
12. Inohaya K, Takano Y, Kudo A (2007) The teleost intervertebral region acts as a growth center of the centrum: In vivo visualization of osteoblasts and their progenitors in transgenic fish. Dev Dyn 236: 3031–3046.
13. Kinoshita M, Murata K, Naruse K, Tanaka M (2009) Medaka: Biology, management and experimental protocol, Chapter 6, Wiley-Blackwell publishers 165–275.
14. To TT, Witten E, Renn J, Bhattacharya D, Huysseune A, et al. (2012) Rankl-induced osteoclastogenesis leads to loss of mineralization in a medaka osteoporosis model. Development 139: 141–150.
15. Lerner UH (2000) Osteoclast formation and resorption. Mat Biol 19: 107–120.

16. Naruse K, Tanaka M, Takeda H (eds) (2011) Medaka: A Model for Organogenesis, Human Disease, and Evolution, Medaka chapter 6: 81–93.

17. Inohaya K, Kudo A (2000) Temporal and spatial patterns of cbfa1 expression during embryonic development in the teleost, *Oryzias latipes*. Dev Genes Evol 210: 570–574.

18. Wagner TU, Renn J, Riemensperger T, Volff JN, Koster RW, et al. (2003) The teleost fish medaka (*Oryzias latipes*) as genetic model to study gravity dependent bone homeostasis in vivo. Adv Space Res 32: 1459–1465.

19. Yasutake J, Inohaya K, Kudo A (2004) Twist functions in vertebral column formation in the medaka, *Oryzias latipes*. Mech Dev 121: 883–894.

20. Hatakeyama H, Nakamura K, Izumiyama-Shimomura N, Ishii A, Tsuchida S, et al. (2008) The teleost *Oryzias latipes* shows telomere shortening with age despite considerable telomerase activity throughout life. Mech Age Dev 129: 550–557.

21. Au DWT, Mok HO, Elmore LW, Holt SE (2009) Japanese medaka: a new vertebrate model for studying telomere and telomerase biology. Comp Biochem Physiol C: Toxicol Pharmacol 149: 161–167.

22. Ding L, Kuhne WW, Hinton DE, Song J, Dynan WS (2010) Quantifiable biomarkers of normal aging in the Japanese Medaka fish (*Oryzias latipes*). PLoS One 5 (10).

23. Thorpe KL, Cummings RI, Hutchinson TH, Scholze M, Brighty G, et al. (2003) Relative potencies and combination effects of steroidal estrogens in fish. Environ Sci Technol 37: 1142–1149.

24. Ternes TA, Kreckel P, Meller J (1999) Behaviour and occurrence of estrogens in municipal sewage treatment plants-II. Aerobic batch experiments with activated sludge. Sci Total Environ 225: 91–99.

25. Kong RYC, Giesy JP, Wu RSS, Chen EXH, Chiang MWL, et al. (2008) Development of a marine fish model for studying in vivo molecular responses in ecotoxicology. Aquat Toxicol 86: 131–141.

26. Parfitt AM, Drezner MK, Glorieux FH, Kanis JA, Malluche H, et al. (1987) Bone histomorphometry: Standardization of nomenclature, symbols, and units. J Bone Min Res 2: 595–610.

27. Chatani M, Takano Y, Kudo A (2011) Osteoclasts in bone modeling, as revealed by in vivo imaging, are essential for organogenesis in fish. Dev Biol 360: 96–109.

28. Zhang XW, Hecker M, Jones PD, Newsted J, Au DWT, et al. (2008) Responses of the medaka HPG axis PCR array and reproduction to prochloraz and ketoconazole. Environ Sci Technol 42: 6762–6769.

29. Turner RT, Riggs BL, Spelsberg TC (1994) Skeletal effects of estrogen. End Rev 15: 275–300.

30. Prestwood KM, Kenny AM, Unson C, Kulldorff M (2000) The effect of low dose micronized 17β-estradiol on bone turnover, sex hormone levels, and side effects in older women: a randomized, double blind, placebo-controlled study. J Clinical Endocrinol Met 85: 4462–4469.

31. Zhou S, Turgeman G, Harris SE, Leitman DC, Kmomm BS, et al. (2003) Estrogens activate bone morphogenetic protein-2 gene transcription in mouse mesenchymal stem cells. Mol Endocrinol 17: 56–66.

32. Padilla S, Cowden J, Hinton DE, Johnson R, Flynn K, et al. (2009) Use of medaka in toxicity testing. Curr Protocol Toxicol doi:10.1002/0471140856.tx0110s39.

33. Au DWT (2004) The application of histo-cytopathological biomarkers in marine pollution monitoring: A review. Mar Poll Bull 48: 817–834.

34. Riggs BL, Khosla S, Melton LJ (2002) Sex steroids and the construction and conservation of the adult skeleton. End Rev 23: 279–302.

35. Turner RT, Rickard DJ, Iwaniec UT, Spelsberg TC (2008) Estrogens and Progestins in 'Principles of Bone Biology 3rd edition' (Bilezikian J.P, et al. eds.): Academic Press, San Diego. 855–879.

36. Boyce BF, Xing L (2008) Functions of RANKL/RANK/OPG in bone modeling and remodeling. Arch Biochem Biophys 473: 139–146.

37. Li J, Sarosi I, Yan XQ, Morony S, Capparelli C, et al. (2000) RANK is the intrinsic hematopoietic cell surface receptor that controls osteoclastogenesis and regulation of bone mass and calcium metabolism. Proc Natl Acad Sci U S A 97: 1566–1571.

38. Khosla S (2001) Minireview: The OPG/RANKL/RANK system. Endocrinol 142: 5050–5055.

39. Ralston SH, Uitterlinden AG (2010) Genetics of osteoporosis. End Rev 31: 629–662.

40. Nakamura T, Imai Y, Matsumoto T, Sato S, Takeuchi K, et al. (2007) Estrogen prevents bone loss via estrogen receptor alpha and induction of Fas ligand in osteoclasts. Cell 130: 811–23.

41. Krum SA, Miranda-Carboni GA, Hauschka PV, Carroll JS, Lane TF, et al. (2008) Estrogen protects bone by inducing Fas ligand in osteoblasts to regulate osteoclast survival. The EMBO J 27: 535–545.

42. Imai Y, Kondoh S, Kouzmenko A, Kato S (2010) Minireview: Osteoprotective action of estrogens is mediated by osteoclastic estrogen receptor-alpha. Mol Endocrinol 24: 877–85.

43. Shevde NK, Bendixen AC, Dienger KM, Pike JW (2000) Estrogens suppress RANK ligand-induced osteoclast differentiation via a stromal cell independent mechanism involving c-Jun repression. Proc Natl Acad Sci U S A 97: 7829–7834.

Permissions

List of Contributors

Jen-Hau Chen
Department of Geriatrics and Gerontology, National Taiwan University Hospital, No. 1, Taipei, Taiwan
Department of Internal Medicine, National Taiwan University Hospital, No. 7, Taipei, Taiwan
Institute of Epidemiology and Preventive Medicine, College of Public Health, National Taiwan University, Taipei, Taiwan

Keh-Sung Tsai
Department of Geriatrics and Gerontology, National Taiwan University Hospital, No. 1, Taipei, Taiwan
Department of Internal Medicine, National Taiwan University Hospital, No. 7, Taipei, Taiwan
Department of Laboratory Medicine, National Taiwan University Hospital, No. 7, Taipei, Taiwan

Yen-Ching Chen and Chien-Lin Mao
Institute of Epidemiology and Preventive Medicine, College of Public Health, National Taiwan University, Taipei, Taiwan

Jeng-Min Chiou
Institute of Statistical Science, Academia Sinica, Nankang, Taipei, Taiwan

Chwen Keng Tsao
MJ Health Management Institution, 12F., No. 413, Section 4, Taipei, Taiwan

Giovanni Cizza, Vi T. Nguyen, Farideh Eskandari and Sara Torvik
Section on Neuroendocrinology of Obesity, National Institutes of Diabetes and Digestive Kidney Diseases (NIDDK), National Institutes of Health, Bethesda, Maryland, United States of America

Sima Mistry
Tulane University Internal Medicine-Pediatrics Residency Program, Tulane University School of Medicine, New Orleans, Louisiana, United States of America

Pedro Martinez and Philip W. Gold
Behavioral Endocrinology Branch, National Institute of Mental Health, National Institutes of Health, Bethesda, Maryland, United States of America

James C. Reynolds, Ninet Sinai and Gyorgy Csako
Clinical Center, National Institutes of Health, Bethesda, Maryland, United States of America

Ching-Lan Wu
Department of Radiology, Taipei Veterans General Hospital, Taipei, Taiwan

Hung-Ta H. Wu, Hong-Jen Chiou and Cheng-Yen Chang
Department of Radiology, Taipei Veterans General Hospital, Taipei, Taiwan
School of Medicine, National Yang-Ming University, Taipei, Taiwan

Wen-Cheng Huang
Department of Neurosurgery, Neurological Institute, Taipei Veterans General Hospital, Taipei, Taiwan
School of Medicine, National Yang-Ming University, Taipei, Taiwan

Jau-Ching Wu and Henrich Cheng
Department of Neurosurgery, Neurological Institute, Taipei Veterans General Hospital, Taipei, Taiwan
School of Medicine, National Yang-Ming University, Taipei, Taiwan
Institute of Pharmacology, National Yang-Ming University, Taipei, Taiwan

Laura Liu
Department of Ophthalmology, Chang Gung Memorial Hospital, Taoyuan, Taiwan
College of Medicine, Chang Gung University, Taoyuan, Taiwan

Yu-Chun Chen
Department of Medical Research and Education, National Yang-Ming University Hospital, I-Lan, Taiwan

Tzeng-Ji Chen
Institute of Hospital and Health Care Administration, National Yang-Ming University School of Medicine, Taipei, Taiwan

Kenneth E. S. Poole and Paul M. Mayhew
Department of Medicine, University of Cambridge, Cambridge, Cambridgeshire, United Kingdom

Graham M. Treece and Andrew H. Gee
Department of Engineering, University of Cambridge, Cambridge, Cambridgeshire, United Kingdom

Jan Vaculík and Pavel Dungl
Department of Orthopaedics, Faculty of Medicine, Charles University Prague and Bulovka Hospital, Prague, Czech Republic

Martin Horák
Department of Radiology, Homolka Hospital, Prague, Czech Republic

Jan J. Štěpán
Department of Rheumatology, Faculty of Medicine 1, Charles University Prague and Institute of Rheumatology, Prague, Czech Republic

Reeva Aggarwal, Jingwei Lu, Suman Kanji, Matthew Joseph, Manjusri Das, Vincent J. Pompili and Hiranmoy Das
Cardiovascular Stem Cell Research Laboratory, Davis Heart and Lung Research Institute, The Ohio State University Medical Center, Columbus, Ohio, United States of America

Garrett J. Noble and Richard T. Hart
Department of Biomedical Engineering, College of Engineering, The Ohio State University, Columbus, Ohio, United States of America

Brooke K. McMichael and Beth S. Lee
Department of Physiology and Cell Biology, College of Medicine, The Ohio State University, Columbus, Ohio, United States of America

Sudha Agarwal and Zongyang Sun
Division of Oral Biology, Department of Orthopedics, College of Dentistry, The Ohio State University, Columbus, Ohio, United States of America

Thomas J. Rosol
Department of Veterinary Clinical Sciences, College of Veterinary Medicine, The Ohio State University, Columbus, Ohio, United States of America

Rebecca Jackson
Division of Endocrinology, Diabetes and Metabolism, College of Medicine, The Ohio State University, Columbus, Ohio, United States of America

Hai-Quan Mao
Department of Materials Science and Engineering, John's Hopkins University, Baltimore, Maryland, United States of America

Tyler J. O'Neill and Laura Rivera
Dalla Lana School of Public Health, University of Toronto, Toronto, Ontario, Canada,

Hla-Hla Thein
Dalla Lana School of Public Health, University of Toronto, Toronto, Ontario, Canada
Ontario Institute for Cancer Research/Cancer Care Ontario, Toronto, Ontario, Canada

Vladi Struchkov
Dalla Lana School of Public Health, University of Toronto, Toronto, Ontario, Canada,
Faculty of Medicine, University of Toronto, Toronto, Ontario, Canada

Ahmad Zaheen
Faculty of Medicine, University of Toronto, Toronto, Ontario, Canada

Mary B. Pierce, Andrew Wong, Marcus Richards, Rebecca Hardy and Diana Kuh
MRC Unit for Lifelong Health & Ageing, London, England

Richard J. Silverwood and Dorothea Nitsch
Department of Non-Communicable Disease Epidemiology, London School of Hygiene and Tropical Medicine, London, England

Judith E. Adams
Manchester Academic Health Science Centre, University of Manchester, Manchester, England,

Alison M. Stephen and Wing Nip
MRC Human Nutrition Research, Elsie Widdowson Laboratory, Cambridge, England,

Peter Macfarlane
Electrocardiology Section, Royal Infirmary, University of Glasgow, Glasgow, Scotland

Wen-Jun Zhang, Yi-Kai Li, Wen-Rui Lan and Chao Chen
Department of Orthopedics, School of Traditional Chinese Medicine, Southern Medical University, Guangzhou, China

Hua-Jun Wang
Department of Orthopedics, School of Traditional Chinese Medicine, Southern Medical University, Guangzhou, China
Biomechanics Laboratory, Division of Orthopedic Research, Mayo Clinic, Rochester, Minnesota, United States of America

Hugo Giambini, Chunfeng Zhao and Kai-Nan An
Biomechanics Laboratory, Division of Orthopedic Research, Mayo Clinic, Rochester, Minnesota, United States of America

Gan-Hu Ye
Chang Ping Hospital, Dongguan, China

Jian-You Li and Xue-Sheng Jiang
Orthopedic Department, Huzhou Central Hospital, Huzhou, China

Qiu-Lan Zou and Xiao-Ying Zhang
You-Hao Residential Care Home, Guangzhou, China

Stine Marit Moen and Elisabeth Gulowsen Celius
Department of Neurology, Oslo University Hospital Ullevål, Oslo, Norway

Leiv Sandvik
Section of Epidemiology and Biostatistics, Oslo University Hospital Ulleva°l, Oslo, Norway

Magritt Brustad
Department of Community Medicine, University of Tromsø, Tromsø, Norway

Lars Nordsletten
Orthopedic Department, Oslo University Hospital Ulleva°l, Oslo, Norway

Erik Fink Eriksen
Department of Endocrinology, Oslo University Hospital, Oslo, Norway

Trygve Holmøy
Department of Neurology, Akershus University Hospital, Lørenskog, Norway
Institute of Clinical Medicine, University of Oslo, Oslo, Norway

Smita Nayak
Section of Decision Sciences and Clinical Systems Modeling, Division of General Internal Medicine, Department of Medicine, University of Pittsburgh School of Medicine, Pittsburgh, Pennsylvania, United States of America

Mark S. Roberts
Section of Decision Sciences and Clinical Systems Modeling, Division of General Internal Medicine, Department of Medicine, University of Pittsburgh School of Medicine, Pittsburgh, Pennsylvania, United States of America

Department of Health Policy and Management, University of Pittsburgh Graduate School of Public Health, Pittsburgh, Pennsylvania, United States of America

Susan L. Greenspan
Division of Endocrinology and Metabolism and Division of Geriatric Medicine, Department of Medicine, University of Pittsburgh School of Medicine, Pittsburgh, Pennsylvania, United States of America

Wei Yi
Department of Mechanics, Huazhong University of Science and Technology, Wuhan, Hubei, China

Qing Tian
Tongji Medical College, Huazhong University of Science and Technology, Wuhan, Hubei, China

Zhipeng Dai
Tongji Medical College, Huazhong University of Science and Technology, Wuhan, Hubei, China

Xiaohu Liu
Department of Mechanics, Huazhong University of Science and Technology, Wuhan, Hubei, China

Wen-Hung Huang, Shen-Yang Lee, Cheng-Hao Weng and Ping-Chin Lai
Department of Nephrology, Chang Gung Memorial Hospital, Linkou, Taiwan, Republic of China
Chang Gung University College of Medicine, Taoyuan, Taiwan, Republic of China

Magnus P. Ekström
Department of Respiratory Medicine & Allergology, Institution for Clinical Sciences, University of Lund, Lund, Sweden

Claes Jogréus
Department of Mathematics and Science, School of Engineering, Blekinge Institute of Technology, Karlskrona, Sweden

Kerstin E. Ström
Department of Respiratory Medicine & Allergology, Institution for Clinical Sciences, University of Lund, Lund, Sweden

Song Yao, Lara E.Sucheston, Warren Davis and Christine B. Ambrosone
Department of Cancer Prevention and Control, Roswell Park Cancer Institute, Buffalo, New York, United States of America

Shannon L. Smiley, Philip L. McCarthy Jr. and Theresa Hahn
Department of Medicine, Roswell Park Cancer Institute, Buffalo, New York, United States of America

Jeffrey M. Conroy
Department of Cancer Genetics, Roswell Park Cancer Institute, Buffalo, New York, United States of America

Norma J. Nowak
Department of Cancer Genetics, Roswell Park Cancer Institute, Buffalo, New York, United States of America
Department of Biochemistry, University at Buffalo, Buffalo, New York, United States of America

Yi-Jie Kuo
Department of Orthopaedic, Taipei Medical University Hospital, Taipei, Taiwan, Republic of China
Institute of Clinical Medicine, National Yang Ming University, Taipei, Taiwan, Republic of China

Fon-Yih Tsuang
Division of Neurosurgery, Department of Surgery, National Taiwan University Hospital, Taipei, Taiwan, Republic of China

Jui-Sheng Sun
Department of Orthopaedic Surgery, National Taiwan University Hospital-Hsin Chu, Hsin-Chu, Taiwan, Republic of China
Graduate Institute of Clinical Medicine, College of Medicine, Taipei Medical University, Taipei, Taiwan, Republic of China

Chi-Hung Lin and Chia-Hsien Chen
Institute of Microbiology and Immunology, National Yang Ming University, Taipei, Taiwan, Republic of China

Jia-Ying Li and Wei-Yu Chen
Department of Biology and Anatomy, National Defense Medical Center, Taipei, Taiwan, Republic of China

Jia-Fwu Shyu
Department of Biology and Anatomy, National Defense Medical Center, Taipei, Taiwan, Republic of China
Department of Psychiatry, Tri-Service General Hospital, Taipei, Taiwan, Republic of China

Yi-Chian Huang
Institute of Anatomy and Cell Biology National Yang Ming University, Taipei, Taiwan, Republic of China

Chin-Bin Yeh
Department of Psychiatry, Tri-Service General Hospital, Taipei, Taiwan, Republic of China

Longxiang Shen, Xuetao Xie, Yan Su, Congfeng Luo, Changqing Zhang and Bingfang Zeng
Department of Orthopedic Surgery, Shanghai Sixth People's Hospital, Shanghai Jiaotong University, Shanghai, People's Republic of China

Jin-Kang Zhang, Liu Yang, Guo-Lin Meng, Zhi Yuan, Jing Fan, Dan Li, Tian- Hui-Min Hu, Bo-Yuan Wei, Zhuo-Jing Luo and Jian Liu
Institute of Orthopedic Surgery, Xijing Hospital, Fourth Military Medical University, Xi9an, People's Republic of China

Jian-Zong Chen
Research Center of Traditional Chinese Medicine, Xijing Hospital, Fourth Military Medical University, Xi9an, People's Republic of China

Tian-Yao Shi
Department of Pharmacology, School of Pharmacy, Fourth Military Medical University, Xi'an, People's Republic of China

Yufeng Zhang and Lingfei Wei
The State Key Laboratory Breeding Base of Basic Science of Stomatology (Hubei-MOST) & Key Laboratory of Oral Biomedicine Ministry of Education, Wuhan University, Wuhan, People's Republic of China

Richard J. Miron
The State Key Laboratory Breeding Base of Basic Science of Stomatology (Hubei-MOST) & Key Laboratory of Oral Biomedicine Ministry of Education, Wuhan University, Wuhan, People's Republic of China
Faculté de medecine dentaire, Université Laval, Québec, Canada

Chengtie Wu
State Key Laboratory of High Performance Ceramics and Superfine Microstructure, Shanghai Institute of Ceramics, Shanghai, People's Republic of China

Pu-Hyeon Cha, Wookjin Shin, Muhammad Zahoor, Hyun-Yi Kim and Kang-Yell Choi
Translational Research Center for Protein Function Control, College of Life Science and Biotechnology, Yonsei University, Seoul, Korea
Department of Biotechnology, College of Life Science and Biotechnology, Yonsei University, Seoul, Korea

Do Sik Min
Translational Research Center for Protein Function Control, College of Life Science and Biotechnology, Yonsei University, Seoul, Korea
Department of Molecular Biology, College of Natural Science, Pusan National University, Pusan, Korea

Jer-Yuarn Wu, Wei-Ru Li, Li-Ying Chen, Li-Fen Shen and Jeffrey J. Y. Yen
Institute of Biomedical Sciences, Academia Sinica, Taipei, Taiwan

I-Wen Song
Institute of Biomedical Sciences, Academia Sinica, Taipei, Taiwan
Graduate Institute of Life Sciences, National Defense Medical Center, Taipei, Taiwan

Kai-Ming Liu
Institute of Biomedical Sciences, Academia Sinica, Taipei, Taiwan
Institute of Clinical Medicine, National Yang-Ming University, Taipei, Taiwan

Yuan-Tsong Chen
Institute of Biomedical Sciences, Academia Sinica, Taipei, Taiwan
Graduate Institute of Life Sciences, National Defense Medical Center, Taipei, Taiwan
Department of Pediatrics, Duke University Medical Center, Durham, North Carolina, United States of America

M. T. Michael Lee
Institute of Biomedical Sciences, Academia Sinica, Taipei, Taiwan
Laboratory for International Alliance on Genomic Research, RIKEN Center for Integrative Medical Sciences, Yokohama, Japan
Graduate Institute of Chinese Medical Science, China Medical University, Taichung, Taiwan

Yi-Ju Chen and Yu-Ju Chen
Institute of Chemistry, Academia Sinica, Taipei, Taiwan

Virginia Byers Kraus
Department of Medicine, Division of Rheumatology, Duke University Medical Center, Durham, North Carolina, United States of America

Mei Li, Yingying Hu and Weibo Xia
Department of Endocrinology, Key Laboratory of Endocrinology of Ministry of Health, Peking Union Medical College Hospital, Peking Union Medical College, Chinese Academy of Medical Sciences, Beijing, China

Yan Li
Department of Laboratory, People's Hospital, Hubei Province, Wuhan, China

Weimin Deng
Department of Geriatrics, General Hospital of Guangzhou Military Command, Guangzhou, China

Zhenlin Zhang
Department of Osteoporosis, Sixth People's Hospital, Shanghai Jiaotong University, Shanghai, China

Zhongliang Deng
Department of Orthopedics, Second Affiliated Hospital of Chongqing Medical University, Chongqing, China

Ling Xu
Department of Obstetrics and Gynecology, Chinese Academy of Medical Sciences, Peking Union Medical College, Peking Union Medical College Hospital, Beijing, China

Charlotte Salter, Lisa McDaid, Richard Holland and Amanda Howe
Norwich Medical School, Faculty of Medicine & Health Science, University of East Anglia, Norwich, Norfolk, United Kingdom

Debi Bhattacharya
School of Chemistry and Pharmacy, University of East Anglia, Norwich, Norfolk. United Kingdom

Tarnya Marshall
Rheumatology Department, Norfolk & Norwich University Foundation Trust Hospital. Norwich, Norfolk. United Kingdom

Jessica Bon, Rehan Kahloon, Yingze Zhang, Jianmin Xue, Jiangning Tan, Mathew Burger, Daniel J Kass, Divay Chandra, Arpit Bhargava, Joseph M. Pilewski, G, Frank C. Sciurba and Steven R. Duncan
Department of Medicine, University of Pittsburgh, Pittsburgh, Pennsylvania, United States of America

Carl R. Fuhrman
Department of Radiology, University of Pittsburgh, Pittsburgh, Pennsylvania, United States of America

Eva Csizmadia and Leo Otterbein
Department of Surgery, Beth Israel Deaconess Medical Center, Harvard Medical School, Boston, Massachusetts, United States of America

David Roodman
Department of Medicine, Indiana School of Medicine, Indianapolis, Indiana, United States of America

Masashi Muramatsu
Laboratory of Genomics and Proteomics, National Center for Geriatrics and Gerontology (NCGG), Aichi, Japan

Sawako Moriwaki and Shumpei Niida
Laboratory of Genomics and Proteomics, National Center for Geriatrics and Gerontology (NCGG), Aichi, Japan
Biobank Omics Unit, National Center for Geriatrics and Gerontology (NCGG), Aichi, Japan

Keiko Suzuki
Department of Pharmacology, School of Dentistry, Showa University, Tokyo, Japan

Atsushi Nomura and Fumihide Inoue
Nihon Seiyaku Kogyo, Co., Ltd., Aichi, Japan

Takeshi Into
Department of Oral Bacteriology, Division of Oral Infections and Health Sciences, Asahi University School of Dentistry, Gifu, Japan

Yuji Yoshiko
Department of Oral Growth and Developmental Biology, Hiroshima University Graduate School of Biomedical Sciences, Hiroshima, Japan

Luai A. Ahmed, Åshild Bjørnerem, Lone Jørgensen and Nina Emaus
Department of Health and Care Sciences, Faculty of Health Sciences, UiT – The Arctic University of Norway, Tromsø, Norway

Nguyen D. Nguyen and Dana Bliuc
Osteoporosis & Bone Biology Program, Garvan Institute of Medical Research, Sydney, Australia

Jacqueline R. Center
Osteoporosis & Bone Biology Program, Garvan Institute of Medical Research, Sydney, Australia
Department of Endocrinology, St Vincent's Hospital, Sydney, Australia
St. Vincent's Clinical School, UNSW Australia, Sydney, Australia

John A. Eisman
Osteoporosis & Bone Biology Program, Garvan Institute of Medical Research, Sydney, Australia
Department of Endocrinology, St Vincent's Hospital, Sydney, Australia

School of Medicine Sydney, University of Notre Dame Australia, Sydney, Australia
St. Vincent's Clinical School, UNSW Australia, Sydney, Australia

Tuan V. Nguyen
Osteoporosis & Bone Biology Program, Garvan Institute of Medical Research, Sydney, Australia
St. Vincent's Clinical School, UNSW Australia, Sydney, Australia
School of Public Health and Community Medicine, University of New South Wales, Sydney, Australia
Centre for Health Technologies, University of Technology, Sydney, Australia

Ragnar M. Joakimsen
Department of Clinical Medicine, Faculty of Health Sciences, UiT – The Arctic University of Norway, Tromsø, Norway
Medical Clinic, University Hospital of Northern Norway, Tromsø, Norway

Jan Størmer
Department of Radiology, University Hospital of Northern Norway, Tromsø, Norway

Admane H. Shanthanagouda, Rui R. Ye, Michael W. L. Chiang, Gopalakrishnan Singaram, Napo K. M. Cheung and Doris W. T. Au
State Key Laboratory in Marine Pollution, Department of Biology and Chemistry, City University of Hong Kong, Hong Kong

Bao-Sheng Guo, Liang Chao and Ge Zhang
Institute for Advancing Translational Medicine in Bone & Joint Diseases, School of Chinese Medicine, Hong Kong Baptist University, Hong Kong

Index

www.ingramcontent.com/pod-product-compliance
Lightning Source LLC
Chambersburg PA
CBHW080933240326

41458CB00143B/4113